Sleep Apnea

LUNG BIOLOGY IN HEALTH AND DISEASE

Executive Editor

Claude Lenfant

Former Director, National Heart, Lung, and Blood Institute
National Institutes of Health
Bethesda, Maryland

For information on volumes 25–182 in the *Lung Biology in Health and Disease* series, please visit www.informahealthcare.com

The opinions expressed in these volumes do not necessarily represent the views of the National Institutes of Health.

Sleep Apnea

Implications in Cardiovascular and Cerebrovascular Disease

Second Edition

Edited by

T. Douglas Bradley
Toronto Rehabilitation Institute
University Health Network and Mount Sinai Hospital
University of Toronto
Toronto, Ontario, Canada

John S. Floras
Mount Sinai Hospital and University Health Network
University of Toronto
Toronto, Ontario, Canada

informa
healthcare

New York   London

Informa Healthcare USA, Inc.
52 Vanderbilt Avenue
New York, NY 10017

© 2010 by Informa Healthcare USA, Inc.
Informa Healthcare is an Informa business

International Standard Book Number-10: 0-8493-4150-7 (Hardcover)
International Standard Book Number-13: 978-0-8493-4150-2 (Hardcover)

Library of Congress Cataloging-in-Publication Data

Sleep apnea : implications in cardiovascular and cerebrovascular disease / edited by T. Douglas Bradley, John S. Floras — 2nd ed.
    p. ; cm. — (Lung biology in health and disease ; 231)
    Includes bibliographical references and index.
    ISBN-13: 978-0-8493-4150-2 (hardcover : alk. paper)
    ISBN-10: 0-8493-4150-7 (hardcover : alk. paper) 1. Sleep apnea syndromes—Complications. 2. Cardiological manifestations of general diseases.
3. Neurologic manifestations of general diseases. 4. Cardiovascular system—Diseases. 5. Cerebrovascular disease. I. Bradley, T. Douglas, 1951- II. Floras, John S., 1953- III. Series: Lung biology in health and disease ; v. 231.
    [DNLM: 1. Sleep Apnea Syndromes—physiopathology. 2. Cardiovascular Physiological Phenomena. 3. Cerebrovascular Disorders—complications.
4. Heart Failure—complications. 5. Hypertension—complications. 6. Respiratory Physiological Phenomena.   W1 LU62 v.231 2009 / WF 143 S631 2009]
    RC737.5.S53 2009
    616.2—dc22

                                                                    2009025967

For Corporate Sales and Reprint Permissions call 212-520-2700 or write to: Sales Department, 52 Vanderbilt Avenue, 7th floor, New York, NY 10017.

Visit the Informa Web site at
www.informa.com

and the Informa Healthcare Web site at
www.informahealthcare.com

Introduction

The publication of this volume, the second edition of *Sleep Apnea: Implications in Cardiovascular and Cerebrovascular Disease*, edited by T. Douglas Bradley and John S. Floras, is an important event in the history of the series of monographs Lung Biology in Health and Disease. It appears on the 25th anniversary of the publication of the first volume on sleep, *Sleep and Breathing* (volume 21 in the series) edited by N. A. Saunders and C. E. Sullivan.

Since the publication of volume 21 in 1984, the series has presented a total of 13 volumes on various aspects of sleep, and a 14th volume will appear shortly. In the Preface of volume 21, the editors noted that "In the space of a few years, sleep research has moved from relative obscurity (from the physician's viewpoint) of psychological literature to become a well-tested tool in clinical practice," including care of patients with common cardiorespiratory problems. Indeed, in the mid-1960s, significant publications linking sleep (disorders) and cardiovascular diseases began to appear, but the main focus of these publications was mostly about the Pickwick syndrome and its cardiovascular consequence, primarily hypertension.

In 1969, a fundamental publication (1) demonstrated a relationship—not to say interdependence—between sleep disturbances and angina. In the following years, many research projects were implemented to further study the associations between sleep and cardiovascular disorders. The preface of the first edition of this volume (volume 146, published in 2000) stated that "Our overall objective was to assemble the experimental and clinical literature on the topic of sleep disorders, apnea, and cardiovascular disease into a single authoritative and timely monograph useful to basic and clinical scientists interested in these concepts, and to practicing physicians managing such patients."

In the years following the publication of this first edition, a body of strong scientific evidence has emerged documenting the interrelationship between sleep disorders and heart disease. Mechanisms of this interrelationship have been investigated and described, and therapeutic clinical investigations have established the indications and effectiveness of therapeutic approaches. Furthermore, it is now clear that the public health burden of the association of sleep disorders and cardiovascular disease is enormous. In the United States, millions suffer from sleep disorders, tens of millions have cardiovascular disease, and it is now estimated that more than 60 million Americans have hypertension, many reporting troubled sleep patterns.

The agreement of Drs T. Douglas Bradley and John S. Floras to edit a second edition of their volume was wonderful news as the field has markedly advanced. This second edition "ensures a critical synthesis" of all the new available data to facilitate the work of the practicing physicians. As the executive editor of this series of monographs, I am most grateful to the editors and their contributors for this volume and for the benefit it will provide to patients suffering from sleep disorders and cardiovascular diseases.

Claude Lenfant, MD
Vancouver, Washington, U.S.A.

Reference

1. Karacan I, Williams RL, Taylor WJ. Sleep characteristics of patients with angina pectoris. Psychosomatics 1969; 10:280–284.

Preface

Sleep, most gentle sleep.

Ovid, *Metamorphosis*, II l. 624

I sleep, but my heart waketh.

Song of Solomon, ch 5 v 2

As Ovid proclaims, the onset of sleep should herald relaxation of the heart and the cardiovascular system. However, when this pacific state is disrupted by pauses in breathing, the heart and the sympathetic nervous system "waketh," denying the slumberer the full restorative effects of sleep. When apnea, a condition common in patients with cardiovascular and cerebrovascular disease, disrupts sleep, it places direct mechanical and neurohumoral stresses on the heart and vasculature. In some instances, these forces can exceed those experienced during vigorous mental and physical activity. However, until recently, the adverse implications of these pathophysiological effects of sleep apnea on the cardiovascular system have received little attention. Indeed, current evidence-based guidelines for the investigation and therapy of conditions such as hypertension and heart failure focus on the patient with hypertension or heart failure as he or she presents, in clinic, while awake. This clinical approach presupposes that any mechanisms that might contribute to the pathophysiology or progression of such conditions are quiescent during sleep.

Over the last decade, the concerted efforts of many integrative physiologists, epidemiologists, and clinical investigators worldwide have transformed our understanding and appreciation of the many mechanisms by which apneas during sleep may contribute to the pathophysiology or complications of cardiovascular and cerebrovascular disease. These are the most common life-threatening and debilitating diseases affecting the adult Western population; as life expectancy in developed and developing countries extends, the number of individuals suffering from one or more of these conditions will increase greatly. Over the same period there has been increasing recognition of the limitations of conventional drug-based approaches to the therapy of cardiovascular conditions that fail to specifically address and treat coexisting sleep-related breathing disorders. As a result there has been a renewal of interest in concepts such as "refractory hypertension" and "limits to neurohumoral blockade in heart failure" in the cardiovascular literature.

These several considerations underscored the compelling need for a comprehensive reference text on the topic of sleep apnea and its implications for cardiovascular and cerebrovascular disease. For the last two decades, the editors, a respirologist and cardiologist, respectively, have shared the concern that cardiovascular turmoil triggered by sleep-related breathing disorders may participate in the initiation or progression of common and debilitating conditions such as heart failure, hypertension, stroke, arrhythmias, and nocturnal angina. We therefore accepted with great enthusiasm the invitation from Dr Claude Lenfant to develop and edit a comprehensive monograph specifically addressing the cardiovascular and cerebrovascular consequences of sleep apnea. We undertook this project with the confidence that transmission of this information to a broader readership would ultimately benefit patients who suffer from sleep apnea and its complications.

Our objective in the first edition of this text was to assemble the available experimental and clinical literature on this topic into a single authoritative and timely monograph useful to basic and clinical scientists interested in these concepts, and to practicing physicians managing such patients. We addressed, in turn, the influence of normal sleep and respiration on the cardiovascular system, the effects of sleep apnea on blood pressure, the relationship of sleep apnea to coronary and cerebrovascular disease, and the pathophysiological interactions between sleep apnea and congestive heart failure. We were gratified by the enthusiastic response to our first edition, in 2000, and by the subsequent acceleration of interest, among the broader medical research and clinical communities in this entire topic, and in related public health issues such as interactions between sleep apnea, obesity, and the metabolic-cardiovascular syndrome. With this success came the responsibility to ensure that important new advances in this field were not overlooked.

Our objective in preparing the second edition of this text was to ensure the critical synthesis, into the existing literature, of new information linking sleep apnea to the major disease burdens facing developed and developing nations. This includes both new basic and epidemiological data linking sleep apnea to inflammation, the metabolic syndrome, and stroke, in addition to hypertension and heart failure and, importantly, the results of recently published clinical trials. The majority of the studies reviewed in the first edition of this text were mechanistic or interventional studies, comprising small numbers of experimental or human subjects, performed in single centers. These investigations have since stimulated a number of single and multicenter randomized controlled trials of interventions specifically addressing the treatment of sleep apnea on clinically important outcomes. Because these trials have important implications for clinical practice, they therefore merit particular attention. Our contributors were invited to review critically the current literature in their area of expertise and encouraged to highlight, whenever possible, those novel observations and important concepts arising from their laboratories with the greatest impact. Our role as editors was to ensure that our readers would consider this volume transformative rather than simply evolutionary.

We thank our authors for the quality, comprehensiveness, and the timeliness of their contributions, and Dr Claude Lenfant of the World Hypertension League and Ms Sandra Beberman at Informa Healthcare for their patience and good humor during the editing and publishing process. We have enjoyed the opportunity to create this second edition and trust that our readers and the patients we treat will benefit from its contents.

T. Douglas Bradley
John S. Floras

Contributors

Michael Arzt University of Regensburg, Regensburg, Germany

Claudio L. Bassetti Department of Neurology, University Hospital of Zurich, Zurich, Switzerland

T. Douglas Bradley Toronto Rehabilitation Institute, University Health Network and Mount Sinai Hospital, University of Toronto, Toronto, Ontario, Canada

Luciano F. Drager University of São Paulo, São Paulo, Brazil

John S. Floras Mount Sinai Hospital and University Health Network, University of Toronto, Toronto, Ontario, Canada

Oded Friedman Samuel Lunenfeld Research Institute, Mount Sinai Hospital, Division of Nephrology, Mount Sinai Hospital and University Health Network, and Department of Medicine, University of Toronto, Toronto, Ontario, Canada

Apoor S. Gami Midwest Heart Specialists, Elmhurst, Illinois, U.S.A.

John Garvey St. Vincent's University Hospital and University College Dublin, Dublin, Ireland

Patrice G. Guyenet University of Virginia School of Medicine, Charlottesville, Virginia, U.S.A.

Richard L. Horner University of Toronto, Toronto, Ontario, Canada

Michael C. K. Khoo University of Southern California, Los Angeles, California, U.S.A.

Fatima H. Sert Kuniyoshi Mayo Clinic, Rochester, Minnesota, U.S.A.

Paola A. Lanfranchi University of Montreal, Montreal, Quebec, Canada

Richard S. T. Leung   University of Toronto, Toronto, Ontario, Canada

Yamini S. Levitzky   Heart and Vascular Center, MetroHealth Campus, Case Western Reserve University and University Hospitals, Case Medical Center, Cleveland, Ohio, U.S.A.

Alexander G. Logan   Samuel Lunenfeld Research Institute, Mount Sinai Hospital, Division of Nephrology, Mount Sinai Hospital and University Health Network, and Department of Medicine, University of Toronto, Toronto, Ontario, Canada

Geraldo Lorenzi-Filho   University of São Paulo, São Paulo, Brazil

Sheldon Magder   McGill University Health Centre, Montreal, Quebec, Canada

Tami A. Martino   Department of Biomedical Sciences, OVC, University of Guelph, Guelph, Ontario, Canada

Kenneth R. McGaffin   University of Pittsburgh Medical Center, Pittsburgh, Pennsylvania, U.S.A.

Walter T. McNicholas   St. Vincent's University Hospital and University College Dublin, Dublin, Ireland

Krzysztof Narkiewicz   Medical University of Gdansk, Gdansk, Poland

Matthew T. Naughton   Alfred Hospital and Monash University, Melbourne, Australia

Christian L. Nicholas   University of Melbourne, Parkville, Victoria, Australia

Christopher P. O'Donnell   University of Pittsburgh Medical Center, Pittsburgh, Pennsylvania, U.S.A.

Bradley G. Phillips   College of Pharmacy, University of Georgia, Athens, Georgia, U.S.A.

Naresh M. Punjabi   Johns Hopkins University School of Medicine, Baltimore, Maryland, U.S.A.

Susan Redline   Heart and Vascular Center, MetroHealth Campus, Case Western Reserve University and University Hospitals, Case Medical Center, Cleveland, Ohio, U.S.A.

Clodagh M. Ryan   University of Toronto, Toronto, Ontario, Canada

Silke Ryan   St. Vincent's University Hospital and University College Dublin, Dublin, Ireland

Massimiliano M. Siccoli   Department of Neurology, University Hospital of Zurich, Zurich, Switzerland

Michael J. Sole   Toronto General Hospital Research Institute, University Health Network, Heart and Stroke, Richard Lewar Centre of Excellence, University of Toronto, Toronto, Ontario, Canada

Virend K. Somers   Mayo Clinic, Rochester, Minnesota, U.S.A.

Dan Sorajja   Mayo Clinic, Scottsdale, Arizona, U.S.A.

Cormac T. Taylor   St. Vincent's University Hospital and University College Dublin, Dublin, Ireland

John Trinder   University of Melbourne, Parkville, Victoria, Australia

Dai Yumino   Toronto Rehabilitation Institute, University of Toronto, Toronto, Ontario, Canada; Tokyo Women's Medical University, Tokyo, Japan

Contents

1

Diurnal Molecular Rhythms: Unrecognized Critical Determinants of Cardiovascular Health and Disease

MICHAEL J. SOLE
Toronto General Hospital Research Institute, University Health Network, Heart and Stroke, Richard Lewar Centre of Excellence, University of Toronto, Toronto, Ontario, Canada

TAMI A. MARTINO
Department of Biomedical Sciences, OVC, University of Guelph, Guelph, Ontario, Canada

Prior to the 20th century, human activity was synchronized to natural light/dark rhythms and adequate sleep was a cornerstone of the therapy of disease. Contemporary society appears to have lost interest in these physiological foundations of good health as it focuses on 24/7 schedules and the therapies of modern medicine.

I. Introduction

Physicians have recognized for centuries that both homeostasis and biological rhythms, although apparent antonyms, are the keystones of normal physiology. Two giants of physiology, Claude Bernard in France and Walter Cannon in the United States, championed the importance of homeostasis in modern medicine. This concept of maintenance of biological steady state so dominated medical thinking that the importance of biological rhythms fell into the shadows. In recent years, the measurement of neurohormonal rhythms and the subsequent discovery of actual molecular clocks have renewed interest in the importance of these circadian or diurnal rhythms—the genetic heritage of our evolution under the earth's 24-hour day/night cycle.

II. Rhythms in Cardiovascular Physiology and Disease

Circadian clocks allow us to entrain to environmental cues and hence anticipate the differing physiological and behavioral demands of daily events. We observe the output of these entrained clocks as daily rhythms such as sleep-wake cycles, body temperature cycles, and cyclic variations in heart rate and blood pressure. Neurohormones with anabolic or catabolic activity relevant to the cardiovascular system, such as plasma catecholamines, growth hormone, atrial natriuretic peptide (ANP), aldosterone, cortisol, renin, and melatonin, exhibit diurnal variations (1–3); these cycles are profoundly disrupted in heart failure (4,5). Rhythms have also been documented for vasomotor tone, platelet aggregability, and blood viscosity.

The occurrence of pathological cardiovascular events also exhibits diurnal variations. Acute myocardial infarction, ischemic and hemorrhagic stroke, sudden arrhythmic death, pulmonary embolism, and rupture or dissection of aortic aneurysms all show a peak incidence in the morning hours, just prior to and after awakening (3,6,7). Nocturnal myocardial infarcts are larger, exhibiting a greater risk of heart failure than those experienced during the day (8). The primary role of the intrinsic clock as opposed to the actual "stress" of awakening is illustrated by a study of 535 consecutive coroner's autopsies of sudden death over 11 years on the Hawaiian Island of Kauai (9). The number of cases of sudden death peaked at 6 a.m. to noon in Kauaians but noon to 4 p.m. in visitors, early morning in Japan; visitors were younger and had an incidence of sudden death nearly four times that of Kauaians. Obstructive sleep apnea may profoundly disrupt normal physiological diurnal rhythms; cardiac sudden death in these patients peaks during sleeping hours in contrast to the nadir in these events seen in the general population (10).

III. The Circadian System and Molecular Body Clock

The master or central clock resides in the suprachiasmatic nuclei (SCN); a pair of small nuclei, each a network of about 10,000 neurons, which reside in the anterior hypothalamus of the brain just above the optic chiasm. This clock normally entrains to periodic environmental cues, or zeitgebers, of which the 24-hour day/night or light/dark cycle is the most important; the day/night entrained circadian cycle is referred to as diurnal. The SCN is considered to play a key role because ablation of the SCN in hamsters has been shown to result in the loss of nearly all circadian rhythms, while transplantation of fetal SCN into these arrhythmic animals is restorative with the cycle of the donor tissue (11). The primary photoreceptors for the system are intrinsically photosensitive melanopsin containing retinal ganglionic cells that depolarize in response to light (12). Glutamate is a principal neurotransmitter conveying photic input from the eyes through the retinohypothalamic tract to the SCN. Output from the SCN synchronizes or coordinates biochemistry, physiology, and behavior primarily through neurohormonal outputs via the hypothalamic-pituitary pathways and the autonomic nervous system.

The core clockwork mechanism is based on a group of genes and protein products that positively or negatively interact and feedback in an oscillatory or circadian cycle of approximately 24 hours. Two main components are the genes *clock* and *bmal1*; their respective proteins CLOCK and BMAL1 heterodimerize and bind to E-box enhancers in the DNA as part of a positive loop. This in turn activates the transcription of genes involved in the negative feedback loop: period known as *per* (actually three paralogs *per1, per2, per3*), and cryptochrome, known as *cry* (*cry1* and *cry2*). CLOCK:BMAL1 heterodimers also activate the transcription of the nuclear receptor gene *Rev-Erba;* this protein in turn represses *bmal1* transcription. The protein products PER and CRY heterodimerize. Casein kinase-I ε (CKIε) phosphorylates and stabilizes these proteins; PER:CRY then translocates to the nucleus and negatively regulates the transcription (repress) of their parent genes by interacting with CLOCK:BMAL1 heterodimers. Inhibition of CLOCK:BMAL1–mediated transcription also represses *Rev-Erba* production, derepressing (activating) *bmal1* transcription. CLOCK:BMAL1 heterodimers increase again and another 24-hour clock cycle begins. There is an approximately 6 hours delay between peak protein and gene expression contributing to the rhythm of the feedback loops. There are many excellent reviews of the molecular mechanism of the mammalian circadian clock (13–15); however, relationships of critical components of the clockwork mechanism are illustrated in Figure 1.

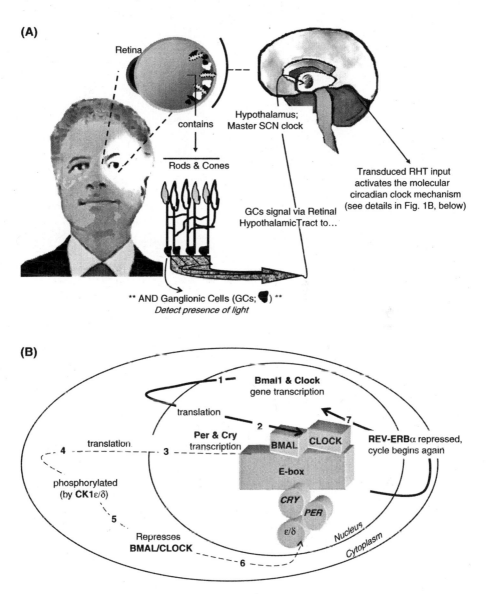

Figure 1 (**A**) The basic signal pathway of the circadian system. The presence or absence of light is detected by dedicated retinal ganglionic cells. Neurotransmitters such as glutamate transmit the signal from the ganglionic cells via a retinal-hypothalamic tract. Input is received by the supra-chiasmatic nucleus (SCN) of the hypothalamus, and used to set or reset the molecular circadian clock mechanism. Peripheral clocks are coordinated through neural and hormonal outputs. (**B**) The Molecular Circadian Clock Mechanism is in Virtually all Cells. The basic clockwork mechanism is illustrated here. It consists of a positive arm (black line) and negative arm (dashed line) of a transcriptional/translational autoregulatory feedback loop that cycles every 24 hours to keep "body time." The detailed pathway is described in the text.

In vitro and in vivo studies have demonstrated the molecular components of the 24-hour circadian clock in all tissues and cells except the testes (16–18). The clocks in peripheral (non-SCN) tissues are not directly exposed to photic input but may respond to behavioral cues such as feeding and exercise; however, their oscillations are primarily coordinated or synchronized by autonomic and neurohormonal outputs originating from the rhythms of the SCN. This is supported by observations such as light activation of the sympathetic nervous system and vagal suppression as measured by changes in arterial blood pressure and heart rate in anaesthetized mice; conversely, SCN lesioning ablates this response. There are likely different mechanisms downstream of neural or hormonal pathways that are key to regulating cross talk between the central clock and peripheral clocks in different tissues. Several bioactive peptides such as prokineticin 2, transforming growth factor-α, vasopressin, vasoactive intestinal peptide, and neurotensin are believed to be important mediators in differentially regulating peripheral clocks in different tissues.

Cell culture is a valuable tool for investigating regulation of peripheral cell clocks. Unlike cultured SCN cells, which cycle continuously, peripheral cells in culture appear unable to maintain coordinated rhythms after a few cycles, unless in the presence of a surrogate SCN signal. For example, circadian periodicity can be demonstrated in vascular smooth muscle cells in culture, maintained by neurohormonal influences such as angiotensin II (19). Circadian oscillators in the liver, kidney, heart, and cultured rat-1 fibroblasts may be controlled by glucocorticoids. Noradrenergic stimulation resets cardiomyocyte gene oscillations in vitro.

Clocks in peripheral tissues, though synchronized within the given tissue, may have a rhythm that runs hours behind that in the SCN. Circadian physiology is presumably coordinated in this manner so that each tissue is best able to meet specific demands for the organism. For example, local tissue oscillators in the heart coordinate clock-dependent physiology such as heart rate and blood pressure. Similarly, local tissue oscillators in vascular smooth muscle cells coordinate clock-dependant vasodilatory responses and within the endothelium they regulate thrombolytic activity. Circadian rhythms coordinate perhaps thousands of biochemical and biophysical pathways and responses daily, ensuring the process occurs during a biologically optimal time of day.

IV. Melatonin and the Cardiovascular System

The pineal gland, with its neuroendocrine effector, melatonin, is a principal target for SCN signaling and possibly regulates cardiac clocks as well. Melatonin is synthesized and released during the dark phase in both diurnal and nocturnal animals (20) and is thus a leading neuroendocrine contender connecting light/dark cycling and peripheral organ circadian activity. The SCN contains high levels of melatonin receptors (MT1, MT2). These are G protein–coupled receptors, with MT1 inhibiting adenylate cyclase activity, while MT2 inhibiting soluble guanylate cyclase and stimulating protein kinase C.

MT1 receptors have also been discovered in human coronary arteries and MT2 in the heart, coronary arteries, and aorta. Experimentally, melatonin administered mice has a marked effect on the myocardial transcriptome (21). Also, melatonin administered to the anterior hypothalamus in rats decreases blood pressure and heart rate; this effect appears to be mediated by MT1 receptors (22). Orally administered melatonin increases cardiac vagal tone, decreases blood pressure, and vascular reactivity in spontaneously hypertensive rats. Cardiomyopathic hamsters show a loss of melatonin cycling as their heart disease progresses (5); relevance to the pathophysiology of this disease may be worthy of further investigation. A possible mechanism for melatonin is through its potent antioxidant and free-radical scavenger activity. It has been shown to markedly reduce ischemia-reperfusion injury in the hearts of pinealectomized rats (which produce minimal endogenous melatonin) in vivo and protect against ischemia-reperfusion arrhythmias ex vivo (23). It also protects rats against cardiac damage from doxorubicin toxicity. Patient studies are limited; however, endogenous melatonin production has been shown to be reduced in patients with coronary artery disease and also during acute myocardial infarction (24,25).

V. Diurnal Molecular Biology of Cardiovascular Tissues

In contrast to the well-documented day/night variations in cardiovascular physiology and pathology, little was known about the temporal control of the underlying molecular mechanisms until recently. In 2002, Storch and colleagues demonstrated circadian gene expression in liver and heart under constant conditions of dim light (17). Real life exists under diurnal conditions; thus it was also important that expression of the genes of the heart be examined under normal diurnal light:dark (L:D) cycling. We used normal C57Bl/6 mice and collected heart tissue over 24-hour diurnal cycles, extracted the mRNA cycling transcriptome, and analyzed this using high-density oligonucleotide microarrays, semiquantitative PCR, and COSOPT, an analytical algorithm specifically designed to identify significant rhythms and corresponding phase optima (16).

We found (16) that greater than 13% of genes in the normal heart exhibited significant changes in gene expression over regular 24-hour day/night cycles; gene expression was remarkably different during day versus night. There were two principal rhythmic expression peaks—one in the light phase and a second peak in the dark (Fig. 3A). Interestingly, a third subset of genes showed remarkably abrupt changes in expression only at the light:dark transition times (Fig. 2). Genes exhibiting diurnal profiles were classified using the Gene Ontology Consortium and map to key biological processes including cardiac metabolism, growth and remodeling, transcription/translation, and molecular signal pathways.

Gene expression in the aorta was similarly examined by microarray and bioinformatics analyses (26). This revealed two major peaks in rhythmic gene expression (one in the light phase and other in the dark phase), though notably these peaks occurred at slightly different times than those in the heart (Fig. 3B). There was also a third minor peak in the aorta that occurred in the dark. Like an advancing wave coordinating body physiology, there is master control by the SCN, organ-to-organ synchrony, and tissue-specific rhythmic profiles over the 24-hour diurnal cycle.

We then examined diurnal gene expression in compensatory cardiac remodeling. For this study (26), we used a model of pressure-overload myocardial hypertrophy produced by transverse aortic constriction (TAC) in the mouse. Hearts and aortae were collected from the TAC mice (and sham-operated controls) every four hours over the diurnal cycle, the mRNA was purified, and rhythmic gene expression evaluated using a microarray and bioinformatics approach (16). Rhythmic gene expression in the TAC mice was virtually superimposable in time (Fig. 3). That is, the cycling transcriptome in TAC hearts showed the same period and phase as normal or sham-operated heart. Similarly, for TAC aorta subject to high pressure (above the ligature) or low pressure (below the ligature), the transcriptome maintained the same rhythmic cycling profile as in normal (or

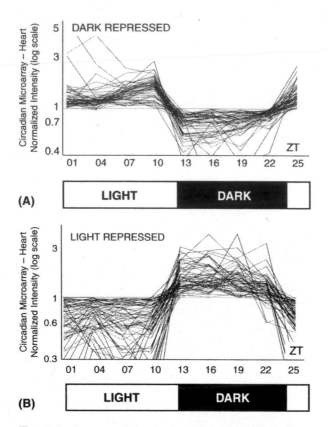

Figure 2 Gene expression in the normal heart is remarkably different day versus night. The subset of genes shown here showed remarkably abrupt changes in expression only at the light:dark transition times. (**A**) Dark repressed genes: these exhibited upregulated expression in the light, they were downregulated across the entire dark period, and upregulated again as soon as the lights returned on. (**B**) Light repressed genes: these exhibited the opposite profile, Down-regulated expression in the light, up-regulated across the entire dark period, and downregulated again as soon as the lights returned on.

sham-operated) vasculature. Thus, global gene rhythms in murine TAC heart and aorta are conserved even in the presence of myocellular remodeling.

Previous studies support the concept that diurnal variation plays a fundamental role in myocyte maintenance and growth. Ornithine decarboxylase, the rate-limiting enzyme in polyamine biosynthesis, and acid phosphatases, lysosomal enzymes important in intracellular metabolism, show significant circadian variation within the myocardium (27). Also, differential incorporation of labeled leucine into rat myocardial protein over 24 hours indicates that myocardial protein may be synthesized at the greatest rate late in the light period (rats asleep) with the least synthesis occurring 12 hours later (rats active) (28).

CLOCK protein has been found recently within the myofilament Z-disc colocalizing with α-actinin; also, myocyte contractility can directly alter the subcellular

Time of day

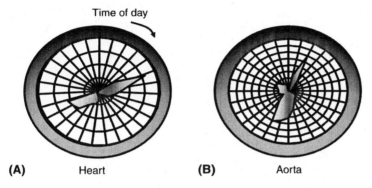

(A)   Heart   **(B)**   Aorta

Figure 3 Bioinformatic analyses of diurnal gene expression in the normal heart and aorta. Rhythmic gene expression in normal heart and aorta is examined by microarray and bioinformatics (COSOPT) analyses, and plotted on a radar diagram. Global gene expression in the heart shows a biphasic pattern with two major peaks, one in the light phase, and one in the dark phase (**A**, *left*). The aorta similarly reveals two major peaks in gene cycling, one in the light and one in the dark, though notably these peaks occur at slightly different times than those for the heart (**B**, *right*). There is also a third minor peak in the aorta that occurs in the dark. Rhythmicity helps coordinate thousands of biochemical and biophysical pathways and responses daily. Presumably the specificity of peak and phase helps ensure that processes occur during a biologically optimal time of day for each tissue/organ as needed.

distribution of CLOCK (29). CLOCK is also implicated in chromatin remodeling and acetylation. Indeed there is a growing belief that many hundreds of genes may be under the direct regulation of the local molecular clockwork. Another link between cardiac hypertrophy or remodeling and the circadian clockwork may be through glycogen synthase kinase-3β (GSK3-β). GSK3-β has recently been discovered to be an integral component of the mammalian circadian clock perhaps promoting the nuclear translocation of PER2 advancing (GSK3-β increased) or delaying (GSK3-β decreased) clock phase (30). It is of particular interest for the current discussion that GSK3-β also negatively regulates cardiac hypertrophy; activation of GSK3-β by phosphorylation at the serine 9 residue antagonizes the cardiac hypertrophic response to stimuli such as pressure overload or catecholamine stimulation (31).

There is also substantive evidence, largely established through Young and coworkers, that the cardiac circadian clock synchronizes cardiac metabolism to the environment (32,33). Using the isolated working rat heart they demonstrated that cardiac contractile performance, carbohydrate utilization, and oxygen consumption were greatest during the night when rats are normally active. There was little day/night variation in oleate oxidation. As the authors noted, this may be considered an example of an important role of the clock—anticipating environmental demands; in this case, clock-synchronized metabolism prepared the heart for an increase in the animal's physical activity; if the animal was unable to find food (a source of carbohydrate), the fatty acid metabolic pathway was readied to utilize fat from body stores.

Recently, these metabolic data were confirmed and extended in isolated adult rat cardiomyocytes (34). Fasting rats resulted in the induction of fatty acid responsive genes; disruption of the cardiac circadian clock through overexpression of a dominant negative clock mutant severely attenuated this response. Reversal of the day/night cycle leads to metabolic desynchrony—reestablishment of normal metabolic synchronization took between five and eight days. Such data would suggest that hearts of shift workers, travelers crossing many time zones, or those suffering chronic sleep disturbance such as obstructive sleep apnea may require several days for appropriate metabolic entrainment to their new day/night environment. Though beyond the scope of this review, these data also suggest that day/night or sleep disturbances may predispose to obesity, not only through disruption of relevant rhythmic neuroendocrine pathways such as leptin and grehlin, but also through impaired metabolic responses of target tissues.

VI. Diurnal Rhythms and Cardiovascular Diagnostic Testing and Therapy

Diurnal rhythms are an important consideration in some diagnostic tests. For example, exercise tolerance in patients with angina is reduced in early morning and again at night, relative to the afternoon (3). Ambulatory ECG monitoring of ischemia in stable patients with coronary artery disease also shows a morning peak (35). This reflects circadian variation of coronary tone with a morning exaggeration of vasoconstrictor tone seen in diseased segments (36).

Normal blood pressure across the diurnal cycle exhibits a 10% decrease at night with a pressure surge in the morning just prior to and upon awakening. Patients with hypertension fall into two primary groups of blood pressure profile (37). One group parallels the cyclic variation in pressure exhibited by normotensives, including the nocturnal drop or "dip" in blood pressure but at an overall elevated level; a small subgroup may exhibit an exaggerated drop. A second group, known as "non-dippers," shows a failure to decrease blood pressure by 10% with a few even exhibiting a nocturnal increase; the non-dipper group exhibits an increased risk of target organ damage, with greater left ventricular hypertrophy and an increased risk of cardiovascular and renal disease (37).

The above data strongly suggest that circadian rhythms are relevant to the effectiveness of some therapies. For example, epidemiological studies indicate that circadian variation has a clinically significant effect on the outcome of primary angioplasty (38). Patients treated in "off-hours" have a significantly worse outcome following angioplasty than those treated during the normal working day; this does not appear to be due to differences in "quality of care." A second example is patients with implantable cardioverter defibrillators. There is a diurnal variation in defibrillation energy requirements with an increase in the early morning—a time when patients are most likely to have a catastrophic event; thus, the estimation of energy requirements in the operating room at the time of implantation must account for diurnal time of day (39). A third example follows conversion from conventional hemodialysis to nocturnal hemodialysis, which results in significant regression of left ventricular hypertrophy in patients with endstage renal disease (40). This could be considered analogous to the long-term reverse remodeling benefits that ensue from the treatment of obstructive sleep apnea—continuous positive airway pressure (CPAP) therapy (41) applied only at night yields long-term benefits for ventricular reverse remodeling. These results may be considered the converse of the increase in target organ damage seen in non-dipper hypertensive patients.

The MILIS ISAM and BHAT databases demonstrate that β-blockade markedly attenuates the morning increase in myocardial infarction and sudden death (3). Interestingly no such decrease in the usual morning peak of ventricular tachycardia was seen in a study of β-blocked patients with implanted cardioverter defibrillators (42); this may reflect the morning increase in human ventricular refractoriness induced by β-blockers (43).

Chronotherapeutic strategies in clinical medicine have been employed on a largely empirical basis or on drug clearance and metabolism data. For example, there are several chronotherapeutic formulations of the calcium channel blockers—some appear to be primarily motivated by patent extension. Low-dose evening aspirin has been shown to have a mild antihypertensive effect and less gastric irritability than the same dose taken in the morning (44). Most statins are more effective when taken in the evening. Discovery of tissue clocks has paved the way for more basic studies. For example, a recent study has demonstrated a link between tissue sensitivity to cyclophosphamide chemotherapy and the molecular state of the tissue circadian clock (45).

Our analysis of gene expression cycling in the heart and aorta in murine TAC (26) showed phase conservation of normal cardiac and vascular diurnal cycling but with upregulation of the genes involved in cardiac responses such as blood pressure homeostasis, myocyte hypertrophy, and tissue remodeling including angiotensin-converting enzyme (ACE). This provided a molecular rationale for the temporal targeting of remodeling. Thus, we investigated the diurnal efficacy of the short-acting ACE inhibitor therapy—captopril, given by intraperitoneal injection—on cardiac remodeling in TAC mouse (46). Captopril, given when the mice normally slept, significantly improved cardiovascular function and reduced adverse remodeling. Conversely, captopril administered during waking active hours did not have this effect; indeed cardiac outcome was as poor as in TAC mice given vehicle alone. Thus, timing of Captopril was most beneficial when administered in coordination with molecular diurnal physiology, at a time when the rhythmic cycling of ACE gene expression levels was highest.

Assessment of all of the molecular, physiological, and therapeutic data described above are consistent with our hypothesis that myocardial renewal and growth is diurnal, with significant activity occurring during sleep when heart rate and blood pressure are at their lowest and physiological stress is at minimum. Cell energy and resources then can be turned from coping with external physiological demands toward cellular repair and growth. This would be also supported by the increased prevalence of adverse cardiovascular events found in shift workers, transmeridian flight crews, patients with sleep apnea, and other sleep disturbances (47). For example, a prospective study of 79,109 U.S. female nurses from the Nurses Health Study Cohort, 42- to 67-year-olds and initially free of diagnosed coronary artery or cerebrovascular disease, revealed that shift work increased the risk of coronary heart disease (48). The data was corrected for multiple risk factors such as smoking, hypertension, diabetes, obesity, hypercholesterolemia, family history, aspirin use, menopausal status, and hormone use, etc. Similar data for males were found in a 14-year follow-up study of 504 Swedish paper mill workers (49). Obstructive sleep apnea, discussed elsewhere in this volume, has been clearly linked as a culprit in the pathogenesis of cardiac arrhythmias, high blood pressure, and coronary artery disease. Sleep disruption itself appears to have broad pathological consequences in humans; studies have demonstrated increases in plasma C–reactive protein an inflammatory risk marker for coronary heart disease (50), profound abnormalities in fat and glucose metabolism, an increased prevalence of hypertension, obesity, and diabetes (51,52).

Certainly this portends a much broader range of public health issues from sleep and day/night schedule disruption than just impaired cognitive function or degraded job performance due to fatigue, the primary foci of contemporary thought to date.

VII. Diurnal Rhythms as Etiological Factors in the Pathogenesis of Cardiovascular Disease

Despite all of the epidemiological, physiological, and molecular data above, circadian disorganization has never been directly shown as a direct causal risk factor in cardiovascular or indeed organ disease. It has been inferred from earlier studies, for example mice exposed to phase advances of the light/dark cycle that mimic chronic jet-lag, exhibit higher mortality than unshifted control mice or even those exposed to phase delays (53). Also, repeated phase shifts in the light/dark cycle reduce longevity in the cardiomyopathic Syrian hamster (54).

Using our murine TAC model of pressure overload hypertrophy, described above (26), we examined the effects of a rhythm-disruptive environment on cardiac pathophysiology. The "rhythm-disrupted" TAC mice housed in an altered light:dark environment (20 hours versus the normal 24-hour diurnal cycle) exhibited increased left ventricular end-systolic and end-diastolic diameters and reduced contractility with an increase in blood pressure compared to "non-rhythm-disrupted" TAC mice. Histology was strikingly abnormal. In spite of the increased pressure load, myocyte hypertrophy in both blood vessels and heart was markedly constrained; fibrous tissue accretion in both vessels (perivascular) and heart, however, was significantly increased. Effectively both heart and blood vessel walls were inappropriately thin relative to the blood pressure burden. The molecular clock was also disrupted in this altered environment, as demonstrated by abnormal cycling of *bmal1* and *per2* in the heart and SCN. Key genes in the hypertrophic pathways such as *BNP, ACE ANF,* and *collagen* were inappropriately downregulated. When the external rhythm was allowed to correspond to the animals' innate 24-hour internal rhythm, the clock normalized, blood pressure fell to that seen in control TAC mice, and there was a dramatic and paradoxical increase in myocyte hypertrophy along with upregulation of hypertrophic gene expression. The data demonstrate that desynchronization between external and internal rhythms can prevent an appropriate tissue histological and genetic response to a rise in blood pressure; thus, in hypertensive humans, desynchronization should augment cardiovascular target organ damage.

We also explored the direct long-term effects of rhythm desynchronization on normal organ physiology, such as might occur in humans with recurrent jet lag, chronic sleep disturbance, or shift work. In spite of the epidemiological data, we did not know if circadian desynchronization, alone, was sufficient to cause disease. We used a prototypic model of circadian rhythm disruption that had been linked with reduced longevity: hamsters carrying a mutation in casein kinase-1ε (*tau* mutants). The mutant allele reduces the free-running circadian period from approximately 24 hours in the wild type to approximately 22 hours in *tau*/+ heterozygotes. When *tau*/+ (22 hours) hamsters are entrained to a 24-hour day, there is early onset and significant fragmentation of activity. We demonstrated that these animals, although normal when young, develop significant cardiac and renal pathology over the long term (55). Ultimately, they die prematurely with severe dilated cardiomyopathy and renal failure. For hamsters on light cycles appropriate for their genotype behavior patterns, life expectancy and heart and renal structure and function are normal. Pathology does not develop in homozygous *tau/tau* hamsters because their extremely short intrinsic (20 hours) circadian period is able to dominate the external environment with little conflict. Similarly, abnormal cardiorenal pathology is not seen in *tau/+* raised in darkness or in those with their SCN removed. In these latter models, no conflict develops between internal and external rhythms—in the former, rhythm is dictated internally and in the latter, by the external environment. Thus, in animals bearing the heterozygote *+/tau* mutation organ pathology arises when normal internal circadian rhythmicity is disrupted or conflicted. In this case and in the case of the TAC, mouse organ pathology develops when there is a conflict between the endogenous tissue clock and diurnal signals coming from the SCN. Thus, circadian dysregulation can be profoundly important in the etiology or exacerbation of cardiovascular and renal disease. Undoubtedly, our observations will be extended by others to other tissues including the central nervous system.

VIII. Summary

Gene expression in the heart is dramatically different in the day as compared to the night. Cardiovascular metabolism, growth, and renewal is dynamic and does not occur uniformly over the day/night cycle; growth and renewal appear to occur during sleep. The risk/benefit ratio of a therapeutic intervention is not uniform across the 24-hour cycle but occurs in a diurnal fashion. Synchrony between intrinsic and extrinsic diurnal/circadian rhythms is integral to healthy organ growth and renewal. Disruption of this synchrony has a devastating effect on the heart, kidney, and possibly other organs.

Unfortunately, awareness of the importance of chronobiology including chronotherapeutics has not substantively penetrated clinical medicine. As noted in Nature as recently as December 2005 (56), sleep is regarded as "of the brain, by the brain and for the brain." Sleep may be "of" the brain but biological rhythms are found in all organs ("by" all organs), and our studies show that the integrity of biological rhythms are likely "for" all organs—certainly for the health and integrity of the cardiovascular system. Modern hospitals, particularly intensive and cardiac care units still use multibedded rooms ignoring the importance of undisturbed diurnal rhythms for the healing process even in critically ill. Finally, save for possible inquiry regarding sleep apnea, clinicians and society largely disregard regular day/night schedules or sleep as a risk factor for disease, yet this aspect of human physiology and behavior is as crucial to our well being as are exercise, nutrition, and hygiene.

> Our body is like a clock; if one wheel be amiss, all the rest are disordered, the whole fabric suffers: with such admirable art and harmony is a man composed.

> Robert Burton (1621)

Acknowledgments

We are grateful for the support of the Abraham and Malka Green Foundation, the A. Ephraim and Shirley Diamond Cardiomyopathy Research Fund, and the Heart and Stroke Foundation of Ontario. We also thank Professors Martin Ralph and Denise Belsham for their support and continuous collaboration in our research.

References

1. Charloux A, Gronfier C, Lonsdorfer-Wolf E, et al. Aldosterone release during the sleep-wake cycle in humans. Am. J. Physiol. 1999; 276:E43–E49.
2. Nicolau HE, Lakatua DJ, Sackett-Lundeenl, et al. Circadian rhythm parameters of endocrine functions in elderly subjects during the seventh to ninth decade of life. Chronobiologia 1989; 16:331–352.
3. Muller JE, Tofler GH, Stone PH. Circadian variation and triggers of onset of cardiovascular disease. Circulation 1989; 79:733–743.
4. Giustina A, Lorusso R, Borghetti V, et al. Impaired spontaneous growth hormone secretion in severe dilated cardiomyopathy. Am Heart J 1996; 131:620–622.
5. Reiter RJ, White T, Lerchl A, et al. Attenuated nocturnal rise in pineal and serum melatonin in a genetically cardiomyopathic Syrian hamster with a deficient calcium pump. J Pineal Res 1991; 11:156–162.
6. Guo Y-F, Stein PK Circadian rhythm in the cardiovascular system: chronocardiology. Am Heart J 2003; 145:779–786.
7. Manfredini R, Boari B, Gallerani M, et al. Chronobiology of rupture and dissection of aortic aneurysms. J Vasc Surg 2004; 40:382–388.
8. Mukamal KJ, Muller JE, Maclure M, et al. Increased risk of congestive heart failure among infarctions with nighttime onset. Am Heart J 2000;140:438–442.
9. Couch RD. Travel, time zones, and sudden cardiac death. Emporiatric pathology. Am J Forensic Med Path 1990; 11:106–111.
10. Gami AS, Howard DE, Olsen EJ, et al. Day-night pattern of sudden death in obstructive sleep apnea. N Engl J Med 2005; 352:1206–1214.
11. Ralph MR, Foster RG, Davis FC, et al. Transplanted suprachiasmatic nucleus determines circadian rhythms. Science 1990; 247:975–978.
12. Guller AD, Ecker JL, Lall GS, et al. Melanopsin cells are the principal conduits for rod-cone input to non-image forming vision. Nature 453(7191):102–105 [Epub April 23, 2008].
13. King DP, Takahashi JS. Molecular genetics of circadian rhythms in mammals. Annu Rev Neurosci 2000; 23:713–742.
14. Reppert SM, Weaver DR. Coordination of circadian timing in mammals. Nature 2002; 418:935–941.
15. Shearman LP, Sriram S, Weaver DR, et al. Interacting molecular loops in the mammalian circadian clock. Science 2000; 288:1013–1019.
16. Martino TA, Arab S, Straume M, et al. Day/night rhythms in gene expression of the normal murine heart. J Mol Med 2004; 82:256–264.
17. Storch KF, Lipan O, Leykin I, et al. Extensive and divergent circadian gene expression in liver and heart. Nature 2002; 417:78–83.
18. James FO, Boivin DB, Charbonneau S, et al. Expression of clock genes in peripheral human blood mononuclear cells throughout the sleep/wake and circadian cycles. Chronobiol Int 2007; 24:1009–1034.
19. Nonaka H, Emoto N, Ikeda K, et al. Angiotensin II induces circadian gene expression of clock genes in cultured vascular smooth muscle cells. Circulation 2001; 104:1746–1748.
20. Pando MP, Sassone-Corsi P. Signaling to the mammalian circadian clocks: in pursuit of the primary mammalian circadian photoreceptor. Sci STKE 2001;107:1–8.
21. Anisimov SV, Boheler KP, Anisimov VN. Microarray technology in studying the effect of melatonin on gene expression in the mouse heart. Doklody Biol Sci 2002; 383:90–93.
22. Ding CN, Cao YX, Zhou L, et al. Effects of microinjection of melatonin and its receptor antagonists into anterior hypothalamic area on blood pressure and heart rate in rats. Acta Phamacol Sin 2001; 22:997–1002.

23. Sahana E, Acet A, Ozer MK, et al. Myocardial ischemia-reperfusion in rats: reduction of infarct size by either supplemental physiological or pharmacological doses of melatonin. J Pineal Res 2002; 33:234–238.
24. Yaprak M, Altun A, Vardar A, et al. Decreased nocturnal synthesis of melatonin in patients with coronary artery disease. Int J Cardiol 2003; 89:103–107.
25. Dominguez-Rodriguez A, Abreu-Gonzolez P, Garcia MJ, et al. Decreased nocturnal melatonin levels during acute myocardial infarction. J Pineal Res 2002; 33:248–252.
26. Martino TA, Tata N, Belsham DD, et al. Disturbed diurnal rhythm alters gene expression and exacerbates cardiovascular disease with rescue by resynchronization. Hypertension 2007; 49:1–10.
27. Waldrop RD, Saydjari R, Arnold JR, et al. Twenty-four-hour variations in ornithine decarboxylase and acid phosphatase in mice. Proc Soc Exp Biol Med 1989; 191:420–424.
28. Rau E, Meyer DK. A diurnal rhythm of incorporation of L-[3H] leucine in myocardium of the rat. In: Harris P, Bing RJ, Fleckenstein A, eds. Recent Advances in Studies on Cardiac Structure and Metabolism. Vol 7. Baltimore: University Park Press, 1975:105–110.
29. Boateng SY, Goldspink PH. Assembly and maintenance of the sarcomere night and day. Cardiovasc Res 2008; 77:667–675.
30. Iitaka C, Miyazaki K, Akaike T, et al. A role for glycogen synthase kinase-3β in the mammalian circadian clock. J Biol Chem 2005; 280:29297–29402.
31. Hardt SE, Sadoshima J. Glycogen synthase kinase-3β: a novel regulator of cardiac hypertrophy and development. Circ Res 2002; 90:1055–1063.
32. Young ME. The circadian clock within the heart: potential influence on myocardial gene expression, metabolism and function. Am J Physiol 2006; 290:H1–H16.
33. Young ME, Razeghi P, Cedars AM, et al. Intrinsic diurnal variations in cardiac metabolism and contractile function. Cic Res 2001; 89:1199–1208.
34. Durgan DJ, Trexler N, Egbejimi O, et al. The circadian clock within the cardiomyocyte is essential for responsiveness of the heart to fatty acids. J Biol Chem 2006; 281:24254–24269.
35. Krantz DS, Kop WJ, Gabbay FH, et al. Circadian variation of ambulatory myocardial ischemia. Circulation 1996; 93:1364–1371.
36. El Tamimi H, Mansour M, Pepine CJ, et al. Circadian variation in coronary tone in patients with stable angina. Circulation 1995; 92:3201–3205.
37. Piexoto AJ, White WB. Circadian blood pressure: clinical implications based on the pathophysiology of its variability. Kidney Int 2007; 71:855–860.
38. Henriques JPS, Haasdjik AP, Zijlstra F, et al. Outcome of primary angioplasty for acute myocardial infarction during routine duty hours versus during off-hours. J Am Coll Cardiol 2003; 41:2138–2142.
39. Venditti FJ, John RM, Hull M, et al. Circadian variation in defibrillation energy requirements. Circulation 1996; 94.1607–1612.
40. Chan CT, Floras JS, Miller JA. Regression of left ventricular hypertrophy after conversion to nocturnal hemodialysis. Kidney Int 2002; 61:2235–2239.
41. Bradley TD, Logan AG, Floras JS, for the CANPAP investigators. Rationale and design of the Canadian Continuous Positive Airway Pressure Trial for Congestive Heart Failure Patients with Central Sleep Apnea—CANPAP. Can J Cardiol 2001; 17:677–684.
42. Nanthakumar K, Newman D, Paquette M, et al. Circadian variation of sustained ventricular tachycardia in patients subject to standard adrenergic blockade. Am Heart J 1997; 134: 752–757.
43. Kong TQ, Goldberger JJ, Parker M, et al. Circadian variation in human ventricular refractoriness. Circulation 1995; 92:1507–1516.
44. Hermida RC, Ayal DE, Calvo C, et al. Administration time-dependent effects of aspirin on blood pressure in untreated hypertensive patients. Hypertension 2003; 41:1259–1267.

45. Gorbacheva VY, Kondrakov RV, Zhang R, et al. Circadian sensitivity to the chemotherapeutic agent cyclophosphamide depends on the functional status of the CLOCK/BMAL1 transactivation complex. Proc Natl Acad Sci U S A 2005; 103:3407–3412.

46. Tata N, Martino TA, Vanderlaan R, et al. Chronotherapy: diurnal efficacy of captopril. J Cardiac Failure 2005; 11:S99.

47. Knuttson A, Boggild H. Shift work and cardiovascular disease: review of disease mechanisms. Rev Environ Health 2000; 15:359—372.

48. Kawachi I, Colditz GA, Sampfer MJ, et al. Prospective study of shift work and risk of coronary heart disease in women. Circulation 1995; 92:3178–3182.

49. Knutsson A, Akerstedt T, Jonsson BG, et al. Increased risk of ischaemic heart disease in shift workers. Lancet 1986; 2:89–92.

50. Meier-Ewert HK, Ridker PM, Rifai N, et al. Effect of sleep loss on C-reactive protein an inflammatory marker of cardiovascular risk. J Am Coll Cardiol 2004; 43:678–683.

51. Spiegel K, Leproult R, van Cauter E. Impact of sleep debt on metabolic and endocrine function. Lancet 1999; 354:1435–1439.

52. Gangwisch JE, Malaspina D, Boden-Albala B, et al. Inadequate sleep as a risk factor for obesity: analyses of the NHANES I. Sleep 2005; 28:1289–96.

53. Davidson AJ, Sellix MT, Yamazaki S, et al. Chronic jet lag increases mortality in aged mice. Curr Biol 2006; 16:R914–R916.

54. Penev PD, Kolker DE, Zee PC, et al. Chronic circadian desynchronization decreases the survival of animals with cardiomyopthic heart disease. Am J Physiol 1998; 275:H2334–H2337.

55. Martino TA, Oudit GY, Herzenberg AM, et al. Circadian rhythm disorganization produces profound cardiovascular and renal disease in hamsters. Am J Physiol Regul Integr Comp Physiol 2008; 294(5):R1675–1683.

56. Hobson JA. Sleep is of the brain, by the brain and for the brain. Nature 2005; 437:1254–1256.

2

Lower Brainstem Mechanisms of Cardiorespiratory Integration

PATRICE G. GUYENET
University of Virginia School of Medicine, Charlottesville, Virginia, U.S.A.

I. Introduction

This chapter is a brief survey of the lower brainstem network that regulates vasomotor sympathetic nerve activity (SNA) and cardiovagal efferent activity. The emphasis is placed on the control of the heart and the sympathetic outflow by chemoreceptors (central and peripheral) and by lung stretch receptors because of the special relevance of these regulatory mechanisms to obstructive sleep apnea (1).

The sympathetic vasomotor system consists of a large subset of sympathetic efferents that innervate the heart, the arterioles and veins, the adrenal medulla, and the kidneys. These efferents regulate the cardiac output, blood pressure (BP), and regional blood flow in accordance with behavior (2–4). They probably also regulate the 24-hour BP set point by controlling renal sodium excretion. The sympathetic vasomotor efferents are differentially regulated depending on the specific organ or tissue that they innervate (5), but they have several common and distinctive characteristics (2,6). They are usually active to some degree (the so-called sympathetic vasomotor tone); their activity is regulated by the brainstem respiratory network and is strongly synchronized to the arterial pressure pulse. There are a few prominent exceptions to this general rule. Adrenaline release by the adrenal medulla plays an important role in cardiovascular regulation, but the secretion of this hormone is not under baroreceptor control and is primarily regulated by the blood glucose level and by stress or exercise (2,7). Cutaneous blood flow is primarily regulated by fear and emotions and also by skin and core temperature for thermoregulatory purposes (8). Adrenaline release and cutaneous blood flow will not be discussed in this chapter.

II. Medullospinal Network That Controls Sympathetic Vasomotor Tone

A. Spinal Mechanisms

Location and Phenotype of SPGNs That Control the Heart and Blood Vessels

Sympathetic preganglionic neurons (SPGNs) are primarily located in the lateral horn (also known as the intermediolateral cell column, or IML) from the lower cervical to the upper lumbar level (e.g., caudal C8 to L3–L5 in rats) (9). Myocardial control originates from SPGNs located in the upper thoracic segments (T1–T3 in rats), and the innervation is somewhat lateralized (10,11). The right side of the spinal cord controls rate preferentially, while ventricular contractility is regulated preferentially by SPGNs located on the left side (10,11). Vasoconstrictor SPGNs that control skin or muscle blood flow are presumably dispersed throughout the IML. Splanchnic, renal, and adrenal SPGNs are confined to specific albeit overlapping sets of thoracic segments. All SPGNs, regardless of function, are cholinergic, and the vast majority contains high levels of nitric oxide (NO) synthase. NO released by the soma or dendrites of SPGNs probably serves as a retrograde signal that enhances the presynaptic release of both excitatory and inhibitory transmitters (12). SPGNs display considerable phenotypical heterogeneity, and at least four different neuropeptides (enkephalin, somatostatin, neurotensin, and substance P) have been detected in mammalian SPGNs by immunohistochemistry (13). SPGNs are also heterogeneous in their expression of several calcium-binding proteins (14,15).

Major Inputs to SPGNs

In neonates, SPGNs are electrically coupled and can be autoactive (16). In adulthood, SPGNs are presumed to need synaptic input to be active. All SPGNs receive monosynaptic input from the same general regions of the brain, albeit in variable proportion and presumably from different subsets of neurons within each region (17,18). Schematically, these inputs can be divided into two broad categories. The first type of input probably targets very broad classes of SPGNs and conveys information of a general modulatory nature often linked to the state of vigilance. The noradrenergic (A5), serotonergic, and, perhaps, the orexinergic inputs fit this definition best (19–22). The second category of input presumably transmits more specialized and discriminative information to specific functional subsets of SPGNs. All the latter inputs probably use a fast transmitter that acts via ionotropic receptors (gamma-aminobutyric acid [GABA], glycine, glutamate primarily), but they also often release other signaling molecules (e.g., peptides, biogenic amines) that operate via metabotropic transmission. These specialized inputs originate from various levels and laminae of the spinal cord, the ventrolateral medulla (VLM), the midline medulla, and several hypothalamic regions, most prominently the parvocellular subdivision of the paraventricular nucleus (17,23). Projections from the dorsolateral pons (Kölliker-Fuse) may also exist but are less convincingly demonstrated (23).

Vasoconstrictor, adrenal, renal, and cardioaccelerator SPGNs receive their dominant excitatory input from the rostral ventrolateral medulla (RVLM) (Fig. 1A). This connection is critical for BP stability and blood gas regulation (2). The rest of the excitatory input to vasomotor SPGNs probably originates from spinal cord interneurons, the caudalmost portion of the medulla oblongata, the raphe, and the hypothalamus (17,24). The major inhibitory input to these neurons probably originates from GABA and glycinergic neurons located in the ventromedial medulla, the raphe, and the spinal cord (17,25,26). The role of the spinal interneurons in vasomotor control may be underrated in our present understanding. These interneurons obviously mediate spinal reflexes, but they may also mediate some of the effects of descending inputs from the medulla oblongata and elsewhere. For example, some evidence suggests that baroreceptor-mediated inhibition of SPGNs in vivo could be partly mediated by the activation of spinal glycinergic or GABAergic interneurons (27). Although vasomotor SPGNs are typically described as solely controlled by monosynaptic inputs from supraspinal structures, these supraspinal inputs may in fact control a spinal sympathetic network consisting of the SPGNs and spinal interneurons antecedent to the latter (28).

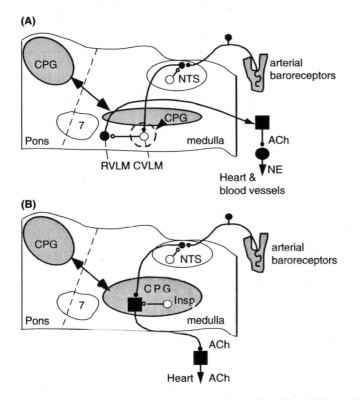

Figure 1 Barorcflexes. (A) Sympathetic baroreflex. The CPG consists of a pontine and a medullary component that are linked reciprocally (*double arrows*). Transmission between baroreceptors and second-order neurons is regulated by interneurons. Transmission between second-order neurons and the CVLM is regulated by the respiratory network. RVLM presympathetic neurons are glutamatergic and express additional transmitters. Those that synthesize catecholamines are called C1 neurons. (B) Cardiovagal baroreflex. Second-order baroreceptor neurons may not synapse directly on the cardiovagal preganglionic neurons as shown but through local interneurons. CVMs are inhibited during insp. In **A** and **B**, *black circles* are excitatory neurons or their terminals. *Open circles* are inhibitory neurons; 7: facial motor nucleus. *Abbreviations*: CPG, central respiratory pattern generator; CVLM, caudal ventrolateral medulla; RVLM, rostral ventrolateral medulla; CVM, cardiovagal motor neuron; insp, inspiration.

Cutaneous vasoconstrictors derive their main excitatory drive from presympathetic cells located in the rostral ventromedial medulla (raphe pallidus and its vicinity) (29). These efferents are primarily involved in thermoregulation and emotional responses (29,30). This vascular bed is little involved in BP and blood gas homeostasis.

B.   The Rostral Ventrolateral Medulla
Contribution of the RVLM to Vasomotor Sympathetic Tone
The VLM is subdivided into several regions according to the location of the major cell groups that participate in the regulation of breathing and circulation (2,31). Its rostral

third, the RVLM, contains bulbospinal catecholaminergic neurons, the C1 neurons, that express all the enzymes required for the synthesis of epinephrine (32). These cells target the IML very selectively and establish monosynaptic connections with SPGNs (33) (Fig. 1A). These neurons also innervate multiple regions of the medulla oblongata, pons, and midbrain. More caudal regions of the VLM also contain C1 neurons, but this group innervates the hypothalamus instead of the spinal cord. These cells regulate the hypo-thalamo-pituitary axis in the context of various physical stresses (infection, hemorrhage, hypotension) (34).

The C1 presympathetic cells express a vesicular glutamate transporter 2 (VGLUT2) isoform that confers neurons the ability to release glutamate by exocytosis (35). These cells belong to a larger ensemble of RVLM presympathetic neurons that utilize glutamate as an ionotropic transmitter (35) and express various combinations of other neuromediators (e.g., neuropeptide Y, enkephalin, pituitary adenylate cyclase activating peptides, substance P, cocaine- and amphetamine-related transcript, or CART, etc.) (36–38). Adrenaline, which defines the C1 cells, may be viewed as one among these many ancillary transmitters.

RVLM presympathetic neurons have discharge properties that are highly reminiscent of that of individual pre- or postganglionic neurons, although their mean activity is much greater than that of SPGNs (2–35 Hz vs. 1–4 Hz in rats) (2,39). RVLM presympathetic neurons have lightly myelinated or unmyelinated axons. The noncatecholaminergic part of the pathway has myelinated axons and appears to excite SPGNs, primarily by releasing glutamate (40). C1 neurons are either myelinated or unmyelinated, and their action seems to be mediated by both glutamate and catecholamines acting via α1-adrenergic receptors (40).

The contribution of RVLM presympathetic neurons to sympathetic vasomotor tone generation is presumed to be equally important in the absence of anesthesia, but this is not proven. The evidence relies on the ability of certain viruses to decrease BP for some time after their administration into the RVLM (41). It also relies on the obser-vation that extensive lesions of the C1 cells reduce BP and attenuate the ability of animals to regulate their BP when they are subjected to a hemorrhage or to the administration of a vasodilator (42). However, massive lesions of the C1 cells only produce a modest drop in resting BP (10 mmHg) (42). This result does not exclude the possibility that sympathetic vasomotor tone might have been massively reduced by these lesions because volume expansion could have compensated for the sympathetic tone deficit, but this interpretation has yet to be tested experimentally.

Functional Heterogeneity of RVLM Presympathetic Neurons: The Organotopy Hypothesis

Physiological evidence suggests that subgroups of RVLM presympathetic neurons control preferentially specific functional subsets of sympathetic efferents. The organization has been characterized as organotopic (43,44). To illustrate this concept, the SPGNs that control muscle arterioles would receive input from a subset of presympathetic RVLM neurons that play no role in controlling the splanchnic vasculature or the heart. A more complicated pattern of convergence and divergence between various classes of RVLM neurons and their SPGN targets is suggested by the result of tract-tracing experiments. For example, experiments using the pseudorabies virus suggest that some of the RVLM C1 neurons may actually be widely branching neurons that may be capable of triggering a generalized activation of SNA, as envisioned by Cannon (18).

What Drives the RVLM Presympathetic Neurons at Rest?

Given the presumed importance of RVLM presympathetic neurons in the generation of SNA, understanding what controls their activity is fundamentally important. In humans, muscle sympathetic tone at rest is very low and is turned off by a very small increase in systemic pressure. In contrast, SNA is massively increased by lowering BP. Thus, in humans at rest, most of the dynamic range of sympathetic vasomotor tone is revealed when pressure falls. This is also the case in animals anesthetized with chloralose, although less so with most other anesthetics (urethane, halothane) (45). Animal experiments suggest that the bulk of this sympathetic "reserve," which is independent of the level of respiration, is caused by disinhibition of RVLM excitatory presympathetic neurons, more specifically by the withdrawal of the continuous GABAergic inhibition that these cells receive from neurons located in a more caudal region of the VLM, called the caudal ventrolateral medulla (CVLM) (23) (Fig. 1A). The latter neurons play a key role both in the baroreflex and in cardiorespiratory integration. They will be considered in detail later.

Excitation of RVLM presympathetic neurons by disinhibition presupposes the existence of a tonic, respiration-independent source of excitation to these neurons that is capable of generating their activity when the inhibitory input from the CVLM is suppressed. Despite intense research, the nature of this excitatory drive is still elusive (2,46,47). It does not originate from structures rostral to the pons and does not originate from the dorsolateral pontine regions involved in cardiorespiratory control (48). Even a complete transection between the pons and the medulla fails to reduce it, suggesting that it may originate entirely within the medulla oblongata (49). In anesthetized cats, up to 50% of the excitatory drive to the RVLM seems to be glutamatergic and may originate from a more dorsal and medial segment of the reticular formation called the lateral tegmental field (50). However, in anesthetized rats, conventional ionotropic glutamate transmission seems to play little or no role in driving RVLM neurons under resting conditions (2,46,51). Alternative hypotheses include a nonglutamatergic ionotropic drive (e.g., acetylcholine, adenosine triphosphate), metabotropic transmission (peptides, serotonin, and glutamate via mGLU receptors), or the intrinsic cellular properties of RVLM presympathetic neurons (autoactivity). In vivo, the action potentials of RVLM sympathoexcitatory neurons typically ride on top of large depolarizing events that have been interpreted as fast excitatory postsynaptic potentials PSPs (52). These events could conceivably be cholinergic or purinergic (53,54). Autoactivity could account for the ongoing activity of C1 neurons recorded in slices (55,56), but the ramp depolarizations observed in slices are no longer observed in mechanically isolated C1 cells (57). The interspike depolarizations observed in slices may therefore be a predominantly dendritic property or a non–cell autonomous property (e.g., release of a neurotransmitter or glial or blood vessel–derived autacoid, pH, hypoxia, etc.). RVLM presympathetic neurons express a vast number of metabotropic receptors (e.g., metabotropic receptors to angiotensin, serotonin, glutamate, ACh, vasopressin, orexin opiates, etc.) (51,58–61), and all the cognate agonists have been identified within the surrounding neuropil. However, no single substance, especially the much investigated angiotensin, has yet been found responsible for a significant fraction of the tonic excitatory drive of presympathetic neurons in vivo (46). Conceivably, the excitatory drive of RVLM presympathetic neurons results from a combination of all the mechanisms listed above, and none dominates.

Role of RVLM Presympathetic Neurons in Sympathetic Vasomotor Reflexes

RVLM presympathetic neurons contribute to all the sympathetic reflexes that have been tested so far, be they of somatic or visceral origin. Invariably, the sympathoinhibitory reflexes are mediated by the release of GABA in the RVLM, and the sympathoexcitatory reflexes are mediated by the release of glutamate. For example, the increase in sympathetic tone caused by stimulation of peripheral chemoreceptors or by activation of somatosensory or vagal afferents is blocked by microinjection of a glutamate receptor antagonist into the RVLM (3,62,63). The efficacy of these blockers in the context of these reflexes renders their inability to reduce the basal activity of RVLM neurons and resting SNA all the more puzzling. Conversely, sympathoinhibitory reflexes such as the baroreflex are severely attenuated by introducing GABA antagonists into RVLM (4). RVLM presympathetic neurons (C1 and non-C1) are also an important though not exclusive relay for many of the descending pathways that originate in more rostral regions of the neuraxis and control circulation [e.g., periaqueductal gray (PAG) and hypothalamus] (39,64,65).

C. The Ventromedial Medulla

Anatomical evidence based on the retrograde transsynaptic propagation of the pseudorabies virus indicates that the rostral ventromedial medulla contains a large and phenotypically diverse population of presympathetic neurons (17). Some of these neurons release GABA and glycine (26); others are serotonergic (17) and/or glutamatergic (66,67). While this region is better known for its control of skin blood flow and thermogenic fat (29), it also controls the heart (68) and probably many other aspects of circulation via its large input from the PAG matter (69). A monosynaptic inhibitory input from the ventral rostral medulla to SPGNs has been well documented by electrophysiology in vitro (70). Furthermore, in cats, neurons whose role seems to be functionally sympathoinhibitory have been recorded in or close to the raphe pallidus and their axonal projections have been traced to the IML region (71,72). The transmitter used by these particular cells has not been ascertained, and homologous neurons have not been identified in rodents.

Electrical stimulation or microinjection of excitatory amino acids in several regions of the brainstem (caudal raphe, gigantocellular depressor area) can also produce decreases in arterial pressure and sympathoinhibition (73–76). The pathways recruited by these manipulations involve RVLM presympathetic neurons in many cases.

In brief, the rostral ventromedial medulla provides mixed inhibitory and excitatory input to various subsets of vasomotor SPGNs (cardiac and cutaneous in particular). This input appears to be recruited in the context of thermoregulation and various emotional responses, especially those that originate from the PAG matter (66,77,78). Although the rostral ventromedial medulla can influence many aspects of circulation, it does not appear to be important for BP stabilization or blood gas homeostasis. These aspects of homeostasis seem to be mainly the purview of the RVLM.

D. The Baroreflex

Stimulation of arterial baroreceptors inhibits the sympathetic outflow to the heart, the kidney, and most of the vasculature (muscle and splanchnic). Baroreceptor stimulation also activates the cardiovagal outflow (cardiovagal baroreflex) and depresses the phrenic nerve discharge (barorespiratory reflex) (2,23,79–81). The pathway of the barorespiratory reflex is unknown.

The Sympathetic Baroreflex

This polysynaptic reflex involves three stages: the nucleus of the solitary tract (NTS), the VLM (specifically the intermediate part here called the CVLM), and the RVLM (2) (Fig. 1A). The circuit includes an excitatory, presumably glutamatergic projection from the NTS to the CVLM, which drives inhibitory GABAergic neurons projecting to RVLM presympathetic neurons. The central role of the CVLM in the baroreflex is inferred from four types of congruent information (2,23,23,79–81). Inhibiting neurons in this region of the VLM blocks the baroreflex. Sustained elevations of BP cause neuronal expression of c-Fos in GABAergic neurons located in the CVLM. Most importantly, the CVLM contains GABAergic propriomedullary interneurons that display the expected properties (excitatory response to baroreceptor stimulation, pulse-modulated firing, and bilateral projections to the RVLM). Finally, the inhibition of single RVLM presympathetic neurons by baroreceptor stimulation is blocked by juxtacellular application of the GABA receptor antagonist bicuculline (4).

According to Bailey and his colleagues, every NTS neuron that projects to the CVLM receives monosynaptic glutamatergic input from the solitary tract (82). It is therefore quasi certain that arterial baroreceptors establish monosynaptic excitatory synapses with second-order neurons that relay the information to the VLM. These second-order neurons are located dorsomedial to the tractus solitarius and caudal to the area postrema level, and they are, appropriately, glutamatergic (80,83,84). However, more indirect routes between arterial baroreceptors and CVLM GABAergic neurons probably also exist, since many types of NTS neurons respond to baroreceptor stimulation at variable latencies or by a sequence of excitation and inhibition (85). Transmission between the baroreceptors and their second-order neurons is regulated by GABAergic interneurons (Fig. 1A). This important regulation enables BP to rise when behaviorally appropriate, such as during exercise (86).

The previous description accounts for the well-established disfacilitation portion of the baroreflex. An inhibitory component of the reflex working by the activation of a bulbospinal inhibitory input to SPGNs may also exist (27,87).

The Cardiovagal Baroreflex

The chronotropic, dromotropic, and negative inotropic controls of the heart seem to operate through largely distinct postganglionic parasympathetic neurons clustered within separate cardiac ganglia (88,89). These postganglionic neurons also appear to be controlled by separate populations of cardiovagal motor neurons (CVMs) (cardiac preganglionic neurons located in the medulla oblongata) located mostly in nucleus ambiguus (90). The neuronal inputs to CVMs are best known from the pattern of retrograde labeling that follows the infection of cardiac ganglia with pseudorabies virus (90,91). This work suggests that a majority of the monosynaptic inputs to CVMs originates from interneurons located in the VLM (Fig. 1B). These anatomical data suggest that the pathway between second-order baroreceptor neurons and the CVMs may not be direct as represented in Figure 1B but may involve an interneuron located in the VLM. These interneurons must be excitatory, since baroreceptor activation produces chloride-independent depolarizing potentials in CVMs (92). In some preparations, the cardiac baroreflex requires the integrity of the pons, which also argues somewhat against the possibility that CVMs are activated by baroreceptors via a monosynaptic input from second-order baroreceptor neurons (49). On the other hand, in slices, electrical stimulation of the NTS activates a monosynaptic glutamatergic input to CVMs (93). Unfortunately, this experimental model cannot establish that the monosynaptic input from the NTS region originates from baroreceptor-related neurons.

CVMs are inhibited during the phrenic nerve discharge (central inspiration) via a postsynaptic chloride-dependent increase in membrane conductance, which shunts the depolarizing effect of the baroreceptor input (92,94) (Fig. 1B). This inspiratory-related inhibition is mediated by GABA or glycine and contributes to the respiratory fluctuations of the heart rate, called sinus arrhythmia. These respiratory neurons are, in turn, under some form of cholinergic control (94).

In summary, CVMs receive a glutamatergic, mono- or possibly disynaptic, excitatory input from NTS second-order barosensory neurons (Fig. 1B). This excitatory input is probably a major contributor to the basal activity of CVMs, the so-called vagal tone, and it accounts for the pulse-related discharge of these cells. The second major input to CVMs is inhibitory and originates from ventrolateral medullary interneurons that are active during inspiration. CVMs, like many central nervous system (CNS) neurons, also receive inputs from brainstem serotonergic and substance P–containing neurons (95).

III. Control of Sympathetic Efferents By Respiration

A. Respiratory Fluctuations of Sympathetic Tone

In all mammals, including humans, SNA fluctuates in synchrony with the breathing cycle. This phenomenon is due in part to fluctuations of the discharge of cardiopulmonary sensory afferents that regulate the sympathetic tone, predominantly arterial baroreceptors and slowly adapting lung stretch receptors (96). The second major cause of respiratory fluctuations in SNA is central cardiorespiratory coupling (96). This phenomenon refers to the fluctuations of SNA that are observed in anesthetized animals in whom baroreceptors and sensory afferents from the lungs have been surgically eliminated. These sympathetic fluctuations are synchronized with the central respiratory pattern generator (CPG) (the lower brainstem network that generates the respiratory rate and the pattern of the various respiratory motor outflows) as monitored by the phrenic nerve discharge but are no longer synchronized with lung ventilation and chest movements (97). These respiratory fluctuations denote the existence of inputs from the central respiratory controller to the neurons that generate sympathetic vasomotor tone. Typically, the respiratory oscillations of SNA are superimposed on a component of SNA that resists hyperventilation to phrenic apnea, and the amplitude of the respiratory oscillations of SNA is roughly proportional to that of the phrenic nerve discharge (98,99).

B. Role of RVLM Presympathetic Neurons in Sympathorespiratory Coupling

Under anesthesia, central coupling probably operates mostly via the presympathetic neurons of the RVLM. This view derives from the close similarity between the discharge probability of these RVLM cells and that of individual postganglionic units during the central respiratory cycle (98,100). Several respiratory patterns are observed in a given preparation, which indicates that the respiratory network can differentially modulate various classes of sympathetic efferents (98,101). Finally, the fact that RVLM presympathetic neurons retain a high basal level of discharge even when the activity of the central respiratory network is silenced by hyperventilation also demonstrates that vasomotor neurons receive only a portion of their excitatory input from the respiratory network. The non-respiratory-related excitatory drive of RVLM neurons has been discussed previously. Its main function is to maintain BP, regardless of breathing intensity.

C. CVLM GABAergic Neurons and Central Sympathorespiratory Coupling

The CVLM GABAergic neurons that mediate the baroreflex are also essential for central cardiorespiratory coupling (Fig. 1A). These neurons have very pronounced and varied respiratory patterns (102), several of which are, appropriately, the mirror image of those exhibited by RVLM presympathetic neurons. This observation suggests that the respiratory fluctuations of the discharge of RVLM presympathetic neurons may occur mainly via disinhibition, that is, via cyclical variations of the inhibitory input that these neurons receive from the CVLM. Second, RVLM presympathetic neurons receive inputs from defined subgroups of CVLM neurons, perhaps in an extended form of organotopic arrangement.

The respiratory modulation of CVLM GABAergic neurons explains satisfactorily the well-described respiratory fluctuations in the strength of the baroreflex (101,103) and may explain why sympathetic efferents with the most pronounced respiratory modulation are also those under the strongest influence from baroreceptors. It could also account for the puzzling respiration-dependent phase shift between the activity of baroreceptor afferents and SNA (104,105).

CVLM neurons reside, on average, slightly below the pre-Bötzinger complex and the immediately adjacent rostral-ventral respiratory group (45). These two regions are essential components of the CPG (106) and presumably contain the respiratory neurons that regulate the CVLM (Fig. 1A). Lesions of the dorsolateral pons or transection of the brain at the pontomedullary junction does not alter the respiration-independent component of the vasomotor SNA, but these lesions disrupt its respiratory entrainment (48,49). Baekey et al. also showed that removal of the pons eliminates the respiratory gating of the sympathetic baroreflex (49). This evidence indicates that pontine neurons somehow participate in the respiratory entrainment of SNA. Pontine neurons could conceivably do so via direct projections to the CVLM or to RVLM neurons, but many other interpretations are possible, since the activity of the medullary portion of the CPG is profoundly affected by pontine lesions.

D. Alternate Potential Mechanisms of Central Sympathorespiratory Coupling

Other potential sources of respiratory-modulated input to the vasomotor SNA have been proposed (107–111). The possibilities include an input from some form of expiration-related Bötzinger neurons to RVLM presympathetic neurons, a contribution of A5 noradrenergic neurons, direct or oligosynaptic inputs from bulbospinal inspiratory neurons to SPGNs (in cats only), and a possible respiratory modulation of sympathoinhibitory neurons located in the midline medulla (112,113). These possibilities should be kept in mind, but the evidence that supports them is incomplete.

IV. Central Chemoreceptors: Effects on Breathing and on the Sympathetic Outflow

SNA is activated by stimulating either central or peripheral chemoreceptors. The effects produced by the activation of each separately are roughly additive, and in both cases, SNA is activated in bursts that are synchronized with the central respiratory cycle (6,97,114). The way in which central chemoreceptors activate respiration and SNA is intimately related to the previously discussed issue of central coupling because central coupling is a phenomenon that is primarily observed in anesthetized or reduced preparations in which the activity of the respiratory centers is driven by CO_2, that is, by central chemoreceptors.

A. Central Respiratory Chemoreception

In the absence of carotid bodies, a rise in arterial PCO_2 produces a vigorous stimulation of breathing and a rise in BP (the central chemoreflex). The central chemoreflex operates as a feedback loop that stabilizes arterial CO_2. CO_2 triggers the chemoreflex by acidifying the brain parenchyma or some portion thereof ("reaction theory") (115). The central chemoreflex has a relatively slow time constant (over one minute) probably because brain pH equilibrates slowly in response to a change in arterial CO_2. The time constant of the peripheral chemoreflex is about three times faster (116).

Brain PCO_2 depends on the level of arterial PCO_2 and on the rate of production of this gas by the brain parenchyma (117). Brain PCO_2 is also influenced by brain blood flow (117). In many, possibly most, regions of the brain, interstitial fluid (ISF) pH appears to be protected against changes in arterial PCO_2 (117,118). This buffering may involve the active secretion of bicarbonate from the blood to the brain ISF by the blood-brain barrier in response to a rise in arterial PCO_2 (117). If correct, this theory implies that central respiratory chemoreceptors must reside in specialized regions of the brainstem where this buffering mechanism is reduced or absent and, therefore, where changes in arterial PCO_2 can readily acidify the ISF. Finally, central respiratory chemoreceptors must be more than just pH responsive (chemosensitive); they must also be connected to the CPG to be able to contribute to its activation when arterial PCO_2 rises.

Three types of neurons are presently considered the most plausible central chemoreceptors: the retrotrapezoid nucleus (RTN), raphe serotonergic neurons, and the locus coeruleus. This review emphasizes the role of the RTN, but other opinions have been expressed. These alternative theories will be briefly considered at the end of the section.

B. Ventral Medullary Surface Chemoreceptors

The notion that the central chemoreceptors reside near the ventral surface of the medulla oblongata originates from the 1960's experiments in which acidification of the ventral surface of the brain of anesthetized animals was shown to stimulate breathing (115). These early investigators proposed that respiratory chemoreception relies on a limited number of specialized neurons that are not part of the CPG but drive this network synaptically. The recently described RTN contains neurons with a superficial location and physiological properties that are generally consistent with the scheme proposed by these early investigators (119–121) (Fig. 2). RTN neurons are acid sensitive in slices, vigorously activated by raising arterial CO_2 in vivo; they innervate selectively the lower brainstem regions that

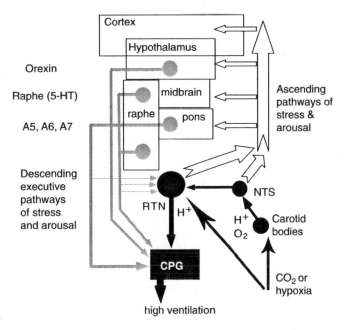

Figure 2 Chemoreceptors and chemoreflexes. This tentative scheme assumes that, under normal circumstances, the central chemoreflex and the peripheral chemoreflex operate through a common respiratory controller located in the retrotrapezoid nucleus (RTN). This pathway is in *black*. RTN neurons are excitatory and stimulate the CPG. RTN is excited by local acidification and hence serves as a central respiratory chemoreceptor. The same neurons receive excitatory input from the carotid bodies and thus also mediate the peripheral chemoreflex. This core is assumed to be selectively engaged when small corrections of breathing intensity are needed for CO_2 homeostasis, that is, under normal circumstances. When blood gases are seriously out of line because of airway obstruction or because of artificially imposed large and abrupt changes in arterial PO_2 and/or PCO_2, an extreme degree of central and/or peripheral chemoreceptor stimulation ensues, which triggers a strong alerting response. This alerting response is assumed to recruit the general executive pathways of stress and arousal, including noradrenergic, orexinergic, serotonergic, and histaminergic neurons. High levels of CO_2 may also directly activate a subset of these aminergic neurons in vivo, as well as certain components of the CPG. *Abbreviations*: RTN, retrotrapezoid nucleus; CPG, central respiratory pattern generator.

contain the CPG, and lesion or inhibition of the region that harbors them reduces breathing at rest and the stimulation of breathing by CO_2 (122). RTN neurons also receive powerful excitatory inputs from the carotid bodies via a short, presumably disynaptic pathway (119) (Fig. 2). RTN neurons express Phox2b, the transcription factor whose mutation causes the congenital central hypoventilation syndrome (CCHS) (119). The CCHS is characterized by reduced or absent respiratory automaticity during sleep and a large reduction of the central chemoreflex (123). The fact that RTN neurons degenerate selectively in a mouse model of the disease (124) suggests that these neurons could indeed be critically important for breathing in general and for central respiratory chemoreception in particular. RTN neurons are probably intrinsically chemosensitive, but their activation by CO_2 in vivo may also be due to the release of substances such as ATP by surrounding glial or other nonneuronal cells (121,125,126).

C. Brainstem Monoaminergic Neurons as Central Chemoreceptors

The activity of brainstem aminergic neurons (serotonergic, noradrenergic) facilitates the central chemoreflex, the principal evidence being that lesion or genetic deletion of these systems attenuates this reflex in animals (127,128). These neurons may also be able to detect increases in arterial PCO_2 via local changes in pH because they are typically activated by acidification in slices or in cell culture (129). Furthermore, serotonin overflow increases with hypercapnia in the hypoglossal nucleus in vivo (130). On the basis of this evidence, it has been proposed that all serotonergic neurons are CO_2 detectors (129) and that the direct activation of these cells by acidification causes an increase in breathing and general brain arousal. However, whereas locus coeruleus neurons are slightly activated by hypercapnia in vivo, few serotonergic neurons respond to this stimulus, even in unanesthetized animals (121,131,132). Furthermore, the CO_2 response of these serotonergic cells is absent or reduced during sleep, which argues against the view that it is an intrinsic response to pH (132).

Sudden stimulation of central chemoreceptors with CO_2 is aversive in humans and is presumably so in animals (133,134). Thus, central chemoreceptor stimulation probably activates to some degree all the classic descending wake-promoting systems, which include locus coeruleus and serotonergic neurons (22,133). This notion is illustrated in Figure 2, although the pathways responsible for the effects of hypercapnia on arousal are entirely hypothetical. Chemoreceptor-mediated arousal is a plausible explanation of the increased neuronal activity that has been detected in the locus coeruleus and a subset of raphe neurons in response to strong hypercapnia in vivo. Intense, brief stimulation of peripheral chemoreceptors produces an equally strong alerting response in animals and also recruits these monoaminergic systems (22,133,135). On the other hand, moderate and sustained hypoxia produces hypothermia and sleepiness, which would be expected to reduce the activity of pontine noradrenergic neurons and the serotonergic system.

D. Other Theories of Central Chemoreception

Many additional regions may also contain neurons that contribute to central respiratory chemoreception. The list includes a variety of CPG neurons and neurons located in the NTS, the cerebellum, and the hypothalamus (126). The evidence implicating these various regions in central respiratory chemoreception is essentially the same for all: These regions contain neurons that respond to acidification in vitro, and acidification of these regions via implanted cannulae in vivo produces some measure of breathing stimulation. The limitations of the evidence are discussed in more detail elsewhere (126).

E. Central Chemoreceptors and Cardiorespiratory Integration

Hypercapnia activates SNA in bursts that are synchronized with the phrenic nerve (97,136). The classic interpretation of this phenomenon assumes the following sequence of events: CO_2 activates central chemoreceptors, central chemoreceptors activate the CPG, and the CPG activates the neurons that generate sympathetic vasomotor tone. However, this linear sequence of events is at odds with the observation that silencing CPG and CVLM neurons simultaneously does not reduce the overall rise of SNA and

RVLM neuron activity by central chemoreceptors (137). This intervention only suppresses the respiratory entrainment of SNA. A plausible and already evoked mechanism for respiratory entrainment is the respiratory modulation of RVLM presympathetic neurons by CVLM GABAergic neurons (Fig. 3A), but the overall activation of RVLM neurons and SNA caused by a rise in CNS PCO_2 must have other explanations (137). Hypothetically, RVLM neurons could be directly activated by acidification in vivo, as

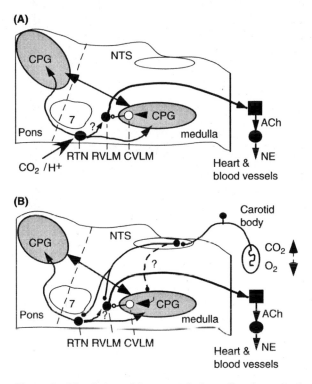

Figure 3 Stimulation of the sympathetic outflow by activation of central or peripheral chemoreceptors. (**A**) Sympathetic nerve activation by central chemoreceptors. SNA is increased primarily through the RVLM. The activation occurs in bursts synchronized with the breathing rhythm. This synchronization is probably mediated via CVLM neurons. RVLM neurons are also activated independently of the effect of CO_2 on the CPG. This second mechanism is incompletely understood and, in theory, could involve a direct stimulation of RVLM neurons by acid or an excitatory input from the nearby RTN chemoreceptors. (**B**) SNA activation by peripheral chemoreceptors. SNA activation is also mediated primarily through the RVLM. RVLM neurons most likely receive a direct excitatory input from the NTS and may also receive an indirect input through the RTN. Carotid body stimulation activates the CPG, which, presumably via the CVLM, produces a strong entrainment of SNA to the breathing rhythm. Very strong stimulation of central or peripheral chemoreceptors may also engage the descending executive pathways of stress and arousal described in Figure 2. These neuronal systems may further stimulate SNA via their projections to the RVLM and the sympathetic preganglionic neurons. *Abbreviations*: SNA, sympathetic nerve activity; RVLM, rostral ventrolateral medulla; CVLM, caudal ventrolateral medulla; CPG, central respiratory pattern generator; RTN, retrotrapezoid nucleus; NTS, nucleus of the solitary tract.

may be the case with other catecholaminergic neurons such as those in the locus coeruleus. Another possibility, evoked previously, is that hypercapnia produces some arousal and activates descending wake-promoting systems (orexin, noradrenergic, serotonin, and cholinergic). These systems release substances already known to activate SPGNs (orexin, NE, 5-HT) and RVLM neurons (orexin, serotonin, and ACh). Lastly, RVLM presympathetic neurons could be directly activated by bona fide central chemoreceptors such as the RTN (119,138) (Fig. 3A).

V. Peripheral Chemoreceptors and Peripheral Chemoreflexes

Peripheral chemoreceptors detect hypoxia and changes in $PaCO_2$ to which they respond with a faster time constant than central chemoreceptors (116,139). Peripheral chemoreceptor stimulation activates most sympathetic barosensitive efferents, including those to the heart (140), although the heart slows initially because of an initial rise in vagal tone. The bradycardia is quickly reversed by the resumption or activation of breathing because central coupling and the activity of lung stretch receptors have vagolytic effects.

A. Carotid Receptor Stimulation: Effects on Breathing

When subjected to hypoxia and/or acidification, the principal cells of the carotid bodies, the glomus cells, release ACh and ATP, which depolarize the sensory afferents (141). The carotid body is also under the control of parasympathetic and sympathetic efferents (142). Carotid body afferents travel via the glossopharyngeal nerve (23,143). They innervate principally the caudal aspect of the nucleus tractus solitarius (nucleus commissuralis), although projections outside this region have also been described (23,143,144) (Fig. 3B). Under anesthesia, the breathing stimulation and the rise in SNA caused by carotid body stimulation are blocked by administering antagonists of glutamate transmission into the nucleus commissuralis, which suggests that the primary afferents are likely to be glutamatergic (143). In the absence of anesthesia, simultaneous blockade of glutamate and P2X receptors within nucleus commissuralis seems to be required to interrupt the autonomic components of the reflex (145). The second-order neurons are also probably glutamatergic (138). They innervate the VLM (146) up to the RTN (138).

Stimulation of the carotid bodies is also a very powerful arousing stimulus, which, in awake animals, causes Fos expression in brainstem noradrenergic, adrenergic, and selected serotonergic neurons (133,147). Thus, depending on the intensity of the stimulation of the carotid bodies, the central respiratory controller and SNA are probably activated by a hierarchy of pathways.

B. Carotid Receptor Stimulation: Effects on the Sympathetic Outflow

In anesthetized animals, carotid body stimulation activates barosensitive SNA in bursts that are synchronized to the phrenic nerve discharge (6,96). In any given species, the respiratory patterns of SNA produced by carotid body stimulation are roughly the same as those elicited by central chemoreceptor stimulation, indicating that the responses share pathways. The activation of RVLM neurons and SNA by carotid body stimulation persists after manipulations that silence the CPG or impair its function, but this activation becomes tonic (48,49). Similar results are obtained when stimulation of central chemoreceptors is performed (137). The similarity of these results indicates that, in both cases (central or peripheral chemoreceptor stimulation), the respiratory fluctuations of SNA and the overall activation of this outflow are partially separable processes. The respiratory fluctuations are likely to be mediated via the CVLM in both cases (Fig. 3), but there is a major difference between the two reflexes: RVLM presympathetic neurons are no longer activated by carotid body stimulation after local blockade of glutamate receptors (148), whereas the central effect of hypercapnia on these cells persists after the same treatment (137). An interpretation that has considerable anatomical support is that carotid body stimulation activates RVLM neurons via a direct glutamatergic projection that originates from the caudal NTS (138,146,149) (Fig. 3B). This interpretation is compatible with results obtained in awake humans, where muscle SNA stimulation caused by peripheral chemoreceptor activation seems to be largely mediated independently of an increase in central respiratory motor output (150).

Very strong stimuli such as those caused by the interruption of airway patency or asphyxia probably also recruit pathways involved in arousal and/or stress (noradrenergic, adrenergic, serotonergic, orexinergic systems). Unit recording and other data suggest that activation of the A5 noradrenergic neurons of the ventrolateral pons may be required for full expression of the sympathoactivation (151). These neurons probably contribute to the rise in SNA via their facilitatory actions at multiple levels of the neuraxis, including the SPGNs.

C. Carotid Receptor Stimulation: Effects on the Cardiovagal Outflow

The primary bradycardia caused by intense carotid body stimulation is due to the activation of cardiovagal preganglionic neurons. The classic mechanism of respiratory arrhythmia (increased inhibition of cardiovagal preganglionic neurons during inspiration and late expiration) is clearly not responsible for this effect because carotid body stimulation increases central inspiratory drive, which should inhibit cardiovagal preganglionic neurons and cause tachycardia, not bradycardia. The primary bradycardia could conceivably involve a direct excitatory input from some of the second-order NTS neurons that are activated by carotid body stimulation to the cardiovagal motoneurons. This mechanism could be a form of nonspecific defensive reflex because a similar bradycardic response occurs in response to the activation of cardiopulmonary vagal C-fiber afferents, which normally respond to bronchial irritation, and all these stimuli appear to converge on a common set of NTS neurons that do not respond to cardiovascular and lung mechanoreceptors (152). The primary parasympathetically mediated bradycardia, elicited by chemoreceptor stimulation, rapidly converts to tachycardia when ventilation increases. The tachycardia may be due to the activation of lung stretch receptors, whose role is examined next.

VI. Regulation of the Circulation by Lung Afferents

The reflexes triggered by slowly adapting lung stretch receptors are briefly reviewed here because of their presumed contribution to the BP surge that accompanies the resumption of breathing following an obstructive apnea (for reviews on lung afferents see Refs. 103,153–156).

A. Effect of Slowly Adapting Receptors on Breathing

Slowly adapting receptors (SARs) are myelinated slowly adapting mechanoreceptors that encode the volume of the lungs (155). These cells are glutamatergic, their cell bodies are located in the nodose ganglia, and they innervate very specific subnuclei of the NTS (e.g., interstitial and ventrolateral nuclei) (157). Within the NTS, SARs contact several types of neurons, in particular the so-called pump cells, which are located in the interstitial subnucleus (155). These neurons innervate more caudal regions of the NTS and large tracts of the VLM, the dorsolateral pons, and the caudal portion of the NTS (155). The pump cells are presumed responsible for the Breuer–Hering reflexes (inspiration shortening and expiration prolongation). Most pump cells so far identified are GABAergic (158). These cells also presumably inhibit phrenic nerve amplitude and frequency when high levels of inflation are maintained (159).

B. Effect of SARs on Cardiovagal Neurons

Lung inflation inhibits cardiovagal tone, which increases the heart rate (153,160). This effect also contributes to sinus arrhythmia (153,160). Because many pump cells are inhibitory and innervate the region of the medulla where the cardiovagal preganglionic neurons reside, a monosynaptic input from pump cells to cardiovagal preganglionic neurons could, in theory, mediate the tachycardia elicited by lung inflation, but these cells could also regulate cardiovagal preganglionic activity via their effect on the central respiratory controller.

C. Effect of SARs on Sympathetic Tone

In dogs, increasing pulmonary ventilation while keeping arterial pressure and arterial PCO_2 constant reduces hindquarter vascular resistance, presumably by withdrawing sympathetic tone (154). The sympathoinhibitory effect of lung inflation depends largely, though not completely, on the central respiratory drive (154,161), and lung inflation may exert different effects on different types of sympathetic efferents (161). It is not certain that the effects of lung inflation on SNA are only due to SARs.

In humans, lung inflation is the most important factor that determines the within-breath respiratory fluctuations of SNA (150,162), but opinions differ as to the contribution made by lung stretch afferents, baroreceptors (arterial or volume), and central coupling to these fluctuations (162,163).

In short, the effect of lung inflation on SNA seems to include a respiratory pattern generator–dependent and a respiratory pattern generator–independent mechanism. The relative importance of these two mechanisms may depend on the species and/or on the state of vigilance (awake or anesthetized). The central pathways responsible for these effects are unknown.

VII. Cardiorespiratory Responses to Brainstem Hypoxia

Under conditions of extreme hypoxia or ischemia, the brainstem mechanisms that coordinate respiration and the cardiovascular outflows break down. Arterial pressure and SNA increase markedly, probably because hypoxia depolarizes RVLM presympathetic neurons directly (113,164,165). This phenomenon contributes to the Cushing response, that is, a rise in BP that is elicited when blood flow to the brain is restricted by brain swelling (166). Central hypoxia or ischemia also reconfigures the breathing system, causing a brief period of gasping before the respiratory network fails and breathing stops. Gasping is attributed to the fact that the rhythmogenic neurons of the pre-Bötzinger region acquire intrinsic bursting properties during hypoxia (167).

Both gasping and the ischemic pressor response are observed under hypoxic conditions that may be regarded as extreme. However, there is some evidence that brainstem PO_2 could be a physiological regulator of the cardiorespiratory network in the intact and unanesthetized state. The direct excitatory effect of hypoxia on this circuitry has been regarded as a potential homeostatic mechanism designed to maintain brain perfusion and oxygenation (168), and this concept is still occasionally invoked as a potential explanation for neurogenic hypertension (169,170). There is little evidence that central hypoxia stimulates breathing in mammals when the carotid bodies are denervated (171). However, some evidence in awake goats and in sleeping dogs suggests that mild CNS hypoxia has the ability to stimulate breathing if peripheral chemoreceptors are intact and are exposed to physiological levels of oxygen and CO_2 (171).

In brief, oxygen may have the ability to regulate the cardiorespiratory circuitry by a direct action on the lower brainstem, in addition to its better-known effects via peripheral chemoreceptors. The parallel with the regulation of the same circuitry by PCO_2 is tempting, but it should be stressed that the existence of physiologically relevant central oxygen receptors in the medulla oblongata remains highly controversial (171).

VIII. Summary and Conclusions

The pontomedullary region contains a set of structures that are essential for the reflex stabilization of BP and for coordination of breathing with oxygen delivery to various tissues. These regions also mediate a large fraction of the reflexes that are elicited by alterations of blood gases and by changes in pulmonary ventilation. The NTS is crucial to all these regulations. The regulation of sympathetic tone to the heart and major blood vessels seems to revolve around two nodal points: the RVLM, which provides the bulk of the excitatory drive to the SPGNs, and the CVLM, which may be the main interface between the SNA-generating network and the central respiratory controller. Each of these nodal points is highly regulated by inputs from structures located throughout the neuraxis. The vagal control of the heart is less well understood in network terms.

Chemoreceptor stimulation probably recruits a hierarchy of pathways depending on the intensity of the stimulus and the presence or absence of anesthesia. Very mild stimuli, such as those that regulate CO_2 homeostasis under normal circumstances, probably utilize discrete connections between the chemoreceptors and specific components of the lower brainstem cardiorespiratory network. Strong and acute stimuli, such as those caused by airway blockade and other life-threatening interruptions of lung ventilation, probably also recruit pathways involved in stress and arousal, most notably subsets of noradrenergic, adrenergic, serotonergic, cholinergic, and orexinergic neurons. These pathways probably increase breathing intensity, airway patency, and SNA by facilitating synaptic transmission at multiple sites of the network down to the motoneurons for breathing and the SPGNs for SNA. It is reasonable to assume that these wake-promoting systems make a significant contribution to the cardiorespiratory stimulation associated with obstructive sleep apnea.

References

1. Narkiewicz K, Somers VK. The sympathetic nervous system and obstructive sleep apnea: implications for hypertension. J Hypertens 1997; 15:1613–1619.
2. Guyenet PG. The sympathetic control of blood pressure. Nat Rev Neurosci 2006; 7:335–346.
3. Sun M-K, Reis DJ. NMDA receptor-mediated sympathetic chemoreflex excitation of RVL-spinal vasomotor neurones in rats. J Physiol 1995; 482:53–68.
4. Sun MK, Guyenet PG. GABA-mediated baroreceptor inhibition of reticulospinal neurons. Am J Physiol Regul Integr Comp Physiol 1985; 249:R672–R680.
5. Morrison SF. Differential control of sympathetic outflow. Am J Physiol Regul Integr Comp Physiol 2001; 281:R683–R698.
6. Janig W, Habler HJ. Neurophysiological analysis of target-related sympathetic pathways—from animal to human: similarities and differences. Acta Physiol Scand 2003; 177:255–274.
7. Morrison SF, Cao WH. Different adrenal sympathetic preganglionic neurons regulate epinephrine and norepinephrine secretion. Am J Physiol Regul Integr Comp Physiol 2000; 279:R1763–R1775.
8. Ootsuka Y, McAllen RM. Comparison between two rat sympathetic pathways activated in cold-defense. Am J Physiol Regul Integr Comp Physiol 2006; 291:R589–R595.
9. Cabot JB. Sympathetic preganglionic neurons: cytoarchitecture, ultrastructure, and bio-physical properties. In: Loewy AD, Spyer KM, eds. Central Regulation of Autonomic Functions. London: Oxford University Press, 1990:44–67.
10. Murugaian J, Sundaram K, Krieger A, et al. Relative effects of different spinal autonomic nuclei on cardiac sympathoexcitatory function. Brain Res Bull 1990; 24:537–542.
11. Sundaram K, Murugaian J, Sapru H. Cardiac responses to the microinjections of excitatory amino acids into the intermediolateral cell column of the rat spinal cord. Brain Res 1989; 482:12–22.
12. Wu SY, Dun SL, Förstermann U, et al. Nitric oxide and excitatory postsynaptic currents in immature rat sympathetic preganglionic neurons *in vitro*. Neuroscience 1997; 79:237–245.
13. Krukoff TL, Ciriello J, Calaresu FR. Segmental distribution of peptide-like immunor-eactivity in cell bodies of the thoracolumbar sympathetic nuclei of the cat. J Comp Neurol 1985; 240:90–102.
14. Grkovic I, Anderson CR. Calbindin D28K-immunoreactivity identifies distinct subpopulations of sympathetic pre- and postganglionic neurons in the rat. J Comp Neurol 1997; 386:245–259.
15. Edwards SL, Anderson CR, Southwell BR, et al. Distinct preganglionic neurons innervate noradrenaline and adrenaline cells in the cat adrenal medulla. Neuroscience 1996; 70:825–832.
16. Logan SD, Pickering AE, Gibson IC, et al. Electrotonic coupling between rat sympathetic preganglionic neurones *in vitro*. J Physiol 1996; 495:491–502.
17. Jansen ASP, Wessendorf MW, Loewy AD. Transneuronal labeling of CNS neuropeptide and monoamine neurons after pseudorabies virus injections into the stellate ganglion. Brain Res 1995; 683:1–24.
18. Jansen ASP, Nguyen XV, Karpitskiy V, et al. Central command neurons of the sympathetic nervous system: basis of the fight-or flight response. Science 1995; 270:644–646.
19. Antunes VR, Brailoiu GC, Kwok EH, et al. Orexins/hypocretins excite rat sympathetic preganglionic neurons in vivo and in vitro. Am J Physiol Regul Integr Comp Physiol 2001; 281:R1801–R1807.
20. Geerling JC, Mettenleiter TC, Loewy AD. Orexin neurons project to diverse sympathetic outflow systems. Neuroscience 2003; 122:541–550.
21. Jacobs BL, Martin-Cora FJ, Fornal CA. Activity of medullary serotonergic neurons in freely moving animals. Brain Res Brain Res Rev 2002; 40:45–52.
22. Lu J, Sherman D, Devor M, et al. A putative flip-flop switch for control of REM sleep. Nature 2006; 441:589–594.

23. Blessing WW. The Lower Brainstem and Bodily Homeostasis. New York: Oxford University Press, 1997.
24. Seyedabadi M, Li Q, Padley JR, et al. A novel pressor area at the medullo-cervical junction that is not dependent on the RVLM: efferent pathways and chemical mediators. J Neurosci 2006; 26:5420–5427.
25. Krupp J, Bordey A, Feltz P. Electrophysiological evidence for multiple glycinergic inputs to neonatal rat sympathetic preganglionic neurons in vitro. Eur J Neurosci 1997; 9:1711–1719.
26. Stornetta RL, McQuiston TJ, Guyenet PG. GABAergic and glycinergic presympathetic neurons of rat medulla oblongata identified by retrograde transport of pseudorabies virus and in situ hybridization. J Comp Neurol 2004; 479:257–270.
27. Lewis DI, Coote JH. Mediation of baroreceptor inhibition of sympathetic nerve activity via both a brainstem and spinal site in rats. J Physiol 1994; 481:197–205.
28. Barman SM, Gebber GL. Spinal interneurons with sympathetic nerve-related activity. Am J Physiol Regul Integr Comp Physiol 1984; 247:R761–R767.
29. Blessing WW, Nalivaiko E. Raphe magnus/pallidus neurons regulate tail but not mesenteric arterial blood flow in rats. Neuroscience 2001; 105:923–929.
30. Blessing WW, Yu YH, Nalivaiko E. Raphe pallidus and parapyramidal neurons regulate ear pinna vascular conductance in the rabbit. Neurosci Lett 2001; 270:33–36.
31. Alheid GF, Gray PA, Jiang MC, et al. Parvalbumin in respiratory neurons of the ventro-lateral medulla of the adult rat. J Neurocytol 2002; 31:693–717.
32. Hokfelt T, Fuxe K, Goldstein M, et al. Immunohistochemical evidence for the existence of adrenaline neurons in the rat brain. Brain Res 1974; 66:235–251.
33. Milner TA, Morrison SF, Abate C, et al. Phenylethanolamine N-methyltransferase-containing terminals synapse directly on sympathetic preganglionic neurons in the rat. Brain Res 1988; 448:205–222.
34. Sawchenko PE, Li HY, Ericsson A. Circuits and mechanisms governing hypothalamic responses to stress: a tale of two paradigms. Prog Brain Res 2000; 122:61–78.
35. Stornetta RL, Sevigny CP, Schreihofer AM, et al. Vesicular glutamate transporter DNPI/GLUT2 is expressed by both C1 adrenergic and nonaminergic presympathetic vasomotor neurons of the rat medulla. J Comp Neurol 2002; 444:207–220.
36. Guyenet PG, Stornetta RL, Weston MC, et al. Detection of amino acid and peptide transmitters in physiologically identified brainstem cardiorespiratory neurons. Auton Neurosci 2004; 114:1–10.
37. Li Q, Goodchild AK, Seyedabadi M, et al. Pre-protachykinin A mRNA is colocalized with tyrosine hydroxylase-immunoreactivity in bulbospinal neurons. Neuroscience 2005; 136: 205–216.
38. Dun SL, Ng YK, Brailoiu GC, et al. Cocaine- and amphetamine-regulated transcript peptide-immunoreactivity in adrenergic C1 neurons projecting to the intermediolateral cell column of the rat. J Chemical Neuroanat 2002; 23:123–132.
39. Sun MK. Central neural organization and control of sympathetic nervous system in mammals. Prog Neurobiol 1995; 47:157–233.
40. Huangfu D, Hwang LJ, Riley TA, et al. Role of serotonin and catecholamines in sympa-thetic responses evoked by stimulation of rostral medulla. Am J Physiol Regul Integr Comp Physiol 1994; 266:R338–R352.
41. Kishi T, Hirooka Y, Sakai K, et al. Overexpression of eNOS in the RVLM causes hypo-tension and bradycardia via GABA release. Hypertension 2001; 38:896–901.
42. Madden CJ, Stocker SD, Sved AF. Attenuation of homeostatic responses to hypotension and glucoprivation after destruction of catecholaminergic rostral ventrolateral medulla (RVLM) neurons. Am J Physiol Regul Integr Comp Physiol 2006; 291:R751–R759.
43. McAllen RM, May CN, Campos RR. The supply of vasomotor drive to individual classes of sympathetic neuron. Clin Exp Hypertens 1997; 19:607–618.

44. Sartor DM, Verberne AJ. Phenotypic identification of rat rostroventrolateral medullary presympathetic vasomotor neurons inhibited by exogenous cholecystokinin. J Comp Neurol 2003; 465:467–479.
45. Schreihofer AM, Guyenet PG. Baroactivated neurons with pulse-modulated activity in the rat caudal ventrolateral medulla express GAD67 mRNA. J Neurophysiol 2003; 89:1265–1277.
46. Dampney RA, Horiuchi J, Tagawa T, et al. Medullary and supramedullary mechanisms regulating sympathetic vasomotor tone. Acta Physiol Scand 2003; 177:209–218.
47. Dampney RAL, Tagawa T, Horiuchi J, et al. What drives the tonic activity of presympathetic neurons in the rostral ventrolateral medulla? Clin Exp Pharmacol Physiol 2000; 27:1049–1053.
48. Koshiya N, Guyenet PG. Role of the pons in the carotid sympathetic chemoreflex. Am J Physiol Regul Integr Comp Physiol 1994; 267:R508–R518.
49. Baekey DM, Dick TE, Paton JF. Ponto-medullary transection attenuates central respiratory modulation of sympathetic discharge, heart rate and the baroreceptor reflex in the in situ rat. Exp Physiol 2008; 93:803–816.
50. Barman SM, Gebber GL, Orer HS. Medullary lateral tegmental field: an important source of basal sympathetic nerve discharge in the cat. Am J Physiol Reg Integr Comp Physiol 2000; 278:R995–R1004.
51. Horiuchi J, Killinger S, Dampney RA. Contribution to sympathetic vasomotor tone of tonic glutamatergic inputs to neurons in the RVLM. Am J Physiol Regul Integr Comp Physiol 2004; 287:R1335–R1343.
52. Lipski J, Kanjhan R, Kruszewska B, et al. Properties of presympathetic neurones in the rostral ventrolateral medulla in the rat: an intracellular study 'in vivo'. J Physiol 1996; 490: 729–744.
53. Sun MK, Wahlestedt C, Reis DJ. Action of externally applied ATP on rat reticulospinal vasomotor neurons. Eur J Pharmacol 1992; 224:93–96.
54. Huangfu D, Schreihofer AM, Guyenet PG. Effect of cholinergic agonists on bulbospinal C1 neurons in rats. Am J Physiol Regul Integr Comp Physiol 1997; 272:R249–R258.
55. Kangrga IM, Loewy AD. Whole-cell recordings from visualized C1 adrenergic bulbospinal neurons: ionic mechanisms underlying vasomotor tone. Brain Res 1995; 670:215–232.
56. Li YW, Bayliss DA, Guyenet PG. C1 neurons of neonatal rats: intrinsic beating properties and α_2-adrenergic receptors. Am J Physiol Regul Integr Comp Physiol 1995; 269:R1356–R1369.
57. Lipski J, Kawai Y, Qi J, et al. Whole cell patch-clamp study of putative vasomotor neurons isolated from the rostral ventrolateral medulla. Am J Physiol Regul Integr Comp Physiol 1998; 274:R1099–R1110.
58. Wang WH, Lovick TA. Excitatory 5-HT2-mediated effects on rostral ventrolateral medullary neurones in rats. Neurosci Lett 1992; 141:89–92.
59. Wang WH, Lovick TA. Inhibitory serotonergic effects on rostral ventrolateral medullary neurons. Pflugers Arch 1992; 422:93–97.
60. Li YW, Guyenet PG. Angiotensin II decreases a resting K^+ conductance in rat bulbospinal neurons of the C1 area. Circ Res 1996; 78:274–282.
61. Sun MK, Guyenet PG. Effects of vasopressin and other neuropeptides on rostral medullary sympathoexcitatory neurons 'in vitro'. Brain Res 1989; 492:261–270.
62. Sun MK, Spyer KM. Nociceptive inputs into rostral ventrolateral medulla spinal vasomotor neurones in rats. J Physiol 1991; 436:685–700.
63. Sun MK, Guyenet PG. Arterial baroreceptor and vagal inputs to sympathoexcitatory neurons in rat medulla. Am J Physiol Regul Integr Comp Physiol 1987; 252:R699–R709.
64. Horiuchi J, McAllen RM, Allen AM, et al. Descending vasomotor pathways from the dorsomedial hypothalamic nucleus: role of medullary raphe and RVLM. Am J Physiol Regul Integr Comp Physiol 2004; 287:R824–R832.

65. Verberne AJM, Guyenet PG. Midbrain central gray—influence on medullary sympathoexcitatory neurons and the baroreflex in rats. Am J Physiol Regul Integr Comp Physiol 1992; 263:R24–R33.
66. Nakamura K, Morrison SF. A thermosensory pathway that controls body temperature. Nat Neurosci 2008; 11:62–71.
67. Nakamura K, Matsumura K, Hubschle T et al. Identification of sympathetic premotor neurons in medullary raphe regions mediating fever and other thermoregulatory functions. J Neurosci 2004; 24:5370–5380.
68. Cao WH, Morrison SF. Disinhibition of rostral raphe pallidus neurons increases cardiac sympathetic nerve activity and heart rate. Brain Res 2003; 980:1–10.
69. Farkas E, Jansen AS, Loewy AD. Periaqueductal gray matter input to cardiac-related sympathetic premotor neurons. Brain Res 1998; 792:179–192.
70. Deuchars SA, Spyer KM, Gilbey MP. Stimulation within the rostral ventrolateral medulla can evoke monosynaptic GABAergic IPSPs in sympathetic preganglionic neurons in vitro. J Neurophysiol 1997; 77:229–235.
71. Morrison SF, Gebber GL. Axonal branching patterns and funicular trajectories of raphespinal sympathoinhibitory neurons. J Neurophysiol 1985; 53:759–772.
72. Morrison SF, Gebber GL. Raphe neurons with sympathetic-related activity: baroreceptor responses and spinal connections. Am J Physiol Regul Integr Comp Physiol 1984; 246: R338–R348.
73. Aicher SA, Reis DJ, Nicolae R, et al. Monosynaptic projections from the medullary gigantocellular reticular formation to sympathetic preganglionic neurons in the thoracic spinal cord. J Comp Neurol 1995; 363:563–580.
74. Coleman MJ, Dampney RAL. Powerful depressor and sympathoinhibitory effects evoked from neurons in the caudal raphe pallidus and obscurus. Am J Physiol Regul Integr Comp Physiol 1995; 268:R1295–R1302.
75. McCall RB. GABA-mediated inhibition of sympathoexcitatory neurons by midline medullary stimulation. Am J Physiol Regul Integr Comp Physiol 1988; 255:R605–R615.
76. Aicher SA, Reis DJ, Ruggiero DA, et al. Anatomical characterization of a novel reticulospinal vasodepresoor area in the rat medulla oblongata. Neuroscience 1994; 60:761–779.
77. Henderson LA, Keay KA, Bandler R. The ventrolateral periaqueductal gray projects to caudal brainstem depressor regions: a functional-anatomical and physiological study. Neuroscience 1998; 82:201–221.
78. Blessing WW, Nalivaiko E. Regional blood flow and nociceptive stimuli in rabbits: patterning by medullary raphe, not ventrolateral medulla. J Physiol 2000; 524:279–292.
79. Kumada M, Terui N, Kuwaki T. Arterial baroreceptor reflex: its central and peripheral neural mechanisms. Prog Neurobiol 1990; 35:331–361.
80. Chan RKW, Sawchenko PE. Organization and transmitter specificity of medullary neurons activated by sustained hypertension: implications for understanding baroreceptor reflex circuitry. J Neurosci 1998; 18:371–387.
81. Schreihofer AM, Guyenet PG. The baroreflex and beyond: control of sympathetic vasomotor tone by GABAergic neurons in the ventrolateral medulla. Clin Exp Pharmacol Physiol 2002; 29:514–521.
82. Bailey TW, Hermes SM, Andresen MC, et al. Cranial visceral afferent pathways through the nucleus of the solitary tract to caudal ventrolateral medulla or paraventricular hypothalamus: target-specific synaptic reliability and convergence patterns. J Neurosci 2006; 26: 11893–11902.
83. Weston M, Wang H, Stornetta RL, et al. Fos expression by glutamatergic neurons of the solitary tract nucleus after phenylephrine-induced hypertension in rats. J Comp Neurol 2003; 460:525–541.

84. Deuchars J, Li YW, Kasparov S, et al. Morphological and electrophysiological properties of neurones in the dorsal vagal complex of the rat activated by arterial baroreceptors. J Comp Neurol 2000; 417:233–249.
85. Zhang J, Mifflin SW. Responses of aortic depressor nerve-evoked neurones in rat nucleus of the solitary tract to changes in blood pressure. J Physiol 2000; 529:431–443.
86. Paton JF, Boscan P, Murphy D, et al. Unravelling mechanisms of action of angiotensin II on cardiorespiratory function using in vivo gene transfer. Acta Physiol Scand 2001; 173:127–137.
87. Goodchild AK, Van Deurzen BT, Sun QJ, et al. Spinal GABA(A) receptors do not mediate the sympathetic baroreceptor reflex in the rat. Am J Physiol Regul Integr Comp Physiol 2000; 279:R320–R331.
88. Gatti PJ, Johnson TA, McKenzie J, et al. Vagal control of left ventricular contractility is selectively mediated by a cranioventricular intracardiac ganglion in the cat. J Auton Nerv Syst 1997; 66:138–144.
89. Massari VJ, Johnson TA, Gatti PJ. Cardiotopic organization of the nucleus ambiguus? An anatomical and physiological analysis of neurons regulating atrioventricular conduction. Brain Res 1995; 679:227–240.
90. Standish A, Enquist LW, Escardo JA, et al. Central neuronal circuit innervating the rat heart defined by transneuronal transport of pseudorabies virus. J Neurosci 1995; 15:1998–2012.
91. Standish A, Enquist LW, Schwaber JS. Innervation of the heart and its central medullary origin defined by viral tracing. Science 1994; 263:232–235.
92. Gilbey MP, Jordan D, Richter DW, et al. Synaptic mechanisms involved in the inspiratory modulation of vagal cardio-inhibitory neurones in the cat. J Physiol 1984; 356:65–78.
93. Neff RA, Mihalevich M, Mendelowitz D. Stimulation of NTS activates NMDA and non-NMDA receptors in rat cardiac vagal neurons in the nucleus ambiguus. Brain Res 1998; 792:277–282.
94. Neff RA, Wang J, Baxi S, et al. Respiratory sinus arrhythmia: endogenous activation of nicotinic receptors mediates respiratory modulation of brainstem cardioinhibitory para-sympathetic neurons. Circ Res 2003; 93:565–572.
95. Massari VJ, Johnson TA, Llewellynsmith IJ, et al. Substance P nerve terminals synapse upon negative chronotropic vagal motoneurons. Brain Res 1994; 660:275–287.
96. Habler HJ, Janig W, Michaelis M. Respiratory modulation in the activity of sympathetic neurones. Prog Neurobiol 1994; 43:567–606.
97. Millhorn DE. Neural respiratory and circulatory interaction during chemoreceptor stimulation and cooling of ventral medulla in cats. J Physiol 1986; 370:217–231.
98. Haselton JR, Guyenet PG. Central respiratory modulation of medullary sympathoexcitatory neurons in rat. Am J Physiol Regul Integr Comp Physiol 1989; 256:R739–R750.
99. Millhorn DE, Eldridge FL. Role of ventrolateral medulla in regulation of respiratory and cardiovascular systems. J Appl Physiol 1986; 61:1249–1263.
100. Darnall RA, Guyenet P. Respiratory modulation of pre- and postganglionic lumbar vaso-motor sympathetic neurons in the rat. Neurosci Lett 1990; 119:148–152.
101. Miyawaki T, Pilowsky P, Sun QJ, et al. Central inspiration increases barosensitivity of neurons in rat rostral ventrolateral medulla. Am J Physiol Regul Integr Comp Physiol 1995; 268:R909–R918.
102. Mandel DA, Schreihofer AM. Central respiratory modulation of barosensitive neurones in rat caudal ventrolateral medulla. J Physiol 2006; 572:881–896.
103. Daly M.de Burgh. Interactions between respiration and circulation. In: Cherniack NS, Widdicombe JG, eds. Handbook of Physiology: The Respiratory System. Sect 3. Bethesda: The American Physiological Society, 1986: 529–594.
104. Gebber GL, Das M, Barman SM. Dynamic changes in baroreceptor-sympathetic coupling during the respiratory cycle. Brain Res 2005; 1046:216–223.
105. Macefield VG, Wallin BG. Modulation of muscle sympathetic activity during spontaneous and artificial ventilation and apnoea in humans. J Auton Nerv Syst 1995; 53:137–147.

106. Feldman JL, Del Negro CA. Looking for inspiration: new perspectives on respiratory rhythm. Nat Rev Neurosci 2006; 7:232–242.

107. Jiang C, Lipski J. Extensive monosynaptic inhibition of ventral respiratory group neurons by augmenting neurons in the Botzinger complex in the cat. Exp Brain Res 1990; 81:639–648.

108. Sun QJ, Minson J, Llewellyn-Smith IJ, et al. Botzinger neurons project towards bulbospinal neurons in the rostral ventrolateral medulla of the rat. J Comp Neurol 1997; 388:23–31.

109. Guyenet PG, Darnall RA, Riley TA. Rostral ventrolateral medulla and sympathorespiratory integration in rats. Am J Physiol Regul Integr Comp Physiol 1990; 259:R1063–R1074.

110. Miyawaki T, Goodchild AK, Pilowsky PM. Evidence for a tonic GABA-ergic inhibition of excitatory respiratory-related afferents to presympathetic neurons in the rostral ventrolateral medulla. Brain Res 2002; 924:56–62.

111. Miyawaki T, Minson J, Arnolda L, et al. Role of excitatory amino acid receptors in cardiorespiratory coupling in ventrolateral medulla. Am J Physiol Regul Integr Comp Physiol 1996; 271:R1221–R1230.

112. Barman SM, Gebber GL. Subgroups of rostral ventrolateral medullary and caudal medullary raphe neurons based on patterns of relationship to sympathetic nerve discharge and axonal projections. J Neurophysiol 1997; 77:65–75.

113. Guyenet PG. Neural structures that mediate sympathoexcitation during hypoxia. Respir Physiol 2000; 121:147–162.

114. Hanna BD, Lioy F, Polosa C. Role of carotid and central chemoreceptors in the CO_2 response of sympathetic preganglionic neurons. J Auton Nerv Syst 1981; 3:421–435.

115. Loeschcke HH. Central chemosensitivity and the reaction theory. J Physiol 1982; 332:1–24.

116. Smith CA, Rodman JR, Chenuel BJ, et al. Response time and sensitivity of the ventilatory response to CO_2 in unanesthetized intact dogs: central vs. peripheral chemoreceptors. J Appl Physiol 2006; 100:13–19.

117. Nattie EE. Chemoreceptors, breathing, and pH. In: Alpern RJ, Hebert SC, eds. Seldin and Giebisch's The Kidney: Physiology & Pathophysiology. 4th ed. New York: Elsevier, 2007: 1587–1600.

118. Arita H, Ichikawa K, Kuwana S, et al. Possible locations of pH-dependent central chemoreceptors: intramedullary regions with acidic shift of extracellular fluid pH during hypercapnia. Brain Res 1989; 485:285–293.

119. Guyenet PG. The 2008 Carl Ludwig lecture: retrotrapezoid nucleus, CO_2 homeostasis and breathing automaticity. J Appl Physiol 2008; 105:410–416.

120. Takakura AC, Moreira TS, Stornetta RL, et al. Selective lesions of retrotrapezoid Phox2b-expressing neurons raises the apneic threshold in rats. J Physiol 2008; 586:2975–2991.

121. Mulkey DK, Stornetta RL, Weston MC, et al. Respiratory control by ventral surface chemoreceptor neurons in rats. Nat Neurosci 2004; 7:1360–1369.

122. Nattie EE, Li A. Substance P saporin lesion of neurons with NK1 receptors in one chemoreceptor site in rats decreases ventilation and chemosensitivity. J Physiol 2002; 544:603–616.

123. Spengler CM, Gozal D, Shea SA. Chemoreceptive mechanisms elucidated by studies of congenital central hypoventilation syndrome. Respir Physiol 2001; 129:247–255.

124. Dubreuil V, Ramanantsoa N, Trochet D, et al. A human mutation in Phox2b causes lack of CO_2 chemosensitivity, fatal central apnoea and specific loss of parafacial neurons. Proc Natl Acad Sci U S A 2008; 105:1067–1072.

125. Gourine AV, Llaudet E, Dale N, et al. ATP is a mediator of chemosensory transduction in the central nervous system. Nature 2005; 436:108–111.

126. Guyenet PG, Stornetta RL, Bayliss DA. Retrotrapezoid nucleus and central chemoreception. J Physiol 2008; 586:2043–2048.

127. Hodges MR, Tattersall GJ, Harris MB, et al. Defects in breathing and thermoregulation in mice with near-complete absence of central serotonin neurons. J Neurosci 2008; 28:2495–2505.

128. Li A, Nattie E. Catecholamine neurones in rats modulate sleep, breathing, central chemoreception and breathing variability. J Physiol 2006; 570:385–396.
129. Richerson GB. Serotonergic neurons as carbon dioxide sensors that maintain pH homeostasis. Nat Rev Neurosci 2004; 5:449–461.
130. Kanamaru M, Homma I. Compensatory airway dilation and additive ventilatory augmentation mediated by dorsomedial medullary 5-hydroxytryptamine 2 receptor activity and hypercapnia. Am J Physiol Regul Integr Comp Physiol 2007; 293;R854–R860.
131. Veasey SC, Fornal CA, Metzler CW, et al. Single-unit responses of serotonergic dorsal raphe neurons to specific motor challenges in freely moving cats. Neuroscience 1997; 79: 161–169.
132. Veasey SC, Fornal CA, Metzler CW, et al. Response of serotonergic caudal raphe neurons in relation to specific motor activities in freely moving cats. J Neurosci 1995; 15:5346–5359.
133. Marshall JM. Peripheral chemoreceptors and cardiovascular regulation. Physiol Rev 1994; 74:543–594.
134. Moosavi SH, Banzett RB, Butler JP. Time course of air hunger mirrors the biphasic ventilatory response to hypoxia. J Appl Physiol 2004; 97:2098–2103.
135. Erickson JT, Millhorn DE. Hypoxia and electrical stimulation of the carotid sinus nerve induce c-Fos-like immunoreactivity within catecholaminergic and serotinergic neurons of the rat brainstem. J Comp Neurol 1994; 348:161–182.
136. Lioy F, Hanna BD, Polosa C. Cardiovascular control by medullary surface chemoreceptors. J Auton Nerv Syst 1981; 3:9–24.
137. Moreira TS, Takakura AC, Colombari E, et al. Central chemoreceptors and sympathetic vasomotor outflow. J Physiol 2006; 577:369–386.
138. Takakura AC, Moreira TS, Colombari E, et al. Peripheral chemoreceptor inputs to retrotrapezoid nucleus (RTN) CO2-sensitive neurons in rats. J Physiol 2006; 572:503–523.
139. Nattie E. Why do we have both peripheral and central chemoreceptors? J Appl Physiol 2006; 100:9–10.
140. Paton JF, Boscan P, Pickering AE, et al. The yin and yang of cardiac autonomic control: vago-sympathetic interactions revisited. Brain Res Brain Res Rev 2005; 49:555–565.
141. Nurse CA. Neurotransmission and neuromodulation in the chemosensory carotid body. Auton Neurosci 2005; 120:1–9.
142. Campanucci VA, Nurse CA. Autonomic innervation of the carotid body: role in efferent inhibition. Respir Physiol Neurobiol 2007; 157:83–92.
143. Sapru HN. Carotid chemoreflex. Neural pathways and transmitters. Adv Exp Med Biol 1996; 410:357–364.
144. Blessing WW, Yu YH, Nalivaiko E. Medullary projections of rabbit carotid sinus nerve. Brain Res 1999; 816:405–410.
145. Braga VA, Soriano RN, Braccialli AL, et al. Involvement of L-glutamate and ATP in the neurotransmission of the sympathoexcitatory component of the chemoreflex in the commissural nucleus tractus solitarii of awake rats and in the working heart-brainstem preparation. J Physiol 2007; 581:1129–1145.
146. Koshiya N, Guyenet PG. NTS neurons with carotid chemoreceptor inputs arborize in the rostral ventrolateral medulla. Am J Physiol Regul Integr Comp Physiol 1996; 270:R1273–R1278.
147. Erickson JT, Millhorn DE. Fos-like protein is induced in neurons of the medulla oblongata after stimulation of the carotid sinus nerve in awake and anesthetized rats. Brain Res 1991; 567:11–24.
148. Sun MK, Reis DJ. Central neural mechanisms mediating excitation of sympathetic neurons by hypoxia. Prog Neurobiol 1994; 44:197–219.
149. Aicher SA, Saravay RH, Cravo S, et al. Monosynaptic projections from the nucleus tractus solitarii to C1 adrenergic neurons in the rostral ventrolateral medulla: comparison with input from the caudal ventrolateral medulla. J Comp Neurol 1996; 373:62–75.

150. Dempsey JA, Sheel AW, St Croix CM, et al. Respiratory influences on sympathetic vasomotor outflow in humans. Respir Physiol Neurobiol 2002; 130:3–20.
151. Koshiya N, Guyenet PG. A5 noradrenergic neurons and the carotid sympathetic chemoreflex. Am J Physiol Regul Integr Comp Physiol 1994; 267:R519–R526.
152. Paton JFR. Pattern of cardiorespiratory afferent convergence to solitary tract neurons driven by pulmonary vagal C-fiber stimulation in the mouse. J Neurophysiol 1998; 79:2365–2373.
153. Coleridge HM, Coleridge JC. Afferent innervation of lungs, airways, and pulmonary artery. In: Zucker IH, Gilmore JP, eds. Reflex Control of the Circulation. Boca Raton: CRC Press, 2001: 579–607.
154. Daly MdeB, Ward J, Wood LM. Modification by lung inflation of the vascular responses from the carotid body chemoreceptors and other receptors in dogs. J Physiol 1986; 378:13–30.
155. Kubin L, Alheid GF, Zuperku EJ, et al. Central pathways of pulmonary and lower airway vagal afferents. J Applied Physiol 2006; 101:618–627.
156. Vatner SF, Uemura N. Integrative cardiovascular control by pulmonary inflation reflexes. In: Zucker IH, Gilmore JP, eds. Reflex Control of the Circulation. Boca Raton: CRC Press, 2001: 609–626.
157. Kalia M, Richter D. Morphology of physiologically identified slowly adapting lung stretch receptor afferents stained with intra-axonal horseradish peroxidase in the nucleus of the tractus solitarius of the cat. I. A light microscopic analysis. J Comp Neurol 1985; 241:503–520.
158. Ezure K, Tanaka I. GABA, in some cases together with glycine, is used as the inhibitory transmitter by pump cells in the Hering-Breuer reflex pathway of the rat. Neuroscience 2004; 127:409–417.
159. Hayashi F, Coles SK, McCrimmon DR. Respiratory neurons mediating the Breuer-Hering reflex prolongation of expiration in rat. J Neurosci 1996; 16:6526–6536.
160. Coleridge HM, Coleridge JC. Pulmonary reflexes: neural mechanisms of pulmonary defense. Annu Rev Physiol 1994; 56:69–91.
161. Bachoo M, Polosa C. The pattern of sympathetic neurone activity during expiration in the cat. J Physiol 1986; 378:375–390.
162. Eckberg DL. The human respiratory gate. J Physiol 2003; 548:339–352.
163. Seals DR, Suwarno NO, Joyner MJ, et al. Respiratory modulation of muscle sympathetic nerve activity in intact and lung denervated humans. Circ Res 1993; 72:440–454.
164. Guyenet PG, Brown DL. Unit activity in nucleus paragigantocellularis lateralis during cerebral ischemia in the rat. Brain Res 1986; 364:301–314.
165. Sun MK. Pharmacology of reticulospinal vasomotor neurons in cardiovascular regulation. Pharmacol Rev 1996; 48:465–494.
166. Cushing H. Concerning a definitive regulatory mechanism of the vaso-motor centre which controls blood pressure during cerebral compression. Bull Johns Hopkins Hosp 1901; 12: 290–292.
167. Paton JF, Abdala AP, Koizumi H, et al. Respiratory rhythm generation during gasping depends on persistent sodium current. Nat Neurosci 2006; 9:311–313.
168. Reis DJ, Golanov EV, Galea E, et al. Central neurogenic neuroprotection: central neural systems that protect the brain from hypoxia and ischemia. Ann N Y Acad Sci 1997; 835: 168–186.
169. Osborn JW, Jacob F, Guzman P. A neural set point for the long-term control of arterial pressure: beyond the arterial baroreceptor reflex. Am J Physiol Regul Integr Comp Physiol 2005; 288:R846–R855.
170. Levy EI, Scarrow AM, Jannetta PJ. Microvascular decompression in the treatment of hypertension: review and update. Surg Neurol 2001; 55:2–10.
171. Curran AK, Rodman JR, Eastwood PR, et al. Ventilatory responses to specific CNS hypoxia in sleeping dogs. J Appl Physiol 2000; 88:1840–1852.

3
Mechanical Interactions Between the Respiratory and Circulatory Systems

SHELDON MAGDER
McGill University Health Centre, Montreal, Quebec, Canada

I. Introduction

Mammalian species evolved with a four-chambered heart and two lungs. The evolutionary advantages of these structures are that they prevent mixing of fully oxygenated and deoxygenated blood in the gas-exchange units and allow low pressures in the delicate alveolar capillaries. However, there is a price to pay. The passage of flow between the two halves of the heart becomes subject to the pressure and volume swings associated with the generation of airflow in the lungs. When lung mechanics are optimal and ventilatory demands are small, the changes in pleural pressure required for airflow are small and thus their effect on cardiac chambers is also small. However, when ventilatory demands increase or the mechanics of the ventilatory system are altered by disease, the effects can become large and significantly impact on circulatory flow. This chapter will review the basics of the interaction between the respiratory and cardiovascular systems. There are numerous components to circulatory-ventilatory interactions, which can make the analysis very complex. However, a few components quantitatively dominate the interactions, and these will be emphasized in this review. I will also discuss only mechanical factors and not the neural-humeral responses to lung inflation that can impact on the circulation (1–7). Before discussing circulatory-ventilatory interactions, it is necessary to review some of the basics of the determinants of cardiac output.

II. Determinants of Cardiac Output

As described by Arthur Guyton, cardiac output is determined by the interaction of two functions: a cardiac function and a return function (Fig. 1) (8–11). The four determinants of cardiac function are preload, afterload contractility, and heart rate. The preload sets the initial length of the sarcomeres, and as expressed in the Frank–Starling relationship there is a linear increase in cardiac output with increases in initial sarcomere length when the afterload contractility and heart rate are kept constant (12). A function curve for the whole heart can be produced by plotting the cardiac output (flow) against the preload for the whole heart as a unit; the preload for the whole heart is given by the right atrial pressure [In this discussion, I will use right atrial pressure (Pra) and central venous pressure (CVP) interchangeably for they are essentially the same under most conditions.] Increasing afterload, decreasing contractility, or decreasing heart rate depress the cardiac function curve and opposite changes shift the cardiac function curve upward.

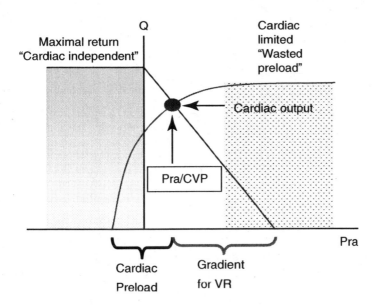

Figure 1 Graph of return (venous) and cardiac function curves. The intersection of these two functions give the working cardiac output (Q), venous return, and right atrial pressure. The shaded area to the right indicates "cardiac limitation," and increases in preload (by giving volume) will not increase cardiac output. The shaded area on the right indicates a limitation of the venous return. Lowering right atrial pressure (Pra or CVP, central venous pressure) in this region will not increase venous return (VR) and therefore will not increase cardiac output. See text for further details.

Around 70% of the total blood volume resides in the small veins and venules at a low pressure, and this region serves as a reservoir or a capacitance region. The capacitance region functions much like a bathtub (8,13). The flow out of a bathtub is determined by the height of the water above the hole at the bottom but is not affected by the pressure in the tap flowing into the tub. The flow from the tap only alters flow out of the tub by increasing the volume of the tub, which increases the height of water, and the consequent increase in hydrostatic pressure increases outflow from the tub. The volume of the bathtub is very large relative to the inflow, and large changes in volume are needed to change the height of the tub. Similarly, small veins and venules store a large volume at a low pressure. Elastic structures that are filled with volume develop an elastic recoil pressure. If the circulation is stopped and the vascular volume from the aortic valve to the entry to the right atrium is isolated, this volume produces a pressure that is called mean systemic filling pressure (MSFP); this pressure is equivalent to the height of the water in a bathtub. Because most of the blood volume resides in the small venules and veins, MSFP is dominated by the elastic characteristics (compliance) of this region. Furthermore, MSFP is relatively unchanged under normal flow conditions because there is no other significant stores of volume that can be recruited from other regions to increase MSFP. The only other significant volume reservoir is in the pulmonary venous circulation but the compliance of these vessels is only about one-seventh of the systemic venous compliance. Thus, there is little volume to be recruited, and improved left ventricular function can only increase MSFP by a small amount by this mechanism (14,15).

When MSFP is equal to the pressure in the right atrium, there is no flow. Flow can only occur when right atrial pressure is lower than the upstream pressure in the venules and veins. Thus, the heart generates cardiac output by lowering right atrial pressure and allowing blood to come back to the heart. Since the bulk of blood volume starts in the venules and veins and as already noted, there is not much volume that the heart can recruit to pass to the venules and veins, MSFP is relatively independent of cardiac function. An exception to this is under conditions of severe left ventricular dysfunction with maintained right ventricular function. Under this extreme condition, the right heart can transfer peripheral volume to the pulmonary vessels and MSFP can significantly fall. In summary, the role of the heart in the circulation is "permissive" by allowing blood to drain from the veins and "restorative" by putting the blood back to where it has come from. Although arterial pressure does not determine cardiac output, it does determine regional flows.

The determinants of the return function that account for the return of blood from the peripheral venous reservoir to the heart are the volume in the vasculature that stretches the vascular walls, which is called stressed vascular volume, venous compliance, venous resistance, and right atrial pressure. The return function (also called venous return curve) can also be represented graphically by plotting blood flow against right atrial pressure. Since the heart can only put out what it receives, in the steady state cardiac output and venous return must be equal. An increase in total volume shifts the venous return curve in parallel to the right. The curve can also be shifted to the right by a decrease in vascular capacitance, which occurs when venous smooth muscles contract for this converts unstressed volume into stressed volume (13,16,17). This too produces a parallel shift to the right, which is identical to the effect of an increase in volume. Venous compliance (the slope of the pressure-volume relationship) does not usually decrease under physiological conditions, but if it decreased it would shift the venous return curve to the right. A decrease in venous resistance rotates the venous return curve upward with the same x-intercept.

Since the cardiac function curve and venous return curve are plotted with the same axes, they can be plotted together on the same graph and their interaction analyzed. However, it is necessary to make an adjustment. The preload-cardiac output relationship is based on the pressure across the wall of the heart, which is called transmural pressure. The pressure outside the wall of the heart is pleural pressure and not atmospheric pressure, and therefore the pressure outside the heart varies relative to atmospheric pressure throughout the ventilatory cycle. On the other hand, the "surrounding" pressure for the return function is atmospheric pressure and does not change during ventilation (leaving out for the moment changes in abdominal pressure). The cardiac function and return curves thus have different reference systems. This is dealt with in the graphical analysis by having the cardiac function curve start with a zero flow-pressure point that is at the value of the pleural pressure. When a person breaths in from atmospheric pressure, the pleural pressure at functional residual capacity (FRC) and pre-inspiration is slightly negative. Thus, the cardiac function curve is shifted to the left of the venous return curve and starts at a negative value. The intersection point of the cardiac and return functions gives the "working" cardiac output, "working" venous return, and "working" right atrial pressure. The distance from the x-intercept of the cardiac function curve to the working right atrial pressure gives the transmural right atrial pressure. The distance from the x-intercept of the return curve to the working right atrial pressure gives the gradient for venous return. An increase in cardiac function with no change in return function produces a rise in cardiac output and fall in right atrial pressure. In contrast, an increase in the return function with no change in cardiac function results in an increase in cardiac output with a rise in right atrial pressure.

An important feature of the cardiac and return functions is that they have limits (Fig. 1). The cardiac function curve has a plateau at values of right atrial pressure that normally occurs at less than 10 to 12 mmHg (referenced at 5 cm below the sternal angle) (18) and when the plateau is reached, further volume loading will not increase cardiac output by the Frank–Starling mechanism (19). This limit of right heart filling normally occurs because of physical constraint by the noncompliant pericardium (19–21), but even occurs without a pericardium by restricting effects of the cardiac cytoskeleton. Constraint can also be produced by hyperinflated lungs, masses in the mediastinum, or large pleural effusions. There is also a limit to the return function that occurs when the pressure in the great veins falls below the surrounding pressure. This results in collapse of venous vessels as they enter the thorax in what has been called a "vascular waterfall" (22). Under this condition pressure in downstream vessels, in this case the right atrium, is no longer the outflow pressure for venous return, and venous return is determined by the gradient from the peripheral veins to the collapse pressure. During spontaneous breathing venous collapse occurs when CVP is less than atmospheric pressure but collapse of veins occurs at positive values relative to atmosphere when breathing with a positive pressure source (23). The collapse of veins entering the thorax brings up an interesting insight into the function of the limits of cardiac output. The best the heart can do is lower the right atrial pressure to the collapse point; right atrial pressures above that value simply impede flow. Thus, if the heart is removed and the great veins are allowed to drain to atmospheric pressure, for that instant blood flow will be maximal and the heart can never do better (24). Of course, the volume in the reservoir will be quickly dissipated and flow will fall. Thus, as already stated, a key role of the heart is to "restore" the volume in the veins and venules, and it is the initial volume and the elastic recoil that it produces is the key determinant of the maximum possible cardiac output for a given set of circuit parameters (10).

III. Basics of Circulatory-Ventilatory Interactions

The primary mechanical interactions between the ventilatory and circulatory systems occur through changes in pleural pressure or alveolar pressures, although there are some direct effects from changes in lung volume that also will be discussed. The analysis can be broken down into the effects of negative pressure breathing (spontaneous breathing) versus positive pressure breathing and then the effects on inflow and outflow to the right heart and the inflow and outflow to the left heart. I will begin with the effects of changes in pleural pressure on inflow to the right heart.

IV. Effects of Pleural Pressure Changes on Output from the Right Heart

As already pointed out above, the pressure environment around the heart is different from that of the rest of the body and changes throughout the ventilatory cycle. The failure to recognize this point initially produced confusion about the mechanical interactions of the circulatory and ventilatory systems. For example, once it was possible to measure cardiac pressures and outputs it was observed that positive pressure breathing produces a fall in cardiac output with a rise in right and left atrial pressures. This was interpreted as indicating depressed cardiac function (25). It turns out that this was an artifact produced by not appreciating that it is the transmural atrial pressure that is critical in the Frank–Starling relationship and when atrial values were corrected for the change in pleural pressure, which is the pressure outside the heart, cardiac function curves were superimposable before and after the application of positive pressure (26,27).

V. Fall In Pleural Pressure During Spontaneous Breathing

Although the cardiac function curve is not altered by changes in pleural pressure, the cardiac output is usually affected. Changing pleural pressure produces the physical equivalent of lifting or lowering the heart relative to the peripheral venous reservoir (venous capacitance bed) (28,29). This shift of the cardiac function relationship relative to the rest of the body plays a key role in circulatory-ventilatory interactions because the normal gradient for venous return is only in the range of 4 to 8 mmHg and small changes in right atrial pressure relative to the venous reservoir can have large effects on blood flow back to the heart. This is clearly seen in Guyton's graphical analysis of the interaction of cardiac and return function (Fig. 2). A spontaneous inspiration lowers the pressure in the heart relative to the rest of the body, and the cardiac function curve intersects the return curve at a lower right atrial pressure relative to atmosphere. However, the cardiac output is higher because the cardiac transmural pressure is increased. When the cardiac function curve intersects the flat part of the venous return curve, further decreases in negative pleural pressure do not augment cardiac volumes and consequently output. This has clinical importance. Normally, right atrial pressure is close to atmospheric pressure or even below. Under these conditions the inspiratory increase in right heart filling is small. However, if the person starts with a high initial CVP, the inspiratory increase in right heart filling is much larger. Thus, a patient's initial blood volume is a very important determinant of the magnitude of the cyclic filling of the right ventricle during spontaneous breathing.

In the previous discussion, the assumption was that the return function intersects the ascending portion of the cardiac function curve. The response is very different when the return curve intersects the plateau of the cardiac function curve (Fig. 2). In this condition, right atrial pressure and cardiac output do not change during spontaneous inspirations. However, the transmural right atrial pressure rises considerably, which could have effects on coronary flow as well as left heart function by causing a shift of the septum into the left ventricle and compromising the diastolic compliance of the left heart (30). We successfully used this observation to develop a bedside diagnostic test, which also gives some good insight into what happens in general with pleural pressure swings (31). The reasoning is as follows. When CVP falls with the fall in pleural pressure of a spontaneous inspiration, this indicates that the return function intersects the ascending portion of the cardiac function curve. Since a volume infusion increases cardiac output by shifting the venous return curve to the right and up the cardiac function curve, in this condition volume infusion could increase cardiac output. I could say because if the return function intersects the cardiac function near the plateau of the cardiac function curve, a volume infusion will produce only a small increase in cardiac

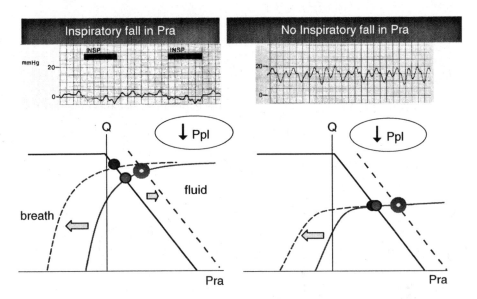

Figure 2 The use of respiratory variation in Pra/CVP to predict fluid responsiveness. The tracings at the top of the figure show Pra (right atrial pressure) over time. On the left, there is a fall in Pra with the inspiratory fall in pleural pressure (Ppl) (marked by thick line), whereas on the right there is no change with inspiration. The bottom part of the figure shows the venous return-cardiac function curves for the two conditions. With an inspiration the pressure in the environment of the heart falls relative to atmosphere and the cardiac function moves to the left to account for this and this results in a higher intersection point for the venous return-cardiac function curves and a rise in cardiac output (Q). Giving fluid to this person and shifting the venous return curve to the right (*dotted line*) will increase cardiac output. When the venous return curve intersects the flat part of the cardiac function curve, there is no change in Pra or Q. Giving volume will not change cardiac output.

output although there is a significant fall in CVP with inspiration. However, when there is no inspiratory fall in CVP, the return function must be intersecting the flat part of the cardiac function curve. In this condition, volume infusion should not increase cardiac output because cardiac function is already volume limited. Indeed, this is what was observed. This test is useful in the negative sense. That is, if there is no fall in CVP with an adequate inspiratory effort to sufficiently lower pleural pressure, the test predicts with a high sensitivity that a volume infusion will not increase cardiac output. However, if there is an inspiratory fall in pleural pressure, the person may or may not respond to fluids depending on how close the intersection of the return curve and cardiac function curve is to the plateau of the cardiac function curve. This cannot be discerned by the test in advance.

A potential misuse of the test brings up another circulatory-ventilatory interaction. Normally, expiration is passive so that there should be no increase in pleural pressure during expiration. However, critically ill patients frequently have active recruitment of expiratory muscles. This results in a rise in abdominal pressure, which is transmitted to

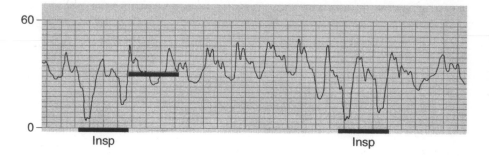

Figure 3 Example of CVP tracing in subject with spontaneous breaths and forced expiration. There is rise in CVP throughout the expiratory phase. Inspiration (Insp) is marked with lines. Note the increase in the 'y' descent with inspiration that helps identify the event.

pleural pressure and CVP. Recruitment of expiratory muscles can occur with both spontaneous, negative pressure ventilation and with positive pressure ventilation. The increase in pleural pressure that is produced from the contracting expiratory muscles must rapidly fall at the start of inspiration for airflow to occur and so does the CVP. It may then appear that there was an inspiratory fall in CVP whereas in reality there was only a loss of positive pressure at the end of expiration and a return to baseline pressure (Fig. 3). This is not predictive of fluid responsiveness. The rise in CVP in these patients could simply be due to transmission of abdominal and pleural pressure to the heart, but in patients who are sufficiently volume replete, it may represent true translocation of abdominal venous volume to the chest and represent an increase in cardiac transmural pressure. This inspiratory increase in right-sided filling can potentially add to ventilator-induced oscillations in cardiac output (32,33). It can also lead to important errors in the assessment of the value of the CVP (9).

Increased abdominal pressure during inspiration also is responsible for what is known as Kussmaul's sign, which is a rise in right atrial pressure relative to atmosphere with inspiration instead of the usual fall. What happens when Kussmaul's sign is present is that the descending diaphragm presses on the venous reservoir in the splanchnic bed and transiently increases the return of blood to the heart. Two factors are required for this sign. The splanchnic reservoir must be sufficiently replete so that there is enough volume to recruit, and right ventricular filling has to be limited so that the increase in filling pressure does not change sarcomere length and allow the dissipation of the volume increase by the Starling mechanism (34,35).

VI. Rise in Pleural Pressure During Positive Pressure Breathing

An increase in pleural pressure does the opposite of a fall in pleural pressure. It effectively lifts the heart relative to the rest of the body (Fig. 4) and in the graphical analysis of return and cardiac functions, an increase in pleural pressure shifts the cardiac function curve to the right (Fig. 5). If the return function intersects the ascending portion of the cardiac function curve, the rightward shift of the cardiac function curve increases right atrial pressure for the intersection of the return curve moves up the cardiac function

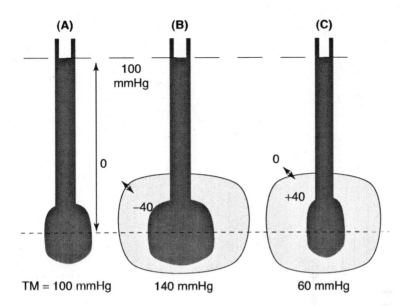

(A)   **(B)**   **(C)**

100 mmHg

0   0

−40   +40

TM = 100 mmHg   140 mmHg   60 mmHg

Figure 4 Schematic representation of the effects of pleural pressure on the afterload of the heart. The figures show hearts (round ball at the bottom) pumping into straight tubes as is used in a Langendorff preparation. In the example on the left, the heart is surrounded by atmosphere and the transmural pressure of the heart (TM = $P_{inside} − P_{outside}$) is 100 mmHg. In the middle example, the pressure around the heart is 40 less than atmosphere so that if the same pressure is generated relative to atmosphere (dotted line at the top), but the TM is 140 mmHg. In the example on the right, the pressure around the heart is 40 mmHg greater than atmosphere so that if the generated pressure relative to atmosphere is 100 mmHg, the TM is 60 mmHg.

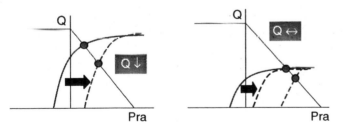

Figure 5 Graphical representation of the return-cardiac function curves with positive inspiration. Labels are the same as in Figures 1 and 2. With positive pressure ventilation the cardiac function curve moves to the right. When the venous return curve intersects the ascending part of the cardiac function curve a positive pressure inspiration results in a rise in Pra and fall in cardiac output. When the venous return curve intersects the flat part of the cardiac function curve there is no change in Q until the cardiac function curve moves sufficiently to the right to again intersect the ascending part of the cardiac function curve.

curve. This decreases the gradient for venous return and cardiac output decreases. However, if the return function intersects the flat part of the cardiac function curve, the rightward shift does not change right atrial pressure or cardiac output until the cardiac function curve moves far enough to the right so that the return function again intersects the ascending portion of the cardiac function curve (Fig. 5) (36). An additional mechanism can also contribute to the fall in cardiac output with positive pleural pressure. Increased lung inflation pushes the diaphragm down, and this has been shown in dogs to compress the inferior vena cava and increase venous resistance, which will also decrease cardiac output (37).

Since the gradient for venous return is only in the range of 4 to 8 mmHg, an increase in pleural pressure of 4 to 5 mmHg can markedly reduce the gradient for venous return and thus cardiac output. In normal lungs, a little less than half of the increase in airway pressure is transmitted to the pleural space so that an increase of airway pressures greater than 10 cmH$_2$O could potentially decrease cardiac output by more than half: Not only is cardiac output reduced but maximum possible cardiac output also is reduced (38). This is because venous collapse occurs when the pressure inside a vein is less than the pressure outside a vein and when pleural pressure becomes positive, the collapse of veins as they enter the thorax occurs at the positive pleural pressure instead of atmospheric pressure.

How then are patients able to survive with positive pressure ventilation and the application of positive end-expiratory pressure (PEEP)? There are a number of mechanisms that make this possible. These are not given in the order that is necessarily the most probable. The first is reflex adjustments. Contraction of vascular smooth muscle in the walls of small veins and venules recruits unstressed volume into stressed volume and thereby raises MSFP (Fig. 6) (39). This is called a decrease in vascular capacitance. The consequent shift to the right of the venous return curve relative to the cardiac function

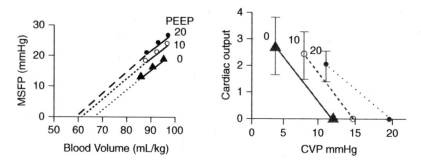

Figure 6 Graphical analysis of adaptations of the circulation to positive end-expiratory pressure (PEEP). The left side shows a plot of MSFP and total blood volume in milliliter per kilogram. With increases in PEEP from 0 to 20 cmH$_2$O, the pressure-volume relationship of the vasculature moves to the left, which indicates a decrease in capacitance. However, the compliance (inverse of the slope of the line) does not change. The result is an increase in MSFP for any given total volume. The effect on the return-cardiac function relationship is shown on the right. The increase in MSFP in PEEP means that the return curve shifts to the right. This allows maintenance of cardiac output (*triangle, closed* and *open circles*). There is a small decrease in the slope of the relationship indicating an increase in venous resistance. *Source*: From Ref. 38.

curve restores cardiac output if the venous return curve intersects the ascending part of the cardiac function curve and increases the maximum cardiac output (that is the plateau of the venous return curve). However, for there to be recruitment of unstressed volume there must be sufficient vascular reserves of unstressed volume to be recruited. This will not happen if the patient's intravascular volume is reduced and the veins are already contracted for there is a limit to smooth muscle shortening and the amount of reserves in unstressed volume that can be recruited. This means that the cardiac response to an increase in pleural pressure is very dependent on the initial volume status and the magnitude of the unstressed volume in particular. Unfortunately, the magnitude of unstressed volume cannot be measured in an intact person and can only be surmised from the volume history of the patient and a sense of their sympathetic tone. Unstressed volume also bears no relationship to CVP. This unfortunately means that capacitance reserve, a key variable in studies on the effects of positive pleural pressure on heart, cannot be measured. As an approximation, from animal studies the expected maximum recruitment of unstressed volume by a decrease in capacitance is around 10 mL/kg. If the venous compliance is around 100 to 120 mL/mmHg in a 70 kg male this would mean that a maximum decrease in capacitance could only increase MSFP by around 6 mm. If the starting CVP is around 6 mmHg then MSFP would only increase to 12 mmHg. Larger increases in MCFP require the infusion of exogenous volume and higher starting values.

Although the baseline CVP does not give an indication of the reserves in the vascular capacitance, it still can give an indication of the cardiac response to an increase in pleural pressure. The higher the initial CVP the more likely it is that the heart is functioning on the flat part of the cardiac function curve in which case the pleural pressure can increase to some extent without there being a decrease in cardiac output (36).

It also needs to be appreciated that patients who have a degree of intrinsic PEEP will only have a fall in cardiac output when the externally applied PEEP is greater than their intrinsic PEEP. However, they still will have an inspiratory assistance from the PEEP because they do not need to lower pleural pressure to the same degree on inspiration as would be necessary if they had to inspire from atmospheric pressure. This reduction of the need for a large inspiratory fall in pleural pressure reduces the inspiratory increase in venous return and the consequent oscillations in stroke volume.

VII. Effects of Lung Inflation on the Right Heart

It was initially thought that lung inflation results in an increase in pulmonary vascular resistance (40) and a consequent increase in right ventricular afterload. The reasoning was that for lungs to inflate, alveolar pressure must rise more than pleural pressure. The heart and larger pulmonary vessels are surrounded by pleural pressure, whereas capillaries situated in alveolar walls are surrounded by alveolar pressure. Therefore, during lung inflation the vessels passing between alveoli would be compressed because the outside pressure would rise relative to the inside pressure and their resistance would increase. Animal experiments seem to support this with a small fall in pulmonary vascular resistance at low levels of lung inflation, which was thought to be due to tethering open vessels and then a progressive increase in pulmonary vascular resistance with increases in lung volume (40).

It turns out that the measured change in pulmonary vascular resistance is an artifact induced by the method of measurement and error in reasoning. First, vessels filled with fluid are not very compressible and lung inflation would not be expected to change their diameter sufficiently to alter the resistance. In the original experiment (40), pulmonary vascular resistance was calculated from the difference between the pressure in pulmonary artery and left atrium. However, as pointed out by Permutt and coworkers (22,41), when lungs are sufficiently inflated, the alveolar pressure rises above the downstream venous pressures. In lung regions where this occurs, pulmonary vessels become flow limited in what is called West Zone II conditions, and flow is determined by the pressure drop from the pulmonary artery to the critical pressure at which there is flow limitation and not to the left atrial pressure. An error in the calculation is thus produced that gets progressively larger the lower the pulmonary arterial pressure and flow because the error becomes a progressively larger proportion of the pressure drop. At each level of lung inflation a greater proportion of the lung is in West Zone II and the pressure-flow relationship of the pulmonary vasculature moves in parallel upward (42) (Fig. 7). Maintenance of constant flow then requires the right ventricle to increase its force of contraction to counter the rise in afterload. This can occur through an increase in end-diastolic pressure (preload) or an increase in contractility, which can occur reflexively.

    The question arises as to which is more important for the decrease in cardiac output with positive pressure ventilation. Is it the effect of lung inflation and the consequent rise in pulmonary critical closing pressures and loading of the right heart or is it the rise in pleural pressure and an inhibition of venous return? In an attempt to address this question Scharf et al. used an elegant experimental preparation that allowed analysis

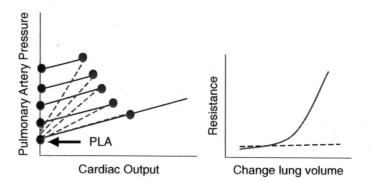

Figure 7 Graphical representation of changes in pulmonary artery resistance with changes in lung inflation. The graph on the left shows the relationship of pulmonary arterial pressure to cardiac output. The lowest line represents the resistance line when the lung is in West Zone I in which case the downstream pressure is the left atrial pressure (Pla). When the lung is in West Zone II, the outflow pressure is alveolar pressure and not Pla and the P-Q relationship moves upward in parallel. If pulmonary vascular resistance is still calculated from the mean pulmonary artery pressure to Pla, it will appear as if the resistance increased when in fact there was no change. The relationship of pulmonary artery pressure to increases in lung inflation with positive pressure and consequent increases in alveolar pressure (Palv) are shown on the right side. When Palv is used as the outflow pressure, the P-Q relationship is flat (i.e., no change in resistance) but appears to increase if Pla is used.

of the effect of an increase in pleural pressure with or without lung inflation (43). To remove the effect of lung inflation and to keep transpulmonary pressure constant, they placed chest tubes in the pleural space and connected them to the endotracheal tube so that the change in airway pressure was directly transmitted to the pleural space. They found that the fall in cardiac output with increases in pleural pressure were similar with the two conditions, but cardiac output fell with less of a rise in pleural pressure in the condition with increases in transpulmonary pressure. This can be explained by the combined condition producing both an increase in afterload from the zone II conditions as well as a decrease in preload because of the inhibition of venous return which reduced the compensatory increase in preload.

The problem also was addressed in patients with a different approach by Vieillard-Baron and coworkers (44–47). They assessed inflow and outflow from the right heart simultaneously in ventilated patients by making Doppler measurements across the tricuspid (inflow) and pulmonary (outflow) valves and found that during lung inflation pulmonary flow decreased before there was a fall in tricuspid inflow. This indicates that in these patients, the primary event was the increase in inspiratory load on the right ventricle. Besides the fact that timing is very difficult because of the different frequencies of the involved events including the cardiac frequency, ventilator frequency, and measurement frequency, the base line conditions are important determinants for the generalizability of the phenomena. An important element is the initial vascular volume of the patient for if vascular volume is high enough such that the heart is functioning on the flat part of the cardiac function curve, pleural pressure can increase over a range with no effect on venous return. Another critical determinant is the status of the right ventricle. If right ventricular systolic function is normal and the end-systolic elastance curve is relatively steep, there should be little effect on right ventricular stroke volume from an increase in afterload except for single beats during the transitions in pressure, whereas the afterload effect should be very important in patients with decreased right ventricular function. A critical factor is the relative values of the initial left atrial pressure and the change in transpulmonary pressure for zone II conditions only occur when alveolar pressure is greater than left atrial pressure. The afterload effect is also dependent on the mode of ventilation, and the relationship of cardiac to ventilator frequency for the effect is greatest during inspiration. Thus, the inspiratory pause and relatively larger tidal volumes used by these investigators would have magnified the phenomena. Finally, the type of patient and their potential to develop intrinsic PEEP that would increase zone II condition is another important consideration for when there is a baseline increase in zone II the effects of lung inflation with positive pressure ventilation could be quite marked.

When comparing the work of Scharf et al. and Vieillard-Baron et al., it is also important to appreciate that Scharf et al. studied sustained increases in pleural pressure which is more reflective of the application of PEEP, whereas the studies of Vieillard-Baron are related to the ventilatory cycle where the pleural pressure and afterload effects are transient and vary depending on the matching of the peak changes in airway pressure to the cardiac cycle with afterload effects being greatest in systole and the effects on venous return more significant in diastole (32). It also still affects venous return by increasing right atrial pressure so that except for transient effects, the change in right heart output with inspiration is still primarily determined by whether or not the right heart is functioning on the flat part of the cardiac function curve.

VIII.   Series Effect

The right and left hearts lie together in the pericardium and share a common wall, the septum. Even without a pericardium, the cardiac cytoskeleton produces an interaction between the two sides of the heart (Fig. 8) (48). An early-recognized issue was the leftward shift of the intraventricular septum with increases in right-sided pressure (30,49,50). This leads to distortion of the left ventricle and changes its diastolic compliance and systolic function. Thus, the afterload effects on the right heart due to lung inflation discussed in the last section could also contribute to cyclic variations in cardiac output by altering left ventricular output. Although ventricular interaction seems obvious and can be demonstrated by putting balloons in the two ventricles and studying the effects of increasing the volume of the right heart on force production of the left heart, the magnitude of the effect is small. It seems to me that the much more significant issue is the "series" effect (51). By this I mean that flow through the right and left hearts are in series, which implies that the left ventricle can only pump out what the right ventricle has pumped except for some small transient shifts. Thus, the transient decreases that are observed in right heart output must be subsequently seen in the left heart, and failure to control for this can lead one to assume that some independent factor is occurring in the left heart. This is especially a problem when trying to assess cardiopulmonary interactions with echocardiography for the technique measures left ventricular function well but does not assess right heart function very well. Thus, it is hard to know whether a respiratory-induced change in left ventricular output is a true direct effect on the left heart or simply a result of cycling of right ventricular output because of changes in its preload or afterload. Nuclear magnetic resonance studies that include measurements of volume shifts in the pulmonary vasculature may be one way to potentially sort this out in the future but studies of ventricular volumes alone will be insufficient.

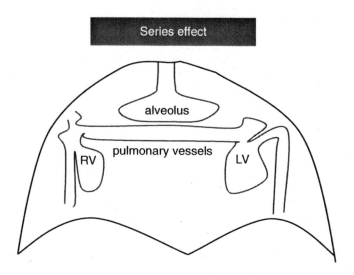

Figure 8   Representation of the "series" effect indicating that in the steady state, the left-heart output must match the right-heart output (LV, left ventricle; RV, right ventricle).

The direct interaction between right and left ventricles can become important under certain pathological conditions. When the right heart is volume limited (maximally filled) and the pericardium constrains both the right and left ventricles, increases in right atrial pressure are accompanied by increases in left atrial pressure. Since the left atrial pressure is the downstream pressure for the pulmonary vasculature, the increase in left atrial pressure leads to an increase in pulmonary artery pressure and a consequent increase in right atrial pressure. Because the right heart volume is limited, the increase in right atrial pressure does not increase right ventricular volume and allow compensation for the increase in right heart afterload so that right heart stroke volume falls. In this situation, the "right-sided preload" becomes "right-sided afterload."

IX. Left Side

In a chapter in the 1965 version of the *Handbook of Physiology* section on effects of respiratory acts on the circulation, Sharpey-Schaffer wrote a long analysis of why the left heart gets smaller on inspiration (52). Unfortunately, his analysis was based on the observation of the inspiratory fall in left atrial pressure, which he assumed to mean that left atrial volume falls on inspirartion and that volume accumulates in the pulmonary vessels. However, this observation occurs because of the error in using atmosphere as the reference pressure for cardiac pressures instead of the pressure surrounding the heart, which is pleural pressure. In a normal breath, the left atrial pressure usually falls less than the pleural pressure (both relative to atmospheric pressure) so that transmural left atrial pressure (inside minus outside) and thus left atrial volume actually get larger, which is what he needed to explain! This is true with both negative (spontaneous) and positive pressure ventilation. An explanation for this phenomena comes from the work of Permutt and coworkers (53). They showed that the lung has two functionally different vascular compartments (Fig. 9). One area is situated between alveoli and gets squeezed with lung inflation and ejects volume into the left heart; the other region is situated in the corners between alveoli and gets stretched with lung inflation and can take up volume and decrease the flow to the left heart during inspiration. These investigators found in isolated lungs that when the left atrial pressure was above around 3 mmHg, the vessels in the corners of the lung are fully filled and therefore cannot take up more volume during lung inflation, whereas those between alveoli always lose volume with lung inflation and the net effect is increased filling of the left heart. Thus, lung inflation would be expected to increase left atrial filling in most people.

Inspiration also has an interesting effect on ejection from the left heart. The fall in pleural pressure that occurs with a spontaneous inspiratory effort effectively lowers the heart relative to the rest of the body, which effectively increases the afterload on the left ventricle (28,54–57). This occurs because if the arterial pressure does not fall as much as pleural pressure, the heart must "lift" the column of blood to atmospheric pressure and then to the pressure measured in the arteries relative to atmospheric pressure (Fig. 4). Two factors determine the significance of this effect; the left ventricular function and the magnitude of the fall in pleural pressure with a breath. With the normal relatively small changes in pleural pressure during spontaneous breaths and with normal ventricular function, the effect is negligible. However, it can become significant when there is decreased left ventricular function or when the inspiratory fall in pleural pressure is large as occurs when there is increased airway resistance or decreased pulmonary compliance.

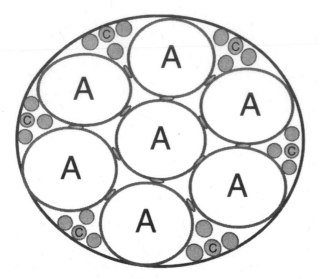

Figure 9 Schematic representation of the two vascular compartments of the lung. The large circles represent alveoli (A). The vessels in the corners (marked with small 'c') can expand and take up volume when the lungs are inflated, whereas the vessels between alveoli are compressed and lose blood volume. The corner vessels only take up volume at low pressure and then become fully distended, whereas the vessels between alveoli are always compressed with lung inflation. The net gain or loss of volume from the lung with inflation is based on the sum of the changes in these two types of vessels. Under most conditions there is a net loss of blood volume in the lungs with inflation.

The effect of inspiration on left ventricular afterload is also compounded by the increase in venous return that occurs when pleural pressure is lowered. An example of this phenomena is seen in the hemodynamics of Mueller maneuver shown in Figure 10 (58). This inspiratory effect is especially important when the patient is volume loaded. When the CVP is elevated there can be a greater fall in venous pressure before the veins collapse as they enter the thorax, which means that there can be a greater inspiratory increase in venous return than normal. Furthermore, when left ventricular end-diastolic pressure starts at a relatively elevated pressure, the left heart is functioning on the steep part of the passive filling curve. This means that small increases in left ventricular volume from either decreased output from the increase in left ventricular afterload or the increased venous return will produce a much more marked rise in pulmonary venous pressure. The combination of increased input and decreased output has a "piston" like effect that compounds the diastolic pressure rise in the left ventricle and pulmonary venous pressures. This process has been shown to produce pulmonary edema in persons with tracheal stenosis or other upper airway obstruction and the pulmonary edema can be relieved by a tracheostomy (59).

Although I have stated that the afterload effect on the normal left ventricle is small, on a beat-to-beat basis it can produce significant changes in left ventricular stroke volume and thus contribute to systolic pressure variations. This occurs because on the

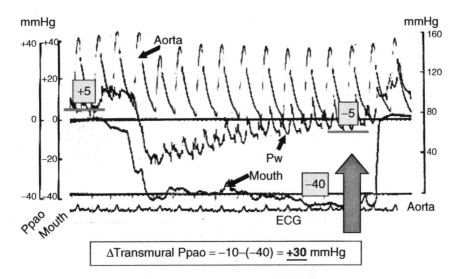

Figure 10 Example of hemodynamic changes during a Mueller maneuver. In this example, the subject breathes against a manometer at the mouth that records the change in mouth pressure and does not allow a change in lung volume. The change in mouth pressure must therefore equal the change in pleural pressure. The zero value for mouth pressure is in the middle of the tracing and the change was −40 mmHg. With the onset of the Mueller there is a transient drop in arterial pressure on the first beat after which the arterial pressure returns to baseline. Since the "outside" pressure fell by 40 mmHg, this means that the transmural arterial pressure rose by 30 mmHg such that left ventricular afterload significantly increased. The pulmonary artery occlusion pressure (P_w, which reflects left atrial pressure) fell but not as much as pleural pressure and then progressively increased during the maneuver so that at the end of the maneuver the P_w is −5 mmHg; the net change in P_w is thus −10 mmHg. The change in the transmural P_w is given at the bottom and based on change in inside minus change in outside, −10−(−40) equals +30 mmHg. When this change is added to the baseline value for P_w actual transmural P_w is 35 mmHg although on the tracing it looks like P_w fell. *Source*: From Ref. 57.

first beat of each breath the ventricular pressure falls with pleural pressure, whereas aortic pressure is unaffected until the aortic valve opens. This produces a sudden large increase in afterload (56). However, on the next beat, aortic pressure will have been reduced and therefore the load is much less.

Positive pressure ventilation obviously has the opposite effect on the left ventricle and produces an inspiratory decrease in left ventricular afterload. It was hoped that this could be used to "aid" left ventricular ejection. However, the magnitude of the effect is very small. For example, if PEEP is 10 cmH$_2$O, and assuming that half the PEEP is transmitted to the pleural space, the reduction in load on the left ventricle is only about 4 mmHg, which is well within the range of the daily fluctuations of life. More importantly, however, the rise in pleural pressure will decrease the gradient for venous return to the right ventricle and decrease cardiac output if the heart is operating on the ascending part of the cardiac function curve. Thus, the effects on input to the heart predominate over any benefits on left ventricular output. The only way that positive pressure ventilation has been shown to aid cardiac output is by first inducing cardiac dysfunction that likely puts the heart on to the flat part of its function curve, and then "gating" the ventilator to the cardiac cycle so that the positive pressure inspiration only occurs during systole (60–62). However, even under these conditions, if the lung inflation is too great the increase in critical closing pressures would increase the load on the right ventricle and nullify the benefit.

Despite the predicted small effect from a reduction of left ventricular afterload, positive airway pressure has been shown to augment stroke volume and cardiac output in patients with poorly controlled heart failure, and this argues for a benefit from the decrease in afterload on the left ventricle (63,64). However, an alternative explanation is that the positive pressure "decompressed" the right ventricle, and thereby allows better filling and function of the left ventricle as demonstrated by Atherton and coworkers (65,66), in which case the dominant action was still through the right ventricle and reduction of venous return. Either explanation can account for some of the beneficial effect of treating acute cardiogenic pulmonary edema by CPAP, and this remains an important therapeutic approach (67).

X. Other Mechanisms of Heart-Lung Interaction

Patients who have a high degree of intrinsic PEEP can develop air trapping and hyperinflation. Besides potentially producing more West Zone II conditions in the lungs and increasing the load on the right ventricular, the hyperinflated lungs can compress the heart and cause some limitation of ventricular filling (68). The late J. Butler used the expression that "the heart is in good hands" to describe this phenomena (69).

XI. Sleep Issues

As I have discussed above, the magnitude of the effect of an inspiratory fall in pleural pressure is influenced by the person's volume status for it determines the potential fall in CVP that can occur before there is flow limitation of the veins entering the thorax and it also determines whether the ventricles are functioning on the steep part of their diastolic passive filling curves. The volume of the heart is increased in the supine position so that this component is greater in almost all sleeping patients, and heart-lung interactions are exaggerated during sleep (unless they are sleeping upright!). Furthermore, vascular volume usually increases over the night because fluid that had accumulated in dependent regions of the body returns to the vasculature when the effect of gravity is removed. This process can progress over two to four hours after going to sleep, which means heart-lung interactions can become exaggerated as the night proceeds and assuming that an upright posture for a period of time can potentially decrease the interactions as is observed in patients with paroxysmal nocturnal dyspnea (PND). Furthermore, along the same lines as PND, as fluid accumulates in the lungs during the night, the lungs become stiffer and airway resistance can also rise. These changes in mechanics require greater inspiratory efforts to produce the same tidal volume, and this will also exaggerate heart lung interactions.

The primary issue for heart-lung interactions is the effect produced by transient obstructions of the airway and its treatment with positive pressure masks. The details of these are covered elsewhere in this monograph but I will highlight some specific issues related to the physiology. Airway obstruction produces the hemodynamics of the Mueller maneuver except that negative pressure is not sustained. However, as discussed in the section on decreased pleural pressure, the afterload effect is greatest at the onset of inspiration and with repeated obstructions this effect will occur on each breath. It is likely that the transient increase in right heart filling is more important than the change in load on the left ventricle, and this is amplified by the increase in vascular volume at night as discussed in the previous paragraph.

A mainstay of the treatment of obstructive sleep apnea is the use of a positive pressure mask. A primary benefit of the mask is likely a reduction in the negative inspiratory pressure required for a breath. This occurs through relief of the obstruction as well as by providing a mild inspiratory assistance. The decrease in the required inspiratory effort reduces the magnitude of the transient rise in transmural left ventricular end-diastolic pressure that occurs with the onset of each spontaneous inspiration for ventricular pressures do not fall as much relative to atmosphere and also reduces the swings in right heart filling and ejection during the ventilatory cycle.

XII. Conclusion

The effects of pleural pressure changes on filling and ejection from the heart dominate heart-lung interactions. In patients with increased lung inflation with positive pressure breathing or intrinsic PEEP increases in zone II conditions can also produce significant interactions by increasing the load on the right ventricle during inspiration, especially if right heart function is compromised or if right heart filling is limited. An important issue in heart lung interactions is the "series" effect in that the left heart can only put out what the right heart gives it. Thus, ventilatory effects on the right heart tend to dominate heart-lung interactions unless there is marked left ventricular dysfunction in which case left-sided effects can potentially be more significant.

References

1. Ashton JH, Cassidy SS. Reflex depression of cardiovascular function during lung inflation. J Appl Physiol 1985; 58(1):137–145.
2. Cassidy SS, Ashton JH, Wead WB, et al. Reflex cardiovascular responses caused by stimulation of pulmonary C-fibers with capsaicin in dogs. J Appl Physiol 1986; 60(3):949–958.
3. Kaufman MP, Iwamoto GA, Ashton JH, et al. Responses to inflation of vagal afferents with endings in the lung of dogs. Circ Res 1982; 51(4):525–531.
4. Glick G, Wechsler AS, Epstein SE. Reflex cardiovascular depression produced by stimulation of pulmonary stretch receptors in the dog. J Clin Invest 1969; 48(3):467–473.
5. Greenwood PV, Hainsworth R, Karim F, et al. Reflex inotropic responses of the heart from lung inflation in anaesthetized dogs. Pflugers Arch 1980; 386(2):199–205.
6. Cheng EY, Kay J, Hoka S, et al. Influence of lung inflation reflex on vascular capacitance in the systemic circulation. Am J Physiol 1989; 257(5 pt 2):R1004–R1011.
7. Grindlinger GA, Manny J, Justice R, et al. Presence of negative inotropic agents in canine plasma during positive end-expiratory pressure. Circ Res 1979; 45(4):460–467.
8. Magder S, Scharf SM. Venous return. In: Scharf SM, Pinsky MR, Magder SA, eds. Respiratory-Circulatory Interactions in Health and Disease. New York: Marcel Dekker, 2001:93–112.
9. Magder S. Central venous pressure: a useful but not so simple measurement. Crit Care Med 2006; 34(8):2224–2227.
10. Magder S. Point: the classical Guyton view that mean systemic pressure, right atrial pressure, and venous resistance govern venous return is/is not correct. J Appl Physiol 2006; 101(5): 1523–1525.

11. Guyton AC. Determination of cardiac output by equating venous return curves with cardiac response curves. Physiol Rev 1955; 35:123–129.
12. Starling EH. The Linacre Lecture of the Law of the Heart. London: Longmans, Green & Co., 1918.
13. Magder S, De Varennes B. Clinical death and the measurement of stressed vascular volume. Crit Care Med 1998; 26:1061–1064.
14. Mitzner W, Goldberg H, Lichtenstein S. Effect of thoracic blood volume changes on steady state cardiac output. Circ Res 1976; 38(4):255–261.
15. Magder S, Veerassamy S, Bates JH. A further analysis of why pulmonary venous pressure rises after the onset of LV dysfunction. J Appl Physiol 2009; 106(1):81–90.
16. Deschamps A, Magder S. Baroreflex control of regional capacitance and blood flow distribution with or without alpha adrenergic blockade. J Appl Physiol 1992; 263:H1755–H1763.
17. Deschamps A, Magder S. Effects of heat stress on vascular capacitance. Am J Physiol 1994; 266:H2122–H2129.
18. Magder S, Bafaqeeh F. The clinical role of central venous pressure measurements. J Intensive Care Med 2007; 22(1):44–51.
19. Sarnoff SJ, Berglund E. Ventricular function: Starling's law of the heart studied by means of simultaneous right and left ventricular function curves in the dog. In: Sarnoff SJ, editor. Boston, Mass.: Department of Physiology, Harvard School of Public Health, 1953.
20. Holt JP, Rhode EA, Kines H. Pericardial and ventricular pressure. Circ Res 1960; VIII:1171–1180.
21. Berglund E, Sarnoff SJ, ISAACS JP. Ventricular function: role of the pericardium in regulation of cardiovascular hemodynamics. Circ Res 1955; 3(2):133–139.
22. Permutt S, Riley S. Hemodynamics of collapsible vessels with tone: the vascular waterfall. J Appl Physiol 1963; 18(5):924–932.
23. Fessler HE, Brower RG, Wise RA, et al. Effects of positive end-expiratory pressure on the gradient for venous return. Am Rev Respir Dis 1992; 146:4–10.
24. Permutt S, Caldini P. Regulation of cardiac output by the circuit: venous return. In: Boan J, Noordergraaf A, Raines J, eds. Cardiovascular system dynamics. Cambridge, Massachusetts and London England: MIT Press, 1978: 465–479.
25. Cassidy S, Eschenbacher, Robertson C, et al. Cardiovascular effects of positive-pressure ventilation in normal subjects. J Appl Physiol 1979; 47:453–461.
26. Marini JJ, Culver BH, Butler J. Mechanical effect of lung distention with positive pressure on cardiac function. Am Rev Respir Dis 1981; 124:382–386.
27. Fewell JE, Abendschein DR, Carlson CJ, et al. Continuous positive-pressure ventilation does not alter ventricular pressure-volume relationship. Am J Physiol 1981; 240:H821–H826.
28. McGregor M. Current concepts: pulsus paradoxus. N Engl J Med 1979; 301(9):480–482.
29. Magder S. Invasive intravascular hemodynamic monitoring: technical issues. Crit Care Clin 2007; 23:401–414.
30. Brinker JA, Weiss JL, Lappe DL, et al. Leftward septal displacement during right ventricular loading in man. Circulation 1980; 61:626.
31. Magder SA, Georgiadis G, Cheong T. Respiratory variations in right atrial pressure predict response to fluid challenge. J Crit Care 1992; 7:76–85.
32. Magder S. Clinical usefulness of respiratory variations in arterial pressure. Am J Resp Crit Care Med 2004; 169(2):151–155.
33. Magder S. Predicting volume responsiveness in spontaneously breathing patients: still a challenging problem. Crit Care 2006; 10(5):165.
34. Takata M, Robotham JL. Effects of inspiratory diaphragmatic descent on inferior vena caval venous return. J Appl Physiol 1992; 72(2):597–607.
35. Takata M, Beloucif S, Shimada M, et al. Superior and inferior vena caval flows during respiration: pathogenesis of Kussmaul's sign. Am J Physiol 1990; 262:H763–H770.

36. Magder S, Lagonidis D, Erice F. The use of respiratory variations in right atrial pressure to predict the cardiac output response to PEEP. J Crit Care 2002; 16(3):108–114.
37. Fessler HE, Brower RG, Wise RA, et al. Effects of positive end-expiratory pressure on the gradient for venous return. Am Rev Respir Dis 1991; 143:19–24.
38. Fessler HE, Brower RG, Wise RA, et al. Effects of positive end-expiratory pressure on the canine venous return curve. Am Rev Respir Dis 1992; 146(1):4–10.
39. Nanas S, Magder S. Adaptations of the peripheral circulation to PEEP. Am Rev Respir Dis 1992; 146:688–693.
40. Whittenberg JL, McGregor M, Berglund E, et al. Influence of state of inflation of the lung on pulmonary vascular resistance. J Appl Physiol 1960; 15:878.
41. Permutt S, Bromberger-Barnea B, Bane HN. Alveolar pressure, pulmonary venous pressure, and the vascular waterfall. Med Thoracalis 1962; 19:239–260.
42. Brower R, Wise RA, Hassapoyannes C, et al. Effect of lung inflation on lung blood volume and pulmonary venous flow. J Appl Physiol 1985; 58(3):954–963.
43. Scharf SM, Caldini P, Ingram RH. Cardiovascular effects of increasing airway pressure in the dog. Am J Physiol 1977; 232(1):H35–H43.
44. Vieillard-Baron A, Loubieres Y, Schmitt JM, et al. Cyclic changes in right ventricular output impedance during mechanical ventilation. J Appl Physiol 1999; 87(5):1644–1650.
45. Vieillard-Baron A, Prin S, Chergui K, et al. Echo-Doppler demonstration of acute cor pulmonale at the bedside in the medical intensive care unit. Am J Respir Crit Care Med 2002; 166(10):1310–1319.
46. Charron C, Caille V, Jardin F, et al. Echocardiographic measurement of fluid responsiveness. Curr Opin Crit Care 2006; 12(3):249–254.
47. Jardin F, Vieillard-Baron A. Monitoring of right-sided heart function. Curr Opin Crit Care 2005; 11(3):271–279.
48. Elzinga G, Van Grondelle R, Westerhof W, et al. Ventricular interference. Am J Physiol 1974; 226:941.
49. Jardin F, Farcot JC, Boisante L, et al. Influence of positive end-expiratory pressure on left ventricular performance. N Engl J Med 1981; 304:387–392.
50. Alderman EL, Glantz SA. Acute hemodynamic interventions shift the diastolic pressure-volume curve in man. Circulation 1976; 54(4):662–671.
51. Magder S. The left heart can only be as good as the right heart: determinants of function and dysfunction of the right ventricle. Crit Care Resusc 2007; 9(4):344–351.
52. Sharpey-Schaffer EP. Effects of respiratory acts on the circulation. In: Dowpey H, ed. Handbook of Physiology, sect. 2. Washington, DC: American Physiological Society, 1965:1875.
53. Permutt S, Howell JBL, Proctor DF, et al. Effect of lung inflation on static pressure volume characteristics of pulmonary vessels. J Appl Physiol 1961; 16:64–70.
54. Hausknecht MJ, Brin KP, Weisfeldt ML, et al. Effects of left ventricular loading by negative intrathoracic pressure in dogs. Circ Res 1988; 62(3):620–631.
55. Permutt S. Some physiological aspects of asthma: bronchomuscular contraction and airway caliber. The CIBA Foundation Symposium, Identification of Asthma. Edinburgh, London: Churchill Livingstone, 1974: 63–85.
56. Bromberger-Barnea B. Mechanical effects of inspiration on heart functions. Fed Proc 1981; 40:2172–2177.
57. Robotham JL, Rabson J, Permutt S, et al. Left ventricular hemodynamics during respiration. J Appl Physiol 1979; 47:1295.
58. Magder SA, Lichtenstein S, Adelman AG. Effects of negative pleural pressure on left ventricular hemodynamics. Am J Cardiol 1983; 52(5):588–593.
59. Timby J, Reed C, Zeilender S, et al. "Mechanical" causes of pulmonary edema. Chest 1990; 98(4):974–979.

60. Pinsky MR, Matuschak GM, Klain M. Determinants of cardiac augmentation by elevations in intrathoracic pressure. J Appl Physiol 1985; 58(4):1189–1198.
61. Pinsky MR, Matuschak GM, Bernardi L, et al. Hemodynamic effects of cardiac cycle-specific increases in intrathoracic pressure. J Appl Physiol 1986; 60(2):604–612.
62. Pinsky MR, Summer WR. Cardiac augmentation by phasic high intrathoracic pressure support in man. Chest 1983; 84(4):370–375.
63. Naughton MT, Rahman MA, Hara K, et al. Effect of continuous positive airway pressure on intrathoracic and left ventricular transmural pressures in patients with congestive heart failure. Circulation 1995; 91(6):1725–1731.
64. Bradley TD, Holloway RM, McLaughlin PR, et al. Cardiac output response to continuous positive airway pressure in congestive heart failure. Am Rev Respir Dis 1992; 145(2 pt 1): 377–382.
65. Atherton JJ, Moore TD, Lele SS, et al. Diastolic ventricular interaction in chronic heart failure. Lancet 1997; 349:1720–1724.
66. Atherton JJ, Thomson HL, Moore TD, et al. Diastolic ventricular interaction. A possible mechanism for abnormal vascular responses during volume unloading in heart failure. Circulation 1997; 96:4273–4279.
67. Bersten AD, Holt AW, Vedig AE, et al. Treatment of severe cardiogenic pulmonary edmea with continuous positive airway pressure delivered by face mask. N Engl J Med 1991; 325 (26): 1825–1830.
68. Robotham JL, Badke FR, Kindred MK, et al. Regional left ventricular performance during normal and obstructed spontaneous respiration. J Appl Physiol 1983; 55(2):569–577.
69. Butler J. The heart is in good hands. Circulation 1983; 67(6):1163–1168.

4
Respiratory and Cardiac Activity During Sleep Onset

JOHN TRINDER and CHRISTIAN L. NICHOLAS
University of Melbourne, Parkville, Victoria, Australia

I. Introduction

This chapter is concerned with the regulatory control relationships between sleep and respiratory and cardiac activity. In particular it covers how those relationships are expressed during sleep onset. Greater emphasis is placed on the influence of sleep mechanisms on respiratory and cardiac activity, although we also comment on the concept that cardiac autonomic control influences the occurrence and nature of sleep. Further, we consider whether there are differences as to how sleep onset affects the respiratory system compared to the cardiac system and on this point take a slightly different position than in the original version of this chapter.

Respiratory and cardiac activity during sleep in general and the effect of non–rapid eye movement (NREM) as opposed to rapid eye movement (REM) sleep are not considered in any detail. This material is covered by other chapters in this volume. However, the effects of NREM sleep on respiratory and cardiac activity are summarized to place changes at sleep onset in context. Further, this chapter does not discuss the relationship between presleep levels of physiological functioning and sleep onset—that is, the question of whether high levels of physiological activity delay sleep onset. Rather, the chapter describes the normal changes that occur in respiratory and cardiac activity as one goes to sleep.

II. Respiration and Cardiac Activity During NREM Sleep

Respiration during NREM sleep has been thoroughly investigated, and the basic findings are well understood (1). Ventilation is lower than during wakefulness, and while there is a reduction in the rate of metabolism during sleep, it is insufficient to explain the magnitude of the effect, as there is a rise in arterial carbon dioxide. Sleep is also associated with a reduction in the activity of upper airway muscles, a rise in airway resistance, and the loss of a number of protective reflex mechanisms, such as the reflex compensation for increases in inspiratory load (1,2).

Most authors have interpreted the fall in ventilation as being a consequence of a change in the regulatory control of respiration during sleep, although the precise nature of the change remains uncertain. A widely supported view has been that during wakefulness ventilation is augmented by a tonic excitatory component, referred to as the "wakefulness stimulus," which is inactivated during sleep (3). Neurophysiologically, the effect has been identified with respiratory-related cells in the reticular formation, which are tonically active in wakefulness but are not respiratory cycle dependent. It has been shown that during sleep these cells become inactive, reflecting a fall in respiratory drive with a consequent reduction in ventilation (4).

The pathway through which sleep affects ventilation has been extensively investigated. One view has been that the withdrawal of the wakefulness stimulus directly reduces ventilatory drive to the respiratory pump muscles (1,3). Alternatively, it has been suggested that ventilation falls as a consequence of poor compensation for an increase in airway resistance (5). There are a number of observations indicating that ventilatory drive is lower during sleep. For example, manipulations that have eliminated or minimized the role of the upper airway, as in the case of patients with tracheostomies (6) and normal individuals on continuous positive airway pressure (7), are associated with lower levels of ventilation. Further, the CO_2 threshold at which pump muscle activity is recruited is higher during sleep than wakefulness (8). On the other hand, it is well established that airway resistance is elevated and load compensation reduced during sleep (5). Thus, it is likely that both components contribute, although the relative importance of these two mechanisms is likely to vary between individuals (9).

Important additional features of the concept of the sleep-related withdrawal of the wakefulness stimulus are that it potentially exposes the respiratory system to the disfacilitatory effect of hypocapnia and likely contributes to respiratory instability during sleep (10). As will be discussed in the following section, these effects may be particularly important at sleep onset.

Cardiac output is also decreased during NREM sleep compared to wakefulness. This occurs as a consequence of a fall in heart rate (HR). Blood pressure (BP) also falls, in part because of the decrease in HR and in part because of a decrease in peripheral resistance. The fall in both HR and BP is "permitted" because of resetting of the baroreflex (11). Changes in HR and BP are only partly attributable to the direct effect of sleep mechanisms on cardiac activity. Sleep has indirect effects via changes in activity and posture, while the circadian system also influences HR (12), metabolic rate (13), thermoregulatory mechanisms (14), and possibly BP (15). Nevertheless, laboratory studies have shown that there are both specific sleep (12,16–18) and circadian (12,15,19–21) influences on both HR and BP, which are independent of changes in posture and physical activity.

Sympathovagal balance is a critical concept for understanding both the nature of sleep and the mechanisms by which disorders of sleep result in pathophysiology. There is substantial evidence indicating that during "normal sleep" sympathovagal balance shifts toward parasympathetic dominance (22). This is particularly the case during NREM sleep, but as NREM makes up 75% to 80% of a night's sleep, parasympathetic dominance characterizes the sleep period generally. However, both the nature of the change in autonomic control producing the shift in sympathovagal balance during NREM sleep and its significance remain obscure. For example, it is not completely clear as to whether these changes are due to sympathetic inhibition or vagal excitation (22) or whether the normal sleep-related change is a functional consequence of sleep, endowing the sleeper with benefits that enhance waking activity, or is sleep promoting, acting to facilitate the occurrence, quality, and maintenance of sleep (23).

There is reasonable evidence from both animal and human studies to indicate that parasympathetic activity is increased during NREM sleep. In animals, studies have shown that sympathectomy does not affect the fall in HR from wakefulness to NREM sleep (24), suggesting that the fall in HR is due to increases in parasympathetic activity. Studies in humans using respiratory sinus arrhythmia have also shown increases in parasympathetic activity during NREM sleep (25–28), although this may in part be due to a circadian influence over parasympathetic activity (12).

As indicated in the previous paragraph, animal studies suggest that sympathetic inhibition does not contribute to the fall in HR (24). Further, recordings from renal and cervical sympathetic nerves in cats show only small decreases (29) or no change (30,31) in sympathetic activity during NREM sleep. However, consistent with the fall in BP, there does appear to be a reduction in sympathetic vasomotor tone (32) and direct measures of sympathetic nerve activity to skeletal muscle blood vessels in humans indicate reduced activity during NREM sleep (33–35). These studies provide evidence of a reduction in peripheral sympathetic activity during NREM sleep. Nevertheless, it should be noted that microneurographic techniques are intrusive and the observed sleep-wake differences may reflect elevated sympathetic activity during wakefulness as a consequence of the stressful procedures rather than a fall specifically associated with sleep mechanisms.

Whether central sympathetic influence over cardiac activity falls during sleep remains uncertain as to date there is not an acceptable and specific measure of central sympathetic tone that may be employed in humans. On this point, it should be noted that the frequently employed measure, the 0.1-Hz peak component obtained from period analyses of HR variability, is not a specific measure of sympathetic activity but, rather, in conjunction with total HR variability, reflects sympathovagal balance (22). Thus, there is good evidence that in the sleep of normal healthy individuals, parasympathetic activity is elevated during sleep. Further, there is strong evidence that sympathetic outflow to vascular beds, particularly to skeletal muscles, is reduced, leading to vaso-dilatation and a reduction in BP. However, whether sympathetic activation of the heart is altered remains uncertain.

III. Sleep Onset

Before describing respiratory activity during sleep onset, it would be of value to comment on the nature of the sleep onset process. Two different perspectives may be identified in the literature, although both emphasize that sleep onset is a process rather than a point in time. As will be discussed at length later, a consideration of changes in physiological processes such as respiration and cardiac activity leads one to emphasize the instability in the sleep-wake state over sleep onset. From this perspective, sleep onset does not usually consist of a single transition from wakefulness to sleep but rather involves alternations between transient periods of wakefulness and sleep before stable sleep is obtained (36). Thus, during sleep onset, there is a period during which the sleep-wake state is unstable. This instability often continues after sleep spindles and K complexes are observed in the electroencephalogram (EEG), with brief arousals interrupting stage 2 sleep. Thus, the occurrence of the first sleep spindle or K complex does not necessarily indicate the attainment of stable sleep. In contrast, investigators who have focused on cortical activity have pointed to the relatively smooth and pro-gressive loss of EEG beta activity and the development of delta activity over the sleep onset period (37). The present paper, being concerned with respiratory and cardiac activity, will emphasize the former perspective. As a final point it should be noted that essentially all physiological, cognitive, and behavioral processes are different during sleep compared to wakefulness, with most changing during sleep onset. Further, the timing within the sleep onset period of the change in different processes varies, emphasizing the perspective that sleep onset is not a point in time but a process (36).

Given the complexity of the sleep onset process, it has been found to be useful to divide it into a number of phases in an attempt to characterize the progression from continuous wakefulness to stable sleep (see Ref. 36 for a review of different methods). We have developed a particular classification scheme specifically to study respiratory (38) and cardiac activity (39) over the sleep onset period. The method distinguishes a number of phases based on behavioral and EEG criteria: lights-on relaxed wakefulness (wakefulness being defined as dominant EEG alpha activity); lights-off relaxed wakefulness; alternating periods of predominantly alpha or predominantly theta activity (early in sleep onset); alternations between α and θ, where the periods of θ include sleep spindles and K complexes (late in sleep onset); and finally continuous stable stage 2 sleep. Importantly, the classification also allows the distinction between sleep (θ) and wake (α) states within the major phases.

A. Respiratory Activity During Sleep Onset

The study of respiratory activity during sleep onset contributes to the literature on sleep and respiration in three major ways. First, it describes and comments on the nature of sleep onset itself. Second, it provides information as to the timing of regulatory changes with respect to both sleep and the relationship between variables affected by sleep. Third, changes at sleep onset offer insight into the primary regulatory change relatively independent of subsequent compensatory changes that may mask primary sleep effects in measurements taken during stable sleep. To illustrate this last point, measurements during stable sleep have shown diaphragmatic electromyographic (EMG) activity to be higher than during wakefulness (40–42), indicating that total ventilatory drive is elevated, not reduced, during sleep. However, studies show a reduction in diaphragmatic EMG activity at sleep onset (43). This suggests that a primary reduction in central ventilatory drive occurs immediately upon entry into sleep and is then followed by a compensatory increase in chemical and/or mechanical drive, with the latter components masking the continued absence of the central component.

Investigations of respiration during sleep onset have demonstrated that sleep exerts extraordinarily tight control over respiratory activity. Further, the influence of sleep is manifest very early in sleep onset—indeed, at the first EEG indication of sleep (44,45). As shown in Figure 1, the transition from α to θ EEG activity is associated with a rapid (within a breath) fall in ventilation. The fall over the first breath or two of theta activity is not only abrupt but also substantial (approximately 10% of waking ventilation at transitions into theta early in sleep onset and over 30% at transitions late in sleep onset in normal young individuals) and is larger than the difference between stable wakefulness and stable stage 2 sleep (45). With the return of EEG alpha activity, ventilation immediately increases, overshooting the stable wakefulness level and then returning to this level after several breaths in wakefulness. Further, as indicated in Figure 1, the amplitude of the fluctuation in ventilation increases as sleep onset progresses from early to late. During presleep wakefulness and stable sleep, when the sleep-wake state is stable, ventilation is also stable (44–46).

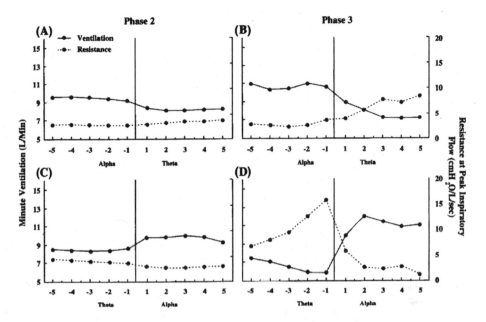

Figure 1 Group transition plots showing mean breath-by-breath changes in minute ventilation (*solid lines*) and resistance at peak inspiratory flow (*dashed lines*) over state transitions. (**A**) Phase 2 (early in sleep onset) alpha (wake) to theta (sleep) transitions, (**B**) phase 3 (late in sleep onset) α to θ transitions, (**C**) phase 2 θ to α transitions, and (**D**) phase 3 θ to α transitions. *Source*: From Ref. 9.

Thus, ventilation is intimately dependent on the sleep-wake state (47) such that if the sleep-wake state is unstable, as it is during sleep onset, ventilation will also be unstable, fluctuating widely with each transient change in state (45). Further, consistent with Phillipson's model of regulatory control (3), the magnitude of state-dependent fluctuations is augmented by secondary fluctuations in chemical drive. Thus, fluctuations in ventilation during sleep onset are larger in individuals with large ventilatory responses to hypoxia (48) and can be reduced by having subjects breathe a hyperoxic gas mixture (48,49). However, Phillipson's model may not fully account for state-related fluctuations, as the magnitude of respiratory activation at arousal from sleep appears to be independent of the intensity of respiratory stimuli (50–53).

Ventilation is not the only respiratory variable to be intimately tied to the sleep-wake state. As indicated in Figure 1, airway resistance increases at the state transition from α to θ EEG activity and returns to waking levels as soon as there is a return to the waking state (9,38). However, the progression of changes in ventilation and upper airway resistance differ. Ventilation falls over sleep onset but is maintained once stable sleep is attained. In contrast, state-dependent changes in airway resistance are very small early in sleep onset, increase markedly late in sleep onset (Fig. 1), and continue to increase during stable sleep as a function of the development of NREM sleep (54), particularly in males (55) (Fig. 2). The differing time course of ventilation and airway

MALES

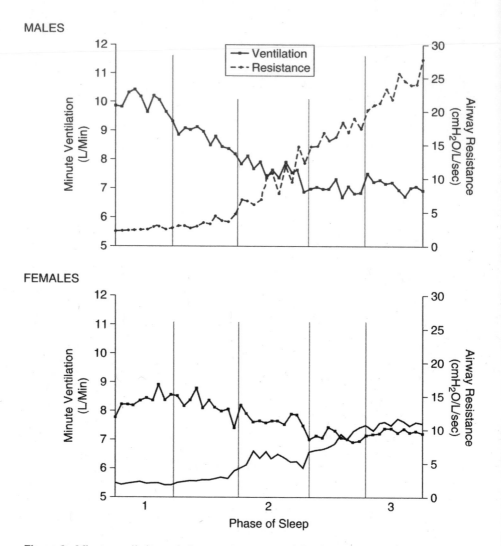

Figure 2 Minute ventilation and airway resistance at peak inspiratory flow over sleep onset and NREM phase of the sleep cycle as a function of gender. The subject's progression from wakefulness to SWS was divided into five phases (see text). To average data over subjects, each phase was divided into 10 equal sections comprising equal numbers of breaths, and a mean value for each section was obtained by averaging data for all breaths within the section. Thus, each point is a mean value representing a variable number of breaths and a 10% progression through the particular phase. The data indicate that minute ventilation falls over sleep onset (phases 1 to 4), while airway resistance rises most markedly toward the end of sleep onset and during stable sleep (phases 3 to 5). These effects were larger in males than females. *Abbreviations*: NREM, non-rapid eye movement; SWS, slow wave sleep. *Source*: Adapted from Ref. 55.

resistance is consistent with the view that an increase in airway resistance is not the only cause of sleep-related hypoventilation.

Reflex compensation for loads is also dependent on the state during sleep onset. Within transient periods of alpha activity during sleep onset, normal waking reflex load compensation is active such that presentation of a load elicits a reflex response (prolongation of inspiration) and ventilation is maintained. However, during transient periods of theta, the reflex response to a load is, as in established sleep, absent. Indeed, the reflex is lost by the first theta breath, and the increase in load that also occurs with the onset of theta is translated into a fall in ventilation (56).

Consistent with changes in ventilation and upper airway resistance, breath-by-breath analysis of muscle EMG activity during sleep onset indicates that both respiratory muscles, such as the diaphragm, and upper airway muscles, such as the genioglossus and tensor palatini, decrease their activity immediately upon a state transition into theta activity (43,57) (Fig. 3). Again, this finding offers support to the view that the state-dependent changes in respiratory control directly affect control of both ventilation and airway resistance.

Diaphragmatic activity shows temporally complex changes over the sleep onset period. The diaphragm initially decreases activity at the α to θ transition (43); then during sustained sleep the diaphragm tends to recover toward waking levels (Fig. 3). Indeed, as briefly mentioned earlier, studies during sustained sleep have suggested that the activity of the diaphragm is at least as high, if not higher, during sleep than wakefulness (40–42). The latter observation has contributed to the view that sleep-related hypoventilation is not a function of reduced ventilatory drive, as pump muscles are, if anything, more active during sleep. However, the observation that diaphragmatic EMG activity falls at α to θ transitions during sleep onset supports the view that a central drive to ventilation is lost at this time and suggests that, during stable sleep, this effect is masked by increased chemical and/or mechanical drive consequent to sleep-related hypoventilation and elevated negative airway pressure.

The behavior of upper airway muscles is equally complex. White and coworkers (58,59) have suggested that upper airway muscles should be distinguished on the basis of whether they are phasic (more active during the inspiratory phase of the respiratory cycle) or tonic (constant activity throughout the respiratory cycle). Analogous with Orem's view (4), they suggest that muscles that are primarily tonic will decrease more during sleep than muscles that are primarily phasic. When assessed by multiunit EMG recordings the behavior of the upper airway muscles tensor palatini and genioglossus during α to θ transitions are consistent with this model (43). Thus, as indicated in Figure 3, the level of activity in the tensor palatini, a primarily tonic upper airway muscle, abruptly decreases with the loss of alpha activity and then continues to fall and to remain low as long as sleep is maintained. In contrast, the genioglossus, a primarily phasic muscle, shows a decrease for several breaths and then rapidly increases its activity above waking levels, presumably under the influence of chemical and/or mechanical drive. It has been suggested that the compensatory activity of the genioglossus is critical in maintaining airway patency during sleep (59,60).

However, the behavior of the genioglossus at sleep onset at the level of individual motor units appears discrepant to predictions from whole-muscle studies. Saboisky et al. (61) have identified a variety of different discharge patterns in genioglossal motor units. These include inspiratory phasic, expiratory phasic, and tonic (absence of respiratory

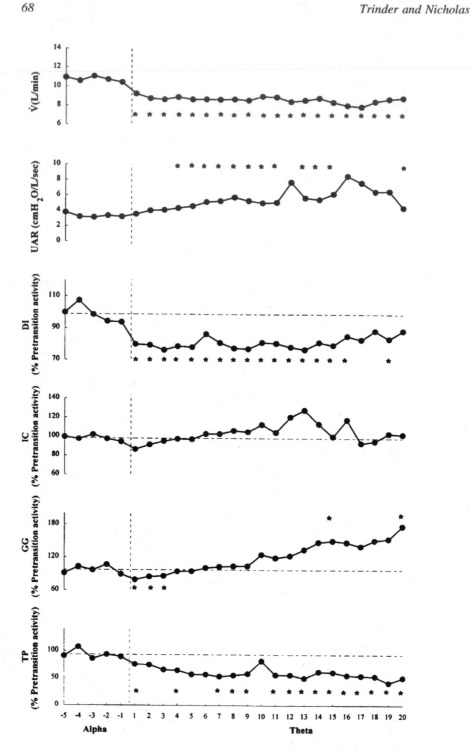

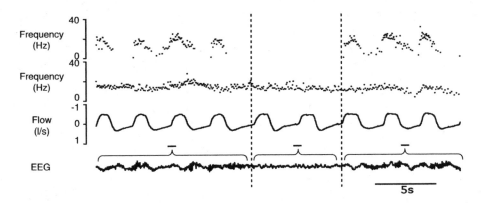

Figure 4 Instantaneous frequency plots for two genioglossus motor units recorded on the same electrode before and after α to θ and θ to α transitions. Also shown are the airflow and EEG recordings. Vertical lines indicate state transitions. The figure illustrates the differential effects of the α to θ transition on inspiratory phasic (*top tracing*) and tonic (*second tracing*) motor units and shows that the cessation of the inspiratory phasic unit was not a consequence of electrode movement. *Abbreviation*: EEG, electroencephalogram.

modulation) patterns. In contrast to the behavior of respiratory-related neurons in the brainstem (4), the fall in total genioglossus activity at sleep onset is due to reductions in inspiratory modulated motor units; indeed, approximately 50% of these units cease activity entirely at the α to θ transition (62). The activity of motor units with a tonic or expiratory phasic pattern is essentially unaffected by the transition into sleep. These contrasting patterns are illustrated in Figure 4. Single-motor-unit activity has not been assessed in the tensor palatini, although such studies will be of considerable interest as the tonic pattern of the whole muscle suggests it is composed of tonic motor units, which in the genioglossus are unaffected by sleep onset, while the activity of the muscle as a whole shows marked reductions at sleep onset.

The activity of all muscles dramatically increases on arousal from sleep during sleep onset such that the level of activity reached is well above waking levels. In the genioglossus the increase is due to recruitment of motor units with an inspiratory phasic pattern and the transient activation of non-respiratory-related units (63). The conventional explanation for respiratory activation at arousal from sleep is that it is

Figure 3 Average breath-by-breath changes in minute V, UAR, and DI, IC, GG, and TP EMG activity over transitions from α to θ EEG activity, extending over 20 posttransition theta breaths. Muscle EMG activity for each data point has been represented as a percentage of the mean of the five pretransition alpha breaths. (*) indicates posttransition values that exceed the 95% confidence intervals derived from the five pretransition alpha breaths. The data illustrate the fall in upper airway (GG and TP) and respiratory pump muscle activity (DI and IC) that occurs at sleep onset. *Abbreviations*: V, ventilation; UAR, upper airway resistance; DI, diaphragm; IC, intercostal; GG, genioglossus; TP, tensor palatini; EMG, electromyographic; EEG, electroencephalogram. *Source*: From Ref. 43.

attributable to the presence of respiratory stimuli that have developed due to hypoventilation during the previous sleep period. However, recent studies have suggested that the activation response is independent of respiratory stimuli present at the time of the arousal and is a consequence of a reflex activation response elicited by the act of arousing (50–53).

To summarize, the study of respiratory activity during sleep onset indicates a very strong state dependence. Respiratory activity and, by inference, respiratory control are dependent on the sleep-wake state such that sleep regulatory control is instituted within a breath of the onset of dominant theta activity and waking control returns immediately upon the return of alpha activity. The rapidity of the sleep-related changes indicates they are not secondary adaptations to the sleep state but rather changes imposed on the respiratory system by sleep mechanisms. Further, the consequences are pervasive, affecting upper airway and pump muscle activity as well as protective reflex mechanisms. The pattern of change identified during sleep onset is broadly consistent with the speculation by earlier authors (3,4,64) that the regulatory change consists of the loss of what has been referred to as the wakefulness stimulus and that the loss of this component affects drive to both upper airway and respiratory pump muscles. However, studies over the sleep onset period have also indicated that the temporal changes in ventilation and airway resistance are different, as are the changes in different muscles. Different temporal patterns over sleep onset raise the possibility that changes in respiration during sleep may not be explainable by a single concept, such as the wakefulness stimulus.

Two further observations should be made about the changes in respiration during sleep onset. The first is that although the magnitude of changes varies widely over individuals, they occur in virtually all individuals. Thus, the influence of sleep on the pattern of respiratory activity appears intrinsic to the normal sleep process. The second is that the association between state and respiratory instability during sleep onset in normal healthy individuals closely matches the pattern of state-related changes in respiratory activity found in patients suffering from sleep-disordered breathing. Studies of the normal changes at α to θ transitions indicate that, for a brief period of time, perhaps 15 seconds or so, there is a reduction in the activity of the diaphragm, both tonic and phasic upper airway muscles, including the protective activity of the genioglossus and protective reflexes, such as the reflex response to inspiratory load. It is during this period that occlusion in the patient with obstructive sleep apnea frequently occurs. Thus, the pattern of change in normal individuals at sleep onset is entirely consistent with the hypothesis that normal sleep-related changes in respiratory activity are one component in the development of sleep apnea, with the disorder developing either because the changes become exaggerated or because normal changes interact with additional factors, such as a narrow airway. Indeed, it is not unreasonable to argue that sleep apnea during NREM sleep, and in particular obstructive sleep apnea, is a disorder of sleep onset, as the attainment of a stable state (either sleep or wakefulness) in patients is typically associated with stabilization of respiratory activity.

B. Cardiac Changes During Sleep Onset

To put cardiovascular changes at sleep onset in context, we begin this section with a discussion of metabolic and thermoregulatory changes during sleep onset. There is a strong influence of the circadian oscillator over the metabolic rate and core body temperature, with heat loss through reduced heat production and distal vasodilatation beginning several hours before the normal time of sleep onset (14). In addition, heat gain, through heat production, begins before morning awakening (65). Recent evidence has suggested that high rates of distal heat loss promote sleep onset (14) via excitation of heat-sensitive neurons in the preoptic area (66). However, the relationship between these thermoregulatory processes and sleep is reciprocal in that sleep onset augments the circadian-determined falls in metabolism (13), core body temperature (67), and peripheral vasodilatation (33), processes that Gilbert et al. (65) have argued facilitate the developing sleep state.

A number of studies have shown that HR and BP have decreased and there have been changes in autonomic control by the time stage 2 sleep has become established (68,69). However, only a small number of studies have specifically measured cardiac activity over the sleep onset process. The initial studies indicated that HR (16,70,71) and BP (16) fall rapidly and progressively over sleep onset, beginning early in the process and possibly before EEG indications of sleep (71). The specificity of the link to sleep onset is indicated by the observation that if sleep onset is experimentally delayed the abrupt reductions in both HR and BP are also delayed (16). BP appears to be more uniquely influenced by sleep onset than HR, as HR is also influenced by the circadian system around the time of normal sleep onset, although this does not negate a role for the circadian system in the control of BP more generally (15). Thus, not surprisingly, the data indicate that during sleep onset HR reflects the change in metabolism, with both circadian and sleep-specific effects (16).

Studies that have divided sleep onset into phases based on behavioral and EEG criteria have indicated a slightly different perspective on the changes in HR and BP over sleep onset. In particular, such studies emphasize the instability in the system before stable sleep is achieved. Neither HR nor BP shows abrupt falls in association with specific EEG features, as occurs in the respiratory system at a transition from α to θ EEG activity. Rather, they show more progressive falls within periods of sleep. However, both show large increases at each arousal from theta activity during sleep onset (70,72). The responses are transient, peaking at approximately four seconds after the arousal for HR and eight seconds for BP, with a rapid return to pre-arousal levels (39,72). Thus, sleep-wake state instability during sleep onset results in instability in both respiratory and cardiovascular systems, although through different combinations of mechanisms. The respiratory and cardiovascular systems have in common an activation response at arousal from sleep (θ to α transition), while the respiratory system is additionally affected by the withdrawal of a tonic drive at α to θ transitions. In the respiratory system, the role of the return of the wakefulness stimulus at arousal from sleep remains unclear.

These observations raise the question of the extent to which the sleep-related falls in HR and BP are modified by state instability during sleep onset. As shown in Figure 5, Carrington et al. (39) have demonstrated that in young normal sleepers the sleep-related falls in HR and BP follow a complex course. Thus, HR and BP fall at two phases. The first is when lights are turned off and the subject is requested to go to sleep. Consistent with an earlier report this occurs before EEG indications of sleep (71). Second, HR and BP fall further once stable stage 2 sleep is attained. In between, while the state is unstable, both HR and BP show activation at each brief rearousal, preventing the attainment of sleep values. In other terms, the dipping profile of BP that characterizes normal sleep does not occur until stable sleep is achieved.

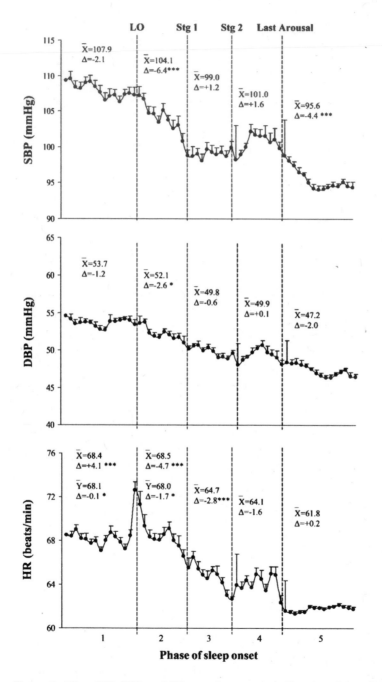

Figure 5 Mean SBP, DBP, and HR over sleep onset as a function of time (2-minute epochs) in phases 1 and 5 and 10% epochs in phases 2, 3, and 4. Standard error bars indicate within-subject

While it is known that variables reflecting cardiovascular autonomic control achieve sleep values very early in NREM sleep (16,69), in this chapter the discussion of cardiovascular function during sleep onset has been limited to HR, BP, and metabolic variables. Autonomic control of the cardiovascular system has not been considered as the available measures either do not have the necessary temporal discrimination (e.g., HR variability analysis) or are confounded by other changes (e.g., pre-ejection period, the period of isovolumetric contraction of the heart, is difficult to interpret when BP is simultaneously changing).

One effect of sleep onset that is at odds with other changes in the cardiovascular system is that cerebral blood flow increases abruptly at the α to θ transition and decreases at the θ to α transition (73). The similarity of these effects to changes in respiratory activity suggests that these changes are instigated by the respiratory system in anticipation of the changes in blood gases that occur secondarily to the hypoventilation that follows the loss of alpha EEG activity.

In summary, metabolic, thermoregulatory, and cardiovascular activities are profoundly affected by the onset of sleep. Some changes anticipate sleep and contribute to its occurrence, particularly metabolic and thermoregulatory changes; other changes are instigated by specific events, such as the reduction in HR and BP at lights-out, or perhaps the cognitive decision to go to sleep, while all components show a reduction in cardiovascular tone in association with the attainment of stable sleep. The progressive changes in HR, BP, and peripheral vasodilatation over sleep onset are perturbed by arousal from sleep, with transient increases in HR and BP and vasoconstriction such that sleep values are not attained until sleep is stable. It may be argued that the relative rapidity of the changes and the specificity of the timing with respect to sleep onset suggests that cardiovascular changes during sleep are not a passive consequence of the sleep state but are actively instigated by sleep mechanisms, perhaps to, as has been previously suggested by others (23,65), promote the continuity of the sleep state.

IV. Conclusion

As has been noted by others (14), the attainment of sleep involves a complex cascade of behavioral and physiological events. In the respiratory and cardiovascular systems, these largely reflect the regulatory influence of sleep mechanisms over respiratory and cardiac activity. The nature of the changes in regulatory control are slightly different in the two systems, with a common activation response at the transition from θ to α EEG activity and abrupt falls in respiration, but not cardiac activity, at α to θ transitions. However, both respiratory and cardiovascular activities are unstable under conditions of sleep-wake state instability, and both attain the stability that characterizes NREM sleep once stable sleep is achieved. Finally, it has been suggested that these, in conjunction with changes in other systems, are necessary to achieve stable, high-quality sleep.

---

variability (variance in the change within subjects over time) *Abbreviations*: SBP, systolic blood pressure; DBP, diastolic blood pressure; HR, heart rate; mmHg, millimeters of mercury; LO, lights-out; $\overline{X}$, overall phase average; $\overline{Y}$, phase average excluding the last value before LO and the first two values following LO (for HR data only); Δ, change from the beginning to the end of the phase; $*p < 0.05$; $***p < 0.001$. $N = 20$ (46 nights).

References

1. Phillipson EA, Bowes G. Control of breathing during sleep. In: Handbook of Physiology: The Respiratory System. Vol 2, sect 3, part 2. Bethesda, MD: American Physiological Society, 1986:649–690.
2. Dempsey JA, Smith CA, Harms CA, et al. Sleep-induced breathing instability. Sleep 1996; 19:236–247.
3. Phillipson EA. Control of breathing during sleep. Am Rev Respir Dis 1978; 118:909–939.
4. Orem J, Osorio I, Brooks E, et al. Activity of respiratory neurones during NREM sleep. J Neurophysiol 1985; 54:1144–1156.
5. Henke KG, Badr MS, Skatrud JB, et al. Load compensation and respiratory muscle function during sleep. J Appl Physiol 1992; 72:1221–1234.
6. Morrell MJ, Harty HR, Adams L, et al. Breathing during wakefulness and NREM sleep in humans without an upper airway. J Appl Physiol 1996; 81:274–281.
7. Morrell MJ, Harty HR, Adams L, et al. Changes in total pulmonary resistance and PCO_2 between wakefulness and sleep in normal human subjects. J Appl Physiol 1995; 78: 1339–1349.
8. Simon PM, Dempsey JA, Landry DM, et al. Effect of sleep on respiratory muscle activity during mechanical ventilation. Am Rev Respir Dis 1993; 147:32–37.
9. Kay A, Trinder J, Kim Y. Individual differences in the relationship between upper-airway resistance and ventilation during sleep onset. J Appl Physiol 1995; 79:411–419.
10. Krimsky WR, Leiter JC. Physiology of breathing and respiratory control during sleep. Semin Respir Crit Care Med 2005; 26:5–12.
11. Bristow JD, Honour AJ, Pickering TG, et al. Cardiovascular and respiratory changes during sleep in normal and hypertensive subjects. Cardiovasc Res 1969; 3:476–485.
12. Burgess HJ, Trinder J, Kim Y, et al. Sleep and circadian influences on cardiac autonomic nervous system activity. Am J Physiol 1997; 273:H1761–H1768.
13. Fraser G, Trinder J, Colrain I, et al. The effect of sleep and circadian cycle on sleep period energy expenditure. J Appl Physiol 1989; 63:2067–2074.
14. Krauchi K, Cajochen C, Werth E, et al. Functional link between distal vasodilation and sleep-onset latency? Am J Physiol Regul Integr Comp Physiol 2000; 278:R741–R748.
15. Trinder J, Kleiman J, Nicholas C, et al. Circadian versus sleep influences on cardiovascular activity. Sleep 2007; 30:A31.
16. Carrington M, Walsh M, Stambas T, et al. The influence of sleep onset on the diurnal variation in cardiac activity and cardiac control. J Sleep Res 2003; 12:213–221.
17. Snyder F, Hobson JA, Morrison DF, et al. Changes in respiration, heart rate, and systolic blood pressure in human sleep. J Appl Physiol 1964; 19:417–422.
18. Van de Borne P, Nguyen H, Biston P, et al. Effects of wake and sleep stages on the 24-h autonomic control of blood pressure and heart rate in recumbent men. Am J Physiol 1994; 266:H548–H554.
19. Kerkhof GA, Van Dongen HP, Bobbert AC. Absence of endogenous circadian rhythmicity in blood pressure? Am J Hypertens 1998; 11:373–377.
20. Krauchi K, Wirz-Justice A. Circadian rhythm of heat production, heart rate and skin and core temperature under unmasking conditions in men. Am J Physiol 1994; 267:R819–R829.
21. Van Dongen HP, Maislin G, Kerkhof GA. Repeated assessment of the endogenous 24-hour profile of blood pressure under constant routine. Chronobiol Int 2001; 18:85–98.
22. Trinder J. Cardiac activity and sympathovagal balance during sleep. Sleep Med Clin 2007; 2:199–208.
23. Otzenberger H, Simon C, Gronfier C, et al. Temporal relationship between dynamic heart rate variability and electroencephalographic activity during sleep in man. Neurosci Lett 1997; 229:173–176.
24. Baust W, Bohnert B. The regulation of heart rate during sleep. Exp Brain Res 1969; 7:169–180.

25. Berlad I, Shlitner S, Ben-Haim S, et al. Power spectrum analysis and heart rate variability in stage 4 and REM sleep: evidence for state-specific changes in autonomic dominance. J Sleep Res 1993; 2:88–90.
26. Burgess HJ, Trinder J. Cardiac parasympathetic nervous system activity does not increase in anticipation of sleep. J Sleep Res 1996; 5:83–89.
27. Orr W, Lin B, Adamson P, et al. Autonomic control of heart rate variability during sleep. J Sleep Res 1993; 22:26.
28. Vanoli E, Adamson PB, Lin B, et al. Heart rate variability during specific sleep stages: a comparison of healthy subjects with patients after myocardial infarction. Circulation 1995; 91:1918–1822.
29. Baust W, Weidinger H, Kirchner F. Sympametic activity during natural sleep and arousal. Arch Ital Biol 1968; 106:379–390.
30. Iwamura Y, Uchino Y, Ozawa S, et al. Spontaneous and reflex discharge of sympathetic nerve during "para-sleep" in decerebrate cat. Brain Res 1969; 16:359–367.
31. Reiner P. Correlational analysis of central noradrenergic neuronal activity and sympathetic tone in behaving cats. Brain Res 1986; 378:86–96.
32. Baccelli G, Guazzi M, Mancia G, et al. Neural and non-neural mechanisms influencing circulation during sleep. Nature 1969; 223:184–185.
33. Hornyak M, Cejnar M, Elam M, et al. Sympathetic muscle nerve activity during sleep in man. Brain 1991; 114:1281–1295.
34. Okada H, Iwase S, Mano T, et al. Changes in muscle sympathetic nerve activity during sleep in humans. Neurology 1991; 41:1961–1966.
35. Somers VK, Dyken ME, Mark AL, et al. Sympathetic-nerve activity during sleep in normal subjects. N Engl J Med 1993; 328:303–307.
36. Ogilvie RD. The process of falling asleep. Sleep Med Rev 2001; 5:247–270.
37. Merica H, Fortune RD. State transitions between wake and sleep, and within the ultradian cycle, with focus on the link to neuronal activity. Sleep Med Rev 2004; 8:473–485.
38. Kay A, Trinder J, Bowes G, et al. Changes in airway resistance during sleep onset. J Appl Physiol 1994; 76:1600–1607.
39. Carrington MJ, Barbieri R, Colrain IM, et al. Changes in cardiovascular function during the sleep onset period in young adults. J Appl Physiol 2005; 98:468–476.
40. Henke KG, Dempsey JA, Badr MS, et al. Effect of sleep-induced increases in upper airway resistance on respiratory muscle activity. J Appl Physiol 1991; 70:158–168.
41. Skatrud JB, Dempsey JA, Badr S, et al. Effect of airway impedance on CO_2 retention and respiratory muscle activity during NREM sleep. J Appl Physiol 1988; 65:1676–1685.
42. Tabachnik E, Muller NL, Bryan AC, et al. Changes in ventilation and chest wall mechanics during sleep in normal adolescents. J Appl Physiol 1981; 51:557–564.
43. Worsnop C, Kay A, Pierce AJ, et al. The activity of respiratory pump and upper airway muscles during sleep onset. J Appl Physiol 1998; 85:908–920.
44. Colrain IM, Trinder J, Fraser G, et al. Ventilation during sleep onset. J Appl Physiol 1987; 63:2067–2074.
45. Trinder J, Whitworth F, Kay A, et al. Respiratory instability during sleep onset. J Appl Physiol 1992; 73:2462–2469.
46. Bulow K. Respiration and wakefulness in man. Acta Physiol Scand Suppl 1963; 209:5–110.
47. Trinder J, Van Beveren J, Smith P, et al. Correlation between ventilation and EEG defined arousal during sleep onset in young subjects. J Appl Physiol 1997; 83:2005–2011.
48. Dunai J, Kleiman J, Trinder J. Individual differences in peripheral chemosensitivity and state related ventilatory instability. J Appl Physiol 1999; 87:661–672.
49. Dunai J, Trinder J, Wilkinson M. Peripheral chemoreceptor contribution to ventilatory instability during sleep onset. J Appl Physiol 1996; 81:2235–2243.

50. Carley DW, Applebaum R, Basner RC, et al. Respiratory and arousal responses to acoustic stimuli. Chest 1997; 112:1567–1571.

51. Catcheside PG, Chiong SC, Orr RS, et al. Acute cardiovascular responses to arousal from non-REM sleep during normoxia and hypoxia. Sleep 2001; 24:895–902.

52. O'Driscoll DM, Meadows GE, Corfield DR, et al. The cardiovascular response to arousal from sleep under controlled conditions of central and peripheral chemoreceptor stimulation in humans. J Appl Physiol 2004; 96:865–870.

53. Trinder J, Ivens C, Kleiman J, et al. The cardiovascular activation response at an arousal from sleep is independent of the level of CO_2. J Sleep Res 2006; 15:174–182.

54. Kay A, Trinder J, Kim Y. Progressive changes in airway resistance as a function of slow wave EEG activity. J Appl Physiol 1996; 81:282–292.

55. Trinder J, Kay A, Kleiman J, et al. Gender differences in airway resistance during sleep. J Appl Physiol 1997; 83:1986–1997.

56. Gora J, Trinder J, Kay A, et al. Load compensation as a function of state during sleep onset. J Appl Physiol 1998; 84:2123–2131.

57. Mezzanotti WS, Tangel DJ, White DP. Influence of sleep onset on upper-airway muscle activity in apnea patients versus normal controls. Am J Respir Crit Care Med 1996; 153: 1880–1887.

58. Tangel DJ, Mezzanotte WS, White DP. The influence of sleep on the activity of tonic vs. inspiratory phasic muscles in normal men. J Appl Physiol 1992; 73:1058–1068.

59. White DP. Pathophysiology of obstructive sleep apnea. Thorax 1995; 50:797–804.

60. Mezzanotti WS, Tangel DJ, White DP. Waking genioglossal EMG in sleep apnea patients versus normal controls (a neuromuscular compensatory mechanism). J Clin Invest 1992; 89:1571–1579.

61. Saboisky J, Butler J, Fogel R, et al. Tonic and phasic respiratory drives to human genioglossus motorneurons during breathing. J Neurophysiol 2006; 95:2213–2221.

62. Wilkinson V, Malhotra A, Nicholas CL, et al. Discharge patters on human genioglossus motor units during sleep onset. Sleep 2008; 31:525–533.

63. Trinder J, Wilkinson V, Nicholas C, et al. Genioglossus motor unit discharge patterns during arousal from sleep. Am J Resp Crit Care Med 2007; 175:A274.

64. Fink BR. Influence of cerebral activity in wakefulness on regulation of breathing. J Appl Physiol 1961; 16:15–20.

65. Gilbert SS, van den Heuvel CJ, Ferguson SA, et al. Thermoregulation as a sleep signaling system. Sleep Med Rev 2004; 8:81–93.

66. Szymusiak R, Gvilia I, McGinty D. Hypothalamic control of sleep. Sleep Med 2007; 8: 291–301.

67. Gillberg M, Ackerstedt T. Body temperature and sleep at different times of day. Sleep 1982; 5:378–388.

68. Burgess HJ, Trinder J, Kim Y. Cardiac autonomic nervous system activity during presleep wakefulness and stage 2 NREM sleep. J Sleep Res 1999; 8:113–122.

69. Trinder J, Kleiman J, Carrington M, et al. Autonomic activity during human sleep as a function of time and sleep stage. J Sleep Res 2001; 10:253–264.

70. Burgess HJ, Trinder J, Kleiman J. Cardiac activity during sleep onset. Psychophysiology 1999; 36:298–306.

71. Pivik RT, Busby K. Heart rate associated with sleep onset in preadolescents. J Sleep Res 1996; 5:33–36.

72. Trinder J, Allen N, Kleiman J, et al. On the nature of cardiovascular activation at an arousal from sleep. Sleep 2003; 26:543–551.

73. Kotajima F, Meadows GE, Morrell MJ, et al. Cerebral blood flow changes associated with fluctuations in alpha and theta rhythm during sleep onset in humans. J Physiol 2005; 568:305–313.

5

Physiological Effects of Sleep on the Cardiovascular System

RICHARD L. HORNER

University of Toronto, Toronto, Ontario, Canada

I. Introduction

This chapter summarizes the effects of wakefulness, non–rapid eye movement (NREM) sleep, and rapid eye movement (REM) sleep on the cardiovascular system. In addition, the changes in autonomic nervous system activities that occur between these sleep-wake states will be reviewed, with particular emphasis placed on the transient effects observed at arousal from sleep. Particular attention will be focused on the cardiovascular responses to arousal because of the increasing realization that arousal mechanisms are important in the acute and chronic cardiovascular consequences of common sleep-related breathing disorders, such as obstructive sleep apnea (OSA) and central sleep apnea (1–3). For example, in OSA patients the repetitive large brief surges in heart rate (HR) and blood pressure (BP) associated with arousal from sleep, and resolution of apneas, are thought to increase the risk for the development of adverse cardiovascular events such as angina, myocardial infarction, stroke, and systemic hypertension (1–3). The presence of nighttime OSA can also produce sustained daytime hypertension (3). Given that the clinical syndrome of OSA affects 2% to 4% of the middle-aged population (4), the cardiovascular effects of arousal from sleep and OSA are a major public health burden (5,6). The adverse impact of sleep-disordered breathing events on the nighttime BP profile is highlighted in Figure 1.

II. Cardiovascular Outputs in Periods of Established Wakefulness and Sleep

Figure 2 illustrates the overall changes in HR and BP between periods of established wakefulness, NREM sleep, and REM sleep. NREM sleep is generally associated with reductions in HR and BP compared to established wakefulness. Tonic REM sleep is associated with further decreases, whereas phasic REM sleep events produce characteristic phasic increases in HR and BP. The direction of these overall changes is generally applicable across species (8,9). It is important to note, however, that whether there is an overall change in the mean levels of HR and BP in REM sleep, compared to NREM sleep or waking, depends in large part on the relative amounts of phasic versus tonic REM sleep and whether both these REM phases are included in the comparison with the other sleep-wake states. The mechanisms involved in producing these overall changes in HR and BP in periods of established sleep and wakefulness are summarized next.

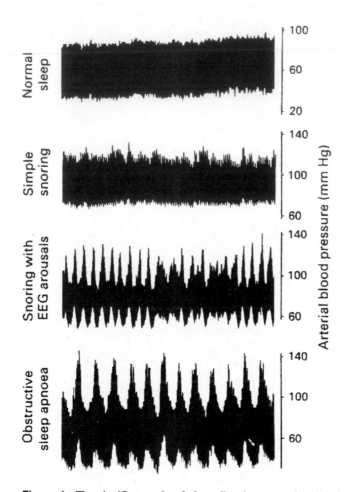

Figure 1 The significant role of sleep disturbance on the nighttime BP profile. Arterial BP profiles are shown in (*i*) a normally sleeping subject, (*ii*) a snorer, (*iii*) a snorer whose sleep is disrupted by repetitive arousals, and (*iv*) a patient with OSA. Each trace shows about 10 minutes of recording. *Abbreviations*: BP, blood pressure; OSA, obstructive sleep apnea. *Source*: From Ref. 7.

A. Hemodynamic Changes Across Sleep-Wake States

Following the pioneering work of Mancia and Zanchetti (8), there has been much progress in delineating the mechanisms underlying the changes in HR and BP in sleep and wakefulness, in large part because animal studies allow the use of invasive techniques to make measurements that are either technically difficult or not feasible in humans. Figure 3 shows data from chronically instrumented, naturally sleeping cats that highlight the major factors contributing to the hemodynamic changes that occur across sleep-wake states. Cardiac output decreases upon progression from wakefulness to NREM and REM sleep, a change primarily caused by a decreased HR because of the

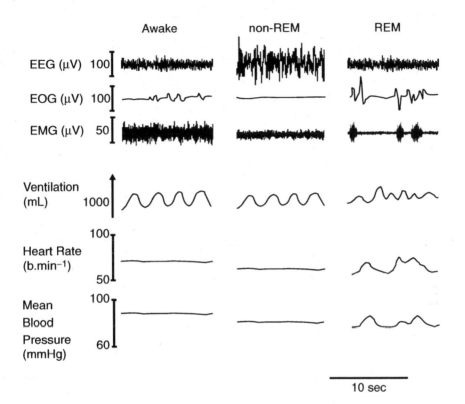

Figure 2 Schema showing overall changes in mean BP, HR, and ventilation between established periods of wakefulness, NREM sleep, and REM sleep. The general changes in appearance of the EEG, EOG, and EMG are also shown for the different sleep-wake states. Note the phasic changes in cardiorespiratory outputs associated with phasic REM events (i.e., eye movements and muscle twitches). *Abbreviations*: BP, blood pressure; HR, heart rate; NREM, non–rapid eye movement; REM, rapid eye movement; EEG, electroencephalogram; EOG, electrooculogram; EMG, electromyogram.

minimal changes in stroke volume (8,9). The minimal change in total peripheral conductance between waking and NREM sleep observed in this, and several other studies (8–11), has been taken to indicate that a decreased HR, and hence cardiac output, is the major factor contributing to the decreased BP in NREM sleep.

In such studies in chronically instrumented cats, REM sleep is associated with increased total peripheral conductance compared to the other states, a change that is indicative of a *net* vasodilatation (Fig. 3D). This net vasodilatation, coupled with a further decrease in cardiac output in REM sleep, is thought to be responsible for the overall decrease in BP. In subsequent studies, however, it was shown that there are *regional* changes in vascular conductance in REM sleep that are not apparent upon inspection of total peripheral conductance. For example, there is vasodilatation in the mesenteric and renal vascular beds in REM sleep but decreased conductance in the ileac

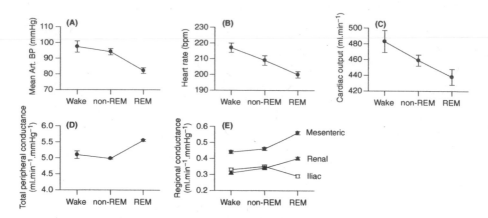

Figure 3 Changes in (A) mean arterial BP, (B) HR, (C) cardiac output, (D) total peripheral conductance, and (E) regional conductances in the mesenteric, renal, and iliac vascular beds across sleep-wake states. Data obtained in chronically instrumented, naturally sleeping cats. *Abbreviations*: BP, blood pressure; HR, heart rate. *Source*: From Ref. 8.

circulation (Fig. 3E). Further experiments attributed this localized decrease in conductance to vasoconstriction in skeletal muscle circulation (8,9). The skeletal muscle vasculature is also thought to play an important role in producing the phasic increases in BP that typically occur during phasic REM events such as eye movements and muscle twitches. Although the autonomic mechanisms producing these transient BP surges in phasic REM sleep are discussed in more detail later, these events are associated with phasic decreases in total peripheral conductance in the skeletal muscle vasculature due to transient vasoconstriction (8,9,12).

It should be noted, however, that the magnitude of the change in BP from NREM to REM sleep observed in Figure 3 is larger than that observed in most other studies (8,9,13). It appears that this larger effect of REM sleep on BP may be related to the time that these chronically instrumented cats were studied postoperatively (13,14). Nevertheless, the mechanisms that affect HR and BP at the transition from NREM to REM sleep are generally applicable across species. Their contribution, however, may vary in magnitude between species and within individuals such that the overall mean levels of HR and BP may change to a varying degree from NREM to REM sleep, although variability is typically increased during REM sleep. The autonomic mechanisms responsible for the overall effects of sleep-wake state on HR, BP, and regional vascular conductances are discussed next.

B. Autonomic Nervous System Changes Across Sleep-Wake States

The changes in HR and BP observed across sleep-wake states are largely dependent on intact vagal and sympathetic innervations (10,15). Determination of the precise autonomic mechanisms involved in mediating these effects of sleep on HR and BP has been facilitated by studies documenting the actual changes in sympathetic and parasympathetic outputs. In some studies, direct recording of autonomic nervous system activity has been performed. For example, microneurography has been used extensively to document sleep-related changes in muscle sympathetic nerve activity in humans (16–18). Chronic recordings of renal sympathetic activity have been performed in animals (19). In contrast, other studies have inferred state-related changes in autonomic activity by observing changes in BP and HR with blockade of one (or other) branch of the autonomic nervous system (20–23). Spectral analysis techniques have also been useful in determining sleep-related changes in autonomic output (24,25).

Although each of these different approaches has yielded valuable information, each technique has its own advantages and disadvantages. For example, interpretation of changes in autonomic nervous system activity from microneurographic recordings from the muscle sympathetic nerve is somewhat limited because only one branch of the autonomic nervous system is recorded and because this branch shows characteristic differences across sleep-wake states compared to the sympathetic output to other vascular beds. For example, in REM sleep, sympathetic nerve output to muscle blood vessels is increased (16–18), whereas sympathetic output to the renal vasculature is decreased (19). Confirmation of this differential effect of REM sleep on vasomotor tone in different vascular beds has been obtained in studies that have recorded blood flow in several vascular beds at the same in time in REM sleep (Fig. 3) (8,9). A differential distribution of sympathetic output to different vascular beds has also been observed in a pharmacological model of REM sleep; in this model, the REM-like state was associated with increased sympathetic output to vasoconstrictor fibers of hind limb skeletal muscle but decreased output to the cardiac, renal, splanchnic, and lumbar sympathetic nerves (26). Depending on the magnitude of this differential distribution of sympathetic output in REM, the overall balance of vasodilatation and vaso-constriction in the major resistance vessels will determine the net change in BP in REM sleep (see earlier).

Spectral analysis of HR variability has also been used to determine the prevailing balance of sympathetic and parasympathetic activities (27,28), and this approach has been applied to sleep (24,25). However, the results of such studies, performed during spontaneous breathing, are somewhat complicated because interpretation relies on the validity of several assumptions, which may be affected by the influences of sleep and its disturbance (28). In particular, changes in the sleep-wake state are associated with changes in other physiological variables, for example, blood gases, lung volume, breathing pattern, and respiratory effort (29,30), each of which can independently influence sympathetic and parasympathetic outflow (28,31–33) and therefore obscure the primary state-dependent effects on autonomic activity. However, most important for studies during sleep, particularly in patients with sleep-related breathing disorders, are the wide fluctuations in respiratory rate that accompany sleep onsets and arousals from sleep. In these cases, interpretation becomes complicated because the large fluctuations in respiratory rate that occur can fully encompass the frequency ranges used to separate the sympathetic and parasympathetic components of HR variability (28), and this is rarely taken into account in the interpretation of spectral analyses.

Despite these caveats, the results of studies using the variety of techniques described earlier, in a variety of species, suggest that established wakefulness exerts a tonic stimulatory effect on sympathetic output to the heart and blood vessels (16–18,20,24,25). This is similar to the tonic stimulating effects on respiratory, and nonrespiratory, motor activity (29,34–36) and may be attributable to the same wakefulness stimulus.

In contrast to the documented effects of wakefulness on sympathetic drive, the effects of waking on parasympathetic activity are less clear-cut. Several studies in animals and humans suggest that established wakefulness is associated with a tonic withdrawal of parasympathetic drive to the heart and that this is an important factor contributing to the increased HR when awake (8,9,13,21,22,24,37). However, a major factor contributing to this parasympathetic withdrawal in established wakefulness is probably secondary to a change in breathing. For example, upper airway resistance typically increases in sleep (30,38–41), leading to increased respiratory efforts in response to the load (30). Increased respiratory efforts themselves can lead to increased vagal contribution to HR variability by the central mechanisms associated with respiratory sinus arrhythmia (42–45). The respiratory slowing observed in some individuals during sleep would also increase the magnitude of the vagal contribution to sinus arrhythmia in these individuals (46,47).

That sleep-related changes in blood gases, breathing pattern, and effort can importantly contribute to the parasympathetic control of HR was demonstrated by a recent study in dogs, in which breathing rate and depth and blood gases were controlled by constant mechanical ventilation while HR changes were monitored during spontaneous fluctuations in the sleep-wake state with blockade of the cardiac sympathetic innervation (20). Under these conditions, there was a minimal change in the parasympathetic influence on HR between NREM sleep and steady-state established wakefulness (Fig. 4), showing that changes in breathing pattern importantly contribute to

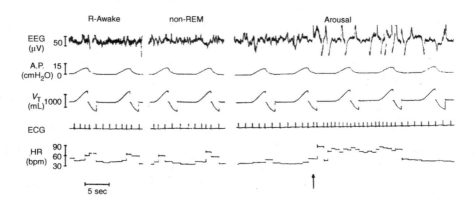

Figure 4 Example showing the differential effects of established wakefulness versus transitions into wakefulness on the parasympathetic control of HR. The traces show changes in HR (*i*) between periods of established relaxed wakefulness (*R-Awake*) and NREM sleep (*left panels*) and (*ii*) at the transition from NREM sleep to wakefulness (*right panels, point of awakening indicated by arrow*). The traces are from a dog undergoing constant mechanical ventilation with blockade of cardiac sympathetic innervation, that is, leaving only the parasympathetic innervation active. The mean HR changed minimally between steady-state wakefulness and NREM sleep, but awakening from sleep produced significant vagal withdrawal and large increases in HR. No body movements or evidence of overt behavioral arousal were noticeable at awakening; the large voltage deflections on the EEG trace are artifacts due to eye movements. The swings in AP are produced by mechanical ventilation. *Abbreviations*: HR, heart rate; NREM, non–rapid eye movement; EEG, electroencephalogram; AP, airway pressure; V_T, tidal volume; ECG, electrocardiogram. *Source*: From Ref. 20.

vagal withdrawal and increased HR when awake (20). However, vagal influences have major contributions to HR acceleration at arousal from sleep, even in the absence of changes in breathing pattern (see next). In addition, bursts of cardiac vagal efferent activity can also contribute to HR deceleration in REM sleep (23).

III. Transient Effects of Arousal from Sleep on the Cardiovascular System

As summarized earlier, there have been several detailed studies on the mechanisms involved in mediating the changes in HR and BP between periods of established sleep and wakefulness. Comparatively little attention, however, has been focused on the mechanisms underlying the large brief surges in HR and BP accompanying arousal from sleep. This neglect is somewhat surprising, given that the repetitive surges in HR and BP at arousal from sleep are thought to predispose patients with sleep-related breathing disorders to increased risk for the development of adverse cardiovascular events (1–3,5,6). This section summarizes the changes in autonomic nervous system activity that occurs at arousal from sleep.

A. Autonomic Nervous System Responses to Arousal from Sleep

One study in intact, chronically instrumented cats has reported that spontaneous arousals from NREM sleep are associated with large increases in renal sympathetic nerve activity (19). In humans the occurrence of K complexes during sleep is associated with transient increases in muscle sympathetic nerve activity, HR, and BP (16–18,48). An example of such a response is shown in Figure 5. Since K complexes during sleep are thought to be markers of an endogenous arousal/alerting response (49), these observations are consistent with the suggestion that arousal-related mechanisms lead to sympathetic activation. The decrease in cardiac vagal activity after presentation of natural arousing stimuli in cats (15) is often taken as evidence that arousal from sleep leads to vagal withdrawal. However, the number and types of stimuli applied to how many cats is unclear in that study, as is whether the stimuli were even applied in wakefulness or sleep.

Overall, these studies show that compared to what is known regarding the effects of established wakefulness and sleep on autonomic nervous system outputs to the cardiovascular system (summarized in sect. II), there are less studies systematically investigating the acute effects of arousal from sleep on sympathetic and parasympathetic activities. Moreover it is not known how the effects observed at arousal from sleep are physiologically different compared to subsequent established wakefulness. Therefore, the aim of a previous study was to systematically determine the effects of arousal from sleep on sympathetic and parasympathetic outputs to the cardiovascular system and compare these effects with those in subsequent periods of established wakefulness (20). Measurements of HR were made in awake and sleeping dogs with, and without, blockade of the cardiac sympathetic and parasympathetic innervations. Studies were performed during spontaneous breathing and when breathing was controlled by constant mechanical ventilation at levels just below resting arterial PCO_2. Mechanical ventilation was used to identify the independent effects of arousal from sleep per se on HR changes, that is, in the absence of confounding influences such as changes in breathing pattern, lung volume, and blood gases, which, in themselves, can lead to changes in cardiac autonomic output and obscure the primary effect of the state change (28,31–33). Under

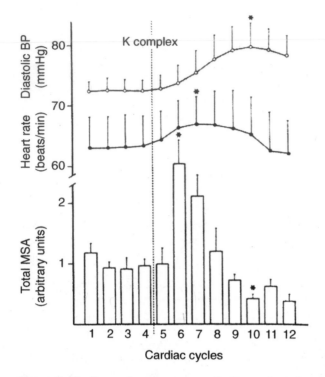

Figure 5 Cardiovascular consequences of a K complex in humans. Mean diastolic BP, HR, and MSA are shown for several cardiac cycles before and after a K complex (indicated by *vertical dashed line*). Note the transient excitation of MSA, HR, and BP after the K complex. *Abbreviations*: BP, blood pressure; HR, heart rate; MSA, muscle sympathetic nerve activity. *Source*: From Ref. 16.

these controlled conditions, wake onset was associated with large transient increases in HR compared to NREM sleep (mean increase = 30%, 20 beats/min), and this was subsequently found to be due to both phasic sympathetic activation and parasympathetic withdrawal (20). However, subsequent periods of established wakefulness (i.e., periods separated by at least 30 seconds from wake onset) were associated with smaller tonic increases in HR (mean increase = 6%, 4 beats/min), and this was due to sympathetic activation with a minimal change in parasympathetic output (20). These changes reflect the primary effects of changes in the sleep-wake state on cardiac sympathetic and parasympathetic outputs because this study was performed with constant mechanical ventilation to hold level the respiratory influences on autonomic activity. In addition, these conditions serve to highlight the profound transient effects of normal spontaneous arousals from sleep on HR and autonomic nervous system outputs. As can be observed in Figure 4, the HR at spontaneous arousal from sleep can even increase to the levels observed during mild exercise, despite no evidence of overt behavioral arousal such as body movements. Overall, the large transient parasympathetic withdrawal to the heart (20) and the increased sympathetic drive to the heart and blood vessels (19,20,48) would explain the large brief HR and BP responses at arousal from sleep.

B. Model to Explain the Large Brief Surges in HR and BP at Arousal from Sleep

Despite the documented effects of arousal from sleep on sympathetic and para-sympathetic activities to the heart and blood vessels (summarized earlier), there is currently no model that has been put forward to explain why such large brief changes in autonomic output occur at wake onset compared to subsequent established wake-fulness. However, a component of these autonomic changes may be explained by a model similar to the one used to account for the stimulatory effects of arousal from sleep on pulmonary ventilation. This ventilatory model is described here briefly to highlight how similar reasoning may apply to the cardiovascular system. In the ven-tilatory model, a component of the surge in ventilation at arousal from sleep is explained by differences in both the set point for $PaCO_2$ and the hypercapnic ven-tilatory response between sleep and wakefulness. In sleep, compared to waking, there is reduced ventilation and increased $PaCO_2$ because of (*i*) an increase in the $PaCO_2$ required to maintain spontaneous breathing (29,50,51), (*ii*) reduced ventilatory responses to the increased $PaCO_2$ (52), (*iii*) increased upper airway resistance (38,53), (*iv*) reduced compensatory responses to this respiratory load (39,54), and (*v*) decreased tonic drive to respiratory neurons (55) and motoneurons (36). However, an important consequence of the increased $PaCO_2$ in sleep is that on arousal, the arterial CO_2 is initially higher than the levels normally encountered in wakefulness. This discrepancy drives ventilation to a level determined by the waking CO_2 response curve and pro-duces a transient surge in ventilation (29,56,57). This homeostatic mechanism, how-ever, cannot fully explain the surge in ventilation at wake onset and accounts for only about 50% of the ventilatory response (58). A significant component of the surge in ventilation is related to arousal mechanisms per se (58,59), and this is discussed in more detail later.

Nevertheless, similar reasoning applied to the control mechanisms for HR and BP may explain a component of the hemodynamic consequences of arousal from sleep. In this scheme, the decreased muscle sympathetic nerve activity observed in NREM sleep compared to wakefulness, in association with decreased HR and BP (16–18), suggests that sleep is associated with a change in baroreceptor function (c.f., the sleep-related changes in the control of ventilation mentioned earlier). Indeed, there are other data suggesting that there is a downward resetting of the baroreflex in NREM sleep compared to wakefulness, and this appears to be accompanied by increased baroreflex sensitivity (60–63), although this latter effect has not been observed consistently (64). Figure 6 illustrates how changes in the set point and sensitivity of the baroreflex between wakefulness and sleep could explain a component of the increased HR and BP at arousal from sleep. In this model, because the set point for mean arterial BP is lower during sleep, and the sensitivity of the baroreflex may be higher (60–63), upon sudden awak-ening from sleep, the BP will initially represent a hypotensive stimulus compared to the levels normally encountered in wakefulness. This inappropriately low BP will drive compensatory mechanisms to increase BP, and there will also be some increase in HR due to differences in the set point of the responses between sleep and wakefulness (Fig. 6). In this model, the transient nature of the BP and HR surge at awakening would be explained in terms of a difference in the baroreflex set point between wakefulness and sleep and possibly an overshoot of the waking set point. The overshoot is likely due to the effects of arousal mechanisms per se acting in addition to the homeostatic corrective

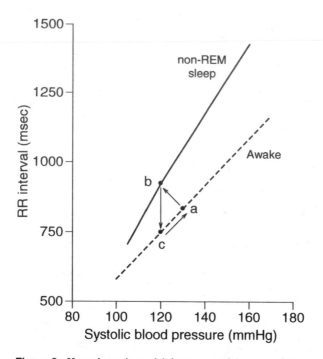

Figure 6 Hemodynamic model that may explain some of the increased HR and BP at awakening from sleep. This model is based on the differences between wakefulness and sleep in the set point and sensitivity of the baroreflex. Points a and b indicate typical changes in HR (plotted as an R-R interval) and BP between wakefulness and NREM sleep, and the *dashed* and *solid lines* represent baroreflex sensitivities in these states (60,61). Systolic pressure is shown on the abscissa because this is typically used to quantify baroreflex responses (60–62,64). On arousal from sleep (at point b), the level of systolic pressure will initially represent a hypotensive stimulus compared to the levels normally encountered in wakefulness, and this inappropriate level will drive compensatory mechanisms to increase blood pressure (i.e., from c to a). There will also be some increase in HR due to differences in the set point of the baroreflex curves between sleep and wakefulness. In this model, the transient nature of the BP and HR change at awakening is explained in terms of a difference in the set point of the baroreflex between wakefulness and sleep and possibly an overshoot of the waking set point due to arousal mechanisms. *Abbreviations*: BP, blood pressure; HR, heart rate; NREM, non–rapid eye movement.

response, that is, a mechanism that similarly contributes to the surge in ventilation at wake onset (58,59).

C.   Limitations of the Hemodynamic Model to Explain the Surge in HR and BP at Arousal from Sleep

Explaining the acute stimulatory effects of arousal from sleep on HR and BP simply in terms of baroreflex responses has certain limitations. Indeed, these limitations (discussed later) make this model unlikely to be able to fully explain the magnitude of the transient surges in HR and BP at arousal. For example, changes in HR and BP occur in baror-eceptor-denervated animals awake and asleep (65), indicating that major state-dependent influences on cardiac autonomic activity and vasomotor tone can occur independently of the baroreflex. Furthermore, that HR and BP changes are larger after baroreceptor denervation than before (65) suggests that the baroreflex normally buffers the hemo-dynamic effects of a change in the sleep-wake state. Moreover, HR increases dramati-cally at arousal from sleep at a time when BP also increases significantly. The large increase in HR, despite the surge in BP, suggests that the baroreflex may even be uncoupled at arousal from sleep. That pharmacologically induced BP increases produce typical baroreflex-induced decreases in HR during sleep, unless sleep is disturbed by a K complex (60,61), supports this suggestion. Indeed, following the K complex, BP con-tinues to increase but is now accompanied by a significant rise in HR. Spontaneous K complexes during sleep themselves often lead to significant increases in HR and BP that occur concomitantly with increased muscle sympathetic nerve activity (16–18,48).

Taken together, these data suggest that phasic arousal reactions may uncouple baroreflex-induced slowing of the heart. Arousals associated with the defense reaction (66,67) and mental activity (62) have a similar effect. This concept is especially relevant because there is evidence of spontaneous activation of a distinct, transiently heightened awake state at wake onset compared to subsequent wakefulness (58,59,68–75). As such, these data suggest that arousal from sleep is likely accompanied by transient uncoupling of the baroreflex, and this contributes to the transient surges in HR and BP at wake onset compared to subsequent wakefulness. These effects would occur via concomitant sympathetic activation and vagal withdrawal described previously. The inhibitory effects of wakefulness on the baroreflex control of HR may explain why only about 15% of spontaneous fluctuations in R-R intervals and arterial pressures follow the directions predicted by the baroreflex (76).

IV. Summary and Unanswered Questions

This chapter describes the autonomic nervous system changes that occur between states of wakefulness and sleep, with particular emphasis placed on the transient effects observed at arousal from sleep. Determination of these mechanisms assumes special importance, given the relevance of the hemodynamic consequences (both transient and chronic) of arousal from sleep in patients with sleep-related breathing disorders that lead to increased risk for angina, myocardial infarction, stroke, left ventricular impairment, and systemic hypertension (1–3).

One of the next challenges is to uncover the nature of the relationship between the changes in activity of sleep-wake-related neurons with effects on autonomic outputs, such as those producing the large, brief surges in HR and BP at arousal from sleep in excess of subsequent wakefulness. For example, it needs to be determined if arousal from sleep, from a neurophysiological viewpoint, represents a state of being "more awake" (i.e., a more intense activation of state-related nuclei at wake onset compared to subsequent wakefulness) or whether there is a transient activation of neural pathways at wake onset (e.g., activation of the fight or flight response), which then become inactive in later periods of wakefulness (73,74).

Although the latter hypothesis has yet to be investigated, the firing patterns on awakening of monoaminergic neurons in the dorsal raphe and locus coeruleus nuclei would support the former hypothesis. These neuronal groups are integral to the ascending activating system, and large transient increases in discharge have been noted for most serotonergic dorsal raphe neurons at spontaneous awakening from REM sleep (70,71) and for most noradrenergic locus coeruleus neurons at awakening from NREM sleep (69), with the levels of discharge far exceeding those in later wakefulness. Given the evidence that locus coeruleus and dorsal raphe neurons are important in modulating sensory (77) and motor responsiveness (78), respectively, their bursts of activity at awakening may serve a protective function by preparing an animal to respond immediately to any potentially threatening stimuli. Viewed in this context, the abrupt changes in the electroencephalogram (EEG) pattern and increases in postural muscle tone, accompanied by the large cardiorespiratory changes at arousal from sleep, would be appropriate physiological responses. Recent studies using the acoustic startle reflex, and its modulation by sensory inputs, also support the hypothesis that the moments just after awakening are neurophysiologically distinct compared to subsequent established wakefulness (68,72). Given the evidence that the wakefulness stimulus exerts powerful stimulatory effects on sympathetic outflow and produces transient vagal withdrawal, a transiently aroused awake state at wake onset would be expected to exert major influences on HR and BP compared to subsequent waking.

As mentioned, the mechanisms and pathways underlying the influence of this transient arousal state on the cardiovascular system at wake onset need to be determined and are at present not well understood (79). For example, although changes in locus coeruleus neuronal activity parallel changes in sympathetic tone across sleep-wake states in cats (80), the nature of this association and its relevance to sleep-related cardiovascular control needs to be established. Similar considerations hold for the postulated influences of sleep-/wake-related serotonergic neurons on sympathetic output (79). Indeed, it has been shown that serotonergic medullary raphe neurons, like the dorsal raphe neurons that are intimately involved in sleep regulation, have higher discharge in wakefulness (71,81–84) and project to sympathetic preganglionic neurons (79,85,86) where 5-hydroxytryptamine depolarizes those neurons and can increase BP (87–89). However, although such effects provide appropriate circuitry and an attractive mechanism to explain state-dependent changes in sympathetic outputs, the actual relevance of these mechanisms to the effects of sleep on BP needs to be established.

It also remains to be determined if the neuronal systems engaged at arousal from sleep are altered by disturbances in the physiological variables that accompany repetitive apneas, for example, hypoxia and hypercapnia, and whether these effects produce long-term sequelae (e.g., chronic sympathetic activation). Indeed, it is relevant to note that exposure to repetitive hypoxia and hypercapnia in humans leads to elevated sympathetic activation after removal of the stimuli (90), and repetitive hypoxia leads to chronic hypertension in rats (91). Discharge of locus coeruleus neurons is increased by increased $PaCO_2$ and decreased Pa_{O2}, and these effects are associated with increased sympathetic output (92,93). Some medullary raphe neurons also increase their firing rates with increased levels of inspired CO_2 (84). Further studies on the basic neuronal mechanisms engaged at arousal from sleep, the modulation of these activities by changes in chemical respiratory stimuli associated with sleep-disordered breathing, and the role of central neuronal processes in modulating autonomic outputs will improve the understanding of the mechanisms underlying the large HR and BP responses at arousal from sleep and the clinical consequences.

References

1. Shepard JW Jr. Hypertension, cardiac arrhythmias, myocardial infarction, and stroke in relation to obstructive sleep apnea. Clin Chest Med 1992; 13:437–458.
2. Bradley TD. Right and left ventricular functional impairment and sleep apnea. Clin Chest Med 1992; 13:459–479.
3. Brooks D, Horner RL, Kozar LF, et al. Obstructive sleep apnea as a cause of systemic hypertension. Evidence from a canine model. J Clin Invest 1997; 99:106–109.
4. Young T, Palta M, Dempsey J, et al. The occurrence of sleep-disordered breathing among middle-aged adults. N Engl J Med 1993; 328:1230–1235.
5. Phillipson EA. Sleep apnea—a major public health problem. N Engl J Med 1993; 328:1271–1273.
6. Dempsey JA. Sleep apnea causes daytime hypertension. J Clin Invest 1997; 99:1–2.
7. Davies RJ, Crosby J, Vardi-Visy K, et al. Non-invasive beat to beat arterial blood pressure during non-REM sleep in obstructive sleep apnoea and snoring. Thorax 1994; 49:335–339.
8. Mancia G, Zanchetti A. Cardiovascular regulation during sleep. In: Orem J, Barnes CD, eds. *Physiology in Sleep.* New York: Academic Press, 1980:1–55.
9. Coote JH. Respiratory and circulatory control during sleep. J Exp Biol 1982; 100:223–244.
10. Baccelli G, Guazzi M, Mancia G, et al. Neural and non-neural mechanisms influencing circulation during sleep. Nature 1969; 223:184–185.
11. Khatri IM, Freis ED. Hemodynamic changes during sleep. J Appl Physiol 1967; 22:867–873.
12. Mancia G, Baccelli G, Adams DB, et al. Vasomotor regulation during sleep in the cat. Am J Physiol 1971; 220:1086–1093.
13. Parmeggiani PL. The auronomic nervous system in sleep. In: Kryger MH, Roth T, Dement WC, eds. *Principles and Practice of Sleep Medicine.* Philadelphia: Saunders, 1994:194–203.
14. Sei H, Sakai K, Kanamori N, et al. Long-term variations of arterial blood pressure during sleep in freely moving cats. Physiol Behav 1994; 55:673–679.
15. Baust W, Bohnert B. The regulation of heart rate during sleep. Exp Brain Res 1969; 7:169–180.
16. Hornyak M, Cejnar M, Elam M, et al. Sympathetic muscle nerve activity during sleep in man. Brain 1991; 114(pt 3):1281–1295.
17. Okada H, Iwase S, Mano T, et al. Changes in muscle sympathetic nerve activity during sleep in humans. Neurology 1991; 41:1961–1966.
18. Somers VK, Dyken ME, Mark AL, et al. Sympathetic-nerve activity during sleep in normal subjects. N Engl J Med 1993; 328:303–307.
19. Baust W, Weidinger H, Kirchner F. Sympathetic activity during natural sleep and arousal. Arch Ital Biol 1968; 106:379–390.
20. Horner RL, Brooks D, Kozar LF, et al. Immediate effects of arousal from sleep on cardiac autonomic outflow in the absence of breathing in dogs. J Appl Physiol 1995; 79:151–162.
21. Zemaityte D, Varoneckas G, Sokolov E. Heart rhythm control during sleep. Psychophysiology 1984; 21:279–289.
22. Kirby DA, Verrier RL. Differential effects of sleep stage on coronary hemodynamic function. Am J Physiol 1989; 256:H1378–H1383.
23. Verrier RL, Lau TR, Wallooppillai U, et al. Primary vagally mediated decelerations in heart rate during tonic rapid eye movement sleep in cats. Am J Physiol 1998; 274:R1136–R1141.
24. Furlan R, Guzzetti S, Crivellaro W, et al. Continuous 24-hour assessment of the neural regulation of systemic arterial pressure and RR variabilities in ambulant subjects. Circulation 1990; 81:537–547.
25. Berlad II, Shlitner A, Ben-Haim S, et al. Power spectrum analysis and heart rate variability in Stage 4 and REM sleep: evidence for state-specific changes in autonomic dominance. J Sleep Res 1993; 2:88–90.
26. Futuro-Neto HA, Coote JH. Changes in sympathetic activity to heart and blood vessels during desynchronized sleep. Brain Res 1982; 252:259–268.

27. Akselrod S, Gordon D, Madwed JB, et al. Hemodynamic regulation: investigation by spectral analysis. Am J Physiol 1985; 249:H867–H875.

28. Novak V, Novak P, de Champlain J, et al. Influence of respiration on heart rate and blood pressure fluctuations. J Appl Physiol 1993; 74:617–626.

29. Phillipson EA, Bowes G. Control of breathing during sleep. In: Cherniack NS, Widdicombe JG, eds. Handbook of Physiology, Sect 3, The Respiratory System, Vol 2, Control of Breathing, part 2. Bethesda, MD: American Physiological Society, 1986:649–689.

30. Henke KG, Badr MS, Skatrud JB, et al. Load compensation and respiratory muscle function during sleep. J Appl Physiol 1992; 72:1221–1234.

31. Kollai M, Koizumi K. Reciprocal and non-reciprocal action of the vagal and sympathetic nerves innervating the heart. J Auton Nerv Syst 1979; 1:33–52.

32. Seals DR, Suwarno NO, Dempsey JA. Influence of lung volume on sympathetic nerve discharge in normal humans. Circ Res 1990; 67:130–141.

33. Somers VK, Mark AL, Zavala DC, et al. Influence of ventilation and hypocapnia on sympathetic nerve responses to hypoxia in normal humans. J Appl Physiol 1989; 67:2095–2100.

34. Glenn LL, Foutz AS, Dement WC. Membrane potential of spinal motoneurons during natural sleep in cats. Sleep 1978; 1:199–204.

35. Orem J. Respiratory neurons and sleep. In: Kryger MH, Roth T, Dement WC, eds. *Principles and Practice of Sleep Medicine*. Philadelphia: Saunders, 1994:177–193.

36. Horner RL, Kozar LF, Kimoff RJ, et al. Effects of sleep on the tonic drive to respiratory muscle and the threshold for rhythm generation in the dog. J Physiol 1994; 474:525–537.

37. George CF, Kryger MH. Sleep and control of heart rate. Clin Chest Med 1985; 6:595–601.

38. Skatrud JB, Dempsey JA. Airway resistance and respiratory muscle function in snorers during NREM sleep. J Appl Physiol 1985; 59:328–335.

39. Hudgel DW, Mulholland M, Hendricks C. Neuromuscular and mechanical responses to inspiratory resistive loading during sleep. J Appl Physiol 1987; 63:603–608.

40. Hudgel DW. The role of upper airway anatomy and physiology in obstructive sleep apnea. Clin Chest Med 1992; 13:383–398.

41. Orem J, Netick A, Dement WC. Increased upper airway resistance to breathing during sleep in the cat. Electroencephalogr Clin Neurophysiol 1977; 43:14–22.

42. Anrep GV, Pascual W, Rossler R. Respiratory variations of the heart rate. II. The central mechanism of the respiratory arrhythmia and the inter-relations between the central and the reflex mechanisms. Proc R Soc Lond B 1936; 119:218–230.

43. De Burgh Daly M. Interactions between respiration and circulation. In: Cherniack NS, Widdicombe JG, eds. *Handbook of Physiology, Sect 3, The Respiratory System, Vol 2, Control of Breathing, part 2*. Bethesda, MD: American Physiological Society, 1986:529–594.

44. Shykoff BE, Naqvi SS, Menon AS, et al. Respiratory sinus arrhythmia in dogs. Effects of phasic afferents and chemostimulation. J Clin Invest 1991; 87:1621–1627.

45. Horner RL, Brooks D, Kozar LF, et al. Respiratory-related heart rate variability persists during central apnea in dogs: mechanisms and implications. J Appl Physiol 1995; 78:2003–2013.

46. Shea SA. Behavioural and arousal-related influences on breathing in humans. Exp Physiol 1996; 81:1–26.

47. Hirsch JA, Bishop B. Respiratory sinus arrhythmia in humans: how breathing pattern modulates heart rate. Am J Physiol 1981; 241:H620–H629.

48. Morgan BJ, Crabtree DC, Puleo DS, et al. Neurocirculatory consequences of abrupt change in sleep state in humans. J Appl Physiol 1996; 80:1627–1636.

49. Halasz P. Arousals without awakening—dynamic aspect of sleep. Physiol Behav 1993; 54:795–802.

50. Skatrud JB, Dempsey JA. Interaction of sleep state and chemical stimuli in sustaining rhythmic ventilation. J Appl Physiol 1983; 55:813–822.

51. Datta AK, Shea SA, Horner RL, et al. The influence of induced hypocapnia and sleep on the endogenous respiratory rhythm in humans. J Physiol 1991; 440:17–33. Erratum in: J Physiol (Lond) 1991; 444:778.

52. Phillipson EA, Murphy E, Kozar LF. Regulation of respiration in sleeping dogs. J Appl Physiol 1976; 40:688–693.

53. Hudgel DW, Martin RJ, Johnson B, et al. Mechanics of the respiratory system and breathing pattern during sleep in normal humans. J Appl Physiol 1984; 56:133–137.

54. Wiegand L, Zwillich CW, White DP. Sleep and the ventilatory response to resistive loading in normal men. J Appl Physiol 1988; 64:1186–1195.

55. Orem J, Osorio I, Brooks E, et al. Activity of respiratory neurons during NREM sleep. J Neurophysiol 1985; 54:1144–1156.

56. Phillipson EA. Sleep disorders. In: Murray JF, Nadel JA, eds. *Textbook of Respiratory Medicine.* Philadelphia: Saunders, 1988:1841–1860.

57. Bradley TD, Phillipson EA. Central sleep apnea. Clin Chest Med 1992; 13:493–505.

58. Horner RL, Rivera MP, Kozar LF, et al. The ventilatory response to arousal from sleep is not fully explained by differences in CO2 levels between sleep and wakefulness. J Physiol 2001; 534:881–890.

59. Trinder J, Padula M, Berlowitz D, et al. Cardiac and respiratory activity at arousal from sleep under controlled ventilation conditions. J Appl Physiol 2001; 90:1455–1463.

60. Smyth HS, Sleight P, Pickering GW. Reflex regulation of arterial pressure during sleep in man. A quantitative method of assessing baroreflex sensitivity. Circ Res 1969; 24:109–121.

61. Pickering GW, Sleight P, Smyth HS. The reflex regulation of arterial pressure during sleep in man. J Physiol 1968; 194:46P–48P.

62. Conway J, Boon N, Jones JV, et al. Involvement of the baroreceptor reflexes in the changes in blood pressure with sleep and mental arousal. Hypertension 1983; 5:746–748.

63. Carrington MJ, Barbieri R, Colrain IM, et al. Changes in cardiovascular function during the sleep onset period in young adults. J Appl Physiol 2005; 98:468–476.

64. Bristow JD, Honour AJ, Pickering TG, et al. Cardiovascular and respiratory changes during sleep in normal and hypertensive subjects. Cardiovasc Res 1969; 3:476–485.

65. Guazzi M, Zanchetti A. Blood pressure and heart rate during natural sleep of the cat and their regulation by carotid sinus and aortic reflexes. Arch Ital Biol 1965; 103:789–817.

66. Hilton SM, The defence-arousal system and its relevance for circulatory and respiratory control. J Exp Biol 1982; 100:159–174.

67. Hilton SM. Ways of viewing the central nervous control of the circulation–old and new. Brain Res 1975; 87:213–219.

68. Horner RL, Sanford LD, Pack AI, et al. Activation of a distinct arousal state immediately after spontaneous awakening from sleep. Brain Res 1997; 778:127–134.

69. Aston-Jones G, Bloom FE. Activity of norepinephrine-containing locus coeruleus neurons in behaving rats anticipates fluctuations in the sleep-waking cycle. J Neurosci 1981; 1:876–886.

70. Trulson ME, Jacobs BL. Raphe unit activity in freely moving cats: correlation with level of behavioral arousal. Brain Res 1979; 163:135–150.

71. Jacobs BL, Azmitia EC. Structure and function of the brain serotonin system. Physiol Rev 1992; 72:165–229.

72. Horner RL. Arousal mechanisms and autonomic consequences. In: Pack AI, ed. *Sleep Apnea: Pathogenesis, Diagnosis and Treatment.* New York: Dekker, 2002:179–216.

73. Horner RL. Arousal from sleep—perspectives relating to autonomic function. Sleep 2003; 26:644–645.

74. Trinder J, Allen N, Kleiman J, et al. On the nature of cardiovascular activation at an arousal from sleep. Sleep 2003; 26(5):543–551.

75. Halasz P, Terzano M, Parrino L, et al. The nature of arousal in sleep. J Sleep Res 2004; 13:1–23.

76. Eckberg DL, Sleight P. Human baroreflexes in health and disease. Monogr Physiol Soc 1992; 43:79–119.
77. Foote SL, Bloom FE, Aston-Jones G. Nucleus locus ceruleus: new evidence of anatomical and physiological specificity. Physiol Rev 1983; 63:844–914.
78. Jacobs BL, Fornal CA. Activation of 5-HT neuronal activity during motor behavior. Semin Neurosci 1995; 7:401–408.
79. Guyenet PG. Role of the ventral medulla oblongata in blood pressure regulation. In: Loewy AD, Spyer KM, eds. *Central Regulation of Autonomic Functions*. Oxford: University Press, 1990:145–167.
80. Reiner PB. Correlational analysis of central noradrenergic neuronal activity and sympathetic tone in behaving cats. Brain Res 1986; 378:86–96.
81. Heym J, Steinfels GF, Jacobs BL. Activity of serotonin-containing neurons in the nucleus raphe pallidus of freely moving cats. Brain Res 1982; 251:259–276.
82. Trulson ME, Trulson VM. Activity of nucleus raphe pallidus neurons across the sleep-waking cycle in freely moving cats. Brain Res 1982; 237:232–237.
83. Fornal C, Auerbach S, Jacobs BL. Activity of serotonin-containing neurons in nucleus raphe magnus in freely moving cats. Exp Neurol 1985; 88:590–608.
84. Veasey SC, Fornal CA, Metzler CW, et al. Response of serotonergic caudal raphe neurons in relation to specific motor activities in freely moving cats. J Neurosci 1995; 15:5346–5359.
85. Loewy AD. Raphe pallidus and raphe obscurus projections to the intermediolateral cell column in the rat. Brain Res 1981; 222:129–133.
86. Coote JH. Bulbospinal serotonergic pathways in the control of blood pressure. J Cardiovasc Pharmacol 1990; 15(suppl 7):S35–S41.
87. McCall RB. Evidence for a serotonergically mediated sympathoexcitatory response to stimulation of medullary raphe nuclei. Brain Res 1984; 311:131–139.
88. Pilowsky PM, Kapoor V, Minson JB, et al. Spinal cord serotonin release and raised blood pressure after brainstem kainic acid injection. Brain Res 1986; 366:354–357.
89. Pickering AE, Spanswick D, Logan SD. 5-Hydoxytryptamine evokes depolarizations and membrane potential oscillations in rat sympathetic preganglionic neurones. J Physiol 1994; 480(pt 1):109–121.
90. Morgan BJ, Crabtree DC, Palta M, et al. Combined hypoxia and hypercapnia evokes long-lasting sympathetic activation in humans. J Appl Physiol 1995; 79:205–213.
91. Fletcher EC, Lesske J, Qian W, et al. Repetitive, episodic hypoxia causes diurnal elevation of blood pressure in rats. Hypertension 1992; 19:555–561.
92. Elam M, Yao T, Thoren P, et al. Hypercapnia and hypoxia: chemoreceptor-mediated control of locus coeruleus neurons and splanchnic, sympathetic nerves. Brain Res 1981; 222:373–381.
93. Guyenet PG, Koshiya N, Huangfu D, et al. Central respiratory control of A5 and A6 pontine noradrenergic neurons. Am J Physiol 1993; 264:R1035–R1044.

6
Sleep Apnea and Alterations in Glucose Metabolism

NARESH M. PUNJABI
Johns Hopkins University School of Medicine, Baltimore, Maryland, U.S.A.

I. Introduction

The past few decades have witnessed a significant increase in the prevalence of obesity worldwide. Although the problem initially gripped industrialized nations, it has rapidly expanded to less developed nations and is having far-reaching public health and economic implications (1). The problem of excess body weight is of concern not only in adults but also in adolescents and young children. Data from the 2000 National Health and Nutrition Examination Survey (NHANES) show that approximately 34% of adults in the United States are overweight and an additional 31% are obese (2). Longitudinal data from the NHANES cohort indicate that the prevalence of obesity in U.S. adults continues to rise (3). It is well established that being overweight or obese increases the risk for a number of chronic conditions, including hypertension, cardiovascular disease, stroke, type 2 diabetes, obstructive sleep apnea, and depression (4,5).

Of the numerous obesity-related complications, the problem of type 2 diabetes has reached epidemic proportions. The International Diabetes Federation estimates that the number of adults with type 2 diabetes worldwide will increase by 122% from 135 million in 1995 to 300 million in 2025 (6,7). Recognizing the enormity of the human and economic costs, the United Nations General Assembly in 2006 declared type 2 diabetes the first noncommunicable disease that threatens world health to the same magnitude as communicable diseases such as HIV infection and tuberculosis (8). Established risk factors for type 2 diabetes include age, obesity, a sedentary lifestyle, and a shift toward a high-energy diet (9,10). Over the last decade, there is a growing recognition that habitual short sleep duration may increase the propensity for metabolic abnormalities (11). Observational and experimental data indicate that disorders of sleep, such as sleep apnea, may also increase the risk for metabolic dysfunction. The possibility of an independent and causal association between sleep apnea and metabolic dysfunction has led to an explosion in research on the mechanisms that may explain the observed association. In fact, a number of comprehensive reviews (12–15) have summarized the evidence for an independent association between sleep apnea and altered glucose metabolism. The purpose of this chapter is to review the available evidence on the potential mechanisms through which sleep apnea could alter glucose metabolism, with a particular emphasis on the independent effects of sleep fragmentation and intermittent hypoxemia. Alterations in autonomic activity, changes in corticotropic function, increase in oxidative stress, activation of inflammatory pathways, and increase in circulating adipokines induced by sleep fragmentation and intermittent hypoxemia are some of the potential processes that could link sleep apnea to adverse metabolic outcomes. While each of the aforementioned mechanisms will be discussed individually, the metabolic effects of sleep apnea are most likely due to a synergistic and interactive network of pathophysiological derangements.

II. Diabetes Mellitus: Definition and Diagnosis

The American Diabetes Association (ADA) consensus guidelines define diabetes mellitus as a group of conditions that are characterized by hyperglycemia resulting either from defects in insulin secretion, insulin action, or both (16). Type 1 diabetes mellitus, which accounts for only 5% of all diabetes cases, results from cell-mediated autoimmune destruction of the pancreatic β cells. Type 2 diabetes mellitus, which accounts for approximately 90% of all diabetes cases, results from a deficit of both insulin sensitivity and insulin secretion. Most patients with type 2 diabetes are obese, and many remain undiagnosed. The third category of diabetes encompasses a group of heterogeneous disorders that include genetic defects of the pancreatic β cells, drug or chemical-induced pancreatic injury, and infections. Finally, the fourth category of diabetes is gestational diabetes, which is defined as any degree of glucose intolerance that develops during pregnancy. The diagnostic criteria for type 2 diabetes are as follows: (a) symptoms of polyuria, polydipsia, or unexplained weight loss and a random glucose level ≥ 200 mg/dL; (b) fasting glucose level ≥ 126 mg/dL; and (c) a two-hour post-challenge glucose level ≥ 200 during an oral glucose tolerance test (OGTT). In addition, the ADA guidelines also define two prediabetic conditions, which include impaired fasting glucose and impaired glucose tolerance. Impaired fasting glucose is defined as a fasting glucose level between 100 and 125 mg/dL. Impaired glucose tolerance is defined as a two-hour postchallenge glucose level between 140 and 200 mg/dL during an OGTT. Although the pathogenesis of type 2 diabetes is beyond the scope of the current discussion, it is important to briefly outline its natural history. It is now well recognized that development of type 2 diabetes is a multistep process along a continuum from normoglycemia to hyperglycemia. This continuum is temporally characterized initially by insulin resistance and compensatory hyperinsulinemia. With increasing duration of insulin resistance, glucose intolerance eventually develops and finally culminates in the expression of type 2 diabetes. Although there has been a great deal of controversy, the body of available data indicates that both insulin resistance and pancreatic β-cell dysfunction are essential in the development of type 2 diabetes. In the following sections, the evidence linking sleep apnea and altered glucose metabolism is reviewed with an emphasis on causal pathways.

III. Sleep Apnea and Abnormalities in Glucose Metabolism

In light of the fact that insulin resistance, even in the absence of overt diabetes, is a risk factor for cardiovascular disease, there is clinical significance in understanding whether sleep apnea causes insulin resistance and glucose intolerance. The first comprehensive analysis of the published literature on this topic was conducted in 2003, and it classified the available studies into three groups (12). The first group of studies examined whether sleep apnea–related symptoms (e.g., snoring, witnessed apneas) were correlated with metabolic dysfunction (17–28). The second group of studies examined whether polysomnographically defined sleep apnea was correlated with metabolic dysfunction (29–50). The third group of studies examined whether treatment with continuous positive airway pressure (CPAP) therapy had favorable effects on glucose metabolism. Based on this comprehensive review, it became evident that many of the initial publications on sleep apnea and glucose metabolism suffered from methodological limitations, including small sample sizes and inadequate consideration for the confounding effects of factors such as obesity. By highlighting major gaps in the field, the review also stimulated additional research in the area, and several studies, which avoided many of the previous methodological pitfalls, were subsequently published.

Studies with overnight polysomnography have found an independent association between sleep apnea, insulin resistance, glucose intolerance, and type 2 diabetes (29–50). Although there are some discrepancies, a majority of publications to date indicate that measures of sleep apnea severity, such as the apnea-hypopnea index (AHI), severity of nocturnal oxyhemoglobin desaturation, and degree of sleep fragmentation, are associated with metabolic dysfunction. Careful consideration of body mass index (BMI) and waist circumference as confounders in these studies has strengthened the notion that metabolic dysfunction may indeed be a consequence of sleep apnea. Longitudinal data correlating symptoms of sleep apnea (21,22) or polysomnographically defined sleep apnea (51,52) also appear to substantiate the possibility of a causal role for sleep apnea in metabolic dysfunction. Studies on the effects of CPAP therapy on metabolic function in sleep apnea, however, have produced mixed results. While some investigators have demonstrated a beneficial effect of CPAP (53–57), others have found no effect (58–65). It is certainly possible that chronic exposure to intermittent hypoxemia and sleep disruption in sleep apnea lead to irreversible changes in glucose metabolism. Alternatively, the lack of a control group and small sample sizes in many of the interventional studies may have limited their ability to detect whether CPAP has favorable effects on insulin resistance or glycemic control. Additional research is clearly needed to determine whether CPAP can improve metabolic function.

Glucose metabolism in sleep apnea has generally been characterized using steady-state measures such as levels of fasting glucose and/or insulin. While these measures have been highly informative, a major drawback is their inability to characterize the dynamic relation between insulin sensitivity and insulin secretion. It is well established that a decrease in peripheral insulin sensitivity is fed back to the pancreatic β cells, which increase insulin output to maintain normal glucose tolerance. A defect in this compensatory response in the face of insulin resistance is central to the pathogenesis of glucose intolerance and type 2 diabetes. The intravenous glucose tolerance test can be used to model in vivo glucose and insulin kinetics and concurrently assess insulin sensitivity and insulin secretion. Using this dynamic approach to examine glucose metabolism, it has been recently shown that patients with sleep apnea demonstrate impairments in insulin-dependent and insulin-independent glucose disposal (66). Moreover, the expected increase in pancreatic insulin secretion, which is necessary to compensate for insulin resistance, appears to be blunted in patients with sleep apnea. These findings indicate that sleep apnea may diminish not only insulin sensitivity but also insulin secretion from the pancreatic β cells.

IV. Mechanistic Links Between Sleep Apnea and Altered Glucose Metabolism

If sufficient evidence eventually implicates sleep apnea as a risk factor for metabolic dysfunction, what then are the potential mechanisms that mediate these effects? Unquestionably, sleep-related hypoxemia and recurrent arousals will have an independent and fundamental role. A number of animal and human studies have shown that exposure to hypoxia (sustained or intermittent) can alter normal glucose homeostasis. Indeed, exposure to sustained hypoxia increases fasting insulin levels in newborn rats (67,68) and calves (69). Similarly, exposure to intermittent hypoxia also increases fasting insulin levels in obese mice (70). Experimental studies in humans corroborate the hypothesis that hypoxia can adversely affect glucose metabolism. Normal subjects demonstrate a decrease in insulin sensitivity and insulin secretion when exposed to either sustained or intermittent hypoxia (71–74).

Sleep apnea–related disruption of sleep continuity may also adversely affect glucose metabolism. Although empirical data on the effects of sleep fragmentation are limited, two independent groups have demonstrated negative effects of sleep fragmentation on insulin sensitivity in normal subjects (75,76). The mechanisms through which intermittent hypoxemia and sleep fragmentation could affect glucose metabolism include (*i*) alterations in sympathetic nervous system activity, (*ii*) changes in activity of the hypothalamic-pituitary-adrenal (HPA) axis, (*iii*) formation of reactive oxygen species, and (*iv*) increases in inflammatory cytokines [i.e., interleukin-6 (IL-6) and tumor necrosis factor α (TNF-α)] and adipocyte-derived factors (i.e., leptin, adiponectin, and resistin).

A. Sympathetic Nervous System Activity as a Causal Intermediate

Compared to normal subjects, patients with sleep apnea exhibit higher levels of sympathetic nervous system activity not just during sleep but also during wakefulness (77). The decrease in oxyhemoglobin saturation and the concurrent increase in carbon dioxide with each disordered breathing event elicit a chemoreflex-mediated surge in sympathetic activity (78,79). Observational and experimental studies have demonstrated that even brief arousals from sleep can lead to a surge in sympathetic activity (80,81). Thus, intermittent hypoxemia and recurrent arousals from sleep can shift autonomic balance in patients with sleep apnea. As described below, an increase in sympathetic nervous activity can alter glucose homeostasis and increase the risk for type 2 diabetes.

Although the exact mechanisms through which sympathetic activation affects insulin sensitivity are not well defined, there is little doubt it has a central role in the regulation of glucose and fat metabolism (82). Catecholamines reduce insulin sensitivity and insulin-mediated glucose uptake (83). Administration of epinephrine in normal subjects can decrease insulin-mediated glycogenesis, increase glycolysis, and dampen the ability of glucose to stimulate its own disposal (84,85). Higher levels of sympathetic activity have lipolytic effects through signaling pathways that activate hormone-sensitive lipase, which can mobilize nonesterified fatty acids (86). An abrupt increase in circulating free fatty acids can worsen insulin sensitivity, while a decrease can improve insulin sensitivity, hyperinsulinemia, and glucose tolerance (87,88).

In addition to the above effects, activation of the sympathetic nervous system can lead to systemic vasoconstriction, which can also affect glucose metabolism. A decrease in vascular lumen size in skeletal muscle from vasoconstriction shunts glucose and insulin to less metabolically active areas of skeletal muscle (89) and thus decreases overall glucose uptake (90). Sympathetic activation can also alter skeletal muscle morphology to a more insulin-resistant type (91), inhibit insulin signaling, and decrease insulin-mediated glucose uptake by adipocytes (92). Thus, there is sufficient basis to speculate that an increase in sympathetic nervous system activity due to recurrent intermittent hypoxemia and sleep fragmentation plays a central role in altering glucose metabolism in sleep apnea.

B. HPA Axis as a Causal Intermediate

The HPA axis is a vital neuroendocrine system not only for maintenance of normal homeostasis but also for the adaptive responses to physiological challenges. Recurrent intermittent hypoxemia and arousals from sleep could alter glucose metabolism by modulating the function of the HPA axis. Specifically, a stress-related increase in HPA activity and cortisol secretion could lead to insulin resistance and hyperglycemia. Observational data from studies of high altitude or of hypobaric conditions indicate that hypoxia modifies the diurnal pattern of the HPA axis and increases circulating cortisol (93–99). Moreover, brief arousals or sustained awakenings from sleep can activate the HPA axis and can further augment corticotropic function (100,101). Despite such robust findings on the effects of hypoxia and sleep fragmentation, conclusive data on HPA dysfunction in sleep apnea are lacking and additional research is clearly needed (102–108). A notable limitation in many of the available studies is that corticotropic function has been assessed with a single measurement of serum cortisol. While convenient, isolated cortisol measurements cannot reveal diurnal changes or the temporal variability in cortisol secretion. Characterizing HPA dysfunction in sleep apnea has scientific and clinical relevance, as it would help clarify its putative role in mediating insulin resistance and glucose intolerance. It is well established that cortisol and other glucocorticoids interfere with glucose metabolism at several different levels (109,110). Cortisol increases hepatic gluconeogenesis and causes protein degradation. It also activates lipoprotein lipase, which mobilizes nonesterified fatty acids, which can greatly diminish insulin sensitivity. Moreover, cortisol inhibits β-cell secretion of insulin and sequentially modifies multiple aspects of the insulin-mediated glucose transport system. Given the myriad of adverse metabolic effects of HPA dysfunction, further research is needed to determine whether sleep apnea affects HPA activity and thus alters normal metabolic function.

C. Oxidative Stress as a Causal Intermediate

Oxidative stress reflects a condition where the production of reactive oxygen species exceeds antioxidant defenses. Reactive oxygen species are free radicals that are associated with oxygen and normally formed during endogenous biochemical reactions. While reactive oxygen species play an important role in an array of biological functions, excess production can have deleterious effects. An increase in reactive oxygen species has been associated with a number of acute and chronic medical conditions, including hypertension, cardiovascular disease, and type 2 diabetes (111). Repetitive cycles of hypoxemia followed by reoxygenation in patients with sleep apnea provide the physiologic milieu for increased reactive oxygen species production similar to that seen with ischemia-reperfusion injury. With acute ischemia, a complex set of pathophysiological events occurs at the cellular level in response to the low levels or complete absence of oxygen. Restoration of blood flow with cellular reoxygenation paradoxically initiates a cascade of events leading to additional cell injury above and beyond that imposed by the initial insult. Measures of reactive oxygen species include susceptibility of low-density lipoprotein to free-radical challenge, red cell glutathione peroxidase and catalase activity, red blood cell fragility, and total cellular thiol levels. Irrespective of the measure used, available data suggest that sleep apnea is associated with higher concentrations of reactive oxygen species (112–121). Differences in lipid peroxidation, isoprostane levels, and markers of DNA oxidation have been documented between patients with sleep apnea and normal subjects. Furthermore, studies examining the effects of treatment have shown a decline in several reactive oxygen species with CPAP therapy (113,114,118).

High concentrations of reactive oxygen species can be potentially damaging to the pancreatic β cells, given their relatively low levels of antioxidant enzymes (122). Reactive oxygen species have been shown to suppress insulin secretion and diminish insulin-stimulated substrate uptake in muscle and adipose tissue (122–125). Furthermore, antioxidants such as vitamin E, vitamin C, and lipoic acid have been associated with improvements in insulin sensitivity and glycemic control (126–129). In light of such findings, abnormalities of glucose metabolism in sleep apnea could well be mediated by the effects of oxidative stress induced by intermittent hypoxemia.

D.   Systemic Inflammation as a Causal Intermediate

There is a growing recognition that low-grade systemic inflammation may be yet another mechanism relating sleep apnea to cardiovascular disease. Inflammation plays an important role in arterial plaque formation, plaque rupture, and vascular thrombosis, thereby increasing the susceptibility to myocardial ischemia and infarction (130). Compared to normal subjects, sleep apnea patients have higher levels of circulating adhesion molecules (131–136) and inflammatory cytokines, including IL-6 and TNF-α, which decrease with CPAP therapy (137–140). Studies examining specific leukocyte populations also reveal that sleep apnea patients exhibit monocyte and lymphocyte activation, which improves with CPAP therapy (141–143). Experimental work in normal subjects has shown that hypoxia increases circulating leukocyte concentration and alters the functional characteristics of lymphocytes (144–146). Sympathetic hyperactivity in sleep apnea may also influence the innate immune response, given that adrenergic stimulation enhances macrophages and lymphocytes activity and alters their proliferation, circulation, and cytokine production (147,148).

Systemic inflammation is now recognized as a key element in the pathogenesis of insulin resistance and type 2 diabetes. Epidemiologic studies are abundant, illustrating that high levels of circulating IL-6, TNF-α, and C-reactive protein (CRP) predict the development of type 2 diabetes (149–156). The availability of longitudinal data in many of these studies strengthens the argument for a causal versus a correlative association between low-grade systemic inflammation and metabolic dysfunction. Additional support for the role of systemic inflammation in the pathogenesis of metabolic dysfunction comes from animal experiments, which show that disruption or transgenic overexpression of inflammatory genes can alter the propensity for insulin resistance and type 2 diabetes (157,158). However, a concern in invoking systemic inflammation as an intermediate between sleep apnea and metabolic dysfunction is the confounding effects of obesity.

Adipose tissue can increase systemic inflammation, as visceral adiposity has an enhanced capacity to produce numerous cytokines including IL-6 and TNF-α. However, it appears that even after considering the effects of BMI and measures of visceral obesity, sleep apnea severity is independently correlated with the degree of inflammatory burden (159). Thus, low-grade systemic inflammation could potentially mediate the adverse metabolic effects of sleep apnea.

E. Adipokines as Causal Intermediates

The adipocyte is a vital endocrine cell that secretes biologically active factors, or adipokines, that influence energy and glucose homeostasis (160). Factors such as leptin, adiponectin, and resistin have a significant role in the genesis of obesity-related abnormalities in glucose metabolism. Leptin regulates hunger and weight gain by increasing anorexigenic and decreasing orexigenic neuropeptides in the hypothalamus (161). Peripherally, leptin appears to be involved in governing glucose homeostasis (162,163). A growing body of literature shows that patients with sleep apnea have higher leptin levels (48,50,164–168), which decrease with CPAP therapy, independent of any changes in body weight (61,62,169,170). Moreover, exposure to hypoxic conditions increases leptin levels in normal subjects (171). Thus, higher leptin levels in sleep apnea could certainly alter glucose metabolism.

Adiponectin is also synthesized by the adipocyte and has been show to have endogenous insulin-sensitizing properties. Animal models lacking adiponectin develop insulin resistance (172,173), and a high adiponectin level in humans has been shown to protect against type 2 diabetes (174). Given that alterations in adiponectin levels influence insulin sensitivity and increase the risk for type 2 diabetes (175), its role in sleep apnea–related metabolic dysfunction is important. Adiponectin in patients with sleep apnea is lower than in normal subjects, and circulating levels appear to correlate with the nadir in oxygen saturation (176–182). Resistin is another adipocytokine that inhibits insulin action and may explain part of the link between obesity and type 2 diabetes (183,184). At present, there are limited data on whether resistin levels differ between sleep apnea patients and control subjects (176,185,186). Clearly, additional work is needed to determine how adiponectin and resistin are affected by intermittent hypoxemia and recurrent arousals and whether these adipocytokines explicate the observation of metabolic dysfunction in sleep apnea.

V. Summary and Directions for Future Research

The above discussion was aimed at examining some of the physiologic processes through which sleep apnea and its concomitants, intermittent hypoxemia and sleep fragmentation, may increase the risk of insulin resistance, glucose intolerance, and type 2 diabetes. Substantial advancements have been made in identifying an independent association between sleep apnea and abnormalities of glucose metabolism. The complex tapestry that interconnects these two conditions is being slowly unraveled through animal and human studies for a detailed understanding of the underlying mechanisms. Nonetheless, many important questions remain. For example, which patient factors (e.g., obesity or age) modify the association between sleep apnea and glucose metabolism? Are insulin resistance, glucose intolerance, and glycemic control in sleep apnea altered by CPAP therapy? Studies aimed at such questions are forthcoming and will provide the

Syndrome X (or Syndrome Zzzz...)

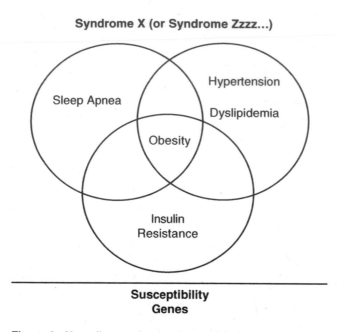

**Susceptibility
Genes**

Figure 1 Venn diagram showing the multiple intersects between obesity, sleep apnea, and the individual components of the metabolic syndrome.

empirical evidence to justify case identification and early intervention to avert some of the metabolic toll imposed by sleep apnea.

   It is also important to note that while much of the focus in this chapter was on how sleep apnea may "cause" altered glucose metabolism, a bidirectional association is likely between these two conditions. That is, while sleep apnea may alter metabolic function, type 2 diabetes may in turn lead to breathing abnormalities during sleep (187–194). Some have also postulated (195–197) that perhaps sleep apnea is a component of metabolic syndrome and that the constellation of central obesity, insulin resistance, dyslipidemia, hypertension, and sleep apnea rests on a common soil of susceptible genes (Fig. 1). Whether this alliance with other known cardiovascular risk factors is of clinical or public health significance remains to be determined. Irrespective of the directionality of causal relations or the metabolic hierarchy in which sleep apnea may eventually find a niche, it is becoming ever increasingly clear that sleep apnea and type 2 diabetes are reaching epidemic proportions. Thus, there is an urgent need for all health care professionals who manage either of these conditions to identify those that are affected by the other disorder but remain undiagnosed.

References

1. World Health Organization. Obesity and overweight. World Health Organization, 2006. Available at: http://www.who.int/dietphysicalactivity/publications/facts/obesity/en/. Accessed January 1, 2007.
2. Flegal KM, Carroll MD, Ogden CL, et al. Prevalence and trends in obesity among US adults, 1999–2000. JAMA 2002; 288(14):1723–1727.

3. Ogden CL, Carroll MD, Curtin LR, et al. Prevalence of overweight and obesity in the United States, 1999–2004. JAMA 2006; 295(13):1549–1555.
4. Field AE, Coakley EH, Must A, et al. Impact of overweight on the risk of developing common chronic diseases during a 10-year period. Arch Intern Med 2001; 161(13):1581–1586.
5. Visscher TL, Seidell JC. The public health impact of obesity. Annu Rev Public Health 2001; 22:355–375.
6. King H, Aubert RE, Herman WH. Global burden of diabetes, 1995–2025: prevalence, numerical estimates, and projections. Diabetes Care 1998; 21(9):1414–1431.
7. Wild S, Roglic G, Green A, et al. Global prevalence of diabetes: estimates for the year 2000 and projections for 2030. Diabetes Care 2004; 27(5):1047–1053.
8. United Nations General Assembly. World Diabetes Day, 61/225, 2006. Available at: http://www.worlddiabetesday.org/files/docs/WDD_Resolution.pdf.
9. DeFronzo RA. Pathogenesis of type 2 diabetes mellitus. Med Clin North Am 2004; 88(4):787–835, ix.
10. Leahy JL. Pathogenesis of type 2 diabetes mellitus. Arch Med Res 2005; 36(3):197–209.
11. Spiegel K, Knutson K, Leproult R, et al. Sleep loss: a novel risk factor for insulin resistance and type 2 diabetes. J Appl Physiol 2005; 99(5):2008–2019.
12. Punjabi NM, Ahmed MM, Polotsky VY, et al. Sleep-disordered breathing, glucose intolerance, and insulin resistance. Respir Physiol Neurobiol 2003; 136(2–3):167–178.
13. Punjabi NM, Polotsky VY. Disorders of glucose metabolism in sleep apnea. J Appl Physiol 2005; 99(5):1998–2007.
14. Tasali E, Ip MS. Obstructive sleep apnea and metabolic syndrome: alterations in glucose metabolism and inflammation. Proc Am Thorac Soc 2008; 5(2):207–217.
15. Tasali E, Mokhlesi B, Van CE. Obstructive sleep apnea and type 2 diabetes: interacting epidemics. Chest 2008; 133(2):496–506.
16. Diagnosis and classification of diabetes mellitus. Diabetes Care 2007; 30(suppl 1):S42–S47.
17. Norton PG, Dunn EV. Snoring as a risk factor for disease: an epidemiological survey. Br Med J (Clin Res Ed) 1985; 291(6496):630–632.
18. Jennum P, Schultz-Larsen K, Christensen N. Snoring, sympathetic activity and cardiovascular risk factors in a 70 year old population. Eur J Epidemiol 1993; 9(5):477–482.
19. Grunstein RR, Stenlof K, Hedner J, et al. Impact of obstructive sleep apnea and sleepiness on metabolic and cardiovascular risk factors in the Swedish Obese Subjects (SOS) Study. Int J Obes Relat Metab Disord 1995; 19(6):410–418.
20. Enright PL, Newman AB, Wahl PW, et al. Prevalence and correlates of snoring and observed apneas in 5,201 older adults. Sleep 1996; 19(7):531–538.
21. Elmasry A, Janson C, Lindberg E, et al. The role of habitual snoring and obesity in the development of diabetes: a 10 year follow up study in a male population. J Intern Med 2000; 248(1):13–20.
22. Al Delaimy WK, Manson JE, Willett WC, et al. Snoring as a risk factor for type II diabetes mellitus: a prospective study. Am J Epidemiol 2002; 155(5):387–393.
23. Renko AK, Hiltunen L, Laakso M, et al. The relationship of glucose tolerance to sleep disorders and daytime sleepiness. Diabetes Res Clin Pract 2005; 67(1):84–91.
24. Shin C, Kim J, Kim J, et al. Association of habitual snoring with glucose and insulin metabolism in nonobese Korean adult men. Am J Respir Crit Care Med 2005; 171(3):287–291.
25. Joo S, Lee S, Choi HA, et al. Habitual snoring is associated with elevated hemoglobin A1c levels in non-obese middle-aged adults. J Sleep Res 2006; 15(4):437–444.
26. Thomas GN, Jiang CQ, Lao XQ, et al. Snoring and vascular risk factors and disease in a low-risk Chinese population: the Guangzhou Biobank Cohort Study. Sleep 2006; 29(7):896–900.
27. Lindberg E, Berne C, Franklin KA, et al. Snoring and daytime sleepiness as risk factors for hypertension and diabetes in women—a population-based study. Respir Med 2007; 101(6):1283–1290.

28. Onat A, Hergenc G, Uyarel H, et al. Obstructive sleep apnea syndrome is associated with metabolic syndrome rather than insulin resistance. Sleep Breath 2007; 11(1):23–30.
29. Levinson PD, McGarvey ST, Carlisle CC, et al. Adiposity and cardiovascular risk factors in men with obstructive sleep apnea. Chest 1993; 103(5):1336–1342.
30. Tiihonen M, Partinen M, Narvanen S. The severity of obstructive sleep apnoea is associated with insulin resistance. J Sleep Res 1993; 2(1):56–61.
31. Davies RJ, Turner R, Crosby J, et al. Plasma insulin and lipid levels in untreated obstructive sleep apnoea and snoring; their comparison with matched controls and response to treatment. J Sleep Res 1994; 3(3):180–185.
32. Strohl KP, Novak RD, Singer W, et al. Insulin levels, blood pressure and sleep apnea. Sleep 1994; 17(7):614–618.
33. Stoohs RA, Facchini F, Guilleminault C. Insulin resistance and sleep-disordered breathing in healthy humans. Am J Respir Crit Care Med 1996; 154(1):170–174.
34. Ip MS, Lam KS, Ho C, et al. Serum leptin and vascular risk factors in obstructive sleep apnea. Chest 2000; 118(3):580–586.
35. Vgontzas AN, Papanicolaou DA, Bixler EO, et al. Sleep apnea and daytime sleepiness and fatigue: relation to visceral obesity, insulin resistance, and hypercytokinemia. J Clin Endocrinol Metab 2000; 85(3):1151–1158.
36. Elmasry A, Lindberg E, Berne C, et al. Sleep-disordered breathing and glucose metabolism in hypertensive men: a population-based study. J Intern Med 2001; 249(2):153–161.
37. De La Eva RC, Baur LA, Donaghue KC, et al. Metabolic correlates with obstructive sleep apnea in obese subjects. J Pediatr 2002; 140(6):654–659.
38. Ip MS, Lam B, Ng MM, et al. Obstructive sleep apnea is independently associated with insulin resistance. Am J Respir Crit Care Med 2002; 165(5):670–676.
39. Manzella D, Parillo M, Razzino T, et al. Soluble leptin receptor and insulin resistance as determinant of sleep apnea. Int J Obes Relat Metab Disord 2002; 26(3):370–375.
40. Punjabi NM, Sorkin JD, Katzel LI, et al. Sleep-disordered breathing and insulin resistance in middle-aged and overweight men. Am J Respir Crit Care Med 2002; 165(5):677–682.
41. Meslier N, Gagnadoux F, Giraud P, et al. Impaired glucose-insulin metabolism in males with obstructive sleep apnoea syndrome. Eur Respir J 2003; 22(1):156–160.
42. Tassone F, Lanfranco F, Gianotti L, et al. Obstructive sleep apnoea syndrome impairs insulin sensitivity independently of anthropometric variables. Clin Endocrinol (Oxf) 2003; 59(3):374–379.
43. Coughlin SR, Mawdsley L, Mugarza JA, et al. Obstructive sleep apnoea is independently associated with an increased prevalence of metabolic syndrome. Eur Heart J 2004; 25(9):735–741.
44. Punjabi NM, Shahar E, Redline S, et al. Sleep-disordered breathing, glucose intolerance, and insulin resistance: the Sleep Heart Health Study. Am J Epidemiol 2004; 160(6):521–530.
45. Gruber A, Horwood F, Sithole J, et al. Obstructive sleep apnoea is independently associated with the metabolic syndrome but not insulin resistance state. Cardiovasc Diabetol 2006; 5:22.
46. Makino S, Handa H, Suzukawa K, et al. Obstructive sleep apnoea syndrome, plasma adiponectin levels, and insulin resistance. Clin Endocrinol (Oxf) 2006; 64(1):12–19.
47. Kono M, Tatsumi K, Saibara T, et al. Obstructive sleep apnea syndrome is associated with some components of metabolic syndrome. Chest 2007; 131(5):1387–1392.
48. McArdle N, Hillman D, Beilin L, et al. Metabolic risk factors for vascular disease in obstructive sleep apnea: a matched controlled study. Am J Respir Crit Care Med 2007; 175(2):190–195.
49. Peltier AC, Consens FB, Sheikh K, et al. Autonomic dysfunction in obstructive sleep apnea is associated with impaired glucose regulation. Sleep Med 2007; 8(2):149–155.

50. Sharma SK, Kumpawat S, Goel A, et al. Obesity, and not obstructive sleep apnea, is responsible for metabolic abnormalities in a cohort with sleep-disordered breathing. Sleep Med 2007; 8(1):12–17.

51. Reichmuth KJ, Austin D, Skatrud JB, et al. Association of sleep apnea and type II diabetes: a population-based study. Am J Respir Crit Care Med 2005; 172(12):1590–1595.

52. Marshall NS, Wong KK, Phillips CL, et al. Is sleep apnea an independent risk factor for prevalent and incident diabetes in the Busselton Health Study. J Clin Sleep Med 2009; 05 (01):15–20.

53. Brooks B, Cistulli PA, Borkman M, et al. Obstructive sleep apnea in obese noninsulin-dependent diabetic patients: effect of continuous positive airway pressure treatment on insulin responsiveness. J Clin Endocrinol Metab 1994; 79(6):1681–1685.

54. Harsch IA, Schahin SP, Bruckner K, et al. The effect of continuous positive airway pressure treatment on insulin sensitivity in patients with obstructive sleep apnoea syndrome and type 2 diabetes. Respiration 2004; 71(3):252–259.

55. Harsch IA, Schahin SP, Radespiel-Troger M, et al. Continuous positive airway pressure treatment rapidly improves insulin sensitivity in patients with obstructive sleep apnea syndrome. Am J Respir Crit Care Med 2004; 169(2):156–162.

56. Babu AR, Herdegen J, Fogelfeld L, et al. Type 2 diabetes, glycemic control, and continuous positive airway pressure in obstructive sleep apnea. Arch Intern Med 2005; 165(4):447–452.

57. Hassaballa HA, Tulaimat A, Herdegen JJ, et al. The effect of continuous positive airway pressure on glucose control in diabetic patients with severe obstructive sleep apnea. Sleep Breath 2005; 9(4):176–180.

58. Saini J, Krieger J, Brandenberger G, et al. Continuous positive airway pressure treatment. Effects on growth hormone, insulin and glucose profiles in obstructive sleep apnea patients. Horm Metab Res 1993; 25(7):375–381.

59. Stoohs RA, Facchini FS, Philip P, et al. Selected cardiovascular risk factors in patients with obstructive sleep apnea: effect of nasal continuous positive airway pressure (n-CPAP). Sleep 1993; 16(8 suppl):S141–S142.

60. Cooper BG, White JE, Ashworth LA, et al. Hormonal and metabolic profiles in subjects with obstructive sleep apnea syndrome and the acute effects of nasal continuous positive airway pressure (CPAP) treatment. Sleep 1995; 18(3):172–179.

61. Saarelainen S, Lahtela J, Kallonen E. Effect of nasal CPAP treatment on insulin sensitivity and plasma leptin. J Sleep Res 1997; 6(2):146–147.

62. Chin K, Shimizu K, Nakamura T, et al. Changes in intra-abdominal visceral fat and serum leptin levels in patients with obstructive sleep apnea syndrome following nasal continuous positive airway pressure therapy. Circulation 1999; 100(7):706–712.

63. Smurra M, Philip P, Taillard J, et al. CPAP treatment does not affect glucose-insulin metabolism in sleep apneic patients. Sleep Med 2001; 2(3):207–213.

64. Czupryniak L, Loba J, Pawlowski M, et al. Treatment with continuous positive airway pressure may affect blood glucose levels in nondiabetic patients with obstructive sleep apnea syndrome. Sleep 2005; 28(5):601–603.

65. West SD, Nicoll DJ, Wallace TM, et al. Effect of CPAP on insulin resistance and HbA1c in men with obstructive sleep apnoea and type 2 diabetes. Thorax 2007; 62(11):969–974.

66. Punjabi NM, Beamer BA. Alterations in glucose disposal in sleep-disordered breathing. Am J Respir Crit Care Med 2009; 179(3):235–240.

67. Raff H, Bruder ED, Jankowski BM. The effect of hypoxia on plasma leptin and insulin in newborn and juvenile rats. Endocrine 1999; 11(1):37–39.

68. Raff H, Bruder ED, Jankowski BM, et al. Effect of neonatal hypoxia on leptin, insulin, growth hormone and body composition in the rat. Horm Metab Res 2001; 33(3):151–155.

69. Cheng N, Cai W, Jiang M, et al. Effect of hypoxia on blood glucose, hormones, and insulin receptor functions in newborn calves. Pediatr Res 1997; 41(6):852–856.

70. Polotsky VY, Li J, Punjabi NM, et al. Intermittent hypoxia increases insulin resistance in genetically obese mice. J Physiol 2003; 552(pt 1):253–264.

71. Larsen JJ, Hansen JM, Olsen NV, et al. The effect of altitude hypoxia on glucose homeostasis in men. J Physiol 1997; 504(pt 1):241–249.

72. Braun B, Rock PB, Zamudio S, et al. Women at altitude: short-term exposure to hypoxia and/or alpha(1)-adrenergic blockade reduces insulin sensitivity. J Appl Physiol 2001; 91(2): 623–631.

73. Oltmanns KM, Gehring H, Rudolf S, et al. Hypoxia causes glucose intolerance in humans. Am J Respir Crit Care Med 2004; 169(11):1231–1237.

74. Louis M, Punjabi NM. Effects of acute intermittent hypoxia on glucose metabolism in normal subjects. J Appl Physiol 2009; 106(5):1538–1544.

75. Stamatakis K, Punjabi N. Effects of experimental sleep fragmentation on glucose metabolism in normal subjects. Chest 2009 (in press).

76. Tasali E, Leproul R, Ehrmann DA, et al. Slow-wave sleep and the risk of type 2 diabetes in humans. Proceedings of the National Academy of Sciences of the United States of America 2008; 105(3):1044–1049.

77. Narkiewicz K, Somers VK. Sympathetic nerve activity in obstructive sleep apnoea. Acta Physiol Scand 2003; 177(3):385–390.

78. Narkiewicz K, van de Borne PJ, Montano N, et al. Contribution of tonic chemoreflex activation to sympathetic activity and blood pressure in patients with obstructive sleep apnea. Circulation 1998; 97(10):943–945.

79. Narkiewicz K, van de Borne PJ, Pesek CA, et al. Selective potentiation of peripheral chemoreflex sensitivity in obstructive sleep apnea. Circulation 1999; 99(9):1183–1189.

80. Loredo JS, Ziegler MG, Ncoli-Israel S, et al. Relationship of arousals from sleep to sympathetic nervous system activity and BP in obstructive sleep apnea. Chest 1999; 116(3): 655–659.

81. Horner RL, Brooks D, Kozar LF, et al. Immediate effects of arousal from sleep on cardiac autonomic outflow in the absence of breathing in dogs. J Appl Physiol 1995; 79(1):151–162.

82. Nonogaki K. New insights into sympathetic regulation of glucose and fat metabolism. Diabetologia 2000; 43(5):533–549.

83. Deibert DC, DeFronzo RA. Epinephrine-induced insulin resistance in man. J Clin Invest 1980; 65(3):717–721.

84. Avogaro A, Toffolo G, Valerio A, et al. Epinephrine exerts opposite effects on peripheral glucose disposal and glucose-stimulated insulin secretion. A stable label intravenous glucose tolerance test minimal model study. Diabetes 1996; 45(10):1373–1378.

85. Raz I, Katz A, Spencer MK. Epinephrine inhibits insulin-mediated glycogenesis but enhances glycolysis in human skeletal muscle. Am J Physiol 1991; 260(3 pt 1):E430–E435.

86. Lafontan M, Berlan M. Fat cell alpha 2-adrenoceptors: the regulation of fat cell function and lipolysis. Endocr Rev 1995; 16(6):716–738.

87. Roden M, Price TB, Perseghin G, et al. Mechanism of free fatty acid-induced insulin resistance in humans. J Clin Invest 1996; 97(12):2859–2865.

88. Santomauro AT, Boden G, Silva ME, et al. Overnight lowering of free fatty acids with Acipimox improves insulin resistance and glucose tolerance in obese diabetic and nondiabetic subjects. Diabetes 1999; 48(9):1836–1841.

89. Julius S, Gudbrandsson T, Jamerson K, et al. The interconnection between sympathetics, microcirculation, and insulin resistance in hypertension. Blood Press 1992; 1(1):9–19.

90. Jamerson KA, Julius S, Gudbrandsson T, et al. Reflex sympathetic activation induces acute insulin resistance in the human forearm. Hypertension 1993; 21(5):618–623.

91. Zeman RJ, Ludemann R, Easton TG, et al. Slow to fast alterations in skeletal muscle fibers caused by clenbuterol, a beta 2-receptor agonist. Am J Physiol 1988; 254(6 pt 1):E726–E732.

92. Klein J, Fasshauer M, Ito M, et al. beta(3)-adrenergic stimulation differentially inhibits insulin signaling and decreases insulin-induced glucose uptake in brown adipocytes. J Biol Chem 1999; 274(49):34795–34802.
93. Moncloa F, Velasco I, Beteta L. Plasma cortisol concentration and disappearance rate of 4-14C-cortisol in newcomers to high altitude. J Clin Endocrinol Metab 1968; 28(3):379–382.
94. Humpeler E, Skrabal F, Bartsch G. Influence of exposure to moderate altitude on the plasma concentraton of cortisol, aldosterone, renin, testosterone, and gonadotropins. Eur J Appl Physiol Occup Physiol 1980; 45(2–3):167–176.
95. Maresh CM, Noble BJ, Robertson KL, et al. Aldosterone, cortisol, and electrolyte responses to hypobaric hypoxia in moderate-altitude natives. Aviat Space Environ Med 1985; 56 (11):1078–1084.
96. Anand IS, Chandrashekhar Y, Rao SK, et al. Body fluid compartments, renal blood flow, and hormones at 6,000 m in normal subjects. J Appl Physiol 1993; 74(3):1234–1239.
97. Obminski Z, Golec L, Stupnicki R, et al. Effects of hypobaric-hypoxia on the salivary cortisol levels of aircraft pilots. Aviat Space Environ Med 1997; 68(3):183–186.
98. Barnholt KE, Hoffman AR, Rock PB, et al. Endocrine responses to acute and chronic high altitude exposure (4300 m): modulating effects of caloric restriction. Am J Physiol Endocrinol Metab 2006; 290(6):E1078–1088.
99. Coste O, Beers PV, Bogdan A, et al. Hypoxic alterations of cortisol circadian rhythm in man after simulation of a long duration flight. Steroids 2005; 70(12):803–810.
100. Follenius M, Brandenberger G, Bandesapt JJ, et al. Nocturnal cortisol release in relation to sleep structure. Sleep 1992; 15(1):21–27.
101. Spath-Schwalbe E, Gofferje M, Kern W, et al. Sleep disruption alters nocturnal ACTH and cortisol secretory patterns. Biol Psychiatry 1991; 29(6):575–584.
102. Grunstein RR, Handelsman DJ, Lawrence SJ, et al. Neuroendocrine dysfunction in sleep apnea: reversal by continuous positive airways pressure therapy. J Clin Endocrinol Metab 1989; 68(2):352–358.
103. Entzian P, Linnemann K, Schlaak M, et al. Obstructive sleep apnea syndrome and circadian rhythms of hormones and cytokines. Am J Respir Crit Care Med 1996; 153(3):1080–1086.
104. Grunstein RR, Stewart DA, Lloyd H, et al. Acute withdrawal of nasal CPAP in obstructive sleep apnea does not cause a rise in stress hormones. Sleep 1996; 19(10):774–782.
105. Bratel T, Wennlund A, Carlstrom K. Pituitary reactivity, androgens and catecholamines in obstructive sleep apnoea. Effects of continuous positive airway pressure treatment (CPAP). Respir Med 1999; 93(1):1–7.
106. Meston N, Davies RJ, Mullins R, et al. Endocrine effects of nasal continuous positive airway pressure in male patients with obstructive sleep apnoea. J Intern Med 2003; 254 (5):447–454.
107. Lanfranco F, Gianotti L, Pivetti S, et al. Obese patients with obstructive sleep apnoea syndrome show a peculiar alteration of the corticotroph but not of the thyrotroph and lactotroph function. Clin Endocrinol (Oxf) 2004; 60(1):41–48.
108. Parlapiano C, Borgia MC, Minni A, et al. Cortisol circadian rhythm and 24-hour Holter arterial pressure in OSAS patients. Endocr Res 2005; 31(4):371–374.
109. Dinneen S, Alzaid A, Miles J, et al. Metabolic effects of the nocturnal rise in cortisol on carbohydrate metabolism in normal humans. J Clin Invest 1993; 92(5):2283–2290.
110. Andrews RC, Walker BR. Glucocorticoids and insulin resistance: old hormones, new targets. Clin Sci (Lond) 1999; 96(5):513–523.
111. Valko M, Leibfritz D, Moncol J, et al. Free radicals and antioxidants in normal physiological functions and human disease. Int J Biochem Cell Biol 2007; 39(1):44–84.
112. Saarelainen S, Lehtimaki T, Jaak-kola O, et al. Autoantibodies against oxidised low-density lipoprotein in patients with obstructive sleep apnoea. Clin Chem Lab Med 1999; 37(5):517–520.

113. Barcelo A, Miralles C, Barbe F, et al. Abnormal lipid peroxidation in patients with sleep apnoea. Eur Respir J 2000; 16(4):644–647.

114. Schulz R, Mahmoudi S, Hattar K, et al. Enhanced release of superoxide from polymorphonuclear neutrophils in obstructive sleep apnea. Impact of continuous positive airway pressure therapy. Am J Respir Crit Care Med 2000; 162(2 pt 1):566–570.

115. Dyugovskaya L, Lavie P, Lavie L. Increased adhesion molecules expression and production of reactive oxygen species in leukocytes of sleep apnea patients. Am J Respir Crit Care Med 2002; 165(7):934–939.

116. Christou K, Markoulis N, Moulas AN, et al. Reactive oxygen metabolites (ROMs) as an index of oxidative stress in obstructive sleep apnea patients. Sleep Breath 2003; 7(3):105–110.

117. Christou K, Moulas AN, Pastaka C, et al. Antioxidant capacity in obstructive sleep apnea patients. Sleep Med 2003; 4(3):225–228.

118. Lavie L, Vishnevsky A, Lavie P. Evidence for lipid peroxidation in obstructive sleep apnea. Sleep 2004; 27(1):123–128.

119. Jung HH, Han H, Lee JH. Sleep apnea, coronary artery disease, and antioxidant status in hemodialysis patients. Am J Kidney Dis 2005; 45(5):875–882.

120. Yamauchi M, Nakano H, Maekawa J, et al. Oxidative stress in obstructive sleep apnea. Chest 2005; 127(5):1674–1679.

121. Tan KC, Chow WS, Lam JC, et al. HDL dysfunction in obstructive sleep apnea. Atherosclerosis 2006; 184(2):377–382.

122. Tiedge M, Lortz S, Drinkgern J, et al. Relation between antioxidant enzyme gene expression and antioxidative defense status of insulin-producing cells. Diabetes 1997; 46 (11):1733–1742.

123. Paolisso G, D'Amore A, Di MG, et al. Evidence for a relationship between free radicals and insulin action in the elderly. Metabolism 1993; 42(5):659–663.

124. Paolisso G, D'Amore A, Volpe C, et al. Evidence for a relationship between oxidative stress and insulin action in non-insulin-dependent (type II) diabetic patients. Metabolism 1994; 43 (11):1426–1429.

125. Rudich A, Tirosh A, Potashnik R, et al. Prolonged oxidative stress impairs insulin-induced GLUT4 translocation in 3T3-L1 adipocytes. Diabetes 1998; 47(10):1562–1569.

126. Paolisso G, Di MG, Pizza G, et al. Plasma GSH/GSSG affects glucose homeostasis in healthy subjects and non-insulin-dependent diabetics. Am J Physiol 1992; 263(3 pt 1): E435–E440.

127. Caballero B. Vitamin E improves the action of insulin. Nutr Rev 1993; 51(11):339–340.

128. Paolisso G, D'Amore A, Balbi V, et al. Plasma vitamin C affects glucose homeostasis in healthy subjects and in non-insulin-dependent diabetics. Am J Physiol 1994; 266(2 pt 1): E261–E268.

129. Jacob S, Ruus P, Hermann R, et al. Oral administration of RAC-alpha-lipoic acid modulates insulin sensitivity in patients with type-2 diabetes mellitus: a placebo-controlled pilot trial. Free Radic Biol Med 1999; 27(3–4):309–314.

130. Libby P, Ridker PM, Maseri A. Inflammation and atherosclerosis. Circulation 2002; 105 (9):1135–1143.

131. Ohga E, Nagase T, Tomita T, et al. Increased levels of circulating ICAM-1, VCAM-1, and L-selectin in obstructive sleep apnea syndrome. J Appl Physiol 1999; 87(1):10–14.

132. Chin K, Nakamura T, Shimizu K, et al. Effects of nasal continuous positive airway pressure on soluble cell adhesion molecules in patients with obstructive sleep apnea syndrome. Am J Med 2000; 109(7):562–567.

133. El-Solh AA, Mador MJ, Sikka P, et al. Adhesion molecules in patients with coronary artery disease and moderate-to-severe obstructive sleep apnea. Chest 2002; 121(5):1541–1547.

134. Ohga E, Tomita T, Wada H, et al. Effects of obstructive sleep apnea on circulating ICAM-1, IL-8, and MCP-1. J Appl Physiol 2003; 94(1):179–184.

135. O'Brien LM, Serpero LD, Tauman R, et al. Plasma adhesion molecules in children with sleep-disordered breathing. Chest 2006; 129(4):947–953.

136. Ursavas A, Karadag M, Rodoplu E, et al. Circulating ICAM-1 and VCAM-1 levels in patients with obstructive sleep apnea syndrome. Respiration 2007; 74(5):525–532.

137. Alberti A, Sarchielli P, Gallinella E, et al. Plasma cytokine levels in patients with obstructive sleep apnea syndrome: a preliminary study. J Sleep Res 2003; 12(4):305–311.

138. Yokoe T, Minoguchi K, Matsuo H, et al. Elevated levels of C-reactive protein and interleukin-6 in patients with obstructive sleep apnea syndrome are decreased by nasal continuous positive airway pressure. Circulation 2003; 107(8):1129–1134.

139. Minoguchi K, Tazaki T, Yokoe T, et al. Elevated production of tumor necrosis factor-alpha by monocytes in patients with obstructive sleep apnea syndrome. Chest 2004; 126 (5):1473–1479.

140. Ryan S, Taylor CT, McNicholas WT. Selective activation of inflammatory pathways by intermittent hypoxia in obstructive sleep apnea syndrome. Circulation 2005; 112(17): 2660–2667.

141. Dyugovskaya L, Lavie P, Hirsh M, et al. Activated CD8+ T-lymphocytes in obstructive sleep apnoea. Eur Respir J 2005; 25(5):820–828.

142. Dyugovskaya L, Lavie P, Lavie L. Phenotypic and functional characterization of blood gammadelta T cells in sleep apnea. Am J Respir Crit Care Med 2003; 168(2):242–249.

143. Dyugovskaya L, Lavie P, Lavie L. Lymphocyte activation as a possible measure of atherosclerotic risk in patients with sleep apnea. Ann N Y Acad Sci 2005; 1051:340–350.

144. Klokker M, Kharazmi A, Galbo H, et al. Influence of in vivo hypobaric hypoxia on function of lymphocytes, neutrocytes, natural killer cells, and cytokines. J Appl Physiol 1993; 74 (3):1100–1106.

145. Facco M, Zilli C, Siviero M, et al. Modulation of immune response by the acute and chronic exposure to high altitude. Med Sci Sports Exerc 2005; 37(5):768–774.

146. Zhang Y, Hu Y, Wang F. Effects of a 28-Day "Living High - Training Low" on T-lymphocyte subsets in soccer players. Int J Sports Med 2007; 28(4):354–358.

147. Madden KS, Sanders VM, Felten DL. Catecholamine influences and sympathetic neural modulation of immune responsiveness. Annu Rev Pharmacol Toxicol 1995; 35:417–448.

148. Elenkov IJ, Wilder RL, Chrousos GP, et al. The sympathetic nerve—an integrative interface between two supersystems: the brain and the immune system. Pharmacol Rev 2000; 52 (4):595–638.

149. Schmidt MI, Duncan BB, Sharrett AR, et al. Markers of inflammation and prediction of diabetes mellitus in adults (Atherosclerosis Risk in Communities study): a cohort study. Lancet 1999; 353(9165):1649–1652.

150. Barzilay JI, Abraham L, Heckbert SR, et al. The relation of markers of inflammation to the development of glucose disorders in the elderly: the Cardiovascular Health Study. Diabetes 2001; 50(10):2384–2389.

151. Pradhan AD, Manson JE, Rifai N, et al. C-reactive protein, interleukin 6, and risk of developing type 2 diabetes mellitus. JAMA 2001; 286(3):327–334.

152. Freeman DJ, Norrie J, Caslake MJ, et al. C-reactive protein is an independent predictor of risk for the development of diabetes in the West of Scotland Coronary Prevention Study. Diabetes 2002; 51(5):1596–1600.

153. Duncan BB, Schmidt MI, Pankow JS, et al. Low-grade systemic inflammation and the development of type 2 diabetes: the atherosclerosis risk in communities study. Diabetes 2003; 52(7):1799–1805.

154. Spranger J, Kroke A, Mohlig M, et al. Inflammatory cytokines and the risk to develop type 2 diabetes: results of the prospective population-based European Prospective Investigation into Cancer and Nutrition (EPIC)-Potsdam Study. Diabetes 2003; 52(3):812–817.

155. Thorand B, Lowel H, Schneider A, et al. C-reactive protein as a predictor for incident diabetes mellitus among middle-aged men: results from the MONICA Augsburg cohort study, 1984–1998. Arch Intern Med 2003; 163(1):93–99.
156. Hu FB, Meigs JB, Li TY, et al. Inflammatory markers and risk of developing type 2 diabetes in women. Diabetes 2004; 53(3):693–700.
157. Uysal KT, Wiesbrock SM, Marino MW, et al. Protection from obesity-induced insulin resistance in mice lacking TNF-alpha function. Nature 1997; 389(6651):610–614.
158. Schafer K, Fujisawa K, Konstantinides S, et al. Disruption of the plasminogen activator inhibitor 1 gene reduces the adiposity and improves the metabolic profile of genetically obese and diabetic ob/ob mice. FASEB J 2001; 15(10):1840–1842.
159. Punjabi NM, Beamer BA. C-reactive protein is associated with sleep disordered breathing independent of adiposity. Sleep 2007; 30(1):29–34.
160. Jackson MB, Ahima RS. Neuroendocrine and metabolic effects of adipocyte-derived hormones. Clin Sci (Lond) 2006; 110(2):143–152.
161. Ahima RS, Flier JS. Leptin. Annu Rev Physiol 2000; 62:413–437.
162. Ceddia RB, Koistinen HA, Zierath JR, et al. Analysis of paradoxical observations on the association between leptin and insulin resistance. FASEB J 2002; 16(10):1163–1176.
163. Margetic S, Gazzola C, Pegg GG, et al. Leptin: a review of its peripheral actions and interactions. Int J Obes Relat Metab Disord 2002; 26(11):1407–1433.
164. Ozturk L, Unal M, Tamer L, et al. The association of the severity of obstructive sleep apnea with plasma leptin levels. Arch Otolaryngol Head Neck Surg 2003; 129(5):538–540.
165. Patel SR, Palmer LJ, Larkin EK, et al. Relationship between obstructive sleep apnea and diurnal leptin rhythms. Sleep 2004; 27(2):235–239.
166. Shimura R, Tatsumi K, Nakamura A, et al. Fat accumulation, leptin, and hypercapnia in obstructive sleep apnea-hypopnea syndrome. Chest 2005; 127(2):543–549.
167. Tatsumi K, Kasahara Y, Kurosu K, et al. Sleep oxygen desaturation and circulating leptin in obstructive sleep apnea-hypopnea syndrome. Chest 2005; 127(3):716–721.
168. Ulukavak CT, Kokturk O, Bukan N, et al. Leptin and ghrelin levels in patients with obstructive sleep apnea syndrome. Respiration 2005; 72(4):395–401.
169. Harsch IA, Konturek PC, Koebnick C, et al. Leptin and ghrelin levels in patients with obstructive sleep apnoea: effect of CPAP treatment. Eur Respir J 2003; 22(2):251–257.
170. Sanner BM, Kollhosser P, Buechner N, et al. Influence of treatment on leptin levels in patients with obstructive sleep apnoea. Eur Respir J 2004; 23(4):601–604.
171. Tschop M, Strasburger CJ, Topfer M, et al. Influence of hypobaric hypoxia on leptin levels in men. Int J Obes Relat Metab Disord 2000; 24(suppl 2):S151.
172. Kubota N, Terauchi Y, Yamauchi T, et al. Disruption of adiponectin causes insulin resistance and neointimal formation. J Biol Chem 2002; 277(29):25863–25866.
173. Maeda N, Shimomura I, Kishida K, et al. Diet-induced insulin resistance in mice lacking adiponectin/ACRP30. Nat Med 2002; 8(7):731–737.
174. Spranger J, Kroke A, Mohlig M, et al. Adiponectin and protection against type 2 diabetes mellitus. Lancet 2003; 361(9353):226–228.
175. Lihn AS, Pedersen SB, Richelsen B. Adiponectin: action, regulation and association to insulin sensitivity. Obes Rev 2005; 6(1):13–21.
176. Harsch IA, Wallaschofski H, Koebnick C, et al. Adiponectin in patients with obstructive sleep apnea syndrome: course and physiological relevance. Respiration 2004; 71(6):580–586.
177. Wolk R, Svatikova A, Nelson CA, et al. Plasma levels of adiponectin, a novel adipocyte-derived hormone, in sleep apnea. Obes Res 2005; 13(1):186–190.
178. Zhang XL, Yin KS, Mao H, et al. Serum adiponectin level in patients with obstructive sleep apnea hypopnea syndrome. Chin Med J (Engl) 2004; 117(11):1603–1606.
179. Masserini B, Morpurgo PS, Donadio F, et al. Reduced levels of adiponectin in sleep apnea syndrome. J Endocrinol Invest 2006; 29(8):700–705.

180. Zhang XL, Yin KS, Wang H, et al. Serum adiponectin levels in adult male patients with obstructive sleep apnea hypopnea syndrome. Respiration 2006; 73(1):73–77.
181. Zhang XL, Yin KS, Li C, et al. Effect of continuous positive airway pressure treatment on serum adiponectin level and mean arterial pressure in male patients with obstructive sleep apnea syndrome. Chin Med J (Engl) 2007; 120(17):1477–1481.
182. Nakagawa Y, Kishida K, Kihara S, et al. Nocturnal reduction in circulating adiponectin concentrations related to hypoxic stress in severe obstructive sleep apnea-hypopnea syndrome. Am J Physiol Endocrinol Metab 2008; 294(4):E778–E784.
183. Steppan CM, Bailey ST, Bhat S, et al. The hormone resistin links obesity to diabetes. Nature 2001; 409(6818):307–312.
184. Asano T, Sakosda H, Fujishiro M, et al. Physiological significance of resistin and resistin-like molecules in the inflammatory process and insulin resistance. Curr Diabetes Rev 2006; 2(4):449–454.
185. Harsch IA, Koebnick C, Wallaschofski H, et al. Resistin levels in patients with obstructive sleep apnoea syndrome—the link to subclinical inflammation? Med Sci Monit 2004; 10(9): CR510–CR515.
186. Tauman R, Serpero LD, Capdevila OS, et al. Adipokines in children with sleep disordered breathing. Sleep 2007; 30(4):443–449.
187. Guilleminault C, Briskin JG, Greenfield MS, et al. The impact of autonomic nervous system dysfunction on breathing during sleep. Sleep 1981; 4(3):263–278.
188. Rees PJ, Prior JG, Cochrane GM, et al. Sleep apnoea in diabetic patients with autonomic neuropathy. J R Soc Med 1981; 74(3):192–195.
189. Catterall JR, Calverley PM, Ewing DJ, et al. Breathing, sleep, and diabetic autonomic neuropathy. Diabetes 1984; 33(11):1025–1027.
190. Mondini S, Guilleminault C. Abnormal breathing patterns during sleep in diabetes. Ann Neurol 1985; 17(4):391–395.
191. Neumann C, Martinez D, Schmid H. Nocturnal oxygen desaturation in diabetic patients with severe autonomic neuropathy. Diabetes Res Clin Pract 1995; 28(2):97–102.
192. Ficker JH, Dertinger SH, Siegfried W, et al. Obstructive sleep apnoea and diabetes mellitus: the role of cardiovascular autonomic neuropathy. Eur Respir J 1998; 11(1):14–19.
193. Bottini P, Dottorini ML, Cristina CM, et al. Sleep-disordered breathing in nonobese diabetic subjects with autonomic neuropathy. Eur Respir J 2003; 22(4):654–660.
194. Resnick HE, Redline S, Shahar E, et al. Diabetes and sleep disturbances: findings from the Sleep Heart Health Study. Diabetes Care 2003; 26(3):702–709.
195. Wilcox I, McNamara SG, Collins FL, et al. "Syndrome Z": the interaction of sleep apnoea, vascular risk factors and heart disease. Thorax 1998; 53(suppl 3):S25–S28.
196. Vgontzas AN, Bixler EO, Chrousos GP. Sleep apnea is a manifestation of the metabolic syndrome. Sleep Med Rev 2005; 9(3):211–224.
197. Coughlin S, Calverley P, Wilding J. Sleep disordered breathing—a new component of syndrome x? Obes Rev 2001; 2(4):267–274.

7
Oxidative Stress, Inflammation, and Vascular Function in Obstructive Sleep Apnea Syndrome

JOHN GARVEY, SILKE RYAN, CORMAC T. TAYLOR, and WALTER T. MCNICHOLAS
St. Vincent's University Hospital and University College Dublin, Dublin, Ireland

I. Introduction

Recent years have seen major developments in our understanding of the pathogenesis of cardiovascular diseases. Endothelial dysfunction crucially contributes to the development of various cardiovascular disease processes, particularly atherosclerosis but also hypertension and congestive cardiac failure. Oxidative stress and inflammation have gained widespread attention as fundamental mechanisms that participate in the initiation and progression of endothelial dysfunction. Intracellular reactive oxygen species (ROS) lead to enhanced oxidative stress in vascular cells and are key mediators of signaling pathways that underlie vascular inflammation in atherogenesis, starting from the initiation of fatty streak development, through lesion progression, to ultimate plaque rupture. Both oxidative stress and inflammation are exaggerated in patients with obstructive sleep apnea syndrome (OSAS) and therefore likely important in the cardiovascular pathogenesis of OSAS.

II. Endothelial Dysfunction in OSAS

The endothelium is the major regulator of vascular homeostasis, maintaining vascular tone and controlling the equilibrium between inhibition and stimulation of smooth muscle cell proliferation, in addition to vascular thrombogenesis and fibrinolysis (1,2). When this balance becomes upset, endothelial dysfunction occurs, causing damage to the endothelial wall. Endothelial dysfunction is considered an early marker for atherosclerosis (3). As well as preceding the development of atherosclerosis, endothelial dysfunction appears to have predictive value for cardiovascular events in patients with established cardiovascular disease (4).

The hallmark of endothelial dysfunction is impairment of endothelial-dependent vasodilatation, which is mediated by nitric oxide (NO). NO is the most potent vascular relaxing factor in the body and plays an important role as a signaling molecule in several biological functions including inflammation and neurotransmission. NO inhibits proinflammatory events such as platelet activation and aggregation, leukocyte adhesion, and low-density lipoprotein oxidation by endothelial macrophages (5,6).

NO is produced by the enzyme nitric oxide synthase (NOS). Three isoforms of NOS have been identified: neuronal NOS (nNOS); endothelial NOS (eNOS), expressed by endothelial cells lining the vasculature; and inducible NOS (iNOS) (7). iNOS is only expressed in response to certain inflammatory stimuli. Both eNOS and nNOS produce NO in relatively low amounts, whereas iNOS can produce large amounts of NO for long periods. It has been suggested that low amounts of NO derived from eNOS and nNOS are beneficial, and NO deficiency has been implicated in the pathogenesis of cardiovascular disease (8). In contrast, the large quantity of NO produced by iNOS is presumed to be harmful, contributing to inflammatory injury through nitrosative stress (9). However, data have also been presented that inhibition of iNOS may exacerbate injury in certain situations, suggesting that iNOS-derived NO may be protective as well (10). There are a number of mechanisms by which NO is known to affect cellular biology, including activation of soluble guanylate cyclase with subsequent formation of cyclic guanosine monophosphate and modulation of cellular respiration, in competition with O_2, through reversible inhibition of the mitochondrial enzyme cytochrome c oxidase (11,12).

There is growing evidence of a critical role of NO as a mediator of endothelial dysfunction in OSAS. Decreased levels of nitrites/nitrates have been found in OSAS patients, and levels increase with continuous positive airflow pressure (CPAP) therapy, suggesting that NO bioavailability is reduced in OSAS (13,14). It has been hypothesized that the unique form of hypoxia with repetitive short cycles of desaturation followed by rapid reoxygenation termed intermittent hypoxia (IH) occurring in OSAS is responsible for the reduction in NO bioavailability and impaired NO-dependent vasodilation by generation of oxygen-free radicals, which subsequently react with NO to produce the damaging free radical peroxynitrite (15,16). However, another case-control study suggested that peroxynitrite formation may not occur in OSAS (17). A recent study demonstrated decreased expression of eNOS and phosphorylated (active) eNOS but increased iNOS expression in patients with OSAS compared with control subjects with reversal of these alterations by CPAP therapy (18). These data indicate the complexity and potential duality of NO metabolism at a molecular level in OSAS.

Various studies have demonstrated impairment in endothelium-mediated vasodilation by acetylcholine (ACh) in OSAS, which acts through an NO-mediated pathway (19,20). Administration of an ACh infusion to OSAS patients results in decreased arm blood flow compared to controls, and vascular function improves following treatment with CPAP. The endothelium also produces vasoconstrictor substances, such as angiotensin II and endothelin-1. Møller et al. demonstrated elevated blood pressure readings in OSAS patients who were associated with elevated plasma levels of angiotensin II and aldosterone. Effective CPAP therapy lowered both blood pressure and renin-angiotensin system activity (21). Studies on endothelin-1 concentrations in OSAS patients before and after CPAP therapy have produced conflicting results (22–24), and as a possible explanation, Jordan et al. suggested that this might be due to the very short half-life of endothelin-1 and measurement of the precursor might be more appropriate in this setting (25).

Increased numbers of circulating apoptotic endothelial cells as a further marker of endothelial dysfunction have also been identified in OSAS. In one study of patients with OSAS, impairment of endothelial-dependent vasodilatation correlated with the degree of endothelial cell apoptosis and CPAP therapy led to a significant decline in circulating apoptotic endothelial cells (26). Furthermore, levels of bone marrow–derived endothelial progenitor cells (EPCs), which are a marker of endothelial repair capacity and inversely correlated with cardiovascular risk, are reduced in OSAS (18). Vascular reactivity as measured by flow-mediated dilation was also decreased in this OSAS patient cohort, and both vascular reactivity and levels of EPCs significantly increased in patients who adhered to CPAP. However, another study has shown no differences in the levels of circulating EPCs between patients with OSAS and controls (27).

In summary, there is a substantial body of evidence supporting a potential causal relationship between OSAS and endothelial dysfunction. Nonetheless, the underlying mechanism(s) of this association remain(s) incompletely understood. However, there is growing evidence of a critical role of oxidative stress and activation of inflammatory pathways in this process.

III. Oxidative Stress in OSAS

Oxidative stress refers to the generation of potentially deleterious products from the cellular metabolism of oxygen. These products, termed ROS, are atoms or small molecules with unpaired valence shell electrons. ROS are therefore primed to react chemically, and they readily accept and donate unpaired electrons. These include superoxide anion ($O_2^{\bullet-}$), hydrogen peroxide (H_2O_2), and the highly aggressive peroxynitrite ($ONOO^-$) and hydroxyl radical ($OH^{\bullet}$). Two ROS molecules reacting with each other result in the formation of a nonradical product, and a single ROS molecule reacting with a nonradical molecule yields a new ROS product, thereby propagating further similar reactions (Fig. 1).

ROS are normal by-products of cellular metabolism, and under physiological conditions, equilibrium is achieved between the rate of ROS production and the rate of ROS elimination. When overproduction of ROS overwhelms antioxidant capabilities, pathogenic oxidative stress occurs, resulting in the inhibition of cellular mechanisms and cellular injury (28). There is a substantial body of evidence linking oxidative stress with vascular injury and cardiovascular disease (29,30).

It has been proposed that the IH occurring in OSAS shares analogies with ischemia-reperfusion injury, thus initiating oxidative stress and potentiating athero-sclerotic sequelae in OSAS (15,16). However, the issue of increased ROS production in OSAS is controversial. Two in vitro studies demonstrated increased ROS production from leucocytes of OSAS patients that was reversed by CPAP therapy (31,32). A number of studies have also shown an increased intensity of lipid peroxidation that improved with CPAP therapy (33–35). Furthermore, there is evidence of decreased antioxidant capacity as an indirect measure of enhanced oxidative stress in OSAS (34,36). In contrast, Svatikova et al. did not detect higher levels of lipid peroxidation biomarkers in exclusively normotensive OSAS patients in comparison to matched control subjects (37), and two further small studies failed to show increased oxidative stress in OSAS (38,39). In support of these findings, another study in children, who are unlikely to be affected by the cardiovascular confounders of adulthood, found no cor-relation between markers of oxidative stress and OSAS (40). A recent cross-sectional study measuring urinary excretion of 8-hydroxy-2-deoxyguanosine as a marker of increased oxidative stress identified an independent correlation of the severity of OSAS with oxidative stress; however, a large percentage of participants in this study were suffering from other cardiovascular diseases and patients with OSAS were significantly more hypertensive than nonapneic subjects (41).

Thus, oxidative stress as the primary injurious stimulus in OSAS remains con-troversial. Oxidative stress may represent a consequence rather than a cause of tissue damage (42,43). Evidence based on ROS-derived factors, such as lipid peroxide levels

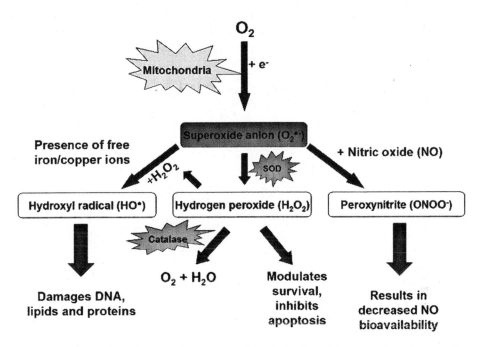

Figure 1 Generation of superoxide anion and its derivatives. The production of superoxide $(O_2^{\bullet-})$ occurs mainly within the mitochondria of cells as a result of premature leakage of electrons to oxygen (O_2) during oxidative phosphorylation. Superoxide dismutase (SOD) catalyzes the dismutation of $O_2^{\bullet-}$ to O_2 and hydrogen peroxide (H_2O_2). As well as causing pathological damage, both $O_2^{\bullet-}$ and H_2O_2 function in normal cell regulation and signaling. H_2O_2 can be eliminated by catalase and glutathione peroxidase or alternatively can react with $O_2^{\bullet}$ in the presence of reduced metals to produce a more aggressive oxidant, the hydroxyl radical $(HO^{\bullet})$. $O_2^{\bullet-}$ can also combine with nitric oxide (NO) to produce peroxynitrite $(ONOO^-)$, thereby modifying the bioavailability of NO.

and thiobarbituric acid–reactive substance (TBARS) formation, and including studies showing improvements with therapy imply association rather than causation. Furthermore, discordance has been demonstrated between the timing of ROS overproduction and tissue injury (44). In addition, damage caused by ischemia-reperfusion in liver tissue has been shown to occur independently of ROS (45).

There is also growing data supporting the role of ROS in the maintenance of homeostasis through both intracellular signaling and intercellular communication (46). ROS, especially at lower concentrations, may signal an adaptive response to injury and mediate tissue healing. ROS have been shown to mediate preconditioning-induced neuroprotection, and antioxidants abolished this adaptive response (47). Thus, generation of ROS in OSAS may reflect an adaptive consequence in order to reestablish homeostasis rather than a causative mechanism of endothelial damage. Furthermore, we lack convincing evidence of a benefit from antioxidant treatment in conditions where oxidative stress is thought to play a pivotal role. In fact, a recent meta-analysis detected increased mortality with antioxidant treatment, suggesting a potential benefit of ROS generation

(48). Therefore, care needs to be exercised in the therapeutic modulation of oxidative stress pathways, as therapy may impair protective responses evoked by ROS as well as attenuate further ROS-mediated damage. We clearly need further research at the bench and beside to more clearly establish the role of oxidative stress in IH-mediated endothelial dysfunction. In particular, further data are required to support the premise that oxidative stress is the de facto oxygen-sensing mechanism that underlies pathogenic processes in OSAS.

IV. Inflammatory Processes in OSAS

The importance of inflammatory processes in the pathogenesis of cardiovascular diseases in OSAS is strongly supported by numerous studies demonstrating elevated levels of circulating proinflammatory cytokines, chemokines, and adhesion molecules in OSAS patients in comparison to matched controls and a significant fall with effective CPAP therapy. In particular, the potent proinflammatory cytokine tumor necrosis factor α (TNF-α) has been evaluated by various case-control studies that have consistently shown elevated levels in OSAS patients in comparison to controls, independent of obesity, and a significant fall with effective CPAP therapy, and both T cells and monocytes have been suggested as potential sources (49–53). Recently, a large prospective study on male subjects without cardiovascular diseases identified a strong association between OSAS severity and TNF-α levels, independent of possible confounders such as body mass index (BMI), age, or sleepiness (50). The chemokine interleukin 8 (IL-8), which plays a key role in the process of adhesion of neutrophils and monocytes to the vascular endothelium (54,55), has also been shown to be elevated in OSAS (50,56). Early preliminary studies have also suggested increased IL-6 levels in OSAS patients (51,57,58); however, some of these reports are limited by relatively small numbers, lack of adequately matched normal control populations, particularly in terms of BMI, and the inclusion of patients with established cardiovascular or metabolic diseases. Furthermore, other recent studies did not detect an association between OSAS and IL-6 (50,59). However, in a large cross-sectional analysis of the Cleveland Family Study, an independent association was found between OSAS severity parameters and soluble IL-6 receptor (59), which appears to be associated with the processes of inflammation and myocardial injury during the acute phase of acute myocardial infarction (60).

A limited number of studies have also examined the levels of various cellular adhesion molecules (CAM) such as intercellular adhesion molecule 1 (ICAM-1), vascular cellular adhesion molecule 1 (VCAM-1), and the family of selectins. The findings consistently suggest an association between OSAS severity and circulating CAM levels, with one report also showing a significant fall after one month of effective CPAP therapy (61–64).

Another potential link between OSAS and inflammation is the acute phase reactant C-reactive protein (CRP). In the high-to-normal range, and when measured with a high-sensitivity assay, CRP levels are widely recognized as potent, independent predictors of future cardiovascular events among apparently healthy subjects as well as in subjects with known cardiovascular disease (65–68). However, recent large-scale studies suggest that the elevated levels may in fact be attributable to the presence of abnormal conventional cardiovascular risk factors, in particular obesity (69–71). The strong relationship between CRP levels and obesity has also influenced various studies investigating CRP levels in adult OSAS patients, and therefore, the role of CRP in OSAS is still under debate. This is reflected in different conclusions obtained from two large cross-sectional studies in OSAS patients. A study on 316 Japanese men detected a significant association between CRP and sleep-disordered breathing; however, the use of overnight oxymetry as a screening tool for OSAS was a significant limitation (72). On the other hand, the Wisconsin Sleep Cohort Study analyzing 907 adults failed to detect an independent association between CRP and OSAS after adjustment for BMI (73). This discrepancy has also been evident in numerous case-control studies where some reports have identified increased levels of CRP in OSAS patients (58,74–76) and others have not (77–79). Furthermore, the impact of CPAP therapy on CRP levels is still unclear (58,79–81).

In addition to elevated inflammatory markers, another line of evidence of inflammatory processes in OSAS comes from investigations in animal models and humans demonstrating interaction between inflammatory cells and the endothelium. Leukocyte accumulation and their adhesion to the endothelium play a central role in the formation of atherosclerotic plaques. Activation of monocytes and T-lymphocytes is among the crucial steps leading to the release of inflammatory mediators and adhesion molecules (82,83). In a rat model, recurrent obstructive apneas led to a significant increase in various leukocyte-endothelial cell interactions such as leukocyte rolling and firm adhesion of leukocytes in comparison to a sham group (84). Monocytes of patients with OSAS adhere more firmly to endothelial cells than those of control subjects, a process that is decreased by the application of CPAP therapy (31). In the same study, OSAS was associated with the upregulation of the adhesion molecules CD15 and CD11c in monocytes. Furthermore, in a cell culture model of repetitive hypoxia and reoxygenation, lipid uptake into macrophages and the expression of various adhesion molecules were significantly increased in comparison to control cells (85). T-lymphocytes are also involved in the pathogenesis of atherosclerosis. In a series of experiments, Dyugovskaya et al. demonstrated that various subpopulations of cytotoxic T cells of OSAS patients acquire an activated phenotype with the downstream consequence of increased cytotoxicity against endothelial cells (31,52,86). Furthermore, this activation process is associated with an increased intracellular content of the proinflammatory mediators TNF-α and IL-8 and a decrease of the anti-inflammatory cytokine IL-10 (52).

A recent in vitro study addressed the involvement of neutrophils in the cardiovascular pathogenesis of OSAS (87). The results demonstrate impaired neutrophil apoptosis and increased adhesion molecule expression by these cells in OSAS, suggesting a further potential pathway in the atherosclerotic process.

The basic mechanisms underlying the inflammatory process in OSAS remain unclear. In addition to sleep fragmentation and sleep deprivation, IH in OSAS is likely to play a significant role in the initiation of the inflammatory process. Utilizing a cell culture model, IH leads to a selective and preferential activation of inflammatory pathways mediated by the transcription factor nuclear factor kappa B (NF-κB) over adaptive, hypoxia-inducible factor 1 (HIF-1)-dependent pathways, which contrasts with sustained hypoxia, where activation of adaptive and protective pathways predominates (49). NF-κB is a key player in inflammatory and innate immune responses and a master regulator of inflammatory gene expression, and genes like TNF-α or IL-8 that are important to the atherosclerotic process, and have also been found upregulated in OSAS, are under the control of this transcription factor. The central role of NF-κB in inflammatory processes in OSAS was furthermore suggested by increased activation in cardiovascular tissues in a mouse model of IH and also in cultured monocytes of OSAS patients (88,89). The p38 mitogen-activated protein kinase (MAPK) plays a major role in the process of IH-induced

NF-κB activation, and pharmacological as well as targeted siRNA inhibition of p38 leads to a significant reduction in NF-κB activity (90). P38 MAPK is a key player in inflammatory processes and necessary for inflammatory cytokine production and signaling (91). Furthermore, p38 is activated in response to environmental stresses and is critically involved in the pathophysiology of a variety of cardiovascular diseases (92–94).

IH also activates other inflammatory transcription factors. Among them is activator protein complex 1 (AP-1), formed by the proteins c-Fos and C-Jun. AP-1 drives transcriptional activation of a variety of genes, including tyrosine hydroxylase, which encodes the key enzyme in catecholamine synthesis (95). C-Fos upregulation by IH has been demonstrated in an animal as well as in a cell culture model (96,97). In a rat model, the activation of inflammatory pathways by IH was associated with an impairment of neurocognitive function, a process that was reversed once the stimulus subsided (98).

The initial sensing and signaling event(s) that occur(s) in response to and the target tissues affected by IH are not yet determined. It has been proposed that ROS production is critical in this process. However, the involvement of ROS in NF-κB signaling is controversial, and experiments by Hayakawa et al. indicate that NF-κB is unlikely to be a sensor of oxidative stress and previous results may have been influenced by cell-type dependency and methodological limitations (99).

Collectively, the activation of inflammatory transcription factors, particularly NF-κB, by IH, the hallmark of OSAS, results in the activation of inflammatory cells, release of inflammatory mediators, and associated vascular pathophysiology (Fig. 2).

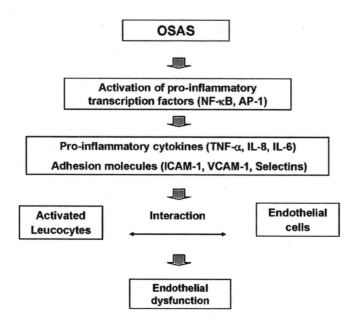

Figure 2 Inflammatory processes in OSAS. Intermittent hypoxia (IH) leads to a preferential nuclear factor kappa B (NF-κB)-dependent inflammatory pathways over adaptive hypoxia-inducible factor 1 (HIF-1)-mediated pathways. This leads to the production of various proinflammatory mediators, which, in turn, mediates the interaction of inflammatory and endothelial cells resulting in endothelial dysfunction.

V. Summary

With growing evidence of an independent association between OSAS and cardiovascular diseases, great effort has been made to identify the mechanisms involved. Given the complexity of OSAS, a multifactorial process appears likely. The classical pattern of IH in OSAS is likely to play a pivotal role leading to the activation of inflammatory pathways and oxidative stress, which, in turn, promote the development of endothelial dysfunction (Fig. 3).

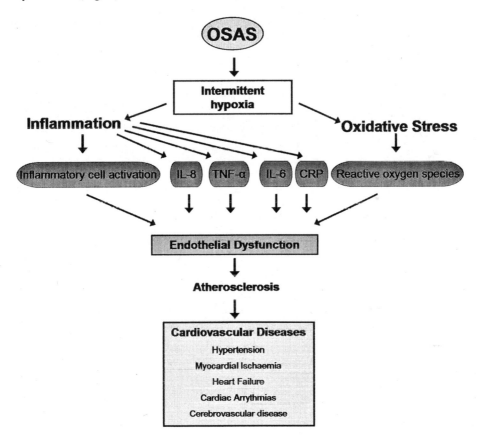

Figure 3 Contribution of inflammation and oxidative stress to the development of cardiovascular disease in OSAS. Proposed mechanisms by which OSAS predisposes to the development of endothelial dysfunction and cardiovascular disease include induction of inflammation and oxidative stress by IH. IH may promote an inflammatory state through the activation of inflammatory cells and increasing levels of inflammatory mediators. Increases in IL-8 and TNF-α are mediated through activation of the transcription factor NF-κB. Increases in CRP and IL-6 levels have also been associated with OSAS. It is proposed that IH is analogous with ischemia-reperfusion injury and can result in the generation of ROS, which can also potentiate cardiovascular damage. Both mechanisms have been linked with the development of endothelial dysfunction, a recognized precursor to atherosclerosis and cardiovascular disease. *Abbreviations*: OSAS, obstructive sleep apnea syndrome; IH, intermittent hypoxia; IL-8, interleukin 8; TNF-α, tumor necrosis factor alpha; NF-κB, nuclear factor kappa B; CRP, C-reactive protein; IL-6, interleukin 6; ROS, reactive oxygen species.

Induction of inflammation, in particular through the NF-κB-mediated pathway, can lead to inflammatory cell activation and increases in inflammatory mediators that have recognized roles in the atherosclerotic process and the development of cardiovascular pathology. Similarly, oxidative stress, through the action of ROS, may contribute to the proatherogenic process. Additional research needs to be undertaken to investigate the detailed molecular mechanisms of these processes. Key questions remaining include elucidating the potential for cross talk between inflammatory and oxidative stress pathways in OSAS and identifying the site(s) of disease in vivo. Expanding our understanding of these pathways, their sites of action, and the interaction between them will yield novel therapeutic targets for the reduction of cardiovascular risk in OSAS.

References

1. Trepels T, Zeiher AM, Fichtlscherer S. The endothelium and inflammation. Endothelium 2006; 13(6):423–429.
2. Kinlay S, Libby P, Ganz P. Endothelial function and coronary artery disease. Curr Opin Lipidol 2001; 12(4):383–389.
3. Ross R. Atherosclerosis—an inflammatory disease. N Engl J Med 1999; 340(2):115–126.
4. Schachinger V, Britten MB, Zeiher AM. Prognostic impact of coronary vasodilator dysfunction on adverse long-term outcome of coronary heart disease. Circulation 2000; 101 (16):1899–1906.
5. Li M, Georgakopoulos D, Lu G, et al. p38 MAP kinase mediates inflammatory cytokine induction in cardiomyocytes and extracellular matrix remodeling in heart. Circulation 2005; 111(19):2494–2502.
6. Hickey MJ, Kubes P. Role of nitric oxide in regulation of leucocyte-endothelial cell interactions. Exp Physiol 1997; 82(2):339–348.
7. Moncada S, Higgs EA. Nitric oxide and the vascular endothelium. Handb Exp Pharmacol 2006; (176 pt 1):213–254.
8. Cohen RA. The role of nitric oxide and other endothelium-derived vasoactive substances in vascular disease. Prog Cardiovasc Dis 1995; 38(2):105–128.
9. Korhonen R, Lahti A, Kankaanranta H, et al. Nitric oxide production and signaling in inflammation. Curr Drug Targets Inflamm Allergy 2005; 4(4):471–479.
10. Grisham MB, Granger DN, Lefer DJ. Modulation of leukocyte-endothelial interactions by reactive metabolites of oxygen and nitrogen: relevance to ischemic heart disease. Free Radic Biol Med 1998; 25(4–5):404–433.
11. Pellegrino D, Shiva S, Angelone T, et al. Nitrite exerts potent negative inotropy in the isolated heart via eNOS-independent nitric oxide generation and cGMP-PKG pathway activation. Biochim Biophys Acta 2009; 1787(7):818–827.
12. Erusalimsky JD, Moncada S. Nitric oxide and mitochondrial signaling: from physiology to pathophysiology. Arterioscler Thromb Vasc Biol 2007; 27(12):2524–2531.
13. Schulz R, Schmidt D, Blum A, et al. Decreased plasma levels of nitric oxide derivatives in obstructive sleep apnoea: response to CPAP therapy. Thorax 2000; 55(12):1046–1051.
14. Ip MS, Lam B, Chan LY, et al. Circulating nitric oxide is suppressed in obstructive sleep apnea and is reversed by nasal continuous positive airway pressure. Am J Respir Crit Care Med 2000; 162(6):2166–2171.
15. Dean RT, Wilcox I. Possible atherogenic effects of hypoxia during obstructive sleep apnea. Sleep 1993; 16(8 suppl):S15–S21; discussion S-2.
16. Lavie L. Obstructive sleep apnoea syndrome—an oxidative stress disorder. Sleep Med Rev 2003; 7(1):35–51.

17. Svatikova A, Wolk R, Wang HH, et al. Circulating free nitrotyrosine in obstructive sleep apnea. Am J Physiol Regul Integr Comp Physiol 2004; 287(2):R284–R287.
18. Jelic S, Padeletti M, Kawut SM, et al. Inflammation, oxidative stress, and repair capacity of the vascular endothelium in obstructive sleep apnea. Circulation 2008; 117(17):2270–2278.
19. Kraiczi H, Hedner J, Peker Y, et al. Increased vasoconstrictor sensitivity in obstructive sleep apnea. J Appl Physiol 2000; 89(2):493–498.
20. Kato M, Roberts-Thomson P, Phillips BG, et al. Impairment of endothelium-dependent vasodilation of resistance vessels in patients with obstructive sleep apnea. Circulation 2000; 102(21):2607–2610.
21. Møller DS, Lind P, Strunge B, et al. Abnormal vasoactive hormones and 24-hour blood pressure in obstructive sleep apnea. Am J Hypertens 2003; 16(4):274–280.
22. Grimpen F, Kanne P, Schulz E, et al. Endothelin-1 plasma levels are not elevated in patients with obstructive sleep apnoea. Eur Respir J 2000; 15(2):320–325.
23. Phillips BG, Narkiewicz K, Pesek CA, et al. Effects of obstructive sleep apnea on endothelin-1 and blood pressure. J Hypertens 1999; 17(1):61–66.
24. Saarelainen S, Seppala E, Laasonen K, et al. Circulating endothelin-1 in obstructive sleep apnea. Endothelium 1997; 5(2):115–118.
25. Jordan W, Reinbacher A, Cohrs S, et al. Obstructive sleep apnea: plasma endothelin-1 precursor but not endothelin-1 levels are elevated and decline with nasal continuous positive airway pressure. Peptides 2005; 26(9):1654–1660.
26. El Solh AA, Akinnusi ME, Baddoura FH, et al. Endothelial cell apoptosis in obstructive sleep apnea: a link to endothelial dysfunction. Am J Respir Crit Care Med 2007; 175(11):1186–1191.
27. Martin K, Stanchina M, Kouttab N, et al. Circulating endothelial cells and endothelial progenitor cells in obstructive sleep apnea. Lung 2008; 186(3):145–150.
28. Valko M, Leibfritz D, Moncol J, et al. Free radicals and antioxidants in normal physiological functions and human disease. Int J Biochem Cell Biol 2007; 39(1):44–84.
29. Lefer DJ, Granger DN. Oxidative stress and cardiac disease. Am J Med 2000; 109(4):315–323.
30. Molavi B, Mehta JL. Oxidative stress in cardiovascular disease: molecular basis of its deleterious effects, its detection, and therapeutic considerations. Curr Opin Cardiol 2004; 19(5): 488–493.
31. Dyugovskaya L, Lavie P, Lavie L. Increased adhesion molecules expression and production of reactive oxygen species in leukocytes of sleep apnea patients. Am J Respir Crit Care Med 2002; 165(7):934–939.
32. Schulz R, Mahmoudi S, Hattar K, et al. Enhanced release of superoxide from polymorphonuclear neutrophils in obstructive sleep apnea. Impact of continuous positive airway pressure therapy. Am J Respir Crit Care Med 2000; 162(2 pt 1):566–570.
33. Barcelo A, Miralles C, Barbe F, et al. Abnormal lipid peroxidation in patients with sleep apnoea. Eur Respir J 2000; 16(4):644–647.
34. Barcelo A, Barbe F, de la Pena M, et al. Antioxidant status in patients with sleep apnoea and impact of continuous positive airway pressure treatment. Eur Respir J 2006; 27(4):756–760.
35. Lavie L, Vishnevsky A, Lavie P. Evidence for lipid peroxidation in obstructive sleep apnea. Sleep 2004; 27(1):123–128.
36. Christou K, Moulas AN, Pastaka C, et al. Antioxidant capacity in obstructive sleep apnea patients. Sleep Med 2003; 4(3):225–228.
37. Svatikova A, Wolk R, Lerman LO, et al. Oxidative stress in obstructive sleep apnoea. Eur Heart J 2005; 26(22):2435–2439.
38. Wali SO, Bahammam AS, Massaeli H, et al. Susceptibility of LDL to oxidative stress in obstructive sleep apnea. Sleep 1998; 21(3):290–296.
39. Ozturk L, Mansour B, Yuksel M, et al. Lipid peroxidation and osmotic fragility of red blood cells in sleep-apnea patients. Clin Chim Acta 2003; 332(1–2):83–88.

40. Montgomery-Downs HE, Krishna J, Roberts LJ II, et al. Urinary F2-isoprostane metabolite levels in children with sleep-disordered breathing. Sleep Breath 2006; 10(4):211–215.

41. Yamauchi M, Nakano H, Maekawa J, et al. Oxidative stress in obstructive sleep apnea. Chest 2005; 127(5):1674–1679.

42. Grossman E. Does increased oxidative stress cause hypertension? Diabetes Care 2008; 31 (suppl 2):S185–S189.

43. Juranek I, Bezek S. Controversy of free radical hypothesis: reactive oxygen species–cause or consequence of tissue injury? Gen Physiol Biophys 2005; 24(3):263–278.

44. Khalid MA, Ashraf M. Direct detection of endogenous hydroxyl radical production in cultured adult cardiomyocytes during anoxia and reoxygenation. Is the hydroxyl radical really the most damaging radical species? Circ Res 1993; 72(4):725–736.

45. Villa P, Carugo C, Guaitani A. No evidence of intracellular oxidative stress during ischemia-reperfusion damage in rat liver in vivo. Toxicol Lett 1992; 61(2–3):283–290.

46. D'Autreaux B, Toledano MB. ROS as signalling molecules: mechanisms that generate specificity in ROS homeostasis. Nat Rev Mol Cell Biol 2007; 8(10):813–824.

47. Ravati A, Ahlemeyer B, Becker A, et al. Preconditioning-induced neuroprotection is mediated by reactive oxygen species and activation of the transcription factor nuclear factor-kappaB. J Neurochem 2001; 78(4):909–919.

48. Bjelakovic G, Nikolova D, Gluud LL, et al. Mortality in randomized trials of antioxidant supplements for primary and secondary prevention: systematic review and meta-analysis. Jama 2007; 297(8):842–857.

49. Ryan S, Taylor CT, McNicholas WT. Selective activation of inflammatory pathways by intermittent hypoxia in obstructive sleep apnea syndrome. Circulation 2005; 112(17):2660–2667.

50. Ryan S, Taylor CT, McNicholas WT. Predictors of elevated nuclear factor-kappaB-dependent genes in obstructive sleep apnea syndrome. Am J Respir Crit Care Med 2006; 174(7): 824–830.

51. Ciftci TU, Kokturk O, Bukan N, et al. The relationship between serum cytokine levels with obesity and obstructive sleep apnea syndrome. Cytokine 2004; 28(2):87–91.

52. Dyugovskaya L, Lavie P, Lavie L. Phenotypic and functional characterization of blood gammadelta T cells in sleep apnea. Am J Respir Crit Care Med 2003; 168(2):242–249.

53. Minoguchi K, Tazaki T, Yokoe T, et al. Elevated production of tumor necrosis factor-alpha by monocytes in patients with obstructive sleep apnea syndrome. Chest 2004; 126(5):1473–1479.

54. Aukrust P, Yndestad A, Smith C, et al. Chemokines in cardiovascular risk prediction. Thromb Haemost 2007; 97(5):748–754.

55. Gerszten RE, Garcia-Zepeda EA, Lim YC, et al. MCP-1 and IL-8 trigger firm adhesion of monocytes to vascular endothelium under flow conditions. Nature 1999; 398(6729):718–723.

56. Ohga E, Tomita T, Wada H, et al. Effects of obstructive sleep apnea on circulating ICAM-1, IL-8, and MCP-1. J Appl Physiol 2003; 94(1):179–184.

57. Vgontzas AN, Papanicolaou DA, Bixler EO, et al. Elevation of plasma cytokines in disorders of excessive daytime sleepiness: role of sleep disturbance and obesity. J Clin Endocrinol Metab 1997; 82(5):1313–1316.

58. Yokoe T, Minoguchi K, Matsuo H, et al. Elevated levels of C-reactive protein and interleukin-6 in patients with obstructive sleep apnea syndrome are decreased by nasal continuous positive airway pressure. Circulation 2003; 107(8):1129–1134.

59. Mehra R, Storfer-Isser A, Kirchner HL, et al. Soluble interleukin 6 receptor: a novel marker of moderate to severe sleep-related breathing disorder. Arch Intern Med 2006; 166(16):1725–1731.

60. Ueda K, Takahashi M, Ozawa K, et al. Decreased soluble interleukin-6 receptor in patients with acute myocardial infarction. Am Heart J 1999; 138(5 pt 1):908–915.

61. Ohga E, Nagase T, Tomita T, et al. Increased levels of circulating ICAM-1, VCAM-1, and L-selectin in obstructive sleep apnea syndrome. J Appl Physiol 1999; 87(1):10–14.

62. Ursavas A, Karadag M, Rodoplu E, et al. Circulating ICAM-1 and VCAM-1 levels in patients with obstructive sleep apnea syndrome. Respiration 2007;74(5):525–532.

63. Zamarron-Sanz C, Ricoy-Galbaldon J, Gude-Sampedro F, et al. Plasma levels of vascular endothelial markers in obstructive sleep apnea. Arch Med Res 2006; 37(4):552–555.
64. El-Solh AA, Mador MJ, Sikka P, et al. Adhesion molecules in patients with coronary artery disease and moderate-to-severe obstructive sleep apnea. Chest 2002; 121(5):1541–1547.
65. Ridker PM, Buring JE, Shih J, et al. Prospective study of C-reactive protein and the risk of future cardiovascular events among apparently healthy women. Circulation 1998; 98(8):731–733.
66. Koenig W, Sund M, Frohlich M, et al. C-Reactive protein, a sensitive marker of inflammation, predicts future risk of coronary heart disease in initially healthy middle-aged men: results from the MONICA (Monitoring Trends and Determinants in Cardiovascular Disease) Augsburg Cohort Study, 1984 to 1992. Circulation 1999; 99(2):237–242.
67. Haverkate F, Thompson SG, Pyke SD, et al. Production of C-reactive protein and risk of coronary events in stable and unstable angina. European Concerted Action on Thrombosis and Disabilities Angina Pectoris Study Group. Lancet 1997; 349(9050):462–466.
68. Heeschen C, Hamm CW, Bruemmer J, et al. Predictive value of C-reactive protein and troponin T in patients with unstable angina: a comparative analysis. CAPTURE Investigators. Chimeric c7E3 AntiPlatelet Therapy in Unstable angina REfractory to standard treatment trial. J Am Coll Cardiol 2000; 35(6):1535–1542.
69. Miller M, Zhan M, Havas S. High attributable risk of elevated C-reactive protein level to conventional coronary heart disease risk factors: the Third National Health and Nutrition Examination Survey. Arch Intern Med 2005; 165(18):2063–2068.
70. Khera A, de Lemos JA, Peshock RM, et al. Relationship between C-reactive protein and subclinical atherosclerosis: the Dallas Heart Study. Circulation 2006; 113(1):38–43.
71. Cao JJ, Arnold AM, Manolio TA, et al. Association of carotid artery intima-media thickness, plaques, and C-reactive protein with future cardiovascular disease and all-cause mortality: the Cardiovascular Health Study. Circulation 2007; 116(1):32–38.
72. Yao M, Tachibana N, Okura M, et al. The relationship between sleep-disordered breathing and high-sensitivity C-reactive protein in Japanese men. Sleep 2006; 29(5):661–665.
73. Taheri S, Austin D, Lin L, et al. Correlates of serum C-reactive protein (CRP)—no association with sleep duration or sleep disordered breathing. Sleep 2007; 30(8).991–996.
74. Shamsuzzaman AS, Winnicki M, Lanfranchi P, et al. Elevated C-reactive protein in patients with obstructive sleep apnea. Circulation 2002; 105(21):2462–2464.
75. Kokturk O, Ciftci TU, Mollarecep E, et al. Elevated C-reactive protein levels and increased cardiovascular risk in patients with obstructive sleep apnea syndrome. Int Heart J 2005; 46 (5):801–809.
76. Can M, Acikgoz S, Mungan G, et al. Serum cardiovascular risk factors in obstructive sleep apnea. Chest 2006; 129(2):233–237.
77. Barcelo A, Barbe F, Llompart E, et al. Effects of obesity on C-reactive protein level and metabolic disturbances in male patients with obstructive sleep apnea. Am J Med 2004; 117(2): 118–121.
78. Guilleminault C, Kirisoglu C, Ohayon MM. C-reactive protein and sleep-disordered breathing. Sleep 2004; 27(8):1507–1511.
79. Ryan S, Nolan GM, Hannigan E, et al. Cardiovascular risk markers in obstructive sleep apnoea syndrome and correlation with obesity. Thorax 2007; 62(6):509–514.
80. Akashiba T, Akahoshi T, Kawahara S, et al. Effects of long-term nasal continuous positive airway pressure on C-reactive protein in patients with obstructive sleep apnea syndrome. Intern Med 2005; 44(8):899–900.
81. Steiropoulos P, Tsara V, Nena E, et al. Effect of continuous positive airway pressure treatment on serum cardiovascular risk factors in patients with obstructive sleep apnea-hypopnea syndrome. Chest 2007; 132(3):843–851.
82. Libby P. Inflammation in atherosclerosis. Nature 2002; 420(6917):868–874.
83. Lusis AJ. Atherosclerosis. Nature 2000; 407(6801):233–241.

84. Nacher M, Serrano-Mollar A, Farre R, et al. Recurrent obstructive apneas trigger early systemic inflammation in a rat model of sleep apnea. Respir Physiol Neurobiol 2007; 155(1): 93–96.

85. Lattimore JD, Wilcox I, Nakhla S, et al. Repetitive hypoxia increases lipid loading in human macrophages-a potentially atherogenic effect. Atherosclerosis 2005; 179(2):255–259.

86. Dyugovskaya L, Lavie P, Hirsh M, et al. Activated CD8+ T-lymphocytes in obstructive sleep apnoea. Eur Respir J 2005; 25(5):820–828.

87. Dyugovskaya L, Polyakov A, Lavie P, et al. Delayed neutrophil apoptosis in sleep apnea patients. Am J Respir Crit Care Med 2008; 177(5):544–554.

88. Greenberg H, Ye X, Wilson D, et al. Chronic intermittent hypoxia activates nuclear factor-kappaB in cardiovascular tissues in vivo. Biochem Biophys Res Commun 2006; 343(2):591–596.

89. Yamauchi M, Tamaki S, Tomoda K, et al. Evidence for activation of nuclear factor kappaB in obstructive sleep apnea. Sleep Breath 2006; 10(4):189–193.

90. Ryan S, McNicholas WT, Taylor CT. A critical role for p38 map kinase in NF-kappaB signaling during intermittent hypoxia/reoxygenation. Biochem Biophys Res Commun 2007; 355(3):728–733.

91. Kotlyarov A, Neininger A, Schubert C, et al. MAPKAP kinase 2 is essential for LPS-induced TNF-alpha biosynthesis. Nat Cell Biol 1999; 1(2):94–97.

92. Cook SA, Sugden PH, Clerk A. Activation of c-Jun N-terminal kinases and p38-mitogen-activated protein kinases in human heart failure secondary to ischaemic heart disease. J Mol Cell Cardiol 1999; 31(8):1429–1434.

93. Behr TM, Nerurkar SS, Nelson AH, et al. Hypertensive end-organ damage and premature mortality are p38 mitogen-activated protein kinase-dependent in a rat model of cardiac hypertrophy and dysfunction. Circulation 2001; 104(11):1292–1298.

94. Cain BS, Meldrum DR, Meng X, et al. p38 MAPK inhibition decreases TNF-alpha production and enhances postischemic human myocardial function. J Surg Res 1999; 83(1):7–12.

95. Shaulian E, Karin M. AP-1 as a regulator of cell life and death. Nat Cell Biol 2002; 4(5): E131–E136.

96. Yuan G, Nanduri J, Bhasker CR, et al. Ca2+/calmodulin kinase-dependent activation of hypoxia inducible factor 1 transcriptional activity in cells subjected to intermittent hypoxia. J Biol Chem 2005; 280(6):4321–4328.

97. Greenberg HE, Sica AL, Scharf SM, et al. Expression of c-fos in the rat brainstem after chronic intermittent hypoxia. Brain Res 1999; 816(2):638–645.

98. Goldbart A, Row BW, Kheirandish L, et al. Intermittent hypoxic exposure during light phase induces changes in cAMP response element binding protein activity in the rat CA1 hippocampal region: water maze performance correlates. Neuroscience 2003;122(3):585–590.

99. Hayakawa M, Miyashita H, Sakamoto I, et al. Evidence that reactive oxygen species do not mediate NF-kappaB activation. EMBO J 2003; 22(13):3356–3366.

8
Obesity, Sleep Apnea, and the Cardiorespiratory Effects of Leptin

KENNETH R. MCGAFFIN and CHRISTOPHER P. O'DONNELL
University of Pittsburgh Medical Center, Pittsburgh, Pennsylvania, U.S.A.

I. Introduction

In the past, adipose tissue was thought of simply as a passive depot for the storage of excess calories. Now, studies have revealed that fat tissue is an active endocrine organ with high metabolic activity. Indeed, excess fat has been shown to synthesize and secrete biologically active molecules that mediate complex respiratory and cardiovascular processes. One such molecule is leptin. In this chapter, we review the link between leptin and cardiorespiratory effects in obstructive sleep apnea (OSA). We discuss the neuromodulators of appetite and metabolism, with particular emphasis on leptin, and review the concept of leptin resistance. We present data that support a stimulatory role for leptin in respiratory function and a protective role for leptin in the development of pathologic cardiac hypertrophy and congestive heart failure (CHF). Finally, we close this chapter with a discussion of how leptin is linked to OSA, obesity hypoventilation syndrome (OHS), and conditions of chronic hypoxia.

II. Obesity as an Epidemic and Risk Factor for Obstructive Sleep Apnea

Both the incidence and prevalence of obesity, classically defined as excess body weight with an abnormally high proportion of body fat (1), have been growing in epidemic proportions worldwide (2). Obesity is the result of chronic positive energy balance (3). Its etiology is complex and involves genetic, environmental, socioeconomic, behavioral, and psychological influences. Whatever the etiology, a lifestyle consisting of low levels of physical activity and the consumption of excess calories plays a dominant role. The genetic defects that seem to govern the development of obesity include those rare genes that directly produce significant obesity and a more common group of genes that underlie the propensity to develop obesity, the so-called "susceptibility" genes (4). Within a permissive environment, these susceptibility genes act to regulate body fat stores, metabolic rate, feeding, and exercise.

Obesity is measured through calculation of the body mass index (BMI), which represents the ratio of body weight (in kilograms) to body height squared (in meters). This measurement has been shown to correlate strongly with total body fat content in adults (1). The National Heart, Lung and Blood Institute task force on the Identification, Evaluation, and Treatment of Overweight and Obesity in Adults has established that overweight individuals have a BMI between 25 kg/m^2 and 30 kg/m^2 and that obesity begins with a BMI of 30 kg/m^2 (1). Recent statistics show that the prevalence of overweight adults in the United States is close to 65%, whereas over 30% are classified as obese (5). Clearly, this represents an important area of public health concern today, as obesity contributes to such disease states as diabetes, hypertension, degenerative joint disease, stroke, coronary atherosclerosis, peripheral vascular atherosclerosis, dyslipidemia, cancer, CHF, and OSA (6).

III. Obesity Associated Pathology and Neuromodulators of Metabolism

A. Obesity, OSA, and the Metabolic Syndrome

In patients with OSA and obesity, both a mechanical substrate (upper airway obstruction) and a neurohormonal milieu coexist to drive disease pathology. Obesity, and more recently OSA, has been linked to the metabolic syndrome. The metabolic syndrome refers to a clustering of specific cardiovascular disease risk factors whose underlying pathophysiology is thought to be related to insulin resistance (7). Traditional cardiovascular risk factors include low serum low-density lipoprotein cholesterol, high serum triglyceride (TG), and elevated blood pressure. However, increased production of plasminogen activator, increased serum C-reactive protein, increased production of tumor necrosis factor alpha (TNFα), increased production of interleukin (IL) 6, left ventricular hypertrophy, microalbuminemia, and insulin resistance have also been added to the list (6). Establishing a definition, the Third Report of the National Cholesterol Education Program's Adult Treatment Panel (ATP III) suggests that individuals with the metabolic syndrome have at least three of the following: waist circumference > 102 cm in men (>88 cm in women), serum TG > 1.7 mmol/L, blood pressure > 130/85, high-density lipoprotein cholesterol < 1.0 mmol/L in men (<1.3 mmol/L in women), and serum glucose > 1.6 mmol/L (8). The World Health Organization definition is similar (9) and incorporates measurements of body weight, blood glucose, TGs, and blood pressure into its determination. In both definitions, obesity is a prominent feature that characterizes the metabolic syndrome, stressing the impact it has on risk factors that contribute to cardiovascular morbidity and mortality.

B. Fat-Derived Cytokines

The neurohormonal control of appetite, body composition, and glucose homeostasis is mediated by hormones and cytokines secreted primarily from adipose tissue and endocrine glands. In contrast to hormones, which are secreted from specific organs into the blood to mediate a biological effect, cytokines are a large group of protein molecules that are produced by many different cell types and act in an autocrine, paracrine, or endocrine manner. Adipose tissue was previously thought to be a passive depot for the storage of excess calories. It is now viewed as an active endocrine organ (10) contributing to an increase in total blood volume and cardiac output seen in obesity (6). Fat is also capable of synthesizing and secreting a variety of biologically active substances (11). Many of these compounds, collectively called cytokines or "adipokines," act as "hormones" regulating energy intake and expenditure. Some, such as levels of adipocyte-derived TNFα, IL6, angiotensinogen, and plasminogen activator inhibitor (PAI)-1, are directly related to BMI (11) and contribute to the proinflammatory milieu that predisposes to coronary events (12). Others, such as adiponectin, resistin, and leptin, have also been linked to the modulation of cardiovascular disease risk factors in a positive way (13). Overall, the association of obesity and insulin resistance with various aspects of the metabolic syndrome seems to be driven at least in part by the biological activity of adipose tissue.

C. Leptin Action and Animal Models of Leptin Resistance

Leptin, a product of the obesity (Ob) gene, is a cytokine derived primarily from fat. First described in terms of its effect on regulating food intake and energy expenditure via its action on the hypothalamus (14), leptin has since been shown to have many additional effects mediated by direct action on peripheral tissues (15). Aside from fat, leptin is also produced, although at lower levels, in other tissues, including skeletal muscle, placenta, brain, and heart (16). The de novo synthesis of leptin in these organs suggests that its action may be autocrine or paracrine mediated. The 167 amino acids of the leptin molecule are relatively conserved among species. Leptin secretion into the blood is mainly constitutive and is present in nanogram concentrations in the systemic circulation (15), but various physiologic and disease states alter leptin levels. For example, leptin levels fall with fasting and increase several hours after eating (17). Leptin is also elevated in states of insulin resistance, obesity, acute infection, glucocorticoid exposure, and proinflammatory cytokine production (16). Mutations in the leptin gene are rare but can be found, including a frameshift mutation in C57Bl/6J mice, resulting in the Ob/Ob mouse (18), and a missense mutation in two human families (19,20), resulting in morbid obesity and its associated sequelae. Thus, a deficiency in the biological action of leptin can result in profound obesity.

Leptin mediates biological responses through membrane-bound leptin receptors (ObRs) that are products of the diabetes (db) gene (16). The gene is alternatively spliced to produce six known receptor isoforms (ObRa–ObRf). All isoforms have identical amino-terminal extracellular domains that bind leptin. ObRa to ObRd and ObRf have transmembrane domains, but only the "long form," ObRb, has a carboxy-terminal intracellular domain that is capable of activating Janus-activated kinase (JAK)-STAT and MAPK signaling (Fig. 1). Collectively, the ObRa, ObRc, ObRd, and ObRf isoforms are known as "short-form" receptors, whereas the ObRe isoform, only having an extracellular domain, is deemed a "soluble ObR" that acts to regulate leptin's bio-availability in the circulation (21). In the lean state, most leptin is bound to ObRc and other serum proteins, whereas in states of obesity, most leptin is found in its free form (22). In addition to the hypothalamus and the central nervous system, the ObR is present in bone marrow, spleen, kidney, lung, and cardiac tissue (23). However, under non-stressful conditions, it has been reported that only 5% to 25% of the total cellular ObR pool is located at the cell surface, the majority otherwise residing in intracellular pools (24). This is physiologically important, as an interaction of leptin with the ObR at the cell membrane is required to initiate downstream biological activity (25).

Although the various cell-associated ObR isoforms are capable of forming heterodimers and homodimers with one another, only the binding of two leptin molecules to a "long-form" homodimer will result in the necessary conformational change for activation of intracellular signaling (25). It is also important to note that the ObR does not form functional heterodimers with other structurally similar cytokine receptors (26). Since the ObR possesses no intrinsic tyrosine kinase activity, signaling events are

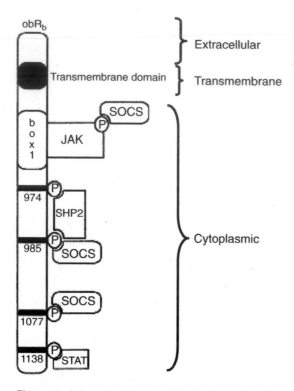

Figure 1 Schematic diagram of the leptin receptor showing extracellular, transmembrane, and cytoplasmic domains and the sites of Janus-activated kinase (JAK) phosphorylation. *Source*: From Ref. 15.

dependent on association with kinases such as JAK-2 (15). Hence, upon ligand binding and ObR oligomerization, JAK-2 phosphorylates the ObR at Y985, Y1077, and Y1138 residues (15). It also phosphorylates itself and a variety of other intracellular substrates, including signal transducer and activator of transcription (STAT)-3 molecules that are recruited to the ObR's Src homology (SH) 2 and SH3 domains containing the Y1138 residue and SH2 molecules that are recruited to the ObR's Y985 residue (27). The phosphorylation of SH2 results in association with growth factor receptor–bound protein 2 (Grb-2) and subsequent activation of the mitogen-activated protein kinase (MAPK) pathway (27). The phosphorylation of STAT results in its activation, dimerization, nuclear translocation, and the increased expression of a number of gene products via promoter element binding (28). The promoter of the suppressor of cytokine signaling (SOCS)-3 molecule is activated by STAT binding (29). SOCS3 has been shown to downregulate cytokine receptor activity by binding not only to JAK kinases but also various phosphorylated tyrosine residues on the ObR itself such as Y985 and Y1077 (15). This allows for a homologous negative feedback loop and creates the potential for cross talk with signaling induced by other receptor/ligand pairs that mediate signal transduction via JAK kinases (15). Further, tightly controlled regulation of SOCS3 expression in this manner may play a role in the development of leptin resistance, as has been postulated for leptin's attenuated effect in Chinese hamster ovary cells (30). Thus, impairment of specific components of the leptin-signaling process can occur at multiple levels and has resulted in many rodent models of genetic obesity (Fig. 2).

There are numerous examples of mutations in the ObR that cause obesity. For example, the db/db mouse has a premature stop codon in the 3' end of the ObR transcript, resulting in only the production of the ObRa isoform (31). However, the phenotype of the db/db mouse is influenced by its genetic background. In the C57BlKS/J background, db/db mice have a shorter life span and early-onset severe diabetes, whereas in the C57Bl/6J background, animals are glucose tolerant and have enhanced longevity (16). Common to both, mice are hyperphagic and obese and do not respond to leptin treatment. In rats, the Zucker (fa/fa) strain has a Gln for Pro substitution in the ObR that results in reduced cell surface expression and leptin binding (32), and the Koletsky strain has a point mutation in the ObR that results in the absence of all cell surface expression (33). Hence, the Koletsky rat is completely unresponsive to leptin treatment, but the Zucker rat will demonstrate blunted leptin action when administered exogenously. As with leptin, mutations in the human ObR gene are rare. However, a reported family having a single nucleotide substitution in the gene that results in absence of transmembrane and intracellular domains of the ObR are, as expected, obese and hyperphagic (34). Since most human obesity is associated with hyperleptinemia, the concept of leptin resistance has emerged to explain its inability to modulate positive metabolic effects.

D. Human Obesity as a State of Leptin Resistance

Animal models of leptin resistance that are well established in the field of obesity research include the db/db mouse and the Zucker rat. In both these models and the majority of humans, obesity can be thought of as a state of central leptin resistance, that is, hypothalamic areas controlling appetite are resistant to the effects of circulating leptin produced by adipose tissue. Experimentally, chronic overexpression of leptin in the central nervous system induces a state of leptin resistance that mimics diet-induced obesity, including decreased ObR expression, reduced ObR signaling, and impaired responsiveness to exogenously administered leptin (35). Additionally, leptin resistance may result from the limitation of leptin movement across the blood-brain barrier, increased soluble ObR reducing leptin bioavailability, and effector molecules downstream of the ObR that downregulate receptor activity. Although hyperleptinemia is common in obesity, it is likely a consequence rather than a cause of impaired central ObR action.

IV. Obesity, Leptin, and Respiratory Control

Obesity can be linked to OSA both mechanically and neurohormonally (36). In particular, the deposition of fat around the neck and submental region makes the upper airway prone to collapse on lying supine (37), whereas circulating levels of various fat-derived cytokines, including TNFα and IL6, are elevated in obesity (38) and contribute to the overall inflammatory milieu that leads to dysfunctional chemoreceptor and sympathetic nervous system responses to hypoxia (39). Experiments in the leptin-resistant Zucker rat and leptin-deficient Ob/Ob mouse have examined the complex

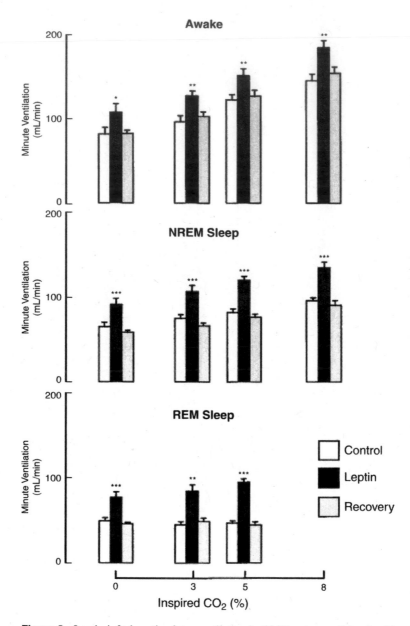

Figure 2 Leptin infusion stimulates ventilation in Ob/Ob mice at all levels of inspired CO_2 and across all sleep/wake states compared with control and recovery conditions. Shown are the mean $\pm$ SEM with statistical significance derived using one-way, within-subject ANOVA with Newman-Keuls post hoc analysis. $*p < 0.05$, $**p < 0.01$, and $***p < 0.001$ compared with control and recovery conditions. From Ref. 42.

relationship between the mechanical and neurohormonal control of respiration in obesity (40,41).

Farkas and Schlenker (40) examined the impact of obesity and leptin resistance in experiments comparing lung volumes, hypercapnic response, diaphragm muscle fiber type, and upper airway collapsibility in lean and obese Zucker rats. Specifically, 32- to 40-week-old obese Zucker rats (weight 698 ± 79 g) exhibited reduced lung volumes compared to lean (weight 304 ± 24 g) controls. Lean rats also showed an appropriate increase in minute ventilation with hypercapnia, whereas obese animals had no change from baseline. The ability of the diaphragm to utilize oxidative metabolism was also examined in lean and obese rats in relationship to muscle fiber type. Compared to their lean counterparts, obese Zucker rats showed an absolute 12% increase in type I high-oxidative fibers, with a proportional decrease in type II low-oxidative fibers. Finally, when upper airway collapsibility was examined, the critical closing pressure in lean rats was slightly, but significantly, lower than in obese animals. Thus, respiratory function in the obese, leptin-resistant Zucker rat is characterized by a derangement in structural, neural, and metabolic function.

Extending the findings from the Zucker rat (40), Tankersley et al. (41) examined mechanical and biochemical aspects of obesity, leptin, and respiratory control using the Ob/Ob mouse as a model. In contrast to the Zucker rat, the Ob/Ob mouse is genetically leptin deficient rather than resistant, so administration of exogenous leptin from birth maintains a lean phenotype into adulthood. To avoid the development of obesity, Tankersley et al. started with 30-day-old (still relatively lean) Ob/Ob mice and age-matched wild-type (+/+) and heterozygous (+/?) mice. At the end of six weeks, the weight of the Ob/Ob group was nearly double (~ 51 g) that of +/+ or +/? lean groups (~ 27 g). Measured lung volumes were significantly reduced in the obese Ob/Ob mouse group compared with the lean groups. Furthermore, in obese Ob/Ob mice, the hypercapnic ventilatory response was depressed relative to lean mice, during wakefulness, non–rapid eye movement (NREM) sleep, and rapid-eye-movement (REM) sleep (42). A significant increase in $PaCO_2$ was also documented in obese Ob/Ob mice (45 mmHg) relative to lean controls (33 mmHg). When diaphragm muscle fiber type was examined in these obese Ob/Ob mice, an absolute 5% increase in type I high-oxidative and an absolute 19% decrease in type II low-oxidative muscle was observed relative to lean controls. Thus, obesity in the Ob/Ob mouse leads to reduced lung volumes, blunted hypercapnic responsiveness, chronically elevated $PaCO_2$, and increased type I oxidative muscle in the diaphragm.

The effect of leptin repletion on respiratory control in the Ob/Ob mouse was also examined in the studies by O'Donnell et al. (42) and Tankersley et al. (41) Specifically, leptin (30 µg/day) was given acutely (daily for 3 days) to obese (~ 60 g) Ob/Ob mice to examine the effect on hypercapnic ventilatory response. Minute ventilation was examined during wake, NREM, and REM periods three days prior to, three days during, and three days after starting leptin therapy. At all concentrations of inspired CO_2 (0%, 3%, 5%, 8%) and under all conditions examined (awake, NREM sleep, REM sleep), leptin repletion stimulated ventilation in the obese Ob/Ob mice relative to three-day pre-repletion and three-day postrepletion values. Longer administration of leptin (six weeks via subcutaneous minipump) was performed to ascertain the effect on lung volumes and diaphragm muscle composition (41). By the end of six weeks, these mice were weight-matched to their +/? and +/+ counterparts. When compared to obese and leptin-deficient Ob/Ob mice at six weeks, leptin replacement partially restored lung volumes but completely reversed the shift in diaphragm muscle type from type I to type II. Thus, these data suggest that restoration of leptin signaling in Ob/Ob mice can stimulate respiration, particularly during sleep, independent of changes in body weight. Moreover, it provides evidence that leptin can reverse pathologic changes in obesity hypoventilation by restoring lung volumes and normalizing diaphragmatic muscle fiber distribution.

V. Obesity, Leptin and Cardiovascular Control

The prevalence of obesity in the world is alarming because of the relationship between obesity and cardiovascular disease. Obesity may affect the cardiovascular system through its influence on known risk factors such as dyslipidemia, hypertension, glucose intolerance, inflammatory markers, and stimulation of the prothrombotic state (43). Additionally, when adipose tissue accumulates in excessive amounts, a variety of adaptations and alterations occur in cardiac structure and function (44). Specifically, obesity has been shown to result in increased total blood volume, increased cardiac output, left ventricular hypertrophy, diastolic dysfunction, and fatty infiltration of the heart (6) all of which predispose to CHF. Also to be considered is the fact that fat produces biologically active molecules, such as TNFα and IL6, that are associated with adverse cardiovascular outcomes (45). Leptin levels have also been reported to be elevated in CHF (46) and after myocardial infarction (MI) (47), independent of weight. Although it is unclear what the cause of hyperleptinemia is in CHF and MI, there are a few key studies in leptin-deficient and leptin-resistant animals that suggest a beneficial effect on the heart and cardiovascular system.

Looking at the cardiovascular effects of obesity and leptin, Barouch et al. (48) were one of the first groups to report on the effect of leptin deficiency on the in vivo development of cardiac hypertrophy. Specifically, Barouch et al. (48) studied myocardial structure and function by echocardiographic and histologic methods in leptin-deficient Ob/Ob and leptin-resistant Db/Db mice at two, four, and six months of age. At the end of six months, the Ob/Ob and Db/Db mice showed a profound weight gain compared to their wild-type, littermate controls (~ 70 g vs. 36 g). By echocardiography, six-month-old obese Ob/Ob and Db/Db mice had developed a significant, approximately 30%, increase in left ventricular wall thickness and calculated mass. These changes were also seen at the cardiomyocyte level on histologic examination of cellular diameters. When these same six-month-old obese mice were then administered exogenous leptin for four weeks, or food restricted to restore a lean phenotype over four weeks, regression of cardiac hypertrophy was seen only in the leptin-repleted group despite equal weight reduction (Fig. 3). Thus, these results strongly support a direct antihypertrophic role for leptin in preventing cardiac hypertrophy, independent of body weight.

Building upon the finding that leptin deficiency results in cardiac hypertrophy, Minhas et al. (49) subsequently demonstrated that leptin repletion restores depressed myocardial β-adrenergic contractility in obese Ob/Ob mice. Specifically, Minhas et al. studied Ob/Ob mice prior to the development of cardiac hypertrophy but after the onset of obesity (at 10 weeks of age). Using isoproterenol, a nonselective β-agonist, and isolated cardiomyocyte preparations from both wild-type and Ob/Ob mice, they observed an attenuation of contractility in the Ob/Ob mice as measured by both degree

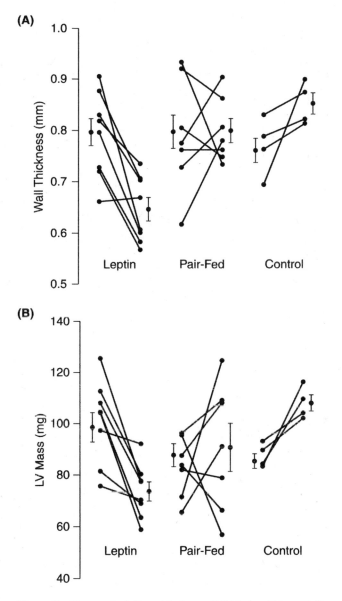

Figure 3 Changes in left ventricular wall thickness (**A**) and left ventricular mass (**B**) in leptin, pair-fed, and control groups of six-month-old Ob/Ob mice before and after four weeks of weight loss. $*p < 0.001$; $†p < 0.05$. *Source*: From Ref. 48.

of sarcomere shortening and magnitude of calcium transients. However, when leptin was given to both wild-type and Ob/Ob mice by minipump for 4 weeks prior to sacrifice at 10 weeks of age, these same isoproterenol-mediated ionotropic responses were restored in Ob/Ob cardiomyocytes compared to age-matched wild-type controls. The authors went on to show depressed sarcoplasmic reticulum calcium stores and protein kinase A activity in Ob/Ob mice relative to wild-type controls, with restoration to normal levels after four weeks of leptin treatment. Thus, these data suggest that leptin is involved in mediating myocardial β-adrenergic contractility independent of left ventricular hypertrophy.

Another series of experiments from the same group addressed the clinical problem of leptin resistance commonly associated with human obesity (50). A reversal of age-related cardiac hypertrophy in leptin-deficient Ob/Ob and leptin-resistant Db/Db mice was demonstrated through activation of the ciliary neurotrophic factor (CNTF) receptor. Similar to leptin, CNTF activates STAT-3 and MAPK signal transduction pathways and has similar effects on body weight and metabolism. In this study, the authors hypothesized that restoring leptin signaling through exogenous leptin would result in reversal of age-related cardiac hypertrophy in only leptin-deficient Ob/Ob mice, whereas CNTF, which acts independently of the ObR, should cause regression of left ventricular size in both leptin-deficient Ob/Ob and leptin-resistant Db/Db mice. Their experimental approach involved using for four weeks six-month-old obese Ob/Ob mice treated with CNTF and six-month-old obese Db/Db mice treated with leptin or CNTF. Myocardial hypertrophy was assessed by echocardiographic and histologic measurements of left ventricular wall thickness and cardiomyocyte size, respectively. At the end of four weeks, regression of myocardial hypertrophy in Ob/Ob mice given CNTF and Db/Db mice given leptin or CNTF were observed. Similar to results with the Ob/Ob mouse in their prior study (48), this regression in left ventricular size occurred independent of weight as parallel groups of food-restricted Ob/Ob and Db/Db mice failed to show any normalization of cardiac wall thickness or myocyte dimensions despite body weights that were matched to their leptin- or CNTF-treated counterparts. These investigators went on to demonstrate activation of cardiac STAT-3 and ERK1/2 signal transduction pathways in response to CNTF in both Ob/Ob and Db/Db mice. Together, these findings support a role for intact cardiac leptin signaling in regulating normal cardiac structure and function. They also suggest that the cardiac pathology associated with obesity and the leptin-resistant state can be overcome by restoring leptin signaling at the post-receptor level.

VI. Obesity, Leptin, and Heart Failure

Along with obesity, CHF has been growing at epidemic proportions over the last decade with nearly 500,000 new cases diagnosed and 5 million people treated in the United States each year (51). By the year 2037, this number is expected to grow to 10 million (52). Despite recent advances in the treatment of CHF, the overall five-year mortality rate is still unacceptably high at greater than 70% (53). This is a mortality rate four to eight times that of the general population of the same age (53). When established clinical criteria are used to define overt CHF, the lifetime risk is one in five for both men and women (54). For CHF occurring in the absence of MI, the lifetime risk is one in nine for men and one in six for women, highlighting a risk that is largely attributable to hypertension (54). The economic burden of CHF is equally impressive, costing $24.3 billion annually for hospital admissions and outpatient treatment of the disease (55). Indeed, CHF represents the most frequent cause of hospital admission in those over the age of 65 years in the United States (56). Clearly, given these statistics, CHF represents a major health concern today, both in terms of its staggering economic impact and in terms of its adverse affect on millions of lives.

There are numerous causes of CHF. Framingham Study data indicate that the most common etiologies include hypertensive, coronary, and valvular heart disease (53), accounting for nearly two-thirds of all cases. There are also unexplained causes, deemed "idiopathic," that comprise a large part of the remaining proportion. Despite varied etiologies, once diagnosed, CHF in general carries a relatively poor prognosis (51). Sudden death is a prominent feature of the mortality in CHF (57). Hypertension has the greatest impact on CHF exacerbations, accounting for 39% of events in men and 59% in women (53). MI also has a high attributable risk in men (34%) and women (13%), whereas valvular heart disease accounts for 7% to 8% of CHF (53). Diabetes has been shown to increase CHF risk up to eightfold, complicating nearly 20% of all CHF cases (53). Dyslipidemia, characterized by a high total/high-density lipoprotein cholesterol ratio, is also a risk factor for CHF development (53). Each of these risk factors for CHF development, including diabetes, hypertension, dyslipidemia, and obesity, are components of the metabolic syndrome (7); as such, an elevated BMI thus predisposes to CHF. Overall, it is estimated that the risk of CHF development increases 5% for men and 7% for women for each one unit increase in BMI, with the existence of a continuous gradient and no evidence of a threshold (58).

In humans, increased serum leptin has been reported after MI (47) and in chronic stable CHF (46). However, it was previously unknown whether ObR signaling is altered in cardiomyocytes in response to CHF or if a deficiency in ObR signaling leads to worse CHF outcomes. To answer these questions, a series of studies were undertaken to examine circulating leptin and cardiac leptin production, and cardiac leptin signaling in C57BL/6J mice at 30 days post experimentally induced MI by coronary artery ligation (CAL) (59). Similar to studies in humans post MI (47) and in CHF (46), there was a statistically significant increase in circulating leptin in C57BL/6J mice at 30 days post-MI, independent of obesity. This was accompanied by an increase in leptin mRNA expression in both whole heart and adipose tissue relative to sham mice (Fig. 4A). In contrast, measured levels of ObR transcript and protein were increased in cardiac tissue, but not in fat, at 30 days post-CAL (Fig. 4B). The observed increase in cardiac leptin production (both mRNA and protein) was found to be localized to the cardiomyocyte by in situ hybridization and immunofluorescence staining of cardiac sections. Finally, increased levels of phosphorylated (active) STAT-3 were also observed in failing mouse cardiomyocytes (Fig. 4C), suggesting activation of leptin signaling in response to increased local leptin production post-MI. Thus, experimental MI leading to CHF causes increases in leptin and ObR expression in cardiac tissue that activates downstream leptin signaling.

Hypothesizing that the increased leptin production and signaling observed in the failing heart plays a protective role in mitigating MI-induced damage, the authors examined post-MI cardiac structure, function, and survival in a separate group of lean and obese leptin-deficient, as well as leptin-repleted, Ob/Ob mice (59). In this set of experiments, seven groups of five- to six-week-old male leptin-deficient Ob/Ob mice and wild-type (littermate control) mice were studied. Shams included (*i*) lean wild-type mice fed ad libitum; (*ii*) obese Ob/Ob mice fed ad libitum; and (*iii*) lean Ob/Ob mice, food restricted. CAL mice included (*i*) lean wild-type mice fed ad libitum; (*ii*) obese Ob/ Ob mice fed ad libitum; (*iii*) lean Ob/Ob mice, food restricted; and (*iv*) lean Ob/Ob mice

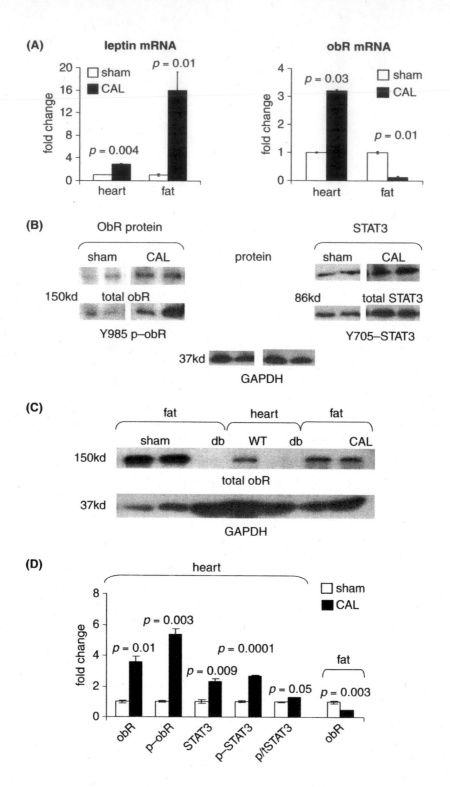

repleted with leptin starting the day prior to the CAL surgery and continuing for four weeks. Survival in all three sham groups (wild-type, Ob/Ob food ad libitum, and Ob/Ob food restricted) was 100% at 30 days (Fig. 5). In lean wild-type mice, survival was significantly reduced to 75% after CAL relative to these three sham groups ($p = 0.009$; log rank Mantel-Cox test). In both lean (food restricted) and obese (food ad libitum) leptin-deficient Ob/Ob mice, survival after CAL was further reduced to 46% and 44%, respectively, relative to all sham groups. In contrast, in lean Ob/Ob mice repleted with leptin, the survival rate was 69%, a value comparable to lean wild-type mice. Similar to its impact on mortality, leptin deficiency in lean and obese Ob/Ob mice resulted in worse morbidity after CAL relative to wild-type and Ob/Ob mice repleted with leptin. Specifically, leptin-deficient mice demonstrated significantly larger decrements in myocardial contractility and markedly greater increases in left ventricular dilation and hypertrophy relative to wild-type and leptin-repleted Ob/Ob mice. Suggesting a mechanism by which leptin deficiency might mediate these effects, the authors examined cardiac leptin signaling and demonstrated an approximately threefold increase in phosphorylated STAT-3 expression and an approximately twofold increase in STAT-3 DNA binding in wild-type and leptin-repleted Ob/Ob mice relative to lean and obese leptin-deficient Ob/Ob mice. Combined, these data suggest that leptin deficiency, independent of obesity, is a key determinant of morbidity and mortality in this animal model of MIs.

VII. Obesity, Leptin, and OSA

As previously discussed, leptin is a powerful stimulant of respiration (41), especially during sleep (42). Even when matched for age and BMI, patients with OSA and OHS demonstrate increased circulating leptin (60,61). The hyperleptinemia associated with OSA and OHS is reduced through the use of continuous positive airway pressure therapy (62–64). Similar to OSA and OHS, which represent various states of hypoxia, leptin is also increased under conditions of chronic hypoxia, as occurs in those living at high altitude (65,66). Chronic hypoxia also increases hypoxia inducible factor (HIF)-1α (67), which is a transcription factor that mediates physiological and pathophysiological

<

Figure 4 Increased leptin and ObR signaling in hearts of mice with experimentally induced heart failure four weeks post-CAL. Graphical data are expressed as fold changes in mean values ± SEM in CAL ($n = 8$) relative to sham ($n = 10$) mice, the latter of which were arbitrarily assigned a value of 1 after statistical calculations (individual two-tailed, unpaired t-tests) were performed. (A) Fold changes in mouse leptin and long-form ObR mRNA in heart and fat from sham/CAL mice as determined by quantitative RT-PCR. (B) Representative western blots showing protein levels of long-form ObR, Y985p-ObR, STAT-3, Y705p-STAT-3, and GAPDH in cardiac tissue from sham/ CAL mice. (C) Representative western blot using antibodies against long-form ObR and GAPDH in fat from wild-type sham (*lanes 2–3*) and CAL (*lanes 4–5*) mice. Also shown on this blot are fat (*lane 1*) and heart (*lane 6*) protein extracts from a db/db mouse; these were included as negative antibody controls, since the Db/Db mouse lacks long-form ObR expression. Lane 7 contains cardiac protein from a wild-type sham mouse, run simultaneously with the Db/Db mouse heart (*lane 6*), as an antibody control. (D) Quantification for group data in panels A and C after normalizing to GAPDH. *Abbreviations*: CAL, coronary artery ligation; RT-PCR, reverse transcriptase polymerase chain reaction; GAPDH, glyceraldehyde-3-phosphate dehydrogenase. *Source*: From Ref. 59.

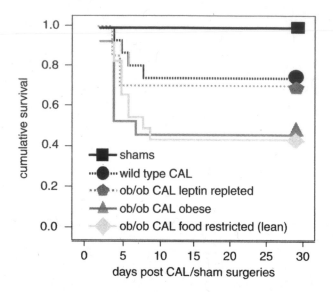

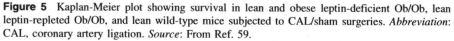

days post CAL/sham surgeries

Figure 5 Kaplan-Meier plot showing survival in lean and obese leptin-deficient Ob/Ob, lean leptin-repleted Ob/Ob, and lean wild-type mice subjected to CAL/sham surgeries. *Abbreviation*: CAL, coronary artery ligation. *Source*: From Ref. 59.

responses to hypoxia (68) and regulates mammalian oxygen homeostasis (69). Specifically, under hypoxic conditions, HIF-1α activates the transcription of genes encoding erythropoietin, glucose transporters, glycolytic enzymes, vascular endothelial growth factor, and other genes whose protein products increase O_2 delivery or facilitate metabolic adaptation to hypoxia (70), including leptin (71). Thus, the hyperleptinemia characterizing chronic hypoxia is directly linked to elevated HIF-1α.

Both chronic and intermittent hypoxia result in increased circulating leptin independent of obesity (65,66,72). However, unlike chronic hypoxia where HIF-1α levels increase (65,66), there are conflicting in vitro data regarding changes in HIF-1α levels in response to intermittent hypoxia. Specifically, Ryan et al. (73) demonstrated no change in Hela (derived from human cervical cancer) cell HIF-1α activation after exposure to intermittent hypoxia, whereas Yuan et al. (74) found that intermittent hypoxia increases HIF-1α expression and activation in adrenal medulla (pheochromocytoma or PC12) cells through a Ca^{2+}/calmodulin kinase–dependent pathway. Extending this in vitro work, Li et al. (75) examined circulating leptin levels after intermittent hypoxia in heterozygous HIF-1α knockout mice that demonstrate partial, but not complete, loss of HIF-1α function. In particular, these authors showed a strong trend for a reduction in the magnitude of hyperleptinemia that occurs with intermittent hypoxia in their partial HIF-1α knockout mice. Thus, evidence suggests that chronic hypoxia, and perhaps intermittent hypoxia, activates HIF-1α and results in increased circulating leptin.

Although hyperleptinemia is found in both OSA and OHS, it is unclear as to what the physiologic relevance of this finding is. Potentially, leptin acts as a respiratory stimulant in OSA and OHS patients and increases ventilation above that found in comparably obese humans without these disorders. Alternatively, if leptin resistance, as occurs with metabolism in the hypothalamus, also occurs with respect to ventilation in obese OSA and OHS patients, then hyperleptinemia may be of limited value. To understand the significance of hyperleptinemia in OSA and OHS, future studies using exogenously administered leptin or, better still, compounds like CNTF that circumvent leptin resistance, in obese OSA and OHS patients, or in animal models of diet-induced obesity, would be most informative.

VIII. Summary and Conclusions

In this chapter, we discussed the link between obesity, the metabolic syndrome, and OSA. We reviewed data suggesting that leptin, an adipokine well known for its control of appetite and metabolism, is a critical neuromodulator of respiratory function. We presented evidence that suggests that leptin plays a protective role in the development of pathologic cardiac hypertrophy and heart failure. Finally, we linked our discussion of OSA and hypoxia to hyperleptinemia that may represent a compensatory response or, alternatively, a leptin-resistant state that may negatively impact long-term cardiovascular and respiratory outcomes.

References

1. Clinical guidelines on the identification, evaluation, and treatment of overweight and obesity in adults: the evidence report. NIH Publication 98-4083, 1998.
2. Eckel RH, York DA, Rossner S, et al. American Heart Association. Prevention Conference VII: obesity, a worldwide epidemic related to heart disease and stroke: executive summary. Circulation 2004; 110:2968–2975.
3. Cummings D, Schwartz MW. Genetics and pathophysiology of human obesity. Annu Rev Med 2003; 54:453 471.
4. Synder EE, Walts B, Perusse L, et al. The human obesity gene map: the 2003 update. Obes Res 2004, 12:369 439.
5. Flegal KM, Carroll MD, Ogden CL, et al. Prevalence and trends in obesity among US adults, 1999–2000. JAMA 2002; 228:1723–1727.
6. Poirier P, Giles TD, Bray GA, et al. AHA scientific statement: obesity and cardiovascular disease: pathophysiology, evaluation, and effect of weight loss. Circulation 2006; 113:1–21.
7. Kahn R, Buse J, Ferrannini E, et al. The metabolic syndrome: time for a critical appraisal: joint statement from the American Diabetes Association and the European Association for the Study of Diabetes. Diabetes Care 2005; 28:2289–2304.
8. National Cholesterol Education Program. Third report of the national cholesterol education program on detection and treatment of blood pressure and cholesterol in adults. Circulation 2002; 106:3143–3421.
9. Alberti K, Zimmet PZ. Definition, diagnosis and classification of diabetes mellitus and its complication part 1: diagnosis and classification of diabetes mellitus provisional report of a WHO consultation. Diabet Med 1998; 15:539–553.
10. Shuldiner AR, Yang R, Dong D-W. Resistin, obesity, and insulin resistance: the emerging role of the adipoctye as an endocrine organ. N Engl J Med 2001; 345:145–146.
11. Vendrell J, Broch M, Vilarrasa N, et al. Resistin, adiponectin, ghrelin, leptin, and proin-flammatory cytokines: relationships in obesity. Obes Res 2004; 12:962–671.
12. Cottam DR, Schaefer PA, Shaftan GW, et al. Effect of surgically-induced weight loss on leukocyte indicators of chronic inflammation in morbid obesity. Obes Surg 2002; 12: 335–342.

13. Lima M, de Correia G, Haynes WG. Leptin, obesity and cardiovascular disease. Curr Opin Nephrol Hypertens 2004;13:251–323.
14. Anand BK, Brobeck JR. Localization of a feeding center in the hypothalamus of the rat. Proc Soc Exp Biol Med 1951; 77:323–324.
15. Sweeney G. Leptin signalling. Cell Signal 2002; 14:655–663.
16. Ahima RS, Oser SY. Leptin signaling. Physiol Behav 2004; 81:223–241.
17. Ahima RS, Prabakaran D, Flier JS. Postprandial leptin surge and regulation of circadian rhythm of leptin by feeding. Implications for energy homeostasis and neuroendocrine function. J Clin Invest 1998; 101:1020–1027.
18. Zhang Y, Proenca R, Maffei M, et al. Positional cloning of the mouse obese gene and its human homologue. Nature 1994; 372:425–432.
19. Rau H, Reaves BJ, O'Rahilly S, et al. Truncated human leptin (delta 133) associated with extreme obesity undergoes proteasomal degredation after defective intracellular transport. Endocrinology 1999; 140:1718–1723.
20. Strobel A, Issad T, Camoin L, et al. A leptin missense mutation associated with hypogonadism and morbid obesity. Nat Genet 1998; 18:213–215.
21. Hegyi K, Fulop K, Kovacs K, et al. Leptin-induced signal transduction pathways. Cell Biol Int 2004; 28:159–169.
22. Sinha MK, Opentanova I, Ohannesian JP, et al. Evidence of free and bound leptin in human circulation. Studies in lean and obese subjects and during short term fasting. J Clin Invest 1996; 98:1277–1282.
23. Fantuzzi G, Faggioni R. Leptin in the regulation of immunity, inflammation and hematopoiesis. J Leukoc Biol 2000; 68:437–446.
24. Barr VA, Lane K, Taylor SI. Subcellular localization and internalization of the four human leptin receptor isoforms. J Biol Chem 1999; 274:21416–21424.
25. Fong TM, Huang RR, Tota MR, et al. Localization of leptin binding domain in the leptin receptor. Mol Pharmacol 1998; 53:234–240.
26. Nakashima K, Narazaki M, Taga T. Leptin receptor (OB-R) oligomerizes with itself but not with its closely related cytokine signal transducer gp130. FEBS Lett 1997; 10403:79–82.
27. Banks A, Davis SM, Bates SH, et al. Activation of downstream signals by the long form of the leptin receptor. J Biol Chem 2000; 275:14563–14572.
28. Darnell J. STATs and gene regulation. Science 1997; 277:1630–1635.
29. Auernhammer CJ, Bousquet C, Melmed S. Autoregulation of pituitary corticotroph SOCS-3 expression: characterization of the murine SOCS-3 promoter. Proc Natl Acad Sci USA 1999; 96:6964–6969.
30. Bjorbaek C, El-Haschimi K, Frantz JD, et al. The role of SOCS-3 in leptin signaling and leptin resistance. J Biol Chem 1999; 274:30059–30065.
31. Lee G, Proenca R, Montez JM, et al. Abnormal splicing of the leptin receptor in diabetic mice. Nature 1996; 379:632–635.
32. Chua S, Chung WK, Wu-Peng XS, et al. Phenotypes of mouse diabetes and rat fatty due to mutations in the OB (leptin) receptor. Science 1996; 271:994–996.
33. Takaya K, Ogawa Y, Hiraoka J, et al. Nonsense mutation of leptin receptor in the obese spontaneously hypertensive Koletsky rat. Nat Genet 1996; 14:130–131.
34. Clement K, Vaisse C, Lahlou N, et al. A mutation in the human leptin receptor gene causes obesity and pituitary dysfunction. Nature 1998; 392:398–401.
35. Scarpace P, Xhang Y. Elevated leptin: consequence or cause of obesity. Front Biosci 2007; 12:3531–3544.
36. Alam I, Lewis K, Stephens JW, et al. Obesity, metabolic syndrome and sleep apnoea: all pro-inflammatory states. Obes Rev 2006; 8:119–127.
37. Hoffstein V, Natekeika S. Differences in abdominal and neck circumferences in patients with and without sleep apnoea. Eur Respir J 1992; 5:377–381.

38. Hatipoglu U, Rubenstein I. Inflammation and obstructive sleep apnoea syndrome pathogenesis: a working hypothesis. Respiration 2003; 70:655–671.
39. Yun A, Lee PY, Bazar KA. Autonomic dysregulation as a basis of cardiovascular disturbances associated with obstructive sleep apnoea and other conditions of chronic hypoxia, hypercapnea, and acidosis. Med Hypotheses 2004; 62:852–856.
40. Farkas G, Schlenker EH. Pulmonary ventilation and mechanics in morbidly obese Zucker rats. Am J Respir Crit Care Med 1994; 150:356–362.
41. Tankersley C, O'Donnell C, Daood MJ, et al. Leptin attenuates respiratory complications associated with the obese phenotype. J Appl Physiol 1998; 85:2261–2269.
42. O'Donnell C, Schaub CD, Haines AS, et al. Leptin prevents respiratory depression in obesity. Am J Respir Crit Care Med 1999; 159:1477–1484.
43. Sowers J. Obesity as a cardiovascular risk factor. Am J Med 2003; 115:37S–41S.
44. Alpert M. Obesity cardiomyopathy: pathophysiology and evolution of the clinical syndrome. Am J Med Sci 2001; 321:225–236.
45. Sharma R, Al-Nasser FO, Anker SD. The importance of tumor necrosis factor and lipoproteins in the pathogenesis of chronic heart failure. Heart Fail Monit 2001; 2:42–47.
46. Schulze P, Kratzsch J, Linke A, et al. Elevated serum levels of leptin and soluble receptor in patients with advanced chronic heart failure. Eur J Heart Fail 2003; 5:33–40.
47. Meisel S, Ellis M, Pariente C, et al. Serum leptin levels increase following acute myocardial infarction. Cardiology 2001; 95:206–211.
48. Barouch L, Berkowitz DE, Harrison RW, et al. Disruption of leptin signaling contributes to cardiac hypertrophy independently of body weight in mice. Circulation 2003; 108:754–759.
49. Minhas K, Khan SA, Raju SVY, et al. Leptin repletion restores depressed B adrenergic contractility in ob/ob mice independently of cardiac hypertrophy. J Physiol 2005; 565:463–474.
50. Raju S, Zheng M, Schuleri KH, et al. Activation of the cardiac ciliary neurotrophic factor receptor reverses left ventricular hypertrophy in leptin-deficient and leptin-resistant obesity. Proc Natl Acad Sci U S A 2006; 103:4222–4227.
51. Jessup M, Brozena S. Heart failure. N Engl J Med 2003; 348:2007–2018.
52. Rich M. Epidemiology, pathophysiology, and etiology of congestive heart failure in older adults. J Am Geriatr Soc 1997; 45:968–974.
53. Kannel W. Incidence and epidemiology of heart failure. Heart Fail Rev 2000; 5:167–173.
54. Lloyd-Jones D, Larson MG, Leip EP, et al., Framingham Heart Study. Lifetime risk for developing congestive heart failure: the Framingham Heart Study. Circulation 2002; 106: 3068–3072.
55. American Heart Association. 2002 heart and stroke statistical update. American Heart Association, Dallas, Texas, 2001.
56. Gehi A, Pinney SP, Gass A. Recent diagnostic and therapeutic innovations in heart failure management. Mt Sinai J Med 2005; 72:176–184.
57. Ho K, Pinsky JL, Kannel W, et al. The epidemiology of heart failure: the Framingham Study. J Am Coll Cardiol 1993; 22:6a–13a.
58. Kenchaiah S, Evans JC, Levy D, et al. Obesity and the risk of heart failure. N Engl J Med 2002; 347:305–313.
59. McGaffin KR, Sun C-K, Rager JJ, et al. Leptin signalling reduces the severity of cardiac dysfunction and remodeling after chronic ischaemic injury. Cardiovasc Res 2008; 77:54–63.
60. Ozturk L, Unal M, Tamer L, et al. The association of the severity of obstructive sleep apnea with plasma leptin levels. Arch Otolaryngol Head Neck Surg 2003; 129:538–540.
61. Phipps P, Starritt E, Caterson I, et al. Association of serum leptin with hypoventilation in human obesity. Thorax 2002; 57:75–76.
62. Yee B, Cheung J, Phipps P, et al. Treatment of obesity hypoventilation syndrome and serum leptin. Respiration 2006; 73:209–212.

63. Sanner B, Kollhosser P, Buechner N, et al. Influence of treatment on leptin levels in patients with obstructive sleep apnoea. Eur Respir J 2004; 23:601–604.
64. Harsch I, Konturek PC, Koebnick C, et al. Leptin and ghrelin levels in patients with obstructive sleep apnoea: effect of CPAP treatment. Eur Respir J 2003; 22:251–257.
65. Tschöp M, Strasburger CJ, Töpfer M, et al. Influence of hypobaric hypoxia on leptin levels in men. Int J Obes Relat Metab Disord 2000; 24(suppl 2):S151.
66. Shukla V, Singh SN, Vats P, et al. Ghrelin and leptin levels of sojourners and acclimatized lowlanders at high altitude. Nutr Neurosci 2005; 8:161–165.
67. Chávez JC, Agani F, Pichiule P, et al. Expression of hypoxia-inducible factor-1alpha in the brain of rats during chronic hypoxia. J Appl Physiol 2000; 89:1937–1942.
68. Semenza G. HIF-1: mediator of physiological and pathophysiological responses to hypoxia. J Appl Physiol 2000; 88:1474–1480.
69. Semenza G. Regulation of mammalian O2 homeostasis by hypoxia-inducible factor 1. Annu Rev Cell Dev Biol 1999; 15:551–578.
70. Semenza G. Expression of hypoxia-inducible factor 1: mechanisms and consequences. Biochem Pharmacol 2000; 59:47–53.
71. Grosfeld A, Andre J, Hauguel-De Mouzon S, et al. Hypoxia-inducible factor 1 transactivates the human leptin gene promoter. J Biol Chem 2002; 2777:42953–42957.
72. Polotsky V, Li J, Punjabi NM, et al. Intermittent hypoxia increases insulin resistance in genetically obese mice. J Physiol 2003; 552:253–264.
73. Ryan S, Taylor CT, McNicholas WT. Selective activation of inflammatory pathways by intermittent hypoxia in obstructive sleep apnea syndrome. Circulation 2005; 112:2660–2667.
74. Yuan G, Nanduri J, Bhasker CR, et al. Ca2+/calmodulin kinase-dependent activation of hypoxia inducible factor 1 transcriptional activity in cells subjected to intermittent hypoxia. J Biol Chem 2005; 280:4321–4328.
75. Li J, Bosch-Marce M, Nanyakkara A, et al. Altered metabolic responses to intermittent hypoxia in mice with partial deficiency of hypoxia-inducible factor-1alpha. Physiol Genomics 2006; 25:450–457.

9

Influence of Sleep and Sleep Apnea on Autonomic Control of the Cardiovascular System

KRZYSZTOF NARKIEWICZ
Medical University of Gdansk, Gdansk, Poland

FATIMA H. SERT KUNIYOSHI and VIREND K. SOMERS
Mayo Clinic, Rochester, Minnesota, U.S.A.

BRADLEY G. PHILLIPS
College of Pharmacy, University of Georgia, Athens, Georgia, U.S.A.

I. Introduction

Sleep-related state changes in central neural activity are accompanied by dynamic and organized modulation of neural circulatory control. In healthy individuals it is possible to observe distinct variations in the cardiovascular system that are related to the sleep stages. During synchronized non–rapid eye movement (NREM) sleep stage, sympathetic activity gradually decreases with a predominance of parasympathetic tone, with consequent slowing of the heart rate and a decrease in blood pressure.

In contrast, during rapid eye movement (REM) sleep, there are periods of profound sympathetic activation and consequent surges in blood pressure. The heart rate is unstable, with abrupt and marked fluctuations in the RR interval. In patients with obstructive sleep apnea (OSA), the normal sleep stage–related variations in sympathetic activity and blood pressure are opposed by chemoreflex-mediated responses to apnea, hypoxemia, and hypercapnia. These chemoreflex-mediated responses frequently overwhelm the modulatory effects of normal sleep on neural circulatory control.

This chapter seeks to review autonomic cardiovascular control during normal sleep and in sleep apnea and the potential links between autonomic responses to OSA and cardiovascular pathophysiology (1).

II. Autonomic Circulatory Responses to Normal Sleep

The physiological variations in heart rate and blood pressure are related to sleep stage. Changes in heart rate and blood pressure during normal sleep are modest. Overall, heart rate and blood pressure decline progressively from stages I through IV of NREM sleep. During REM, blood pressure and heart rate are similar to levels recorded during quiet wakefulness.

Several strategies have been used to study the role of the autonomic nervous system in regulating cardiovascular control during sleep. These include microneurography, a direct intraneural measurement of sympathetic nerve traffic to muscle blood vessels (muscle sympathetic nerve activity, or MSNA) or to the skin (skin sympathetic nerve activity, or SSNA), and spectral analysis of heart rate variability.

A. Microneurography

This technique involves the insertion of a tungsten microelectrode directly into the sympathetic nerve fascicles of a peripheral nerve (usually the peroneal or tibial nerve in the leg and occasionally the median nerve in the arm). These recordings allow direct intraneural measurements of multifiber sympathetic nerve traffic. MSNA measurements are quantifiable, particularly within the same subject during the same session. In contrast to measurements of plasma norepinephrine, MSNA recordings provide a moment-by-moment representation of sympathetic nerve traffic and in a sense serve as a "window" to the sympathetic nervous system. Utilizing these recordings, several investigators have demonstrated similar patterns of changes in MSNA during daytime sleep, after sleep deprivation, and during normal nighttime sleep (2–4).

From stages I through IV of NREM sleep, reductions in heart rate and blood pressure are accompanied by a progressive reduction in MSNA (Fig. 1). During NREM sleep, arousal stimuli elicit K complexes on the electroencephalogram (EEG), which are accompanied by bursts of MSNA and transient increases in blood pressure. This response of MSNA to arousal is strikingly different from the MSNA-arousal relationship during wakefulness. During wakefulness, arousal stimuli do not increase sympathetic nerve traffic to muscle but do increase sympathetic activity involving the skin (5). Arousal stimuli do, however, increase sympathetic traffic to muscle after spinal cord injury (6) or anesthesia of the vagal or glossopharyngeal nerves (which carry baroreceptor reflex afferent impulses) (7). Therefore, during normal sleep, there appears to be a change in the neural processing of auditory and possibly other arousal stimuli.

The synchronous reduction in heart rate, blood pressure, and sympathetic nerve traffic during NREM sleep is suggestive of a profound resetting of the arterial baroreflex. During wakefulness, the baroreflex responds to reductions in blood pressure by increasing both heart rate and MSNA. During NREM sleep, the operating point of the baroreflex is actually "reset" to lower operating pressures, allowing the simultaneous reduction of blood pressure together with a decrease in heart rate and MSNA (8). Because of alterations in absolute levels of blood pressure and heart rate during sleep, studies of baroreflex function during different sleep stages are not easily interpreted. Nevertheless, recent data suggest that the baroreflex resetting is driven by the central nervous system and thus elicits changes in autonomic outflow that occur during NREM sleep (9).

REM sleep is associated with fluctuations in autonomic tone. The increase in MSNA occurs mainly during phasic REM, and is associated with intermittent surges in blood pressure and heart rate fluctuations (Figs. 1 and 2), with occasional irregularity in respiration (10,11). The blood pressure increase due to sympathetic-mediated vasoconstriction in skeletal muscle during REM is opposed by vasodilatation in mesenteric and renal vascular beds. The increase in MSNA during REM appears to be linked to a loss of postural muscle tone, suggesting that the loss of muscle tone during REM is a disinhibitory (excitatory) stimulus to sympathetic activation (4,12).

While studies of MSNA during sleep have demonstrated distinct sleep-related changes, the same is not true for studies of SSNA during sleep. Takeuchi and colleagues (13) measured both muscle and skin sympathetic activity using a double-recording microneurographic technique in eight healthy volunteers during polysomnographic

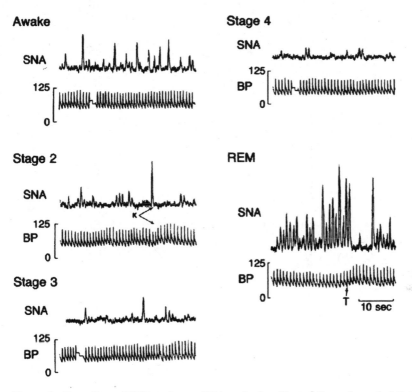

Figure 1 Recordings of SNA and mean BP in a single subject while awake and while in stages 2, 3, 4, and REM sleep. As NREM sleep deepened, SNA gradually decreased and blood pressure gradually reduced. Arousal stimuli elicited K complexes on the EEG (*not shown*), which were accompanied by increases in SNA and BP (*indicated by the arrows*, stage 2 sleep). HR, BP, and SNA increased during REM sleep. *Abbreviations*: SNA, sympathetic nerve activity; BP, blood pressure; REM, rapid eye movement; NREM, non–rapid eye movement; EEG, electroencephalogram; HR, heart rate. *Source*: From Ref. 4.

monitoring during NREM sleep. Their data suggested that both SSNA and MSNA were centrally suppressed during light sleep. Arousal stimuli during sleep induced K complexes and increases in both MSNA and SSNA. Similar multiunit recordings of skin sympathetic activity together with recordings of electrical skin resistance and skin blood flow in sleep-deprived healthy subjects were conducted by Noll and colleagues (14). These investigators reported that NREM sleep was always associated with an increase in skin resistance. Skin blood flow also increased during sleep. No significant difference in mean SSNA was found between wakefulness and NREM sleep, although during REM sleep, SSNA was relatively greater compared to the preceding stage II sleep period. These investigators also found an association between K complexes and bursts of SSNA, followed by transient changes in skin resistance, blood flow, and arterial pressure. Interestingly, they noted that bursts of SSNA were followed by brief increases in skin blood flow within the innervation area of the impaled fascicle, suggesting the existence of specific sympathetic vasodilator fibers in the skin that are activated during sleep.

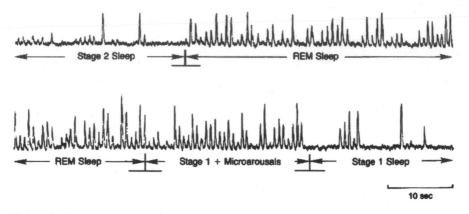

Figure 2 Changes in SNA during the transition from stage 2 sleep to REM sleep (*upper tracing*) and the transition from REM sleep to stage 1 sleep with frequent "microarousals" and then to established stage 1 sleep (*lower tracing*). *Abbreviations*: SNA, sympathetic nerve activity; REM, rapid eye movement. *Source*: From Ref. 4.

B.   Spectral Analysis of Heart Rate Variability

Studies of heart rate variability during different stages of normal sleep have utilized spectral analysis to quantify the oscillatory power of fluctuations in heart rate at low frequency (LF) and high frequency (HF) (15). The LF oscillation lies between 0.04 and 0.1 Hz, and the HF oscillation occurs at the frequency of respiration (usually about 0.25 Hz). It is generally assumed that the LF oscillatory power of heart rate variability increases in association with increased sympathetic modulation of heart rate within the same subject. Similarly, it is thought that within-subject increases in the HF oscillatory power of heart rate variability are associated with an increased vagal modulation of heart rate. To compensate for variations in total power of heart rate variability, a normalization procedure (the LF/HF ratio) is often used.

Using spectral analysis of heart rate variability during quiet wakefulness and during the different sleep stages, a number of studies have consistently demonstrated similar results (16–18). The LF oscillatory component of heart rate variability decreases progressively during NREM sleep, with an associated decrease in the LF/HF of heart rate variability. During REM sleep, however, there is an increase in the LF component of heart rate variability and an increase in the LF/HF ratio. These findings from spectral analysis are consistent with a reduction in sympathetic heart rate modulation during NREM sleep and an increased sympathetic modulation of heart rate during REM sleep. Elsenbruch et al. reported gender differences in autonomic functioning during wakefulness and sleep, with decreased vagal tone during waking and increased sympathetic dominance during REM sleep in the males (19)

The assumption that heart rate during REM is governed exclusively by a dominance of sympathetic activity is challenged by reports of intermittent increases in vagal activity during REM sleep. Verrier et al. (20) have demonstrated that during tonic REM sleep in cats, primary deceleration in heart rate may occur, which is neither preceded nor followed by increases in heart rate or arterial pressure. These brief episodes of heart rate slowing are eliminated by glycopyrrolate, suggesting that the cardiac decelerations are secondary to changes in central regulation of cardiac autonomic control, namely, a bursting or cardiac vagal efferent activity. On the other hand, phases of sustained sympathetic activation occur during NREM sleep, which is characterized by an overall vagal predominance, suggesting that the arterial baroreflex acts to buffer surges of sympathetic activation by means of rapid changes in cardiac vagal circuits throughout the overnight sleep period (21).

Pathophysiological conditions may also significantly alter measurements of heart rate variability during sleep. Vanoli et al. (22) have demonstrated that the heart rate variability patterns described above may be severely disrupted in patients after myocardial infarction (MI). In eight patients, following a recent MI, LF/HF increased during NREM sleep, significantly different from the decrease in LF/HF of RR interval evident during NREM in normal control subjects. During REM, LF/HF increased further in postinfarct patients to levels even greater than those recorded during wakefulness. These investigators suggested that MI was accompanied by a loss of the capacity for cardiac vagal activation during sleep, so sleep in these patients was associated with sympathetic dominance. They hypothesized that the loss of sleep-related vagal activation may be implicated in nocturnal sudden death in patients after MI.

III. Clinical Relevance of Autonomic Circulatory Control During Sleep

There is increasing evidence of a circadian rhythm in cardiovascular events, including sudden death. This concept is covered in greater detail elsewhere (23). The mechanisms underlying the circadian rhythm in cardiovascular events are not clear. The predominance of REM sleep in the early hours of the morning before awakening and the sympathetic and hemodynamic alterations during REM may conceivably be implicated in increased platelet aggregability, plaque rupture, and coronary vasospasm, thus acting as a trigger mechanism for thrombotic events that may present clinically only after arousal (24,25).

While regulation of autonomic function and hemodynamics during sleep may be directly relevant to understanding cardiovascular phenomena, such as circadian rhythms in cardiovascular disease, neural circulatory effects of arousal may also have important implications. Arousal from NREM sleep is accompanied by increases in heart rate, blood pressure, and MSNA (26). Using measurements of blood pressure and RR interval, Van de Borne and colleagues (27) have shown that arterial baroreflex sensitivity is markedly reduced during arousal from sleep and is accompanied by a reduction in the HF oscillatory component of the RR interval and an increase in the LF oscillatory component. Arousal-related surges in blood pressure and heart rate may be potentiated in the setting of baroreflex impairment. Thus, these hemodynamic responses may be linked to the initiation of vascular events in patients with preexisting cardiovascular disease.

Reductions in sympathetic activation during stage IV sleep, with consequent decreases in blood pressure, may be associated with clinically significant hypotension and consequent end-organ ischemia (28,29). This synchronized sleep-related hypotension may be especially relevant in patients with underlying cerebral vascular disease and bilateral carotid artery stenoses and patients on multiple antihypertensive medications who also have coexistent autonomic dysfunction. In these patients, impaired perfusion secondary to iatrogenic nocturnal hypotension may be amplified by stenoses in conduit vessels and impaired autoregulation in parenchymal brain blood vessels. Dysfunctional autonomic regulation—for example, in diabetics—will potentiate nocturnal hypotension in the face of multiple antihypertensive medications.

IV. Neural Circulatory Regulation in OSA

The autonomic effects of OSA reflect an integrated response to several powerful stimuli. These include hypoxia, hypercapnia, apnea, the Mueller maneuver, and the effects of sleep. Direct and reflex effects of these stimuli are further modulated by other reflex mechanisms, such as the baroreflex. Identifying the individual effects of each of the above stimuli helps in understanding the integrated response to obstructive apneas and variations of the response in different pathophysiological conditions.

A. Sympathetic Responses to Sleep Apnea

Both hypoxia and hypercapnia result in local vasodilation (30). The vasodilatory action is opposed by chemoreflex-mediated sympathetic vasoconstriction. Hypoxia acts primarily on peripheral chemoreceptors in the carotid bodies (31,32). Hypercapnia acts primarily on central chemoreceptors in the brainstem (33). These stimuli elicit increases in minute ventilation and efferent sympathetic vasoconstrictor activity. Increased ventilation acts via thoracic afferents to inhibit sympathetic responses to both hypoxia and hypercapnia (34,35). Thus, during apnea, when the inhibitory influence of thoracic afferents is eliminated, the sympathetic neural responses to hypoxia and hypercapnia are potentiated.

During episodes of sleep apnea, subjects are exposed to simultaneous hypoxia, hypercapnia, and apnea. Simultaneous hypoxia and hypercapnia result in synergistic increases in sympathetic traffic. Coexisting apnea further potentiates the sympathetic response. Thus, it would be expected that in patients with OSA, hypoxia, hypercapnia, and the absence of lung inflation will result in marked increases in sympathetic nerve traffic (36). This sympathetic activation would be opposed by the normal mechanisms governing neural circulatory regulation during the different sleep stages, as described earlier (Fig. 3) (37).

Evidence for sympathetic activation in OSA is not restricted only to experimental studies. A population-based study has also shown a strong correlation between OSA and increased urinary normetanephrine and metanephrine, independent of recognized confounding factors, suggesting increased sympathoadrenal activity (38).

B. Responses in Hypertension

There is an increased incidence of hypertension in patients with sleep apnea (39–41). The most compelling evidence linking OSA and hypertension was provided by data from the Wisconsin Sleep Cohort Study. This study has demonstrated a dose-response association between sleep-disordered breathing at the baseline and the presence of de novo hypertension four years later (42).

Hypertensive patients have an increased ventilatory response to hypoxic stress (43). In untreated mild hypertensives, the sympathetic response to hypoxia is about twice that seen in matched controls (44). During apnea, the increase in sympathetic activity in hypertensive patients is about 12-fold the response seen in normal subjects. Thus, in those patients with OSA who also have hypertension, the sympathetic response to obstructive apneas during sleep may be exacerbated.

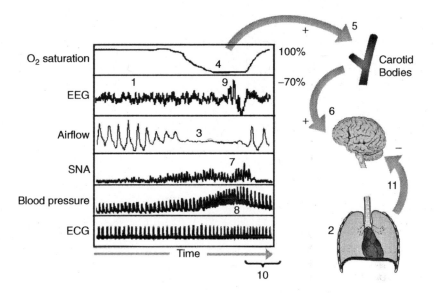

Figure 3 Pathophysiologic events in OSA. Representative polysomnographic data are shown. In the legend, the numbers in parentheses correspond to the numbers in the figure. Sleep onset is heralded by electroencephalography wave slowing (1) and a reduction in minute ventilation (2). In persons with OSA, diminution or cessation of airflow results from progressive collapse of the upper airway (3), which leads to reduced oxyhemoglobin saturation (O_2 *saturation*) (4) and consequent stimulation of peripheral chemoreceptors, the carotid bodies (5). Hypercapnic effects are not shown. Chemoreflex stimulation acts through the central nervous system (6) to increase SNA, which is recorded peripherally as microneurographic bursts (7). BP (8) increases as the apnea progresses. The exact mechanisms are not clear, but the apnea terminates with a central nervous system arousal, which is marked by an increase in electroencephalographic wave frequency (9). The far right portions of the tracings (10) show the cascade of events resulting from the arousal from sleep and restored upper-airway patency, including temporary supranormal ventilation, normalization of oxyhemoglobin saturation, and instantaneous suppression of SNA. During resumption of ventilation, sympathetic outflow is inhibited by afferents originating from thoracic mechanoreceptors, which synapse in the brainstem (11). A subset of patients show signs of the diving reflex, in which marked bradycardia accompanies the vascular sympathetic excitation (not shown here). *Abbreviations*: OSA, obstructive sleep apnea; SNA, sympathetic neural activity; BP, blood pressure. *Source*: From Ref. 37.

C. Baroreflex-Chemoreflex Interactions

The mechanism underlying the potentiated sympathetic response in hypertensives may be linked to baroreflex dysfunction. Baroreflexes exert a powerful inhibitory influence on chemoreflex responses (45). During hypoxia in normal subjects, simultaneous activation of the baroreceptors by intravenous phenylephrine infusion attenuates the sympathetic response to hypoxia (46). In patients with hypertension, in whom there may be underlying baroreflex impairment, the sympathetic response to chemoreflex activation may be increased, with a consequent increase in the pressor response to apneic episodes. A similar consideration is applicable to heart failure patients with sleep apnea, since heart failure is also linked to baroreflex impairment (47,48). Even in the absence of heart failure, it has been shown that the presence of central sleep apnea might contribute to baroreflex dysfunction in the subacute phase of acute MI. This phenomenon might be linked to prognosis in this patient population (49).

D. The Mueller Maneuver

While studies of chemoreflex involvement in sleep apnea have simulated sleep apnea using voluntary apnea together with hypoxia and hypercapnia, actual obstructive apneic events do not involve central apneas but rather consist of repetitive brief periods of inspiration against an obstructed airway. This generates significant changes in intra-thoracic pressure, resulting in distortion of cardiac chamber geometry (50,51). The cardiac distortion during inspiration against an occluded airway (the Mueller maneuver) may itself result in significant neural and circulatory changes. The initial phase (first 10 seconds) of the Mueller maneuver results in marked hypotension and a paradoxical reduction in sympathetic activity. Toward the end of the maneuver, however, sympathetic activity gradually increases, as does blood pressure (52). Changes in atrial hemodynamics and volume during the Mueller maneuver (53) may also modulate autonomic responses. Thus, in seeking to understand sympathetic responses to prolonged obstructive apneic events, the response to the Mueller maneuver (which opposes the initial sympathetic excitatory response to hypoxia) needs to be considered.

E. Bradycardia During Apnea

The primary response to hypoxia is bradycardia. During hyperventilation, the vagally mediated bradycardia is prevented by the vagolytic effects of hyperventilation. However, with apnea during hypoxia, when the effect of ventilation is eliminated, chemoreflex-mediated vagal bradycardia becomes evident. The combined apnea response—consisting of sympathetic-mediated vasoconstriction in peripheral blood vessels (not including the cerebral and coronary circulations) and vagal bradycardia—constitutes part of the diving reflex (54,55).

The intensity of bradycardia during apnea varies considerably between individuals. One important determinant may be the baroreflex sensitivity. As described earlier, the baroreflex has a powerful inhibitory influence on chemoreflex-mediated vasoconstriction. The baroreflex may also influence chemoreflex-mediated bradycardia such that in those clinical conditions where the baroreflex is impaired, vagal bradycardia may be potentiated (56). Neck suction and consequent baroreflex activation during apnea would normally be expected to increase bradycardia during the apnea. However, baroreflex activation during apnea actually prevents chemoreflex-mediated bradyarrhythmias, suggesting that the inhibitory influence of baroreflex activation on chemoreflex responses extends not only to the sympathetic response but also to the vagal bradycardic response.

V. Autonomic Function in Wakefulness in Patients with Sleep Apnea

Several studies have demonstrated consistently that patients with OSA have high levels of norepinephrine (57–59). These patients also have elevated MSNA recorded during quiet normoxic wakefulness (60,61). Increased MSNA is present in OSA patients and is evident even in the absence of hypertension (Fig. 4). Furthermore, high levels of

NORMAL **OSA**

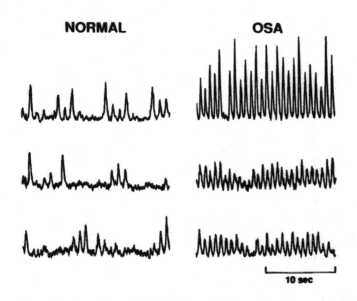

Figure 4 Recordings of SNA during wakefulness in patients with OSA and matched controls showing high levels of SNA in patients with sleep apnea. *Abbreviations*: SNA, sympathetic neural activity; OSA, obstructive sleep apnea. *Source*: From Ref. 61.

sympathetic traffic in patients with OSA are not explained by obesity, since obese patients proven not to have sleep apnea do not have markedly elevated levels of MSNA (62).

In studies of unmedicated and otherwise healthy patients with OSA, in comparison to gender and body mass index–matched healthy subjects in whom sleep apnea has been excluded by overnight polysomnography, several abnormalities in daytime neural circulatory control have become apparent (63). First, patients with severe sleep apnea have faster heart rates. These are associated with a marked reduction in overall heart rate variability but a relative increase in the LF oscillatory component of RR variability (Figs. 5 and 6). In patients with overt cardiovascular disease, reduced heart rate variability may be linked to adverse cardiovascular outcomes. Even though the sleep apnea patients studied were normotensive, with blood pressures very similar to those seen in control subjects, there was a marked increase in blood pressure variability (Fig. 5). Thus, otherwise healthy patients with OSA who are normotensive have faster heart rates, increased LF of RR, decreased RR variability, and increased blood pressure variability (63). Increased blood pressure variability, in hypertensive patients, is associated with an increased likelihood of target-organ damage, independent of the absolute blood pressure level (64,65). These abnormalities of neural control in sleep apnea are strikingly similar to the abnormalities in neural control evident in patients with essential hypertension. Thus, it may be that the abnormalities in neural control described above precede the development of sustained hypertension in sleep-apneic patients.

The mechanism underlying the derangement in neural control in sleep apnea is unknown. Abnormalities in chemoreflex function may be implicated. The arterial

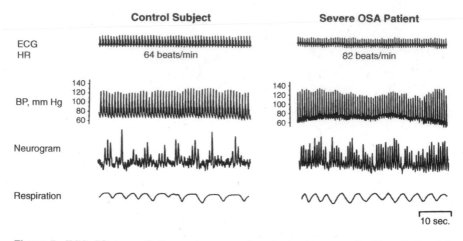

Figure 5 ECG, BP, sympathetic neurograms, and respiration in a control subject (*left*) and in a patient with severe OSA (*right*), showing faster HR, increased blood pressure variability, and markedly elevated MSNA in the patient with OSA. Spectral analysis recordings for these subjects are shown in Figure 6. *Abbreviations*: ECG, electrocardiogram; BP, blood pressure; OSA, obstructive sleep apnea; HR, heart rate; MSNA, muscle sympathetic nerve activity. *Source*: From Ref. 63.

chemoreceptors may exert important influences on neural control even during normoxia. Elimination of the influence of arterial chemoreceptors using room air and 100% oxygen in a double-blind study showed that in patients with sleep apnea, suppression of the chemoreflexes slowed heart rate, lowered blood pressure, and decreased MSNA (Fig. 7) (66). Furthermore, we have shown that autonomic, hemodynamic, and ventilatory responses to peripheral chemoreceptor activation by hypoxia are selectively potentiated in patients with OSA (67). Thus, potentiated chemoreflex function may contribute to the abnormalities in cardiovascular variability.

VI. Autonomic Function During Sleep in Patients with Sleep Apnea
A. Sympathetic and Hemodynamic Responses
We have described the effects of chemoreflex activation on sympathetic activity and that the sympathetic excitatory effect of hypoxia, hypercapnia, and apnea would be expected to oppose the sleep stage–related changes in hemodynamics and sympathetic traffic. Indeed, in patients with sleep apnea, there is a marked disruption of the tightly regulated changes in hemodynamics and sympathetic activity evident during the different stages of normal sleep. By contrast, the sympathetic nerve activity (SNA) and blood pressure profile during sleep in OSA patients is dominated by responses to episodes of obstructive apnea that occur continuously throughout sleep. Apneic episodes result in progressive increases in SNA, these increases being most marked toward the end of apnea (Fig. 8). At cessation of apnea and resumption of breathing, there is an abrupt termination of sympathetic activity and an increase in blood pressure. The duration of

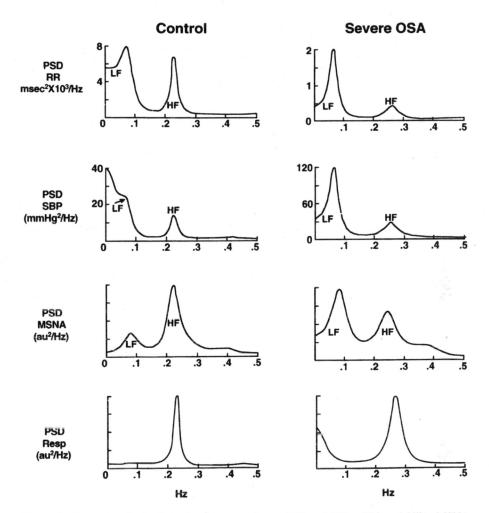

Figure 6 Spectral analysis of simultaneous recordings of RR variability, SBP variability, MSNA variability, and respiration (*Resp*) in the control subject (*left*) and in the patient with OSA (*right*) shown in Figure 4. RR variance is decreased and SBP variance is increased in the patient with OSA compared to the control subject. There is a relative predominance of the LF component over the HF component of the RR interval in the patient with OSA. LF components are clearly present in the MSNA variability profiles of both subjects. *Abbreviations*: SBP, systolic blood pressure; MSNA, muscle sympathetic nerve activity; OSA, obstructive sleep apnea; LF, low frequency; HF, high frequency; PSD, power spectral density; au, arbitrary units. *Source*: From Ref. 63.

apnea and the level of oxygen desaturation are key factors in determining sympathetic activation during episodes of OSA. The surge in blood pressure at the end of apnea are explained in part by the increase in cardiac output, secondary to the increased venous return, which occurs during breathing after apnea. In addition, the severely vaso-constricted peripheral vasculature, together with the increased cardiac output, results in

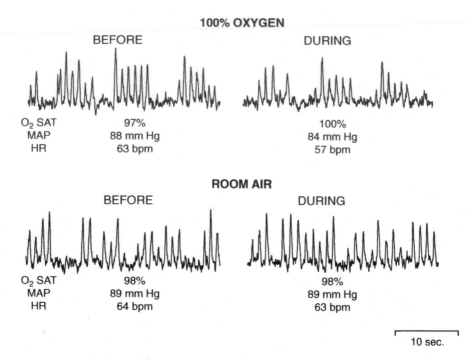

Figure 7 Recordings of MSNA in a single patient with OSA during administration of 100% oxygen (*top*) and room air (*bottom*). MSNA, MAP, and HR decreased during administration of 100% oxygen but did not change during administration of room air. *Abbreviations*: MSNA, muscle sympathetic nerve activity; MAP, mean arterial pressure; OSA, obstructive sleep apnea; HR, heart rate. *Source*: From Ref. 66.

the marked increases in blood pressure. Other factors, such as increased muscle tone and arousal, may also contribute to increased blood pressure at the end of apnea (68,69).

B. Sleep Apnea and Arrhythmias

The chemoreflex-mediated vagal activation described earlier is frequently evident in clinical situations involving patients with sleep apnea. A number of studies have characterized the spectrum of bradyarrhythmic responses to OSA, and these extend from sinus bradycardia to prolonged periods of cardiac asystole (70–72). Atropine prevents sleep apnea–induced bradycardia (73). From a clinical perspective, it is important that patients with nocturnal bradyarrhythmias evident on Holter monitoring be evaluated for OSA, since continuous positive airway pressure (CPAP) rather than pacemaker implantation would be the preferred initial therapy. Furthermore, in those patients in whom bradyarrhythmias are also evident during the daytime, it is important to ensure that these patients do not fall asleep with consequent obstructive apnea during the daytime. While it may be appropriate to exclude thyroid hypofunction in sleep-apneic patients generally, this is particularly true for those with apnea-related bradyarrhythmias.

Both sympathetic and parasympathetic mechanisms may initiate or maintain atrial fibrillation in susceptible individuals. In OSA, relevant mechanisms may include the

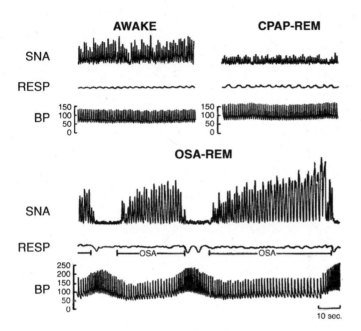

Figure 8 Recordings of sympathetic activity, respiration, and intra-arterial BP in a patient with sleep apnea on no medications and free of other diseases. Measurements were obtained during wakefulness (*top left*), during OSA in REM sleep (*bottom*), and during REM sleep after treatment of OSA with CPAP. During wakefulness, sympathetic activity was high and BP was approximately 130/60 mmHg. During REM sleep, repetitive apnea resulted in hypoxia and chemoreflex stimulation with consequent sympathetic activation. The vasoconstriction resulting from sympathetic activation caused marked surges in BP to levels as high as 250/110 mmHg at the end of apnea because of increases in cardiac output at the termination of apnea. Treatment of sleep apnea and elimination of apneic episodes by CPAP resulted in stabilization and lower levels of both BP and sympathetic activity during REM sleep. *Abbreviations*: BP, blood pressure; OSA, obstructive sleep apnea; REM, rapid eye movement; CPAP, continuous positive airway pressure. *Source*: From Ref. 61.

activation of atrial catecholamine-sensitive ion channels or the effects of vagotonia on atrial conduction properties (74). In addition to the acute autonomic fluctuations during sleep, chronically elevated sympathetic drive, even during wakefulness, may contribute to the initiation and maintenance of atrial tachyarrhythmias and to the difficulty or failure of rate-control strategies in managing atrial fibrillation (75).

C. Sleep Apnea and Acute Cardiovascular Events

In a retrospective study of people who had been evaluated for the presence of sleep apnea and then had sudden death, the pattern of occurrence of sudden death in those who did not have sleep apnea was in accordance with the previous epidemiologic studies, namely, sudden death occurred primarily in the morning around the time of waking. However, in those who had sleep apnea, the majority of sudden-death events occurred during the nighttime (Fig. 9). The mechanisms causing the reversal of distribution of

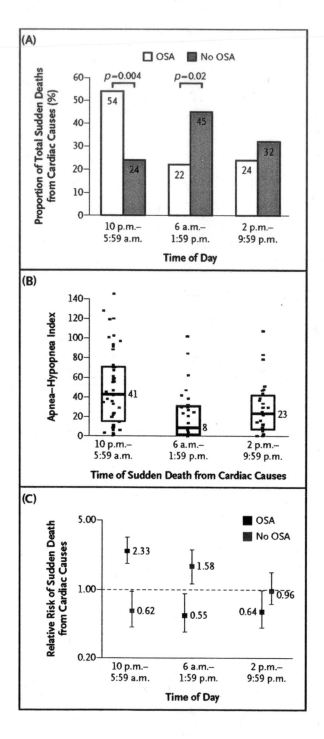

sudden cardiac death are not clear but may relate to the neural, circulatory, and metabolic stresses induced by OSA. Indeed, OSA may be a trigger for nocturnal MI, perhaps because of the acute pathophysiological responses to the apneic events, with hypoxemia-induced increases in sympathetic drive, followed by surges in blood pressure during the sleep hours (76).

Recent evidence has shown that patients with OSA do in fact have an altered diurnal variation in the occurrence of MI (Fig. 10). This observation suggests that nocturnal MI may contribute to the increased likelihood of nocturnal sudden cardiac death observed in OSA patients (77). While sympathetic activation might contribute to the shift in the timing of MI from the morning hours to the night in OSA patients, other mechanisms that increase the risk of nocturnal coronary thrombosis might be involved. These include platelet activation (78), elevated fibrinogen levels (79), and decreased fibrinolytic activity (80), all of which may contribute to an increase in whole-blood viscosity during sleep in OSA patients.

D. Sleep Apnea and "Nondippers"

Blood pressure and sympathetic activity in sleep-apneic patients are highest during REM sleep, since during this sleep stage, the apneas are most prolonged. The reduction in muscle tone during REM may influence muscle tone in the upper airway, thus potentiating the likelihood of airway obstruction. Because of repetitive vasoconstriction and blood pressure surges, blood pressure overall does not fall during sleep in patients with sleep apnea. The blood pressure pattern during sleep in OSA patients may be important in helping explain the absence of nocturnal hypotension in the subgroup of hypertensive patients termed nondippers.

Prevalence of hypertension might be underdiagnosed in OSA patients if blood pressure is assessed by office readings only. Baguet et al (81) have shown that ambulatory blood pressure monitoring might be of particular significance in the hypertension diagnosis of OSA patients. In this study, while 42% of OSA patients demonstrated office hypertension, 58% had daytime hypertension, and 76% had nighttime hypertension.

The nocturnal blood pressure profile in nondipper hypertensive patients is strikingly similar to that described in studies of 24-hour blood pressure measurements in patients with sleep apnea. There is also evidence of high probability of coexisting sleep-disordered breathing in nondipping males with essential hypertension (82).

←——

Figure 9 Sudden death from cardiac causes according to usual sleep-wake cycles. Panel A shows day-night patterns of sudden death from cardiac causes on the basis of eight-hour time intervals for 78 persons with and 34 persons without OSA. Panel B shows the apnea-hypopnea index for persons with sudden death from cardiac causes during eight-hour intervals. The line within each box represents the median apnea-hypopnea index, and the box represents the interquartile range (25th percentile to 75th percentile). The figure includes data from persons with and from persons without OSA ($p = 0.001$) for the comparison of the apnea-hypopnea index according to the time of sudden death. Panel C shows the relative risk of sudden death from cardiac causes during eight-hour intervals, compared with the remaining 16 hours of the day, for 78 persons with and 34 persons without OSA. The squares represent the relative risk point estimates, and the I bars the 95% confidence intervals. *Abbreviation*: OSA, obstructive sleep apnea. *Source*: From Ref. 76.

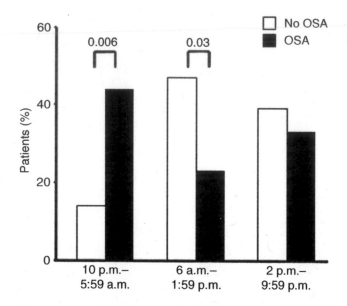

Figure 10 Day-night pattern of MI based on three eight-hour time intervals in OSA (64) and no-OSA (28) patients. *Abbreviations*: MI, myocardial infarction; OSA, obstructive sleep apnea. *Source*: From Ref. 77.

It has been shown that nondipping of nocturnal blood pressure in OSA patients is related to apnea severity (83,84).

Thus, OSA and the consequent cardiovascular effects of repetitive hypoxemia, hypercapnia, respiratory acidosis, and blood pressure surges may be involved in the increased cardiovascular morbidity that characterizes those hypertensive patients in whom there is an absence of a nocturnal blood pressure decline (85,86).

E. Effects of Therapy with CPAP

Effective long-term treatment of OSA by CPAP has been shown to improve 24-hour blood pressure control in hypertensive patients (87,88). CPAP may result in reduction of both systolic and diastolic blood pressure, during both sleep and wakefulness, although several recent meta-analyses suggested that the blood pressure–lowering effect was modest, approximately 2 mmHg (89). The benefit is larger in patients with more severe sleep apnea, is independent of the baseline blood pressure (90), and is especially evident in patients with resistant hypertension. Interestingly, a faster heart rate also predicts a greater CPAP effect on blood pressure (91).

Because nocturnal oxygen therapy improves oxyhemoglobin saturation without affecting blood pressure levels, it seems that improving oxygen saturation, without treating airway obstruction and arousal, may not be enough to lower blood pressure in OSA patients (92).

Treatment with CPAP, when effective, results in a significant acute reduction in sympathetic nerve traffic and blunts blood pressure surges during sleep (Fig. 8) (61). Long-term CPAP treatment has been shown to decrease MSNA (Fig. 11) (93), and

TREATED OSA

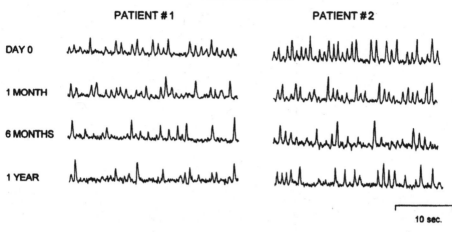

Figure 11 Sympathetic neurograms during repeated measurements in two treated patients with OSA. Measurements were obtained at baseline (day 0) and after one month, six months, and one year of CPAP treatment. Long-term CPAP treatment decreased MSNA, as was evident from the measurements obtained both at six months and one year. *Abbreviations*: OSA, obstructive sleep apnea; CPAP, continuous positive airway pressure; MSNA, muscle sympathetic nerve activity. *Source*: From Ref. 93.

randomized control trials have demonstrated that CPAP therapy can also improve baroreflex function (94) and reduce arterial stiffness in OSA patients (95). Furthermore, treatment of coexisting OSA by nocturnal CPAP in patients with heart failure has been shown to reduce MSNA (96) and improve vagal modulation of heart rate (97). Therefore, CPAP therapy may provide beneficial effects beyond better blood pressure control.

VII. Clinical Relevance of Autonomic Responses to OSA

There is increasing evidence that OSA is linked to cardiovascular morbidity and mortality. High sympathetic drive, baroreflex dysfunction, and abnormalities in cardiovascular variability, evident during sleep and wakefulness, may precede and perhaps predispose to cardiovascular disease, particularly to hypertension, and might increase the cardiovascular risk in hypertensive nondippers. During sleep, repetitive hypoxemia with consequent chemoreflex activation, sympathetic excitation, and blood pressure surges may be involved in nocturnal cardiovascular events such as MI and sudden death in sleep-apneic patients. Abrupt changes in cardiac sympathetic and parasympathetic activation may be implicated in development of atrial fibrillation (98). In the setting of severe hypoxemia, bradyarrhythmias (in particular, prolonged asystole) may predispose to cerebral hypoperfusion as well as to dispersion of cardiac refractoriness and consequent life-threatening arrhythmias.

Randomized trials provided evidence that OSA treatment with CPAP improves surrogates such as sympathetic activation and blood pressure. However, there are presently no data showing whether treatment for OSA can reduce the overall risk of acute cardiac events and cardiac death, and further research is needed to identify the effects of OSA therapy on outcomes such as survival.

Acknowledgments

Krzysztof Narkiewicz was a recipient of an NIH Fogarty International Research Fellowship. Virend Somers is supported by NIH Grants HL65176 and M01-RR00585. Fatima H. Sert Kuniyoshi is supported by American Heart Association grant 06-15709Z and 0920069G; a Perkins Memorial Award from the American Physiological Society.

We also extend our appreciation to those colleagues who contributed to the work described in this chapter.

References

1. Somers VK, White DP, Amin R, et al. Sleep apnea and cardiovascular disease: an American Heart Association/American College of Cardiology Foundation Scientific Statement from the American Heart Association Council for High Blood Pressure Research Professional Education Committee, Council on Clinical Cardiology, Stroke Council, and Council On Cardiovascular Nursing. In collaboration with the National Heart, Lung, and Blood Institute National Center on Sleep Disorders Research (National Institutes of Health). Circulation 2008; 118(10):1080–1111.
2. Hornyak M, Cejnar M, Elam M, et al. Sympathetic muscle nerve activity during sleep in man. Brain 1991; 114(pt 3):1281–1295.
3. Okada H, Iwase S, Mano T, et al. Changes in muscle sympathetic nerve activity during sleep in humans. Neurology 1991; 41(12):1961–1966.
4. Somers VK, Dyken ME, Mark AL, et al. Sympathetic-nerve activity during sleep in normal subjects. N Engl J Med 1993; 328(5):303–307.
5. Mark AL. Regulation of sympathetic nerve activity in mild human hypertension. J Hypertens Suppl 1990; 8(7):S67–S75.
6. Stjernberg L, Blumberg H, Wallin BG. Sympathetic activity in man after spinal cord injury. Outflow to muscle below the lesion. Brain 1986; 109(pt 4):695–715.
7. Fagius J, Wallin BG, Sundlof G, et al. Sympathetic outflow in man after anaesthesia of the glossopharyngeal and vagus nerves. Brain 1985; 108(pt 2):423–438.
8. Conway J, Boon N, Jones JV, et al. Involvement of the baroreceptor reflexes in the changes in blood pressure with sleep and mental arousal. Hypertension 1983; 5(5):746–748.
9. Silvani A. Physiological sleep-dependent changes in arterial blood pressure: central autonomic commands and baroreflex control. Clin Exp Pharmacol Physiol 2008; 35(9):987–994.
10. Khatri IM, Freis ED. Hemodynamic changes during sleep. J Appl Physiol 1967; 22(5):867–873.
11. Snyder F, Hobson JA, Morrison DF, et al. Changes in respiration, heart rate, and systolic blood pressure in human sleep. J Appl Physiol 1964; 19:417–422.
12. Mancia G, Zanchetti A. Cardiovascular regulation during sleep In: Orem J, Barnes C, eds. Physiology in Sleep. Vol 3. New York: Academic Press, 1980:2–55.
13. Takeuchi S, Iwase S, Mano T, et al. Sleep-related changes in human muscle and skin sympathetic nerve activities. J Auton Nerv Syst 1994; 47(1–2):121–129.
14. Noll G, Elam M, Kunimoto M, et al. Skin sympathetic nerve activity and effector function during sleep in humans. Acta Physiol Scand 1994; 151(3):319–329.
15. Heart rate variability: standards of measurement, physiological interpretation and clinical use. Task Force of the European Society of Cardiology and the North American Society of Pacing and Electrophysiology. Circulation 1996; 93(5):1043–1065.
16. Baharav A, Kotagal S, Gibbons V, et al. Fluctuations in autonomic nervous activity during sleep displayed by power spectrum analysis of heart rate variability. Neurology 1995; 45(6): 1183–1187.

17. Shinar Z, Akselrod S, Dagan Y, et al. Autonomic changes during wake-sleep transition: a heart rate variability based approach. Auton Neurosci 2006; 130(1–2):17–27.
18. Vaughn BV, Quint SR, Messenheimer JA, et al. Heart period variability in sleep. Electro-encephalogr Clin Neurophysiol 1995; 94(3):155–162.
19. Elsenbruch S, Harnish MJ, Orr WC. Heart rate variability during waking and sleep in healthy males and females. Sleep 1999; 22(8):1067–1071.
20. Verrier RL, Lau TR, Wallooppillai U, et al. Primary vagally mediated decelerations in heart rate during tonic rapid eye movement sleep in cats. Am J Physiol 1998; 274(4 pt 2):R1136–R1141.
21. Iellamo F, Placidi F, Marciani MG, et al. Baroreflex buffering of sympathetic activation during sleep: evidence from autonomic assessment of sleep macroarchitecture and micro-architecture. Hypertension 2004; 43(4):814–819.
22. Vanoli E, Adamson PB, Ba L, et al. Heart rate variability during specific sleep stages. A comparison of healthy subjects with patients after myocardial infarction. Circulation 1995; 91(7):1918–1922.
23. Muller JE, Tofler GH, Stone PH. Circadian variation and triggers of onset of acute cardio-vascular disease. Circulation 1989; 79(4):733–743.
24. King MJ, Zir LM, Kaltman AJ, et al. Variant angina associated with angiographically demonstrated coronary artery spasm and REM sleep. Am J Med Sci 1973; 265(5):419–422.
25. Tofler GH, Brezinski D, Schafer AI, et al. Concurrent morning increase in platelet aggreg-ability and the risk of myocardial infarction and sudden cardiac death. N Engl J Med 1987; 316(24):1514–1518.
26. Morgan BJ, Crabtree DC, Puleo DS, et al. Neurocirculatory consequences of abrupt change in sleep state in humans. J Appl Physiol 1996; 80(5):1627–1636.
27. Van de Borne P, Nguyen H, Biston P, et al. Effects of wake and sleep stages on the 24-h autonomic control of blood pressure and heart rate in recumbent men. Am J Physiol 1994; 266(2 pt 2):H548–H554.
28. Mancia G. Autonomic modulation of the cardiovascular system during sleep. N Engl J Med 1993; 328(5):347–349.
29. Kario K, Motai K, Mitsuhashi T, et al. Autonomic nervous system dysfunction in elderly hypertensive patients with abnormal diurnal blood pressure variation: relation to silent cer-ebrovascular disease. Hypertension 1997; 30(6):1504–1510.
30. Daugherty RM Jr., Scott JB, Dabney JM, et al. Local effects of O_2 and CO_2 on limb, renal, and coronary vascular resistances. Am J Physiol 1967; 213(5):1102–1110.
31. Wade JG, Larson CP Jr., Hickey RF, et al. Effect of carotid endarterectomy on carotid chemoreceptor and baroreceptor function in man. N Engl J Med 1970; 282(15):823–829.
32. Lugliani R, Whipp BJ, Seard C, et al. Effect of bilateral carotid-body resection on ventilatory control at rest and during exercise in man. N Engl J Med 1971; 285(20):1105–1111.
33. Gelfand R, Lambertsen CJ. Dynamic respiratory response to abrupt change of inspired CO_2 at normal and high PO_2. J Appl Physiol 1973; 35(6):903–913.
34. Somers VK, Mark AL, Zavala DC, et al. Contrasting effects of hypoxia and hypercapnia on ventilation and sympathetic activity in humans. J Appl Physiol 1989; 67(5):2101–2106.
35. Somers VK, Mark AL, Zavala DC, et al. Influence of ventilation and hypocapnia on sympathetic nerve responses to hypoxia in normal humans. J Appl Physiol 1989; 67(5):2095–2100.
36. Somers VK, Abboud FM. Chemoreflexes—responses, interactions and implications for sleep apnea. Sleep 1993; 16(8 suppl):S30–S33; discussion S33–S34.
37. Caples SM, Gami AS, Somers VK. Obstructive sleep apnea. Ann Intern Med 2005; 142(3): 187–197.
38. Elmasry A, Lindberg E, Hedner J, et al. Obstructive sleep apnoea and urine catecholamines in hypertensive males: a population-based study. Eur Respir J 2002; 19(3):511–517.
39. Bixler EO, Vgontzas AN, Lin HM, et al. Association of hypertension and sleep-disordered breathing. Arch Intern Med 2000; 160(15):2289–2295.

40. Young T, Peppard PE, Palta M, et al. Population-based study of sleep-disordered breathing as a risk factor for hypertension. Arch Intern Med 1997; 157(15):1746–1752.
41. Nieto FJ, Young TB, Lind BK, et al. Association of sleep-disordered breathing, sleep apnea, and hypertension in a large community-based study. Sleep Heart Health Study. JAMA 2000; 283(14):1829–1836.
42. Peppard PE, Young T, Palta M, et al. Prospective study of the association between sleep-disordered breathing and hypertension. N Engl J Med 2000; 342(19):1378–1384.
43. Trzebski A, Tafil M, Zoltowski M, et al. Increased sensitivity of the arterial chemoreceptor drive in young men with mild hypertension. Cardiovasc Res 1982; 16(3):163–172.
44. Somers VK, Mark AL, Abboud FM. Potentiation of sympathetic nerve responses to hypoxia in borderline hypertensive subjects. Hypertension 1988; 11(6 pt 2):608–612.
45. Heistad DD, Abboud FM, Mark AL, et al. Interaction of baroreceptor and chemoreceptor reflexes. Modulation of the chemoreceptor reflex by changes in baroreceptor activity. J Clin Invest 1974; 53(5):1226–1236.
46. Somers VK, Mark AL, Abboud FM. Interaction of baroreceptor and chemoreceptor reflex control of sympathetic nerve activity in normal humans. J Clin Invest 1991; 87(6):1953–1957.
47. Rea RF, Berg WJ. Abnormal baroreflex mechanisms in congestive heart failure. Recent insights. Circulation 1990; 81(6):2026–2027.
48. Ferguson DW, Berg WJ, Roach PJ, et al. Effects of heart failure on baroreflex control of sympathetic neural activity. Am J Cardiol 1992; 69(5):523–531.
49. Strassburg A, Majunke B, Notges JK, et al. Central sleep apnea is associated with blunted baroreflex sensitivity in patients with myocardial infarction. Int J Cardiol 2008; 126(3):333–339.
50. Condos WR Jr., Latham RD, Hoadley SD, et al. Hemodynamics of the Mueller maneuver in man: right and left heart micromanometry and Doppler echocardiography. Circulation 1987; 76(5):1020–1028.
51. Scharf SM, Brown R, Warner KG, et al. Intrathoracic pressures and left ventricular configuration with respiratory maneuvers. J Appl Physiol 1989; 66(1):481–491.
52. Somers VK, Dyken ME, Skinner JL. Autonomic and hemodynamic responses and interactions during the Mueller maneuver in humans. J Auton Nerv Syst 1993; 44(2–3):253–259.
53. Orban M, Bruce CJ, Pressman GS, et al. Dynamic changes of left ventricular performance and left atrial volume induced by the mueller maneuver in healthy young adults and implications for obstructive sleep apnea, atrial fibrillation, and heart failure. Am J Cardiol 2008; 102(11):1557–1561.
54. Daly MD, Angell-James JE, Elsner R. Role of carotid-body chemoreceptors and their reflex interactions in bradycardia and cardiac arrest. Lancet 1979; 1(8119):764–767.
55. De Burgh Daly M, Scott MJ. An analysis of the primary cardiovascular reflex effects of stimulation of the carotid body chemoreceptors in the dog. J Physiol 1962; 162:555–573.
56. Somers VK, Dyken ME, Mark AL, et al. Parasympathetic hyperresponsiveness and bradyarrhythmias during apnoea in hypertension. Clin Auton Res 1992; 2(3):171–176.
57. Baruzzi A, Riva R, Cirignotta F, et al. Atrial natriuretic peptide and catecholamines in obstructive sleep apnea syndrome. Sleep 1991; 14(1):83–86.
58. Dimsdale JE, Coy T, Ziegler MG, et al. The effect of sleep apnea on plasma and urinary catecholamines. Sleep 1995; 18(5):377–381.
59. Fletcher EC. Sympathetic over activity in the etiology of hypertension of obstructive sleep apnea. Sleep 2003; 26(1):15–19.
60. Carlson JT, Hedner J, Elam M, et al. Augmented resting sympathetic activity in awake patients with obstructive sleep apnea. Chest 1993; 103:1763–1768.
61. Somers VK, Dyken ME, Clary MP, et al. Sympathetic neural mechanisms in obstructive sleep apnea. J Clin Invest 1995; 96(4):1897–1904.
62. Narkiewicz K, van de Borne PJ, Cooley RL, et al. Sympathetic activity in obese subjects with and without obstructive sleep apnea. Circulation 1998; 98(8):772–776.

63. Narkiewicz K, Montano N, Cogliati C, et al. Altered cardiovascular variability in obstructive sleep apnea. Circulation 1998; 98(11):1071–1077.
64. Frattola A, Parati G, Cuspidi C, et al. Prognostic value of 24-hour blood pressure variability. J Hypertens 1993; 11(10):1133–1137.
65. Parati G, Lantelme P. Blood pressure variability, target organ damage and cardiovascular events. J Hypertens 2002; 20(9):1725–1729.
66. Narkiewicz K, van de Borne PJ, Montano N, et al. Contribution of tonic chemoreflex activation to sympathetic activity and blood pressure in patients with obstructive sleep apnea. Circulation 1998; 97(10):943–945.
67. Narkiewicz K, van de Borne PJ, Pesek CA, et al. Selective potentiation of peripheral chemoreflex sensitivity in obstructive sleep apnea. Circulation 1999; 99(9):1183–1189.
68. Narkiewicz K, Somers VK. The sympathetic nervous system and obstructive sleep apnea: implications for hypertension. J Hypertens 1997; 15(12 pt 2):1613–1619.
69. Pinto JM, Garpestad E, Weiss JW, et al. Hemodynamic changes associated with obstructive sleep apnea followed by arousal in a porcine model. J Appl Physiol 1993; 75(4):1439–1443.
70. Guilleminault C, Connolly S, Winkle R, et al. Cyclical variation of the heart rate in sleep apnoea syndrome. Mechanisms, and usefulness of 24 h electrocardiography as a screening technique. Lancet 1984; 1(8369):126–131.
71. Guilleminault C, Connolly SJ, Winkle RA. Cardiac arrhythmia and conduction disturbances during sleep in 400 patients with sleep apnea syndrome. Am J Cardiol 1983; 52(5):490–494.
72. Tilkian AG, Guilleminault C, Schroeder JS, et al. Sleep-induced apnea syndrome. Prevalence of cardiac arrhythmias and their reversal after tracheostomy. Am J Med 1977; 63(3):348–358.
73. Zwillich C, Devlin T, White D, et al. Bradycardia during sleep apnea. Characteristics and mechanism. J Clin Invest 1982; 69(6):1286–1292.
74. Gami AS, Somers VK. Implications of obstructive sleep apnea for atrial fibrillation and sudden cardiac death. J Cardiovasc Electrophysiol 2008; 19(9):997–1003.
75. Gami AS, Hodge DO, Herges RM, et al. Obstructive sleep apnea, obesity, and the risk of incident atrial fibrillation. J Am Coll Cardiol 2007; 49(5):565–571.
76. Gami AS, Howard DE, Olson EJ, et al. Day-night pattern of sudden death in obstructive sleep apnea. N Engl J Med 2005; 352(12):1206–1214.
77. Kuniyoshi FH, Garcia-Touchard A, Gami AS, et al. Day-night variation of acute myocardial infarction in obstructive sleep apnea. J Am Coll Cardiol 2008; 52(3):343–346.
78. Sanner BM, Konermann M, Tepel M, et al. Platelet function in patients with obstructive sleep apnoea syndrome. Eur Respir J 2000; 16(4):648–652.
79. Chin K, Ohi M, Kita H, et al. Effects of NCPAP therapy on fibrinogen levels in obstructive sleep apnea syndrome. Am J Respir Crit Care Med 1996; 153(6 pt 1):1972–1976.
80. Rangemark C, Hedner JA, Carlson JT, et al. Platelet function and fibrinolytic activity in hypertensive and normotensive sleep apnea patients. Sleep 1995; 18(3):188–194.
81. Baguet JP, Hammer L, Levy P, et al. Night-time and diastolic hypertension are common and underestimated conditions in newly diagnosed apnoeic patients. J Hypertens 2005; 23(3):521–527.
82. Portaluppi F, Provini F, Cortelli P, et al. Undiagnosed sleep-disordered breathing among male nondippers with essential hypertension. J Hypertens 1997; 15(11):1227–1233.
83. Pankow W, Nabe B, Lies A, et al. Influence of sleep apnea on 24-hour blood pressure. Chest 1997; 112(5):1253–1258.
84. Lavie P, Yoffe N, Berger I, et al. The relationship between the severity of sleep apnea syndrome and 24-h blood pressure values in patients with obstructive sleep apnea. Chest 1993; 103(3):717–721.
85. Verdecchia P, Schillaci G, Guerrieri M, et al. Circadian blood pressure changes and left ventricular hypertrophy in essential hypertension. Circulation 1990; 81(2):528–536.

86. Verdecchia P, Schillaci G, Gatteschi C, et al. Blunted nocturnal fall in blood pressure in hypertensive women with future cardiovascular morbid events. Circulation 1993; 88(3):986–992.
87. Wilcox I, Grunstein RR, Hedner JA, et al. Effect of nasal continuous positive airway pressure during sleep on 24-hour blood pressure in obstructive sleep apnea. Sleep 1993; 16(6):539–544.
88. Faccenda JF, Mackay TW, Boon NA, et al. Randomized placebo-controlled trial of continuous positive airway pressure on blood pressure in the sleep apnea-hypopnea syndrome. Am J Respir Crit Care Med 2001; 163(2):344–348.
89. Bazzano LA, Khan Z, Reynolds K, et al. Effect of nocturnal nasal continuous positive airway pressure on blood pressure in obstructive sleep apnea. Hypertension 2007; 50(2):417–423.
90. Pepperell JC, Ramdassingh-Dow S, Crosthwaite N, et al. Ambulatory blood pressure after therapeutic and subtherapeutic nasal continuous positive airway pressure for obstructive sleep apnoea: a randomised parallel trial. Lancet 2002; 359(9302):204–210.
91. Sanner BM, Tepel M, Markmann A, et al. Effect of continuous positive airway pressure therapy on 24-hour blood pressure in patients with obstructive sleep apnea syndrome. Am J Hypertens 2002; 15(3):251–257.
92. Norman D, Loredo JS, Nelesen RA, et al. Effects of continuous positive airway pressure versus supplemental oxygen on 24-hour ambulatory blood pressure. Hypertension 2006; 47 (5):840–845.
93. Narkiewicz K, Kato M, Phillips BG, et al. Nocturnal continuous positive airway pressure decreases daytime sympathetic traffic in obstructive sleep apnea. Circulation 1999; 100 (23):2332–2335.
94. Coughlin SR, Mawdsley L, Mugarza JA, et al. Cardiovascular and metabolic effects of CPAP in obese males with OSA. Eur Respir J 2007; 29(4):720–727.
95. Kohler M, Pepperell JC, Casadei B, et al. CPAP and measures of cardiovascular risk in males with OSAS. Eur Respir J 2008; 32(6):1488–1496.
96. Usui K, Bradley TD, Spaak J, et al. Inhibition of awake sympathetic nerve activity of heart failure patients with obstructive sleep apnea by nocturnal continuous positive airway pressure. J Am Coll Cardiol 2005; 45(12):2008–2011.
97. Gilman MP, Floras JS, Usui K, et al. Continuous positive airway pressure increases heart rate variability in heart failure patients with obstructive sleep apnoea. Clin Sci (Lond) 2008; 114 (3):243–249.
98. Grassi G, Seravalle G, Bertinieri G, et al. Behaviour of the adrenergic cardiovascular drive in atrial fibrillation and cardiac arrhythmias. Acta Physiol Scand 2003; 177(3):399–404.

10

Epidemiological Evidence for an Association Between Sleep Apnea, Hypertension, and Cardiovascular Disease

YAMINI S. LEVITZKY and SUSAN REDLINE
Heart and Vascular Center, MetroHealth Campus, Case Western Reserve University and University Hospitals, Case Medical Center, Cleveland, Ohio, U.S.A.

I. Introduction: Role of Epidemiologic Studies in Assessing Causality

The emergence of obstructive sleep apnea (OSA) as a common health condition associated with substantial expenditures of health care dollars has been accompanied by skepticism over whether this condition represents a "real disease" (1). Although there is irrefutable evidence that OSA contributes to excessive daytime somnolence, there is greater uncertainty over whether OSA contributes to the incidence or progression of the two health conditions of established public health importance, hypertension and cardiovascular disease (CVD). There are several challenges in establishing and evaluating the putative causal associations between OSA and health outcomes, which have fueled criticism of the current evidence base. Inferring causality between an "exposure" such as OSA and outcomes such as hypertension/CVD requires multiple lines of evidence. Data from observational studies, such as case-control or cross-sectional or longitudinal cohort studies, may be useful in quantifying associations and identifying subgroups in which the disease may be especially important. The validity of such inferences relates to the precision of the statistical estimates, which is a function of the sample size, the appropriateness of the study design and analytical methods, including the validity and reliability of the measurements of exposure and outcomes, and the extent to which findings are unexplained by selection, measurement, confounding, or other biases. There is greater confidence in such associations if they are consistent across studies and different populations, if consistent patterns are observed between increasing levels of exposure (severity of OSA) with severity or frequency of adverse outcomes ("dose-response" associations), and if it can be demonstrated from longitudinal assessments that the exposure preceded the outcome. Since data from observational studies may never completely address residual confounding or precisely identify temporal associations, data often are needed from experimental studies, notably randomized controlled trials, that address whether altering the exposure (i.e., treating OSA) leads to a change in the health outcome. The existing epidemiological literature that has addressed OSA and CVD has been limited by intrinsic challenges in designing the large-scale studies required to quantify associations of modest effects, by the complexities in accurately and reliably measuring OSA in large-scale research studies, and by analytical challenges in dissecting the role of confounders. This chapter will review the existing database of moderate- to large-scale studies that have addressed the association of OSA to hypertension and CVD.

II. OSA and Hypertension

A. Snoring

The most extensively studied cardiovascular outcome relating to OSA has been hypertension. The earliest research in this area used self-reported snoring history as a surrogate for OSA. There are several studies that have evaluated the association between snoring and hypertension. Lindberg and colleagues followed 2668 men for 10 years who were habitual snorers (aged 30–69 years at baseline) to determine the risk of incident hypertension. In men aged 30 to 49 years who were persistent snorers (i.e., reported snoring at baseline and also 10 years later), the odds of hypertension were 2.6 times greater [95% confidence internal (CI), 1.5–4.5] after adjusting for age, body mass index (BMI), weight gain, physical inactivity, alcohol, and smoking. In men aged 50 to 69 years at baseline, there were no increased odds of incident hypertension. The authors offered several hypotheses regarding the lack of association in the older age group: first, the cumulative effects of other factors impact the development of hypertension more than habitual snoring; second, older individuals in the study may represent survivor bias; and, possibly, third, the upper airway resistance conferred by snoring may result in especially negative physiological effects in younger individuals (2). In another longitudinal study conducted in women, participants from the Nurses' Health Study cohort who were either occasional snorers or habitual snorers were compared with nonsnorers (self-reported) and followed for eight years. The multivariate-adjusted relative risks (adjusted for age, BMI, waist circumference, smoking, alcohol, and physical activity) for incident hypertension in occasional snorers was 1.29 (95% CI, 1.22–1.37) and in habitual snorers was 1.55 (95% CI, 1.42–1.70) (3). The findings with respect to snoring and incident hypertension have been reproduced, most recently in a prospective study of 8603 normotensive Korean adults aged 40 to 69 with BMI <27.5 [by the World Health Organization (WHO) definition of obesity in Asian individuals] followed for two years for development of incident hypertension. Significantly increased odds of developing hypertension (defined as systolic blood pressure $\geq$140, diastolic blood pressure $\geq$90, or antihypertensive treatment) were reported in habitual snorers (OR 1.49, 95% CI, 1.08–2.05 in men; OR 1.56, 95% CI, 1.07–2.27 in women) in models adjusted for age, BMI, alcohol use, smoking, exercise, triglycerides, and changing rate of body weight over the follow-up period. The odds ratios (ORs) for incident hypertension in habitual snorers were significant for each age stratum, except for those aged $\geq$60, consistent with other studies that have used the apnea-hypopnea index (AHI) as a measure of exposure (4–6). Polysomnographic data were obtained on 457 participants of this latter study, confirming that 55% of habitual snorers had an AHI $\geq$5 and, thus, lending support to the utility of snoring as a surrogate for OSA.

B. Objective Measurements of OSA

While a relationship between objectively measured OSA and hypertension was recognized at least as far back as 1985 (7), most of the studies published before 1995 were limited by small sample sizes and possible confounding by obesity, a factor strongly related to both hypertension and OSA. However, the current evidence base includes data from at least five large cohort studies, including the Wisconsin Sleep Cohort; the Sleep Heart Health Study (SHHS), a cohort in southern Pennsylvania; a Spanish cohort; and the Outcomes of Sleep Disorders in Older Men Study (MrOS), which support an independent associations between OSA and hypertension (Table 1) (4,8–10).

The Wisconsin Sleep Cohort comprises over 1000 state employees, ages 30 to 60 years, who were examined with in-laboratory polysomnography (PSG) on entry into the study. Cross-sectional analyses from this cohort showed that an increasing AHI was linearly associated with increasing systolic, and to a lesser extent, diastolic blood pressure. Compared to individuals with an AHI of 0, those with an AHI $\geq$15 were estimated to have 1.8-fold increased odds of hypertension (11). An interaction with BMI was observed such that the association between OSA and hypertension was stronger in less compared with more obese individuals. A significant association between hypertension and OSA was confirmed in a prospective analysis of 709 Wisconsin study participants who completed a follow-up PSG four years later, and 184 who were also studied eight years after the baseline study, resulting in 893 sets of four-year PSG studies. Logistic regression modeling was used to predict incident hypertension, given the baseline level of OSA, using varying definitions of hypertension ranging from 130/85 to 180/110. Age- and sex-adjusted ORs were similar for all definitions of hypertension, with an OR of 2.71 (95% CI, 1.78–4.14) for the group with an AHI of 5 to 15 and an OR of 4.47 (95% CI, 2.37–8.36) for the group with AHI $\geq$15, compared to the referent group. In models adjusted for age, sex, baseline hypertension, BMI, waist and neck circumference, and alcohol and cigarette use, ORs were attenuated but remained statistically significant at 2.03 (95% CI, 1.29–3.17) for the group with an AHI of 5 to 15 and 2.89 (95% CI, 1.46–5.64) for the group with AHI $\geq$15. No evidence of the absence of an effect was found for lower levels of OSA.

The SHHS represents the largest and most diverse sample studied to date. The SHHS draws its participants from several ongoing cohort studies, including the Atherosclerosis Risk in Communities study, the Cardiovascular Health Study, the Framingham Heart Study, the New York Hypertension cohorts, the Tucson Epidemiologic Study, and the Strong Heart Study, to obtain a total sample of 6441 participants from geographically diverse communities (aged 40–98, 23% ethnic minorities) who had had their risk factors previously measured by their parent cohorts (12). The participants underwent in-home PSG, which provided highly reliable estimates of AHI. In cross-sectional analysis of data from the baseline exam, and after adjusting for age, sex, and ethnicity, compared to the referent group with an AHI <1.5, the OR for the group with an AHI of 5 to 14.9 was 1.57 (95% CI, 1.35–1.81), rising to 2.27 (95% CI, 1.76–2.92) for the group with AHI $\geq$30. In models adjusted for age, sex, ethnicity, alcohol, smoking, and measures of adiposity (BMI, neck circumference, and waist-to-hip ratio), compared to the referent group, the ORs significantly increased across AHI categories of 1.5 to 4.9, 5 to 14.9, 15 to 30 and >30, to 1.07, 1.20, 1.25, and 1.37, respectively. The authors note that the true estimate of the association between hypertension and OSA may fall somewhere between the minimally adjusted ORs and the fully adjusted models, since adjusting for measures of adiposity may be "overadjusting" for a variable potentially in the causal pathway (8). The difference in the magnitude of the estimates between the Wisconsin Sleep Cohort and the SHHS may be in part due to differences in the age and racial composition of the sample. Support for the latter may be derived by examination

Table 1 Summary of Major Trials Evaluating Relation Between Sleep-Disordered Breathing and Hypertension

Cohort	Sample/study design	Groups	Findings	Limitations
Sleep Heart Health Study (8) Cross-sectional cohort study	Healthy individuals sampled from other cohort studies, n = 6132, with interpretable PSGs and complete demographic information[a] Logistic regression to calculate OR of OSA, given HTN	Ref: AHI <1.5 AHI 1.5–4.9 AHI 5–14.9 AHI 15–29.9 AHI ≥30	OSA is associated with HTN even after adjusting for measures of adiposity	Cross-sectional study does not allow inference about causation
Wisconsin Sleep Cohort (9) Prospective cohort study	n = 709 state employees who completed baseline and 4-yr PSG and an additional 187 PSG done 8-yr post baseline, yielding 893 4-yr sleep sets[b] Logistic regression to determine odds of HTN at follow-up based on level of OSA at baseline	Ref: AHI = 0 AHI 0.1–4.9 AHI 5.0–14.9 AHI ≥15	OSA is associated with development of incident HTN, particularly at levels of more severe OSA	Few participants with events >15/hr
Southern Pennsylvania (4)	Randomly selected households with telephones in two counties in Pennsylvania interviewed; 741 men and 1000 women participated in in-hospital PSG[c]	Ref: No OSA Snoring Mild OSA (AHI 0.1–14.9 with snoring) Moderate/severe OSA (AHI ≥15)	Independent association in young and middle-aged individuals at any level of OSA (mild and moderate/severe) OSA and prevalent HTN, even when adjusting for age, BMI, sex, menopause, alcohol, smoking, and race	No normal-weight premenopausal women with OSA in this cohort

Spanish cohort (10)	Randomly selected residents aged 30–70 yr, residing in Basque Country[d] Phase 1 – n = 2148 Phase 2 – n = 555 (390 with OSA, 165 without OSA)	Ref: AHI = 0 AHI 0.1–4.9 AHI 5.0–14.9 AHI ≥ 15.0 Adjusted for age, sex, BMI, neck circumference, alcohol, and smoking	OR of 2.28 (95% CI, 0.92–5.66) for HTN in participants with AHI ≥ 15 compared with AHI = 0	Smaller sample size

Individual Study Definitions: [a]Hypertension—blood pressure 140/90 or current treatment; apnea—complete or almost complete cessation of airflow; hypopnea—decrease in airflow or thoracoabdominal excursion by ≥30% of baseline for 10 seconds with ≥4% oxygen desaturation. [b]Hypertension defined as 140/90 or treatment; apnea—cessation of airflow for at least 10 seconds; hypopnea—discernible reduction in the sum amplitude of the rib cage plus abdominal excursions detected by respiratory inductance plethysmography lasting 10 seconds with at least 4% oxyhemoglobin desaturation. [c]Hypertension—systolic blood pressure >140 or diastolic blood pressure >90 or hypertension treatment at the time of PSG; apnea—breathing cessation for ≥10 seconds; hypopnea—50% reduction of airflow at nose or mouth associated with oxyhemoglobin desaturation of 4%. [d]Hypertension—systolic blood pressure ≥140 or diastolic blood pressure ≥90 or hypertension treatment; apnea—complete cessation of airflow for ≥10 seconds; hypopnea—50% reduction in airflow with ≥4% oxyhemoglobin desaturation and/or electroencephalographic arousal. *Abbreviations:* Ref, Referent group; PSG, polysomnography; OR, odds ratio; CI, confidence interval; OSA, obstructive sleep apnea; HTN, hypertension; AHI, apnea-hypopnea index; BMI, body mass index.

of stratified analyses conducted in the SHHS. A higher OR was observed in younger members of the cohort, in American Indians compared to other ethnic groups, and in men compared to women. In later analyses of SHHS data, Haas and colleagues further explored whether associations of OSA with hypertension varied according to hypertension subtype and age (5). In particular, the study addressed whether different associations with OSA were apparent for essential (systolic and diastolic) hypertension compared to isolated systolic hypertension (ISH). Mechanistically, systolic/diastolic hypertension is thought to reflect the interplay of multiple pathways, with the sympathetic nervous system activation being an important contributor, while ISH is thought to reflect the age-dependent loss of vascular compliance (5,13). Activation of the sympathetic nervous system is hypothesized to be critical in the development of hypertension in OSA (14) and could explain the discrepancy between risks of hypertension in young/middle-aged individuals compared with older individuals in the population-based studies discussed previously. This analysis found that among participants aged 60 and older with AHI $\geq$15, prevalence of systolic/diastolic hypertension was 4.9% versus 28.1% with ISH. In participants aged 40 to 59 with AHI $\geq$15, the distribution was more even, with 13.5% participants with systolic/diastolic hypertension versus 13.8% with ISH, though Haas and colleagues note that only in the younger group did the prevalence of systolic/diastolic hypertension increase with severity of OSA. No significant association was found between OSA occurring in older individuals and either systolic/diastolic hypertension or ISH, while there was a strong association between severe OSA (analyzed as a percentage of sleep time spent with oxyhemoglobin saturation <90%) and systolic/diastolic hypertension in individuals aged 40 to 59 (fully adjusted OR 2.73, 95% CI, 1.45–5.15, $p < 0.001$ for trend). They conclude that studies that aggregate systolic/diastolic hypertension with ISH and include participants over the age of 60 may underestimate the true association between OSA and hypertension (5).

A third large study that has examined OSA and hypertension drew its cohort by randomly selecting households with telephones from two counties in southern Pennsylvania. Potential participants were interviewed and selected if they had risk factors for OSA, resulting in 741 men and 1000 women (mean age 47.4 years) who underwent in-hospital PSG. A broad dose-response association was suggested with the multivariable-adjusted ORs for hypertension of 1.56, 2.29, and 6.85 for snorers, mild OSA (AHI of 0.1–14.9), and moderate OSA (AHI >15) (4). The strongest association between hypertension and OSA was in young and middle-aged individuals of normal weight. In older, normal-weight individuals, the OR for developing hypertension in patients with moderate/severe OSA compared with individuals without OSA was 0.08 (95% CI, 0.02–0.31) (4).

A fourth study examined a large cohort of participants aged 30 to 70 in Basque Country, Spain (10). Subjects were recruited in a two-phase manner. Eligible participants underwent a home interview, limited physical exam, and sleep apnea assessment for one night using a portable system. In the second phase of the study, subjects with OSA and a random sample of participants without OSA completed attended overnight PSG ($n = 555$). A high prevalence of OSA, with almost equal gender distributions, was observed (27% with AHI >5). The researchers found a significantly increased odds of hypertension in participants with an AHI of 0.1 to 4.9 (OR 2.47, 95% CI, 1.06–5.76, adjusted for age, sex, BMI, neck circumference, smoking, and alcohol). However, no evidence of a dose-response relationship was observed, with lower and nonsignificant

ORs at higher AHI categories. The authors note that their relatively small sample size may account for the discrepancy between their findings and those discussed previously.

The MrOS is a more recent multisite U.S. population–based cohort study of 2911 older men (mean age 76 years) studied with in-home polysomonography, using methods similar to that of the SHHS (15). Given the controversy over whether OSA is a distinct disorder in the elderly, an initial cross-sectional report evaluated the distribution of risk factors for OSA. In total, 26% of the sample was classified with moderate or more severe OSA (AHI >15). A history of hypertension increased the odds of OSA by 24% (95% CI, 1.06–1.50). The magnitude of this association is comparable with what was observed in the generally older SHHS study.

C. Relationship to Mechanisms

Several mechanisms have been postulated to explain an increased prevalence of hypertension associated with OSA. Acute surges in sympathetic activation that accompany apnea-related hypoxemia, arousal, or respiratory effort may lead to increased nocturnal systolic and diastolic blood pressure, with elevations in blood pressure persisting into the daytime (16). The extent to which sustained hypertension may be secondary to the effects of intermittent surges in blood pressure on vascular remodeling and altered vasoreactivity, to changes in endothelial function, to salt and water homeostasis, or to other effects of intermittent hypoxemia or sympathetic activation is unclear. Several epidemiological studies have attempted to identify which sleep parameters best predict blood pressure in OSA. Stradling and colleagues measured overnight blood pressure changes in 528 community volunteers and estimated that 5% to 10% of the variance in overnight blood pressure could be explained by respiratory effort and oxyhemoglobin dip rates (17). However, sex-stratified analyses showed that these associations were only present in men. In the Cleveland Family Study, the magnitude of associations between hypertension with three commonly measured indices of OSA—hypoxemia, AHI, and arousal—were compared (18). Of these indices, the arousal index was most strongly associated with hypertension, consistent with the hypothesis that sympathetic activation plays a role in the pathogenesis of OSA-mediated hypertension. However, additional research is needed to systematically and more fully evaluate the relative contribution of different measures of physiological disturbance on hypertension pathogenesis.

D. Intervention Studies

The literature regarding OSA treatment studies and blood pressure response is discussed in more detail in chapter 11. The demonstration of improvement in blood pressure with OSA treatment provides evidence of a potential causal relation between OSA and hypertension. Surprisingly few studies have rigorously assessed the effect of sleep apnea treatment on blood pressure. Existing studies largely have been limited by small sample sizes, did not include a placebo arm, and often addressed changes after only one day to one week of therapy. A meta-analysis of 16 randomized trials with minimal durations of two weeks, including 818 participants, estimated that continuous positive airway pressure (CPAP) led to an average net decrease in systolic blood pressure of 2.46 mmHg (95% CI, −4.31 to −0.62) and a net change in diastolic blood pressure of 1.83 mmHg (95% CI, −3.05 to −0.61) (19). Control treatments have included sham CPAP, usual care, and a placebo pill. Studies that included sham CPAP generally found greater blood pressure–lowering effects in the control arm than did studies that used alternative control interventions, raising a concern that blood pressure–lowering effects of CPAP may have been overestimated in some trials that did not include appropriate control arms. Because of considerable subject heterogeneity, it is not clear whether differential effects on blood pressure occur according to the level of OSA severity, baseline blood pressure, or other subject characteristics.

III. Sleep-Disordered Breathing and CVD

A. Ischemic Heart Disease

Definitions of coronary heart disease (CHD) and CVD vary by investigator, but in general, CHD refers to hard endpoints, such as nonfatal myocardial infarction (MI), while CVD encompasses CHD, stroke, and intermittent claudication and may include less well-defined endpoints such as transient ischemic attack and angina. Similar to hypertension, more epidemiological data addressing these outcomes are available for snoring as a surrogate for OSA than for objectively measured OSA. In a retrospective analysis of Finnish twins from the early 1980s, Koskenvuo and colleagues reported a significant association between habitual snoring and angina (RR 2.01, $p < 0.01$) but not MI or hospitalization for ischemic heart disease (20). While this study was limited by reliance on self-reports for snoring and for the major outcome events, it raised the important question of whether mild OSA has an impact on the risk of CVD. The first prospective study examining the relation between snoring and MI was conducted by the same group and followed over three years 4388 Finnish male participants aged 40 to 69 years with habitual and frequent, occasional, or nonsnorers for self-reported ischemic heart disease. After adjustment for age, BMI, hypertension, smoking, and alcohol use, the relative risk for ischemic heart disease was 1.71 ($p < 0.01$) for habitual and frequent snorers versus nonsnorers (21). Hu and colleagues examined incident CVD in participants of the Nurses' Health Study in 2000. In their work, 121,000 registered nurses were followed with postal questionnaires every two years. Participants were categorized as being either never, occasional, or regular snorers and followed over eight years for incident CVD events (defined as nonfatal MI, fatal CHD, fatal stroke, and nonfatal stroke), ascertained by review of medical records, where available. In the multivariable-adjusted model for total cardiovascular events (CHD + stroke), the RR was 1.33 (95% CI, 1.06–1.67) for regular snorers and 1.20 (95% CI, 1.01–1.43) for occasional snorers compared with never snorers. However, when endpoints were analyzed individually, there was no statistically significant increased risk (22).

Only a few epidemiological studies have examined the relation between objectively measured OSA with CVD (23–26). In a cross-sectional analysis, investigators from the SHHS found relative odds of CVD (self-reported angina, heart attack, heart failure, stroke, or revascularization procedure) of 1.30 (95% CI, 1.01–1.67) in a fully adjusted model comparing the highest quartile of AHI (11.1) with the lowest quartile (Table 2). This association was modestly higher in models that excluded adjustment for factors thought to be in the causal pathway, such as diabetes and hypertension [relative odds 1.42 (95% CI, 1.13–1.78) for the highest quartile of AHI (11.1) compared with the lowest quartile] (26). Of interest was the lack of evidence of increasing risk for the aggregate CVD outcome at levels of AHI greater than 11, suggesting a "plateau" at a level of OSA generally considered only modestly elevated and one that is common in the population. Associations were somewhat higher when the discrete outcomes of heart

Table 2 Summary of Major Prospective Trials Evaluating Relation Between Sleep-Disordered Breathing and Coronary Heart Disease

Cohort	Study design	Sample	Results/conclusions	Strengths/limitations
Nurse's Health Study (22)	Prospective cohort design: 121,700 registered nurses followed by postal questionnaire every 2 yr	Categorized by self-report: regular, occasional, and never snorers, followed for 8 yr for incident CVD events (nonfatal MI, fatal CHD event, nonfatal stroke, fatal stroke)	In the multivariable-adjusted model[a], there was a 33% increased risk of total CVD[b] events in regular snorers, 20% increased risk in occasional snorers. When endpoints were analyzed individually, no longer statistically significant	• Very large sample of women • Excluded prevalent CVD at baseline • Endpoints relied on self-report
Swedish cohort (25)	Prospective cohort design: Consecutive patients with CAD requiring ICU-level care in County Hospital, Skaraborg, Skövde, Sweden, who underwent an overnight sleep study 4–21 mo later, $n = 62$	16 patients with OSA (RDI >10, desat >4%) and 43 patients without, followed for 5 years for MI, stroke, and cardiovascular mortality	Neither MI nor stroke incidence differed significantly between groups, but cardiovascular mortality rate was significantly higher in OSA group	• Included elderly patients (>75-yr-old) • Small sample
Sleep Heart Health Study (26)	$n = 6440$ community-dwelling participants drawn from parent cohorts (see text)	Healthy individuals samples from other large cohort studies	Cross-sectional analyses showed a 30% increased relative odds of CVD in the fully adjusted model at an AHI = 11	• Ethnically and geographically diverse sample • Relied on self-report of CVD

[a]Adjusted for age, time period, BMI, smoking, menopausal status, family history of MI, alcohol, vitamin use, activity, usual sleep position, diabetes, hypercholesterolemia, and average number of sleep hours. [b]CVD defined as positive response to "Has a doctor ever told you that you had angina, heart attack, heart failure, or stroke?" or if the participant reported having undergone coronary bypass surgery or coronary angioplasty. Fully adjusted model accounted for covariates: age, race, sex, smoking status and number of cigarettes smoked per day, self-reported diabetes, self-reported hypertension, use of antihypertensive medication, systolic blood pressure, BMI, total cholesterol, and high-density lipoprotein. *Abbreviations*: CVD, cardiovascular disease; MI, myocardial infarction; CHD, coronary heart disease; CAD, coronary artery disease; OSA, obstructive sleep apnea; AHI, apnea-hypopnea index; BMI, body mass index.

failure or stroke were analyzed, with some evidence that risk of stroke continued to increase at higher levels of AHI.

Marin and coworkers conducted a 10-year longitudinal study in Spain of approximately 1700 men, including individuals referred to a sleep center for evaluation of OSA, and an age- and weight-matched control group from the community for nonfatal and fatal MI or stroke (27). Compared with controls, those with untreated severe OSA (AHI >30 or AHI >5 with associated sleepiness) had increased odds of fatal CVD of 2.87 and increased odds of nonfatal CVD of 3.17. Compared to the severe group, incident CVD was approximately 50% lower in the 372 men who were treated with CPAP, which was approximately equivalent to the relative risk in the snoring group (OR 1.42). Although treatment was not randomized in this observational study, the group undergoing CPAP treatment was generally more severely affected than other individuals and would have been anticipated to have a higher incidence rate, thus providing data consistent with reversibility of CVD risk with OSA treatment.

Smaller studies have found increased odds of incident CVD events in patients with OSA and evidence of nocturnal ischemia detected by ST depressions on the electrocardiogram (EKG) (24,28). Conversely, patients with known coronary artery disease, including survivors of an MI, are more likely to have OSA (23) and are at increased risk of CVD events without treatment (29).

Stroke

The association between AHI with cross-sectional and incident stroke rates was analyzed in the Wisconsin Sleep Cohort. A significant cross-sectional association in adjusted analyses was demonstrated between stroke and moderate OSA [AHI >20 (OR 4.33, 95% CI, 1.32–14.24)). No evidence of a dose-response relationship was observed. In longitudinal analysis, the researchers found that the four-year adjusted risk of incident stroke was elevated, but with only four events in the follow-up of the relatively young OSA group, the association was not statistically significant (OR 3.08, 95% CI, 0.74–12.81) (30).

Yaggi and colleagues analyzed data from a clinic referral sample of patients 50 years and older to better characterize whether OSA was associated with death and incident stroke independent of other cardiovascular risk factors. Overall event rates were higher in this referral sample than in the Wisconsin cohort. At a median follow-up time of 3.4 years, the relative risk of incident stroke or death in fully adjusted models was 1.97 (95% CI, 1.12–3.48), with a significant trend toward increased risk with increasing AHI (31). However, most follow-up events were deaths (22 were strokes), and stroke-specific incidence rate was not reported.

Munoz and colleagues have confirmed that the sex-adjusted risk of incident stroke is significantly increased in elderly (median age 77 years) participants of the Vitoria Sleep Project, with moderate to severe OSA (AHI ≥30) (hazard ratio 2.52, 95% CI, 1.04–6.01) (32). The investigators did not adjust for obesity or for other stroke risk factors, such as age, hypertension, and diabetes, which were not significant in univariate analyses. However, jointly, these factors may have explained a significant portion of the observed relationship with OSA, and thus, the possibility of residual confounding exists.

Heart Failure

Heart failure may be associated with OSA through several mechanisms, as described in chapter 17. Of all cardiac outcomes examined in the SHHS, the strongest cross-sectional association was seen with heart failure. Participants with an AHI >11.1 had increased adjusted odds of heart failure of 2.2 compared with participants in the lowest quartile (26). In this community-based sample, the frequency of central apneas or Cheyne–Stokes respiration was low, supporting an association specifically with OSA. A prospective study of 164 patients with systolic heart failure and untreated OSA (AHI ≥15) suffered significantly worse mortality than patients with systolic heart failure who had mild or no OSA (33). At least two clinical trials have examined the impact of CPAP therapy in patients with heart failure. Kaneko randomized 24 patients with heart failure and OSA to one month of usual care versus CPAP. The left ventricular ejection fraction improved by almost 9% in the CPAP group, with no significant change in the control group (34). Improvement in the ejection fraction was accompanied by reductions in systolic blood pressure, heart rate, and left ventricular end-systolic dimensions. In a longer and slightly larger study, Mansfield and colleagues reported a 5% absolute improvement in left ventricular function in 19 patients with stable congestive heart failure and OSA (mean AHI 28) who underwent three months of CPAP therapy, which was greater than what was observed in 21 control patients (35). Parallel improvements in norepinephrine excretion were observed in the CPAP-treated group, suggesting that CPAP led to reduced sympathetic tone.

B. Arrhythmia and Conduction Disorders

Among healthy individuals free of known CVD, sinus bradycardia, sinus pauses, sinus arrhythmia, and type 1 second-degree atrioventricular block are common during sleep (36). Patients with OSA may also experience increased bradyarrhythmias, tachyarrhythmias, and ventricular premature beats (VPBs) (37). A predisposition to arrhythmias is consistent with the notion that patients with OSA have an electrical milieu that predisposes them to more frequent arrhythmias (38). The best studied association is that between OSA and atrial fibrillation (AF), which is the most prevalent sustained arrhythmia in the United States (39). Mehra and colleagues examined data from the SHHS for prevalent arrhythmias, comparing the frequency of arrhythmias in participants with an AHI ≥30 compared to <5 (40). A four-fold increased odds of AF in OSA was demonstrated, which was not explained by potential confounders. In the first reported study of OSA and development of incident AF, Gami and colleagues followed a sample referred for evaluation of OSA for a mean of 4.7 years and found that in individuals less than 65 years old, the presence of OSA (defined as AHI > 5) predicted incident AF. There was no apparent effect of CPAP therapy on the risk of AF, though a negative finding may have been due to poor compliance with CPAP treatment, which was not objectively measured (41). A small (n = 45) prospective trial conducted by Harbison and colleagues, however, suggested that severe OSA (mean AHI = 50) is associated with clinically significant arrhythmias and that these arrhythmias were improved by nasal CPAP (42). Another study of patients undergoing cardioversion for AF suggested that those with untreated OSA had a higher recurrence rate than those without OSA or those treated for OSA (43).

With respect to ventricular arrhythmias, nonsustained ventricular tachycardia and ventricular bigeminy, trigeminy, and quadrigeminy were observed more frequently in the Sleep Heart Health cohort in participants with severe sleep-disordered breathing (SDB) (AHI ≥30) compared with those without SDB (AHI < 5) (40). There are as yet no large, randomized, controlled trials examining the impact of treating OSA on ventricular arrhythmias, although a small trial ($n = 18$) of patients with OSA and heart failure (medically optimized) randomized to treatment with CPAP or no treatment demonstrated significant reductions in VPBs one month later in the CPAP group (44). The mechanism for the relation between OSA and ventricular arrhythmias is hypothesized to be related to hypoxemia and sympathetic activation, similar to that proposed for atrial arrhythmias, but remains unclear (45).

IV. Summary

In summary, data from several large cohort studies from across the globe provide evidence of an association between hypertension and snoring or OSA. Although prospective data are limited, longitudinal assessments using snoring as a surrogate for OSA as well as prospective data from the Wisconsin Sleep Cohort, where OSA was objectively measured, suggest that even mild OSA is associated with an increased incidence of hypertension. Although much of the association between OSA and hypertension may be explained by confounding with age, sex, and obesity, the data support an independent effect of OSA on increasing the odds of hypertension by 20% to as much as sevenfold. There may be stronger associations for essential compared with isolated systolic hypertension when blood pressure is evaluated using 24-hour or early-morning readings and among relatively younger individuals. Further, in aggregate, clinical trial data suggest that CPAP treatment leads to slight improvement in blood pressure. The literature does not provide consistent data regarding the nature of a dose-response relationship or whether specific threshold or ceiling levels exist. Higher risks are evident in individuals under the age of 50 to 60 years, with some data also indicating a higher risk in men and in less obese individuals. Weaker associations among older individuals may be attributed to a survival bias (4), the higher frequency of isolated systolic hypertension in the elderly, or to differences in the etiology or physiological responses to OSA in individuals of different ages.

Although there are relatively sparse data, the weight of evidence also suggests that OSA is associated with CVD and stroke, although this association is likely partly attributable to confounding factors. Some studies indicate that these associations are not explained by hypertension, suggesting that OSA adversely affects cardiac function through pathways that also include those unrelated to blood pressure regulation. No large-scale, well-controlled study, however, has been conducted that has addressed the impact of treatment of OSA on CVD incidence or mortality. However, uncontrolled studies suggest that CPAP treatment reduces CVD incidence and mortality. Limited data also suggest that treating high-risk patients, such as those with heart failure, also may lead to improved cardiovascular outcomes. Further large-scale prospective trials are needed to address the overall impact of OSA treatment on cardiovascular outcomes and mortality and to better identify which patients are most likely to benefit from intervention.

A. Issues to Consider in the Design of Future Epidemiologic Studies of OSA and Hypertension/CVD

Complexity of Measurement Limiting Sample Size

OSA traditionally has been diagnosed and quantified with the use of overnight monitoring of multiple physiological signals. Monitoring-related expense and participant burden likely have limited the initiation of more research studies, as well as have limited sample sizes of conducted studies. Compared to major CVD studies that enroll thousands to tens of thousands of patients, with only a few exceptions, OSA studies typically have enrolled less than 100 subjects, limiting their power and precision to adjust for confounders and increasing the likelihood of spurious findings. Several studies suggest important subgroup differences in the association between OSA and hypertension/CVD (e.g., stronger effects in younger compared with older individuals.) Most studies have not been designed to formally test for such subgroup differences (or "effect modification"). In addition, participation rates in most community studies of OSA have been only modest, raising concern of selection bias, with preferential participation of individuals who have the highest level of concern about their sleep or health or are otherwise more motivated to participate in research.

B. Accuracy and Reliability of Assessment

A second challenge relates to difficulties in quantifying the relevant OSA exposures. Early large-scale studies of OSA used fairly easily obtainable questionnaire data on snoring or other sleep habits as surrogates for OSA (4,6). In addition to imprecise classification by including individuals across a wide spectrum of disease severity, systematic misclassification may have occurred because of underreporting of snoring and other symptoms in population subgroups, such as the elderly, women, or those of a lower socioeconomic status (46). Most other studies have used various approaches for measuring AHI, or, more simply, the number of oxyhemoglobin desaturations per hour of sleep obtained from overnight recordings. Lack of standard definitions and measurements of exposure (criteria for respiratory event identification, methods of quantifying sleep fragmentation, etc.) likely have contributed to inconsistencies in the literature. Translating clinical approaches for diagnosing OSA, traditionally accomplished with the use of highly sophisticated, multichannel measurements to measurements that are reliable and quantify relevant exposures in large numbers of participants and across research settings also has been hampered by uncertainty over which of the physiological parameters acquired using overnight monitoring contribute etiologically to given health outcomes. Even when such quantitative data have been available, the methods for measuring individual events (most notably hypopneas) have varied, and there has been little consensus on how to apply thresholds for defining disease status (47). Thus, the existing literature does not provide consensus on whether dose-response relationships exist between indices of OSA and hypertension/CVD or if (and what) threshold of OSA severity operates to increase risk.

Confounding

Perhaps the largest challenge relates to dissecting the confounding influences of obesity, age, male gender, and other comorbidities from the effects directly attributable to OSA. Even in a large sample recruited from the community (where selection biases may be less than in clinic samples), Newman and colleagues found that AHI is strongly associated with traditional CVD risk factors: BMI, waist-hip ratio, hypertension, dyslipidemia, and diabetes (48). Because patients with OSA typically have much comorbidity, which places them at higher risk of CHD or CVD events, it can be difficult to separate the impact of OSA on CVD from the influence of CVD risk factors on CVD endpoints. Strategies for addressing the influence of these confounding factors include the following: (*i*) use a case-control design, with attempts to match controls to cases on confounding variables; (*ii*) restrict analyses to individuals without known comorbidities; and (*iii*) recruit from a community sample (where prevalence of comorbidities may be lower than in a clinic-based sample) and rigorously measure confounders and adjust for these analytically. Each strategy, however, has notable limitations. For example, the choice of an appropriate control group may be difficult. For example, studies of patients referred for evaluation of OSA found to have a low AHI on a single study likely may not represent "unexposed" controls. Statistical models that "control" for BMI or other confounders may overadjust for the exposure of interest. For example, if OSA contributed to the development of obesity, controlling for BMI would falsely attenuate a factor in the causal pathway between OSA and hypertension. Too often, statistical multivariable models are developed with scant consideration of biological plausibility.

Validity of Outcome Measurements
Some of the difficulty in assessing the epidemiologic evidence pertaining to OSA and CVD relates to challenges in defining relevant outcomes. Although not unique to studies of OSA, the level of blood pressure or hypertension status, for example, is difficult to ascertain in individuals using antihypertensive medications. In addition, some research suggests markedly different associations between OSA and systolic compared to diastolic blood pressure, as well to differences in whether blood pressure is quantified using morning, evening, or 24-hour measurements. Congestive heart failure is often quantified using self-report data or information from medical records, which may not allow for precise characterization of systolic and diastolic dysfunction. Inconsistencies across studies, or the use of less sensitive outcome measurements, may have contributed to discrepancies in the literature.

Assessing Temporal Patterns
Most of the literature that has addressed associations between OSA and hypertension/ CVD has been based on cross-sectional studies, where the exposure (OSA) and outcome (hypertension or CVD) are assessed concurrently. However, without knowing whether the OSA exposure preceded the health outcome, it is not possible to exclude reverse causality. This may be especially relevant for CVD or stroke, where impaired cardiac function or cerebral circulation may contribute to ventilatory control abnormalities predisposing to OSA. In support of this is the finding of Bassetti et al., who showed an approximately 50% reduction in AHI measured six months compared to immediately after a stroke, with the earlier higher indices presumably associated with greater cardiac-cerebral dysfunction occurring immediately after a stroke (49). Causality may be better inferred from either prospective studies that demonstrate the appropriate temporal associations between OSA and the health outcome or randomized controlled studies that demonstrate that OSA treatment reverses or improves the health parameter more than would be observed in a placebo condition. It is critical that such studies be designed with sufficient power to detect health effects of clinical importance, and allow assessment of subgroup differences, including special vulnerabilities to OSA or its treatment.

References
1. Wright J, Johns R, Watt I, et al. Health effects of obstructive sleep apnoea and the effectiveness of continuous positive airways pressure: a systematic review of the research evidence. BMJ 1997; 314(7084):851–860.

2. Lindberg E, Janson C, Gislason T, et al. Snoring and hypertension: a 10 year follow-up. Eur Respir J 1998; 11(4):884–889.

3. Hu FB, Willett WC, Colditz GA, et al. Prospective study of snoring and risk of hypertension in women. Am J Epidemiol 1999; 150(8):806–816.

4. Bixler EO, Vgontzas AN, Lin HM, et al. Association of hypertension and sleep-disordered breathing. Arch Intern Med 2000; 160(15):2289–2295.

5. Haas DC, Foster GL, Nieto FJ, et al. Age-dependent associations between sleep-disordered breathing and hypertension: importance of discriminating between systolic/diastolic hypertension and isolated systolic hypertension in the Sleep Heart Health Study. Circulation 2005; 111(5):614–621.

6. Kim J, Yi H, Shin KR, et al. Snoring as an independent risk factor for hypertension in the nonobese population: the Korean Health and Genome Study. Am J Hypertens 2007; 20(8): 819–824.

7. Fletcher EC, DeBehnke RD, Lovoi MS, et al. Undiagnosed sleep apnea in patients with essential hypertension. Ann Intern Med 1985; 103(2):190–195.

8. Nieto FJ, Young TB, Lind BK, et al. Association of sleep-disordered breathing, sleep apnea, and hypertension in a large community-based study. JAMA 2000; 283(14):1829–1836.

9. Peppard PE, Young T, Palta M, et al. Prospective study of the association between sleep-disordered breathing and hypertension. N Engl J Med 2000; 342(19):1378–1384.

10. Duran J, Esnaola S, Rubio R, et al. Obstructive sleep apnea-hypopnea and related clinical features in a population-based sample of subjects aged 30 to 70 yr. Am J Respir Crit Care Med 2001; 163(3 pt 1):685–689.

11. Young T, Peppard P, Palta M, et al. Population-based study of sleep-disordered breathing as a risk factor for hypertension. Arch Intern Med 1997; 157(15):1746–1752.

12. Quan SF, Howard BV, Iber C, et al. The Sleep Heart Health Study: design, rationale, and methods. Sleep 1997; 20(12):1077–1085.

13. Lakatta EG, Levy D. Arterial and cardiac aging: major shareholders in cardiovascular disease enterprises: part I: aging arteries: a "set up" for vascular disease. Circulation 2003; 107(1): 139–146.

14. Fletcher EC. Sympathetic over activity in the etiology of hypertension of obstructive sleep apnea. Sleep 2003; 26(1):15–19.

15. Mehra R, Stone KL, Blackwell T, et al. Prevalence and correlates of sleep-disordered breathing in older men: osteoporotic fractures in men sleep study. J Am Geriatr Soc 2007; 55 (9):1356–1364.

16. Davies CW, Crosby JH, Mullins RL, et al. Case-control study of 24 hour ambulatory blood pressure in patients with obstructive sleep apnoea and normal matched control subjects. Thorax 2000; 55(9):736–740.

17. Stradling JR, Barbour C, Glennon J, et al. Which aspects of breathing during sleep influence the overnight fall of blood pressure in a community population? Thorax 2000; 55(5):393–398.

18. Sulit L, Storfer-Isser A, Kirchner HL, et al. Differences in polysomnography predictors for hypertension and impaired glucose tolerance. Sleep 2006; 29(6):777–783.

19. Bazzano LA, Khan Z, Reynolds K, et al. Effect of nocturnal nasal continuous positive airway pressure on blood pressure in obstructive sleep apnea. Hypertension 2007; 50(2):417–423.

20. Koskenvuo M, Kaprio J, Partinen M, et al. Snoring as a risk factor for hypertension and angina pectoris. Lancet 1985; 1(8434):893–896.

21. Koskenvuo M, Kaprio J, Heikkila K, et al. Snoring as a risk factor for ischaemic heart disease and stroke in men. Br Med J (Clin Res Ed) 1987; 294(6572):643.

22. Hu FB, Willett WC, Manson JE, et al. Snoring and risk of cardiovascular disease in women. J Am Coll Cardiol 2000; 35(2):308–313.

23. Hung J, Whitford EG, Parsons RW, et al. Association of sleep apnoea with myocardial infarction in men. Lancet 1990; 336(8710):261–264.

24. Mooe T, Franklin KA, Wiklund U, et al. Sleep-disordered breathing and myocardial ischemia in patients with coronary artery disease. Chest 2000; 117(6):1597–1602.
25. Peker Y, Hedner J, Kraiczi H, et al. Respiratory disturbance index: an independent predictor of mortality in coronary artery disease. Am J Respir Crit Care Med 2000; 162(1):81–86.
26. Shahar EYAL, Whitney CW, Redline SUSA, et al. Sleep-disordered breathing and cardiovascular disease. Cross-sectional results of the Sleep Heart Health Study. Am J Respir Crit Care Med 2001; 163(1):19–25.
27. Marin JM, Carrizo SJ, Vicente E, et al. Long-term cardiovascular outcomes in men with obstructive sleep apnoea-hypopnoea with or without treatment with continuous positive airway pressure: an observational study. Lancet 2005; 365(9464):1046–1053.
28. Peker Y, Hedner J, Norum J, et al. Increased incidence of cardiovascular disease in middle-aged men with obstructive sleep apnea: a 7-year follow-up. Am J Respir Crit Care Med 2002; 166(2):159–165.
29. Milleron O, Pilliere R, Foucher A, et al. Benefits of obstructive sleep apnoea treatment in coronary artery disease: a long-term follow-up study. Eur Heart J 2004; 25(9):728–734.
30. Arzt M, Young T, Finn L, et al. Association of sleep-disordered breathing and the occurrence of stroke. Am J Respir Crit Care Med 2005; 172(11):1447–1451.
31. Yaggi HK, Concato J, Kernan WN, et al. Obstructive sleep apnea as a risk factor for stroke and death. N Engl J Med 2005; 353(19):2034–2041.
32. Munoz R, Duran-Cantolla J, Martinez-Vila E, et al. Severe sleep apnea and risk of ischemic stroke in the elderly. Stroke 2006; 37(9):2317–2321.
33. Wang H, Parker JD, Newton GE, et al. Influence of obstructive sleep apnea on mortality in patients with heart failure. J Am Coll Cardiol 2007; 49(15):1625–1631.
34. Kaneko Y, Floras JS, Usui K, et al. Cardiovascular effects of continuous positive airway pressure in patients with heart failure and obstructive sleep apnea. N Engl J Med 2003; 348 (13):1233–1241.
35. Mansfield DR, Gollogly NC, Kaye DM, et al. Controlled trial of continuous positive airway pressure in obstructive sleep apnea and heart failure. Am J Respir Crit Care Med 2004; 169 (3):361–366.
36. Gula LJ, Krahn AD, Skanes AC, et al. Clinical relevance of arrhythmias during sleep: guidance for clinicians. Heart 2004; 90(3):347–352.
37. Guilleminault C, Connolly SJ, Winkle RA. Cardiac arrhythmia and conduction disturbances during sleep in 400 patients with sleep apnea syndrome. Am J Cardiol 1983; 52(5):490–494.
38. Quan SF, Gersh BJ. Cardiovascular consequences of sleep-disordered breathing: past, present and future: report of a workshop from the National Center on Sleep Disorders Research and the National Heart, Lung, and Blood Institute. Circulation 2004; 109(8):951–957.
39. Braunwald E. Cardiovascular medicine at the turn of the millennium: triumphs, concerns, and opportunities. N Engl J Med 1997; 337(19):1360–1369.
40. Mehra R, Benjamin EJ, Shahar E, et al. Association of nocturnal arrhythmias with sleep-disordered breathing: the Sleep Heart Health Study. Am J Respir Crit Care Med 2006; 173 (8):910–916.
41. Gami AS, Hodge DO, Herges RM, et al. Obstructive sleep apnea, obesity, and the risk of incident atrial fibrillation. J Am Coll Cardiol 2007; 49(5):565–571.
42. Harbison J, O'Reilly P, McNicholas WT. Cardiac rhythm disturbances in the obstructive sleep apnea syndrome: effects of nasal continuous positive airway pressure therapy. Chest 2000; 118(3):591–595.
43. Kanagala R, Murali NS, Friedman PA, et al. Obstructive sleep apnea and the recurrence of atrial fibrillation. Circulation 2003; 107(20):2589–2594.
44. Ryan CM, Usui K, Floras JS, et al. Effect of continuous positive airway pressure on ventricular ectopy in heart failure patients with obstructive sleep apnoea. Thorax 2005; 60(9):781–785.

45. Somers VK, White DP, Amin R, et al. Sleep apnea and cardiovascular disease: an American Heart Association/American College of Cardiology Foundation Scientific Statement from the American Heart Association Council for High Blood Pressure Research Professional Education Committee, Council on Clinical Cardiology, Stroke Council, and Council on Cardiovascular Nursing. J Am Coll Cardiol 2008; 52(8):686–717.
46. Kump K, Whalen C, Tishler PV, et al. Assessment of the validity and utility of a sleep-symptom questionnaire. Am J Respir Crit Care Med 1994; 150(3):735–741.
47. Redline S, Sanders M. A quagmire for clinicians: when technological advances exceed clinical knowledge. Thorax 1999; 54(6):474–475.
48. Newman AB, Nieto FJ, Guidry U, et al. Relation of sleep-disordered breathing to cardiovascular disease risk factors: the Sleep Heart Health Study. Am J Epidemiol 2001; 154(1):50–59.
49. Bassetti CL, Milanova M, Gugger M. Sleep-disordered breathing and acute ischemic stroke: diagnosis, risk factors, treatment, evolution, and long-term clinical outcome. Stroke 2006; 37 (4):967–972.

11

Treatment of Hypertension in Sleep Apnea

ODED FRIEDMAN and ALEXANDER G. LOGAN
Samuel Lunenfeld Research Institute, Mount Sinai Hospital, Division of Nephrology, Mount Sinai Hospital and University Health Network, and Department of Medicine, University of Toronto, Toronto, Ontario, Canada

I. Introduction

The worldwide prevalence of hypertension in 2000 was 26.4% among adults, on the basis of either blood pressure (BP) $\geq 140/90$ or antihypertensive drug use (1). The prevalence of sleep-related breathing disturbances (SRBD) was 15% and 5% among middle-aged men and women, respectively, using an apnea-hypopnea index (AHI) ≥ 10 events/hr (2). Not surprisingly then, the two conditions overlap. In fact, while the reported prevalence of obstructive sleep apnea (OSA) among hypertensive individuals varies depending on the population studied, it approximates 30% to 40% using the same AHI threshold (3). Much work has sought to determine whether a causal and independent association between OSA and sustained hypertension exists that transcends beyond coincidence and shared epidemiological risk factors. Recent large-scale observational studies, conducted in both general (4–14) and sleep or weight loss clinic (15–19) populations, have attempted to address these issues by either using controls well matched for possible confounders or statistically correcting for confounding. Perhaps the most important potential confounder is obesity, which has typically been matched or adjusted for using such crude indices as body mass index (BMI), waist–hip circumference ratio or neck circumference, or other related measures of central obesity (20,21). These epidemiological studies have been instrumental in suggesting a causal relationship. However, evidence from adequately powered interventional studies demonstrating that abolition of OSA, independent of other attendant hypotensive strategies, results in improved and durable BP control would serve as proof of principle.

II. Review of Literature

At present, the mainstay of therapy in OSA remains the nocturnal application of continuous positive airway pressure (CPAP). Nonetheless, the salutary effects of weight loss on BP and possibly OSA cannot be overstated, and it may be a valuable therapeutic option among motivated patients. Additionally, oral appliance therapy is an alternative treatment for CPAP that may be considered for people who cannot tolerate CPAP therapy. However, the effectiveness of these non-CPAP treatments in lowering BP of hypertensive patients has not been critically evaluated in randomized controlled trials.

CPAP acts as a pneumatic splint and thus would be expected to eliminate recurrent upper airway obstruction and its associated acute downstream effects. CPAP per se does not appear to have a BP-lowering effect independent of the eradication of OSA nor does it seem to have a significant pressor effect related to its use. This stems from an interventional study of nightly CPAP use for three weeks by middle-aged men with untreated hypertension that demonstrated a significant reduction of nighttime BP and a similar trend in daytime BP among those with occult SRBD (AHI $\geq$ 5 threshold), but not in nonapneic subjects, adjusted for age and BMI (22). Unfortunately, the existing literature on CPAP therapy in hypertension has many limitations. First, the majority of studies involved small numbers of subjects, usually less than 50. Second, subjects with normotension, prehypertension, and hypertension were often lumped together as were those with variable duration and severity of OSA. Third, the duration of CPAP treatment and follow-up differed but was typically less than three to six months. Fourth, few studies included a control arm such as an oral placebo, subtherapeutic or sham CPAP, or supplemental oxygen. Fifth, concomitant antihypertensive drug and lifestyle changes were often poorly described with antihypertensive drug use varying between studies. Sixth, BP responses were not uniformly determined on the basis of 24-hour ambulatory BP monitoring (ABPM) rather than casual BP measurements nor were daytime values consistently reported. Even among controlled studies using 24-hour ABPM, few provided nighttime BP results, which, along with a nondipping pattern during sleep, have prognostic significance, independent of 24-hour BP (23–26).

Overall, uncontrolled short-term studies have revealed reductions in daytime and nighttime BP readings along with conversion from nondipper to dipper status among normotensive and hypertensive subjects with CPAP therapy applied both acutely and over periods of days to months (27–31). However, such findings were not consistently identified in a few similar studies (32,33). Likewise, short-term analyses of BP responses in patients with drug-resistant or refractory hypertension have demonstrated significant decreases in daytime, nighttime, and 24-hour BP recordings as well as nondipping (34,35). In parallel, uncontrolled long-term studies have shown reductions in 24-hour and daytime BP values following CPAP application over a span of six to thirty six months, particularly among those with hypertension (36–40). Effects on BP have been comparable in response to oral appliance therapy (41,42).

At least three meta-analyses of randomized controlled trials that addressed the impact of CPAP treatment on BP endpoints were published in 2007. The largest identified 16 studies, up to July 2006, that involved at least two weeks (range 2–24 weeks) of therapeutic CPAP (43). Although the trials proved not to be significantly heterogeneous, important differences nonetheless existed. The control arms entailed sham CPAP in eight studies, oral placebo in four studies, and usual care in the remaining four studies; nine of the trials used a parallel design, whereas seven used a crossover design. Of note, sham CPAP, possibly by disturbing sleep, may not be entirely BP neutral as evident in one study that observed a significant increase in nocturnal systolic BP (44,45); however, this effect has not been uniformly demonstrated as has already been mentioned (22). ABPM was utilized in 11 of the studies, with manual recordings employed in the remainder; hypertensive subjects were specifically recruited in 2 trials and excluded in 3 trials. Overall then, data from 818 subjects were analyzed. Baseline characteristics of these subjects were as follows: mean age 51.3 years, 86.3% male, mean AHI 36.2 events/hr, mean BMI 31.7 kg/m², and mean BP 130.9/80.1 mmHg. Of the 15 studies specifically reporting systolic and diastolic BP, the pooled (weighted) reduction in BP with CPAP was significant at 2.46/1.83 mmHg; likewise, of the 7 studies specifically reporting mean BP, the pooled (weighted) reduction in BP with CPAP was 2.22 mmHg. These findings were not significantly different following exclusion of the 2 trials that enrolled patients with comorbid heart failure (46,47) in a sensitivity analysis. In teasing out data from the studies that used ABPM, it remains unclear which specific BP values (daytime, nighttime, 24-hour) from each were analyzed. However, there were no differences in BP reductions with CPAP between day and night using figures from the trials that specifically reported daytime and/or nighttime BP. Planned subgroup analyses demonstrated an increased likelihood of a BP fall in those with a BMI $\geq$ 31.4 kg/m² or baseline BP $\geq$ 129.6/79.9 mmHg. A tendency for systolic BP decline to correlate with nightly CPAP use was also identified (43).

A second meta-analysis identified 10 studies with 587 participants, again up to July 2006, that involved therapeutic CPAP; 9 studies were identical to those in the largest meta-analysis, and 2 studies involved the same patient population (48). Findings included a trend for a BP reduction of 1.38/1.52 mmHg with CPAP; post hoc analyses revealed trends for an association between systolic BP decline and CPAP compliance as well as for a greater BP fall in the trials involving more severe OSA (AHI > 30) (48). The third meta-analysis identified 12 studies with 572 subjects, up to August 2006, that involved therapeutic CPAP and utilized ABPM with an endpoint of 24-hour mean BP; 9 studies were identical to those in the largest meta-analysis (49). Trials that included patients with comorbidities other than hypertension, including heart failure, were excluded from analysis. Significant BP reductions with CPAP were as follows: 1.69 mmHg (24-hr mean), 1.77/1.79 mmHg (24-hr systolic/diastolic), 1.76 mmHg (daytime), and 2.25/2.87 mmHg (daytime systolic/diastolic). Predefined metaregression revealed falls of 24-hour mean BP by 0.89 mmHg per 10 event/hr increment in AHI and 1.38 mmHg per 1 hr/night increment in CPAP use (49). Table 1 (pp. 184 & 185) summarizes the individual data from each of the 19 studies that were included in the above-mentioned meta-analyses and that involved therapeutic CPAP for at least two weeks [one study was therefore not incorporated as it drew its findings from only one week of CPAP use (50)]. Data from three randomized controlled trials published since the meta-analyses were added (51–53).

Although predictors of a CPAP-induced depressor response, such as those already cited, have not been unanimously agreed upon across all studies, a consensus tends to exist in some instances. First, observed BP reductions seem to be associated with OSA severity as determined objectively (e.g., AHI or the desaturation index) (48,49,54,55) or subjectively (e.g., Epworth Sleepiness Scale) (55–58). Second, the observed hypotensive effect seems to relate to the presence of hypertension (39) and/or more difficult-to-control hypertension as indicated by a higher baseline BP (40,43,59,60) or a requirement for antihypertensive drug(s) (55), perhaps suggesting a greater influence of OSA in the latter cases in mediating sustained BP elevation. Third, increased compliance, a significant hurdle with CPAP therapy (61), is strongly coupled with the observed BP fall (27,39,40,43,48,49,52,54); in fact, in one of the controlled trials included in the meta-analyses, no BP reduction was noted despite a fall in AHI of 50% with sham CPAP, unlike therapeutic CPAP, which resulted in a fall in AHI of 95% (62). Given the association between adherence and OSA severity (AHI) (63,64) or symptoms (Epworth Sleepiness Scale) (65,58), it may be difficult, however, to determine the precise independent contributions of either in predicting BP response (49,56,57). Further, the existing literature may be underpowered to detect a significant, albeit attenuated, hypotensive effect of CPAP treatment in those with milder disease.

Despite the utility of ABPM, discontinuous measurements (even with 15- to 30-minute intervals) fail to capture the effect CPAP therapy bears on nightly BP variability as manifested by recurrent surges in BP (66). Although short lived, such fluctuations occur incessantly night after night and likely bear prognostic significance (67). Of course, it may be that some of the OSA-induced mechanisms that continue to perpetuate sustained hypertension, such as vascular remodeling, may be only partially reversed with CPAP (68). If true, one would predict a differential antihypertensive response according to the duration of hypertension among sleep apneics. Moreover, there may be a salutary role of CPAP in preventing death and cardiovascular disease in subjects with OSA that goes beyond any BP effects as determined peripherally (69); not surprisingly, there are no longitudinal, randomized interventional studies in this regard.

Reversal of the purported mechanisms linking OSA to hypertension has been demonstrated in many, but not all, studies. These mechanistic studies, however, often suffer from the same limitations inherent in the clinical trial arena. For example, the great majority of the effects of CPAP on neurohormones and vascular function have been short term with long-term observations therefore relying on animal models; further, such effects are typically not reported in a comparator control group. Without question, the greatest representation of data stems from work examining the sympathetic nervous system in which improvements in baroreflex sensitivity (70–73) and chemoreflex control (74), along with reductions in plasma and urine norepinephrine levels (29,75–78) and muscle sympathetic nerve activity (79–82), have been shown, especially among hypertensive individuals (83). Many other potential and disturbed pathways that have been implicated in mediating hypertension display a return toward normal with CPAP therapy including endothelial dysfunction (decreased nitric oxide [73,84–86] and therefore endothelium-dependent vasorelaxation [82,86,87]), systemic and vascular inflammation (88), elevated endothelin-1 (89) or endothelin-1 precursor (90) levels, increased arterial stiffness (91), insulin resistance particularly in nonobese subjects (65,92,93), amplified oxidative stress (94,95), increased endogenous digitalis-like factor levels (96), elevated erythropoietin levels (97,98), and activation of the renin-angiotensin-aldosterone system (108,109).

Whether specific antihypertensive drug classes exert variable and unique hypotensive effects in hypertensive subjects with OSA (despite persistence of repetitive apnea, hypopnea, and arousal) remains unanswered as studies conducted thus far failed to include a matched control group without OSA. In addition, although biologically plausible, whether a greater BP reduction in hypertensive subjects with OSA follows an equivalent weight loss, secondary to attendant diminution of OSA severity, compared to matched non-OSA subjects is unproven. Finally, there is limited information on the effects of antihypertensive medications on sleep stages and the severity of OSA in hypertensive patients with OSA.

Table 1 Randomized Controlled Trials Involving Therapeutic CPAP for Duration of Two Weeks or More

Primary author's name	Engleman HM(99)	Barbe F (56)	Faccenda JF(54)	Monasterio C(100)	Barnes M(101)	Pepperell JC(55)	Becker HF(62)	Kaneko Y[a](46)	Barnes M(102)	Coughlin SR(103)
Year	1996	2001	2001	2001	2002	2002	2003	2003	2004	2004
Source of publication	Sleep	Ann Int Med	Am J Resp Crit Care Med	Am J Resp Crit Care Med	Am J Resp Crit Care Med	Lancet	Circu- lation	N Engl J Med	Am J Resp Crit Care Med	ATS Conference Abstract
Country of origin	United Kingdom	Spain	United Kingdom	Spain	Australia	United Kingdom	Germany	Canada	Australia	United Kingdom
Sample size	13	54	68	125	28	95	32	24	89	25
Study design	Crossover	Parallel	Crossover	Parallel	Crossover	Parallel	Parallel	Parallel	Crossover	Crossover
Type of control	Pil	Sham CPAP	Pil	Usual care	Pil	Sham CPAP	Sham CPAP	Usual care	Pil	Sham CPAP
Mean AHI (events/hr)	49	55.4	35	20.5	12.9	–	63.8	41.2	21.3	–
Mean age (years)	51	53	50	53.5	45.5	50.6	53.4	55.6	47	–
Male (%)	84.6	90.7	80.9	85.7	85.7	100	90.6	87.5	79.8	–
Mean BMI (kg/m^2)	36	29	30	29.4	30.9	35	33.4	31.4	31.1	–
Mean ESS	–	7	15	12.6	11.2	16.2	14.2	6.2	10.7	–
Mean baseline sBP/dBP (mmHg)	–	124.6/ 78.1	–	128.8/ 82.4	130.3/ 81.6	133.7/ 85.1	136.1/ 82.3	127.0/ 61.0	126.5/ 76.3	–
Hypertensive (%)	31	30	0	–	25	10	66	50	15	–
Method of BP measurement	Ambul- atory	Ambu- latory	Ambu- latory	Manual	Ambu- latory	Ambu- latory	Ambu- latory	Manual	Ambu- latory	Ambu- latory
CPAP duration (weeks)	3	6	4	24	8	4	9	4	12	6
Mean nightly CPAP use (hours)	4.3	5	3.3	4.8	3	4.5	5.5	6.2	3.3	–
Mean CPAP pressure (cm H$_2$O)	–	8	–	7	–	9.8	9.1	8.9	–	–
Mean net sBP/dBP &/or mBP change (mmHg)[c]	−1.0//−2.0 & −1.0	−2.0// −1.0, −3.0// −1.0 (24-hour)	−1.3// −1.5 & −1.0	−2.0// −1.0	+0.5// −0.9 (24-hour)	−4.2, −3.4// −3.3 & −3.3 (24-hour)	−10.3//− 11.2 & −11.3, −10.6// −11.3 & −10.5 (24-hour)	−16.0// −1.0	−0.9// −0.6 (24-hour)	−6.0// −5.2 (24-hour)

[a]Study included patients with comorbid heart failure.
[b]Study also included a control arm of supplemental oxygen in 13 subjects (data not shown).
[c]Daytime BP change unless otherwise indicated.
Abbreviations: CPAP, continuous positive airway pressure; AHI, apnea-hypopnea index; ESS, Epworth Sleepiness Scale; sBP, systolic blood pressure; dBP, diastolic blood pressure; mBP, mean blood pressure.

Ip MS(87)	Mansfield DR[a](47)	Arias MA(104)	Campos-Rodriguez F(105)	Mills PJ(78)	Robinson GV(57)	Usui K[a](106)	Norman D(45)	Arias MA(107)	Coughlin SR(52)	Hui DS(51)	Kohler M(53)
2004	2004	2005	2006	2006	2006	2005	2006	2006	2007	2006	2008
Am J Resp Crit Care Med	Am J Resp Crit Care Med	Circulation	Chest	J Appl Physiol	Eur Resp J	J Am Col Cardiol	Hypertension	Eur Heart J	Eur Resp J	Thorax	Eur Resp J
Hong Kong	Australia	Spain	Spain	USA	United Kingdom	Canada	USA	Spain	United Kingdom	Hong Kong	United Kingdom
27	40	25	68	33	32	17	33[b]	21	34	56	102
Parallel	Parallel	Crossover	Parallel	Parallel	Crossover	Parallel	Parallel	Crossover	Crossover	Parallel	Parallel
Usual care	Usual care	Sham CPAP	Sham CPAP	Sham CPAP	Sham CPAP	Usual care	Sham CPAP	Sham CPAP	Sham CPAP	Sham CPAP	Sham CPAP
46.5	25.8	44.1	58.9	63.1	28.1	40.4	63	44.1	–	31.2	–
42.7	57.6	51	56.7	48.3	54	53.5	50	51	49	50.8	48.4
100	95	96	60.2	84.8	88.5	88	85	96	–	76.8	100
29.4	33.4	30.9	34.8	31.9	33.2	30.6	30.8	30.9	36.1	27.2	35.2
–	9.1	–	14.3	–	5.3	–	12	–	13.8	11.1	15.5
122.5/	–	122.2/	131.2/	152.2/	143.0/	138.2/	129.4/	127.0/	–	123.7/	138.7/
75.6		76.4	78.0	83.4	86.7	68.6	77.8	79.0		80.9	91.1
0	–	0	100	36	75	47	–	0	27	50	23.6
Manual	Manual	Ambulatory	Ambulatory	Manual	Ambulatory	Manual	Ambulatory	Ambulatory	Ambulatory	Ambulatory	Ambulatory
4	12	12	4	2	4	4	2	12	6	12	4
4.2	5.6	6	5	4.7	4.8	6	6.7	6.2	3.9	5.1	4.3
–	8.8	10	9.5	–	–	7.5	–	10	10	10.7	–
−0.3// −8.9	7	0//0	0.9// −0.7 & −0.8 (24-hour)	−8.0// −4.0	+0.7, +0.4// −1.2 & −0.8 (24-hour)	−19.9// −8.5	−7.0 (24-hour)	−1.0//0	−6.7// −4.9 & −5.5	−2.5// −1.8 & −2.2, −0.4// −3.5 & −3.8 (24-hour)	5.6// −4.7 & −5.2, −3.4//−3.2 & −3.2 (24-hour)

III. Conclusions

Epidemiological evidence in support of a causal and independent association between OSA and chronic hypertension is robust. Despite flaws in the existing literature and in accordance with such data, CPAP therapy has been demonstrated, particularly in short-term studies, to effectively and significantly reduce BP among subjects with OSA. Observed falls in BP have been most pronounced among more severe sleep apneics, hypertensives (especially if uncontrolled), and more adherent patients. Such clinical work has also been mirrored in the laboratory with reports that indicate a reversal, following CPAP application, of many of the alleged disturbances that result in hypertension.

References

1. Kearney PM, Whelton M, Reynolds K, et al. Global burden of hypertension: analysis of worldwide data. Lancet 2005; 365(9455):217–223.
2. Young T, Palta M, Dempsey J, et al. The occurrence of sleep-disordered breathing among middle-aged adults. N Engl J Med 1993; 328(17):1230–1235.
3. Baguet JP, Narkiewicz K, Mallion JM. Update on hypertension management: obstructive sleep apnea and hypertension. J Hypertens 2006; 24(1): 205–208.
4. Hla KM, Young TB, Bidwell T, et al. Sleep apnea and hypertension. A population-based study. Ann Intern Med 1994;120(5):382–388.
5. Worsnop CJ, Naughton MT, Barter CE, et al. The prevalence of obstructive sleep apnea in hypertensives. Am J Respir Crit Care Med 1998; 157(1):111–115.
6. Bixler EO, Vgontzas AN, Lin HM, et al. Association of hypertension and sleep-disordered breathing. Arch Intern Med 2000; 160(15):2289–2295.
7. Nieto FJ, Young TB, Lind BK, et al. Association of sleep-disordered breathing, sleep apnea, and hypertension in a large community-based study. Sleep Heart Health Study. JAMA 2000; 283(14):1829–1836.
8. Ohayon MM, Guilleminault C, Priest RG, et al. Is sleep-disordered breathing an independent risk factor for hypertension in the general population (13,057 subjects)? J Psychosom Res 2000; 48(6):593–601.
9. Peppard PE, Young T, Palta M, et al. Prospective study of the association between sleep-disordered breathing and hypertension. N Engl J Med 2000; 342(19):1378–1384.
10. Duran J, Esnaola S, Rubio R, et al. Obstructive sleep apnea-hypopnea and related clinical features in a population-based sample of subjects aged 30 to 70 yr. Am J Respir Crit Care Med 2001; 163(3 pt 1):685–689.
11. Wright JT Jr., Redline S, Taylor AL, et al. Relationship between 24-H blood pressure and sleep disordered breathing in a normotensive community sample. Am J Hypertens 2001; 14 (8 pt 1):743–748.
12. Sjostrom C, Lindberg E, Elmasry A, et al. Prevalence of sleep apnoea and snoring in hypertensive men: a population based study. Thorax 2002; 57(7):602–607.
13. Tanigawa T, Tachibana N, Yamagishi K, et al. Relationship between sleep-disordered breathing and blood pressure levels in community-based samples of Japanese men. Hypertens Res 2004; 27(7):479–484.
14. Hedner J, Bengtsson-Bostrom K, Peker Y, et al. Hypertension prevalence in obstructive sleep apnoea and sex: a population-based case-control study. Eur Respir J 2006; 27(3): 564–570.
15. Kiselak J, Clark M, Pera V, et al. The association between hypertension and sleep apnea in obese patients. Chest 1993; 104(3):775–780.

16. Carlson JT, Hedner JA, Ejnell H, et al. High prevalence of hypertension in sleep apnea patients independent of obesity. Am J Respir Crit Care Med 1994; 150(1):72–77.
17. Grote L, Ploch T, Heitmann J, et al. Sleep-related breathing disorder is an independent risk factor for systemic hypertension. Am J Respir Crit Care Med 1999; 160(6):1875–1882.
18. Lavie P, Herer P, Hoffstein V. Obstructive sleep apnoea syndrome as a risk factor for hypertension: population study. BMJ 2000; 320(7233):479–482.
19. Kraiczi H, Peker Y, Caidahl K, et al. Blood pressure, cardiac structure and severity of obstructive sleep apnea in a sleep clinic population. J Hypertens 2001; 19(11):2071–2078.
20. Grunstein R, Wilcox I, Yang TS, et al. Snoring and sleep apnoea in men: association with central obesity and hypertension. Int J Obes Relat Metab Disord 1993; 17(9):533–540.
21. Vgontzas AN, Papanicolaou DA, Bixler EO, et al. Sleep apnea and daytime sleepiness and fatigue: relation to visceral obesity, insulin resistance, and hypercytokinemia. J Clin Endocrinol Metab 2000; 85(3):1151–1158.
22. Hla KM, Skatrud JB, Finn L, et al. The effect of correction of sleep-disordered breathing on BP in untreated hypertension. Chest 2002; 122(4):1125–1132.
23. Verdecchia P. Prognostic value of ambulatory blood pressure: current evidence and clinical implications. Hypertension 2000; 35(3):844–851.
24. Ohkubo T, Hozawa A, Yamaguchi J, et al. Prognostic significance of the nocturnal decline in blood pressure in individuals with and without high 24-h blood pressure: the Ohasama study. J Hypertens 2002; 20(11):2183–2189.
25. Fagard RH, Van Den Broeke C, De Cort P. Prognostic significance of blood pressure measured in the office, at home and during ambulatory monitoring in older patients in general practice. J Hum Hypertens 2005; 19(10):801–807.
26. Fagard RH, Celis H, Thijs L, et al. Daytime and nighttime blood pressure as predictors of death and cause-specific cardiovascular events in hypertension. Hypertension 2008; 51(1): 55–61.
27. Wilcox I, Grunstein RR, Hedner JA, et al. Effect of nasal continuous positive airway pressure during sleep on 24-hour blood pressure in obstructive sleep apnea. Sleep 1993; 16 (6):539–544.
28. Akashiba T, Kurashina K, Minemura H, et al. Daytime hypertension and the effects of short-term nasal continuous positive airway pressure treatment in obstructive sleep apnea syndrome. Intern Med 1995; 34(6):528–532.
29. Minemura H, Akashiba T, Yamamoto H, et al. Acute effects of nasal continuous positive airway pressure on 24-hour blood pressure and catecholamines in patients with obstructive sleep apnea. Intern Med 1998; 37(12):1009–1013.
30. Akashiba T, Minemura H, Yamamoto H, et al. Nasal continuous positive airway pressure changes blood pressure "non-dippers" to "dippers" in patients with obstructive sleep apnea. Sleep 1999; 22(7):849–853.
31. Voogel AJ, van Steenwijk RP, Karemaker JM, et al. Effects of treatment of obstructive sleep apnea on circadian hemodynamics. J Auton Nerv Syst 1999; 77(2–3):177–183.
32. Hermida RC, Zamarron C, Ayala DE, et al. Effect of continuous positive airway pressure on ambulatory blood pressure in patients with obstructive sleep apnoea. Blood Press Monit 2004; 9(4):193–202.
33. Dursunoglu N, Dursunoglu D, Cuhadaroglu C, et al. Acute effects of automated continuous positive airway pressure on blood pressure in patients with sleep apnea and hypertension. Respiration 2005; 72(2):150–155.
34. Logan AG, Tkacova R, Perlikowski SM, et al. Refractory hypertension and sleep apnoea: effect of CPAP on blood pressure and baroreflex. Eur Respir J 2003; 21(2):241–247.
35. Martinez-Garcia MA, Gomez-Aldaravi R, Soler-Cataluna JJ, et al. Positive effect of CPAP treatment on the control of difficult-to-treat hypertension. Eur Respir J 2007; 29(5): 951–957.

36. Mayer J, Becker H, Brandenburg U, et al. Blood pressure and sleep apnea: results of long-term nasal continuous positive airway pressure therapy. Cardiology 1991; 79(2):84–92.

37. Sanner BM, Tepel M, Markmann A, et al. Effect of continuous positive airway pressure therapy on 24-hour blood pressure in patients with obstructive sleep apnea syndrome. Am J Hypertens 2002; 15(3):251–257.

38. Dhillon S, Chung SA, Fargher T, et al. Sleep apnea, hypertension, and the effects of continuous positive airway pressure. Am J Hypertens 2005; 18(5 pt 1):594–600.

39. Chin K, Nakamura T, Takahashi K, et al. Falls in blood pressure in patients with obstructive sleep apnoea after long-term nasal continuous positive airway pressure treatment. J Hypertens 2006; 24(10):2091–2099.

40. Campos-Rodriguez F, Perez-Ronchel J, Grilo-Reina A, et al. Long-term effect of continuous positive airway pressure on BP in patients with hypertension and sleep apnea. Chest 2007; 132(6):1847–1852.

41. Otsuka R, Ribeiro de Almeida F, Lowe AA, et al. The effect of oral appliance therapy on blood pressure in patients with obstructive sleep apnea. Sleep Breath 2006; 10(1):29–36.

42. Yoshida K. Effect on blood pressure of oral appliance therapy for sleep apnea syndrome. Int J Prosthodont 2006; 19(1):61–66.

43. Bazzano LA, Khan Z, Reynolds K, et al. Effect of nocturnal nasal continuous positive airway pressure on blood pressure in obstructive sleep apnea. Hypertension 2007; 50(2): 417–423.

44. Kuniyoshi FH, Somers VK. Sleep apnea in hypertension: when, how, and why should we treat? Hypertension 2006; 47(5):818–819.

45. Norman D, Loredo JS, Nelesen RA, et al. Effects of continuous positive airway pressure versus supplemental oxygen on 24-hour ambulatory blood pressure. Hypertension 2006; 47 (5):840–845.

46. Kaneko Y, Floras JS, Usui K, et al. Cardiovascular effects of continuous positive airway pressure in patients with heart failure and obstructive sleep apnea. N Engl J Med 2003; 348 (13):1233–1241.

47. Mansfield DR, Gollogly NC, Kaye DM, et al. Controlled trial of continuous positive airway pressure in obstructive sleep apnea and heart failure. Am J Respir Crit Care Med 2004; 169 (3):361–366.

48. Alajmi M, Mulgrew AT, Fox J, et al. Impact of continuous positive airway pressure therapy on blood pressure in patients with obstructive sleep apnea hypopnea: a meta-analysis of randomized controlled trials. Lung 2007; 185(2):67–72.

49. Haentjens P, Van Meerhaeghe A, Moscariello A, et al. The impact of continuous positive airway pressure on blood pressure in patients with obstructive sleep apnea syndrome: evidence from a meta-analysis of placebo-controlled randomized trials. Arch Intern Med 2007; 167(8):757–764.

50. Dimsdale JE, Loredo JS, Profant J. Effect of continuous positive airway pressure on blood pressure: a placebo trial. Hypertension 2000; 35(1 pt 1):144–147.

51. Hui DS, To KW, Ko FW, et al. Nasal CPAP reduces systemic blood pressure in patients with obstructive sleep apnoea and mild sleepiness. Thorax 2006; 61(12):1083–1090.

52. Coughlin SR, Mawdsley L, Mugarza JA, et al. Cardiovascular and metabolic effects of CPAP in obese males with OSA. Eur Respir J 2007; 29(4):720–727.

53. Kohler M, Pepperell JC, Casadei B, et al. CPAP and measures of cardiovascular risk in males with OSAS. Eur Respir J 2008; 32(6):1488–1496.

54. Faccenda JF, Mackay TW, Boon NA, et al. Randomized placebo-controlled trial of continuous positive airway pressure on blood pressure in the sleep apnea-hypopnea syndrome. Am J Respir Crit Care Med 2001; 163(2):344–348.

55. Pepperell JC, Ramdassingh-Dow S, Crosthwaite N, et al. Ambulatory blood pressure after therapeutic and subtherapeutic nasal continuous positive airway pressure for obstructive sleep apnoea: a randomised parallel trial. Lancet 2002; 359(9302):204–210.

56. Barbe F, Mayoralas LR, Duran J, et al. Treatment with continuous positive airway pressure is not effective in patients with sleep apnea but no daytime sleepiness. a randomized, controlled trial. Ann Intern Med 2001; 134(11):1015–1023.

57. Robinson GV, Smith DM, Langford BA, et al. Continuous positive airway pressure does not reduce blood pressure in nonsleepy hypertensive OSA patients. Eur Respir J 2006; 27(6): 1229–1235.

58. Montserrat JM, Garcia-Rio F, Barbe F. Diagnostic and therapeutic approach to nonsleepy apnea. Am J Respir Crit Care Med 2007; 176(1):6–9.

59. Borgel J, Sanner BM, Keskin F, et al. Obstructive sleep apnea and blood pressure. Interaction between the blood pressure-lowering effects of positive airway pressure therapy and antihypertensive drugs. Am J Hypertens 2004; 17(12 pt 1):1081–1087.

60. Malik J, Drake CL, Hudgel DW. Variables affecting the change in systemic blood pressure in response to nasal CPAP in obstructive sleep apnea patients. Sleep Breath 2008; 12(1): 47–52.

61. Malhotra A, Ayas NT, Epstein LJ. The art and science of continuous positive airway pressure therapy in obstructive sleep apnea. Curr Opin Pulm Med 2000; 6(6):490–495.

62. Becker HF, Jerrentrup A, Ploch T, et al. Effect of nasal continuous positive airway pressure treatment on blood pressure in patients with obstructive sleep apnea. Circulation 2003; 107 (1):68–73.

63. McArdle N, Devereux G, Heidarnejad H, et al. Long-term use of CPAP therapy for sleep apnea/hypopnea syndrome. Am J Respir Crit Care Med 1999; 159(4 pt 1):1108–1114.

64. Hui DS, Choy DK, Li TS, et al. Determinants of continuous positive airway pressure compliance in a group of Chinese patients with obstructive sleep apnea. Chest 2001; 120 (1):170–176.

65. Lindberg E, Berne C, Elmasry A, et al. CPAP treatment of a population-based sample— what are the benefits and the treatment compliance? Sleep Med 2006; 7(7):553–560.

66. Marrone O, Romano S, Insalaco G, et al. Influence of sampling interval on the evaluation of nocturnal blood pressure in subjects with and without obstructive sleep apnoea. Eur Respir J 2000; 16(4):653–658.

67. Frattola A, Parati G, Cuspidi C, et al. Prognostic value of 24-hour blood pressure variability. J Hypertens 1993; 11(10):1133–1137.

68. Sharabi Y, Rabin K, Grossman E. Sleep apnea-induced hypertension: mechanisms of vascular changes. Expert Rev Cardiovasc Ther 2005; 3(5):937–940.

69. Phillips CL, Yee B, Yang Q, et al. Effects of continuous positive airway pressure treatment and withdrawal in patients with obstructive sleep apnea on arterial stiffness and central BP. Chest 2008; 134(1):94–100.

70. Bonsignore MR, Parati G, Insalaco G, et al. Continuous positive airway pressure treatment improves baroreflex control of heart rate during sleep in severe obstructive sleep apnea syndrome. Am J Respir Crit Care Med 2002; 166(3):279–286.

71. Ito R, Hamada H, Yokoyama A, et al. Successful treatment of obstructive sleep apnea syndrome improves autonomic nervous system dysfunction. Clin Exp Hypertens 2005; 27 (2–3):259–267.

72. Bonsignore MR, Parati G, Insalaco G, et al. Baroreflex control of heart rate during sleep in severe obstructive sleep apnoea: effects of acute CPAP. Eur Respir J 2006; 27(1):128–135.

73. Noda A, Nakata S, Koike Y, et al. Continuous positive airway pressure improves daytime baroreflex sensitivity and nitric oxide production in patients with moderate to severe obstructive sleep apnea syndrome. Hypertens Res 2007; 30(8):669–676.

74. Imadojemu VA, Mawji Z, Kunselman A, et al. Sympathetic chemoreflex responses in obstructive sleep apnea and effects of continuous positive airway pressure therapy. Chest 2007; 131(5):1406–1413.

75. Baruzzi A, Riva R, Cirignotta F, et al. Atrial natriuretic peptide and catecholamines in obstructive sleep apnea syndrome. Sleep 1991; 14(1):83–86.

76. Hedner J, Darpo B, Ejnell H, et al. Reduction in sympathetic activity after long-term CPAP treatment in sleep apnoea: cardiovascular implications. Eur Respir J 1995; 8(2):222–229.

77. Sukegawa M, Noda A, Sugiura T, et al. Assessment of continuous positive airway pressure treatment in obstructive sleep apnea syndrome using 24-hour urinary catecholamines. Clin Cardiol 2005; 28(11):519–522.

78. Mills PJ, Kennedy BP, Loredo JS, et al. Effects of nasal continuous positive airway pressure and oxygen supplementation on norepinephrine kinetics and cardiovascular responses in obstructive sleep apnea. J Appl Physiol 2006; 100(1):343–348.

79. Somers VK, Dyken ME, Clary MP, et al. Sympathetic neural mechanisms in obstructive sleep apnea. J Clin Invest 1995; 96(4):1897–1904.

80. Waradekar NV, Sinoway LI, Zwillich CW, et al. Influence of treatment on muscle sympathetic nerve activity in sleep apnea. Am J Respir Crit Care Med 1996; 153(4 Pt 1): 1333–1338.

81. Narkiewicz K, Kato M, Phillips BG, et al. Nocturnal continuous positive airway pressure decreases daytime sympathetic traffic in obstructive sleep apnea. Circulation 1999; 100 (23):2332–2335.

82. Imadojemu VA, Gleeson K, Quraishi SA, et al. Impaired vasodilator responses in obstructive sleep apnea are improved with continuous positive airway pressure therapy. Am J Respir Crit Care Med 2002; 165(7):950–953.

83. Heitmann J, Ehlenz K, Penzel T, et al. Sympathetic activity is reduced by nCPAP in hypertensive obstructive sleep apnoea patients. Eur Respir J 2004; 23(2):255–262.

84. Ip MS, Lam B, Chan LY, et al. Circulating nitric oxide is suppressed in obstructive sleep apnea and is reversed by nasal continuous positive airway pressure. Am J Respir Crit Care Med 2000; 162(6):2166–2171.

85. Schulz R, Schmidt D, Blum A, et al. Decreased plasma levels of nitric oxide derivatives in obstructive sleep apnoea: response to CPAP therapy. Thorax 2000; 55(12):1046–1051.

86. Ohike Y, Kozaki K, Iijima K, et al. Amelioration of vascular endothelial dysfunction in obstructive sleep apnea syndrome by nasal continuous positive airway pressure—possible involvement of nitric oxide and asymmetric NG, NG-dimethylarginine. Circ J 2005; 69(2): 221–226.

87. Ip MS, Tse HF, Lam B, et al. Endothelial function in obstructive sleep apnea and response to treatment. Am J Respir Crit Care Med 2004; 169(3):348–353.

88. Ohga E, Tomita T, Wada H, et al. Effects of obstructive sleep apnea on circulating ICAM-1, IL-8, and MCP-1. J Appl Physiol 2003; 94(1):179–184.

89. Phillips BG, Narkiewicz K, Pesek CA, et al. Effects of obstructive sleep apnea on endothelin-1 and blood pressure. J Hypertens 1999; 17(1):61–66.

90. Jordan W, Reinbacher A, Cohrs S, et al. Obstructive sleep apnea: plasma endothelin-1 precursor but not endothelin-1 levels are elevated and decline with nasal continuous positive airway pressure. Peptides 2005; 26(9):1654–1660.

91. Kitahara Y, Hattori N, Yokoyama A, et al. Effect of CPAP on brachial-ankle pulse wave velocity in patients with OSAHS: an open-labelled study. Respir Med 2006; 100(12): 2160–2169.

92. Brooks B, Cistulli PA, Borkman M, et al. Obstructive sleep apnea in obese noninsulin-dependent diabetic patients: effect of continuous positive airway pressure treatment on insulin responsiveness. J Clin Endocrinol Metab 1994; 79(6):1681–1685.

93. Harsch IA, Schahin SP, Radespiel-Troger M, et al. Continuous positive airway pressure treatment rapidly improves insulin sensitivity in patients with obstructive sleep apnea syndrome. Am J Respir Crit Care Med 2004; 169(2):156–162.

94. Barcelo A, Barbe F, de la Pena M, et al. Antioxidant status in patients with sleep apnoea and impact of continuous positive airway pressure treatment. Eur Respir J 2006; 27(4):756–760.
95. Christou K, Kostikas K, Pastaka C, et al. Nasal continuous positive airway pressure treatment reduces systemic oxidative stress in patients with severe obstructive sleep apnea syndrome. Sleep Med 2009; 10(1):87–94.
96. Ehlenz K, Peter JH, Kaffarnik H, et al. Disturbances in volume regulating hormone system—a key to the pathogenesis of hypertension in obstructive sleep apnea syndrome? Pneumologie 1991; 45(suppl 1):239–245.
97. Cahan C, Decker MJ, Arnold JL, et al. Erythropoietin levels with treatment of obstructive sleep apnea. J Appl Physiol 1995; 79(4):1278–1285.
98. Winnicki M, Shamsuzzaman A, Lanfranchi P, et al. Erythropoietin and obstructive sleep apnea. Am J Hypertens 2004; 17(9):783–786.
99. Engleman HM, Gough K, Martin SE, et al. Ambulatory blood pressure on and off continuous positive airway pressure therapy for the sleep apnea/hypopnea syndrome: effects in "non-dippers". Sleep 1996; 19(5):378–381.
100. Monasterio C, Vidal S, Duran J, et al. Effectiveness of continuous positive airway pressure in mild sleep apnea-hypopnea syndrome. Am J Respir Crit Care Med 2001; 164(6):939–943.
101. Barnes M, Houston D, Worsnop CJ, et al. A randomized controlled trial of continuous positive airway pressure in mild obstructive sleep apnea. Am J Respir Crit Care Med 2002; 165(6):773–780.
102. Barnes M, McEvoy RD, Banks S, et al. Efficacy of positive airway pressure and oral appliance in mild to moderate obstructive sleep apnea. Am J Respir Crit Care Med 2004; 170(6):656–664.
103. Coughlin S, Murgaza J, Mawdsley L, et al. Continuous positive airway pressure treatment reduces the cardiovascular risk factors associated with obstructive sleep apnea [abstract]. In: American Thoracic Society 100th International Conference. Orlando, FL, 2004.
104. Arias MA, Garcia-Rio F, Alonso-Fernandez A, et al. Obstructive sleep apnea syndrome affects left ventricular diastolic function: effects of nasal continuous positive airway pressure in men. Circulation 2005; 112(3):375–383.
105. Campos-Rodriguez F, Grilo-Reina A, Perez-Ronchel J, et al. Effect of continuous positive airway pressure on ambulatory BP in patients with sleep apnea and hypertension: a placebo-controlled trial. Chest 2006; 129(6):1459–1467.
106. Usui K, Bradley TD, Spaak J, et al. Inhibition of awake sympathetic nerve activity of heart failure patients with obstructive sleep apnea by nocturnal continuous positive airway pressure. J Am Coll Cardiol 2005; 45(12):2008–2011.
107. Arias MA, Garcia-Rio F, Alonso-Fernandez A, et al. Pulmonary hypertension in obstructive sleep apnoea: effects of continuous positive airway pressure: a randomized, controlled cross-over study. Eur Heart J 2006; 27(9):1106–1113.
108. Saarelainen S, Hasan J, Siitonen S, et al. Effect of nasal CPAP treatment on plasma volume, aldosterone and 24-h blood pressure in obstructive sleep apnoea. J Sleep Res 1996; 5(3):181–185.
109. Moller DS, Lind P, Strunge B, et al. Abnormal vasoactive hormones and 24-hour blood pressure in obstructive sleep apnea. Am J Hypertens 2003; 16(4):274–280.

12

Sleep Apnea and Cardiac Arrhythmias

RICHARD S. T. LEUNG and CLODAGH M. RYAN
University of Toronto, Toronto, Ontario, Canada

I. Introduction

Obstructive sleep apnea (OSA) is a common condition, being present in approximately 2% to 4% of the general middle-aged population (1). Repetitive collapse of the upper airway during sleep leads to ineffectual respiratory efforts and apnea, and causes abnormalities in sleep architecture and excessive daytime sleepiness. In recent years, there has been mounting evidence that OSA can also lead to serious cardiovascular consequences including hypertension, coronary artery disease, stroke, and congestive heart failure (CHF) (2–6). Central sleep apnea (CSA) differs from OSA in that central apneas are characterized by absent respiratory effort and result from instability in the chemoreflex control of breathing. Although rare in the general population, CSA is very common in the setting of heart failure (HF), being present in 30% to 40% of these patients in the two largest reported series (7,8).

Both OSA and CSA have been associated with cardiac arrhythmias (9–11), a relationship thought to be mediated through a number of potential mechanisms. Cardiac rhythm is dependent on an orderly progression of electrical impulses and activation of ion channels. Disruption in either of these components may cause cardiac arrhythmias. However, the initiation of acquired cardiac arrhythmias is a complex interaction between the cardiac substrate (causing increased susceptibility) and triggering factors (12). An in-depth review of the pathogenesis of cardiac arrhythmias is beyond the scope of this chapter. However, in brief, increases in afterload or preload can cause structural changes to the myocardium through stretch and wall stress, facilitating local noradrenaline release and inhibiting vagal activity, predisposing to myocardial fibrosis. This fibrosis may cause electrical remodeling including ion channel and gap junction remodeling and therefore changes in cardiac repolarization. Other important determinants of arrhythmias include neurohormonal factors such as increased sympathetic tone and alterations to the renin-angiotensin-aldosterone system (RAAS). Neurohormonal factors may cause cardiac remodeling either directly through myocyte hypertrophy or indirectly by causing hemodynamic changes. Changes in cardiac repolarization appear to be as a result of abnormal cycling of intracellular calcium ions and downregulation of potassium channels (13–15).

Sudden cardiac death causes 10% to 20% of all deaths among adults and the commonest underlying cause is fatal cardiac arrhythmia (16). The reported occurrence of an excess of sudden deaths during sleep between midnight and 0600 hours in patients with OSA suggests that OSA may trigger lethal nocturnal ventricular arrhythmias (17).

In patients with HF, up to 50% of deaths are sudden and arrhythmic in origin (18). Although as yet unproven, CSA may hasten the acceleration and progression to death in HF through the initiation of lethal cardiac arrhythmias (11,19,20).

In OSA and CSA, there are both acute and chronic effects that may develop over time and both may predispose to the development of cardiac arrhythmias. However, before delving into the deleterious and potentially pro-arrhythmic pathophysiological consequences of sleep-disordered breathing (SDB), it is worthwhile to review the cardiovascular and autonomic milieu of normal sleep.

II. Cardiovascular and Autonomic Milieu of Normal Sleep

Sleep is most commonly divided into two distinct neurophysiological states: non–rapid eye movement (NREM) sleep, and rapid eye movement (REM) sleep (21). The physiological effects of NREM and REM are very different. In NREM sleep, mental activity is minimal or absent, and the respiratory and cardiovascular systems are controlled mainly by chemical-metabolic factors. In contrast, REM sleep is characterized by central nervous system activation associated with a variety of phasic events that are probably related to dream content (22). NREM and REM sleep do not occur randomly during sleep. Rather, periods of NREM and REM sleep alternate in a predictable cycle, each cycle typically lasting 90 to 100 minutes, and there being three to four such cycles per night.

Adults normally spend 85% of their total sleep time in NREM sleep. With the transition from wakefulness to NREM sleep, withdrawal of the nonchemical "wakefulness drive" to breathe results in a slight but abrupt decrease in minute ventilation and increase in $PaCO_2$ (23,24). Subsequently, there is a further progressive reduction in central respiratory drive leading to decreased minute ventilation that is more pronounced in the deeper sleep stages; $PaCO_2$ increases and PaO_2 decreases incrementally from stages 1 through 4 NREM sleep (24). In the deeper stages of NREM sleep, respiration is almost exclusively under chemoreflex control, resulting in a very stable and regular pattern of breathing (24,25). These changes in respiratory control are accompanied by similar changes in cardiovascular and autonomic regulation. As metabolic rate declines progressively from wakefulness through stages 1 to 4 NREM sleep, parasympathetic nervous system tone increases and sympathetic nervous system activity (SNA), heart rate (HR), blood pressure (BP), stroke volume, cardiac output, and systemic vascular resistance decrease (26–31). As a result, the cardiovascular system is in a state of hemodynamic and autonomic quiescence during which myocardial workload is reduced and cardiac electrical stability is enhanced: myocardial refractory period lengthens (32) and ventricular premature beats (VPBs) occur less frequently (33) despite a slower heart rate.

REM normally comprises about 15% of total sleep time. During REM sleep, breathing becomes more irregular, being less dependent on chemoreflexes and more so on behavioral factors and dream content (24,34). Overall, ventilation decreases and $PaCO_2$ rises, owing to a combination of reduced chemosensitivity and skeletal muscle atonia affecting the nondiaphragmatic respiratory muscles (22,35). HR also becomes more irregular, and there are surges in HR, SNA, and BP linked to phasic REM sleep events (36). However, cardiovascular and autonomic regulation during REM sleep differs from ventilation in that overall BP, HR, and SNA during REM are increased relative to NREM, to levels similar to relaxed wakefulness (27,29) (Fig. 1).

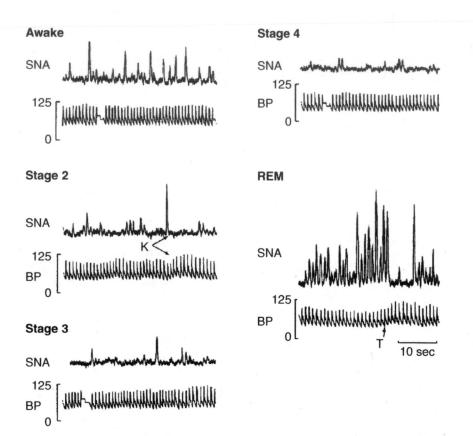

Figure 1 Muscle sympathetic nerve activity measured during wakefulness, stages 2 to 4 NREM sleep and REM sleep. *Abbreviations*: REM, rapid eye movement; NREM, non–rapid eye movement. *Source*: From Ref. 27.

Because the majority of adult sleep time is composed of NREM sleep, sleep is generally a time of cardiovascular relaxation and autonomic quiescence. However, through its acute effects, SDB transforms what is normally a time of enhanced myocardial electrical stability into a milieu in which the heart is under constant strain and arrhythmias provoked rather than protected against. Through the chronic effects of repeated exposure, SDB also has the potential to alter the myocardial substrate, rendering it more susceptible to arrhythmias, during both sleep and wakefulness.

III. Pro-Arrhythmic Effects of SDB: Acute Effects

As a consequence of the repetitive apneas characteristic of OSA and CSA, hemodynamic variables and cardiovascular autonomic activity oscillate between the apneic and ventilatory phases. Surges in HR and BP typically occur five to seven seconds after apnea termination in OSA (37,38), coincident with arousal from sleep, peak ventilation, and the nadir of SaO_2. In CSA, these surges occur not at apnea termination, but during hyperpnea (39). These repetitive surges counteract the usual fall in HR and BP that accompany normal sleep, and there is evidence that the tendency toward cardiac arrhythmias is also accentuated (40,41). Three key pathophyiological features of SDB give rise to these abnormal cardiovascular oscillations: (*i*) hypoxia, (*ii*) arousals from sleep, and (*iii*) generation of negative intrathoracic pressure; in turn, these disturbances give rise to a fourth feature of SDB, i.e., (*iv*) sympathetic activation during sleep.

A. Hypoxia

A hallmark of SDB is recurrent arterial desaturation alternating with normoxia. Hypoxia can reduce myocardial oxygen delivery, directly depress myocardial contractility and increase left ventricular (LV) afterload, and indirectly cause pulmonary vasoconstriction and increase pulmonary arterial pressure (42). Hypoxia can either increase or decrease heart rate dependent on whether parasympathetic or sympathetic influences predominate (43). It is well known that apnea-associated hypoxia can lead to episodes of extreme bradycardia and even heart block (9). Alternatively, the combination of hypoxia and tachycardia further impairs myocardial contractility (42). Hypocapnia, as a result of postapneic hyperventilation, can further exacerbate matters by inducing coronary artery vasoconstriction and a leftward shift of the oxyhemoglobin dissociation curve, reducing oxygen availability to the myocardium (44).

Hypoxia-induced ischemia of myocardial tissue induces electrical, mechanical, and biochemical dysfunction, particularly in those with preexisting cardiac dysfunction. Ischemia-induced activation of nonselective cationic stretch receptors has been demonstrated in animal models to induce arrhythmogenesis (45,46). Ischemia-induced increases in intracellular Ca^{2+} and H^+, accumulation of lipid metabolites, and dephosphorylation of gap junction protein connexin 43 cause electrical uncoupling and trigger arrhythmias (47,48). With these factors in mind, it is unsurprising that severe hypoxia accompanying OSA has been reported to acutely trigger ventricular arrthythmias (49).

B. Arousals

The normal morning transition from sleep to wakefulness is coincident with the highest rates of sudden cardiac death and implanted cardiac defibrillator discharges (50,51). Since arousals from sleep similarly represent sleep-wake transitions with associated cardiac and autonomic effects that can be repeated hundreds of times per night in patients with SDB, the pro-arrhythmic potential of these transient events might be considerable.

Arousals typically accompany each apneic event in both OSA and CSA. In OSA, arousals are critical to the opening of the upper airway and resumption of ventilation; in CSA, they occur after ventilation has resumed and can contribute to ventilatory control instability (22,52,53). Arousals in SDB may contribute to postapneic surges in HR and BP (54–56), sympathetic nervous system activation, and catecholamine release (57,58). Repetitive arousals may contribute to increased oxygen consumption and LV hypertrophy, and promote cardiac remodeling.

C. Negative Intrathoracic Pressure

Futile inspiratory efforts against a closed glottis as occur in OSA result in the generation of negative intrathoracic pressure to as low as -108 mmHg (59). Exaggerated negative intrathoracic pressure of a lesser magnitude is also observed during CSA due to pulmonary congestion and the increased respiratory efforts accompanying hyperpnea. Negative intrathoracic pressure increases venous return to the right heart, leading to distension of the right ventricle and leftward shift of the interventicular septum during diastole (2), which reduces LV preload. Negative intrathoracic pressure also increases LV transmural pressure by increasing the difference between extracardiac and intracardiac pressures (55,60,61). The consequent increase in systolic wall stress increases afterload. In patients with coexistent cardiac disease these effects are magnified (62). The increased mechanical stretch of the myocardium might acutely trigger arrhythmias through mechanoelectrical feedback (63) or predispose to ventricular hypertrophy, itself a predisposing factor for cardiac arrhythmias (14).

D. Increased Sympathetic Activity

Numerous studies have demonstrated enhanced SNA during sleep in patients with OSA compared with controls (64,65), a phenomenon that is attenuated under hyperoxic conditions (66). Elevations in SNA during obstructive apneas are largely responsible for the characteristic surges in HR and BP that typically occur shortly following apnea termination (37,38,65). These repetitive surges in BP oppose the usual fall that accompanies normal sleep and may be responsible in many cases for the phenomenon of "non-dipping" of the nocturnal BP profile (67).

Hypoxia is an obvious candidate for the sympathoexcitation that accompanies OSA. Through stimulation of the peripheral chemoreceptors, sympathetic vasomotor outflow is increased (68). Therefore, despite hypoxia causing vasodilation through local autoregulation, peripheral vasoconstriction actually occurs in most vascular beds (69). The effect of hypoxia on HR is similarly two-pronged. In the absence of the normal ventilatory response to hypoxia, peripheral chemoreceptor stimulation leads to vagally mediated bradycardia (70,71). This response may be relevant to bradycardic episodes during apneas. In contrast, in the presence of the normal ventilatory response to hypoxia, tachycardia is observed, owing to lung inflation reflexes that inhibit cardiac vagal efferents, permitting cardiac sympathetic activity to remain unopposed (72).

While hypoxic stimulation of the peripheral chemoreceptors leads to sympathoexcitation, the act of respiration is itself sympathoinhibitory. The muscle sympathetic nerve activity (MSNA) response to hypoxia is markedly potentiated by the absence of breathing (68). Respiration, while diminishing the sympathetic response to hypoxia, does not eliminate it entirely. Therefore, hypoxia is sympathoexcitatory whether breathing is present or absent, with the magnitude of the effect being greater during apnea. Since patients with HF and CSR display an increased ventilatory response to peripheral chemoreceptor stimulation (73,74), it is possible that they might also have an exaggerated sympathetic response to hypoxia. However, the chemoreflex response to hypoxia cannot be entirely responsible for the acute autonomic effects of sleep apnea, since elimination of hypoxia only modestly dampens the HR and BP oscillations that accompany OSA and CSA (75,76).

The MSNA response to hypoxia and the degree of its inhibition by respiration may be further modified by the level of $PaCO_2$. Hypercapnia itself causes increased ventilation, tachycardia, increased cardiac output, and BP. Sympathetic vasoconstrictor activity is increased, which is opposed by the direct vasodilatory action of CO_2 (77). Indeed, hypercapnia is a more potent stimulus for sympathoexcitation than hypoxia, in the sense that for equivalent increases in minute ventilation, greater MSNA is observed with hypercapnia than hypoxia, and the sympathoinhibitory effect of respiration is less effective (68). This observation suggests that hypoxia and hypercapnia do not cause sympathoexcitation solely through generation of central respiratory drive, but must also be able to influence the vasomotor centers independently. Combined hypoxia and hypercapnia have a synergistic effect on both sympathetic activity and ventilation and result in a more marked rise in BP.

Chemoreceptor reflexes may be of particular importance in the setting of CHF. Patients with CHF and CSA are known to have increased chemoreceptor sensitivity (74,78,79), and an increased sympathetic response to CO_2 has also been observed in CHF (80). Thus, the hyperpneic phase of CSA, which is a manifestation of intense chemostimulation by CO_2, might be expected to exert considerable sympathoexcitatory effects.

IV. Pro-Arrhythmic Effects of SDB: Chronic Effects

Although it seems likely that the acute effects of SDB can provoke cardiac arrhythmias, there has also been an explosion of evidence in recent years that SDB also exerts chronic effects that may increase the myocardium's intrinsic susceptibility to arrhythmias. Most of the postulated mechanisms of cardiac damage will be discussed at length in other chapters of this volume, but three of the most relevant will be briefly reviewed here. They are (*i*) endothelial dysfunction and atherosclerosis, (*ii*) cardiac remodeling, and (*iii*) neurohormonal dysfunction.

A. Endothelial Dysfunction and Atherosclerosis

The cyclic intermittent hypoxia accompanying SDB is akin to a chronic ischemia-reperfusion type injury that may have a direct effect on the myocardium or vasculature, an effect exacerbated by hypercapnia and acidosis (81). Oxygenation/reoxygenation injury is known to initiate oxidative stress via the production of reactive oxygen species and is recognized to play an important role in the genesis of endothelial dysfunction, via inactivation of nitric oxide (NO) (82) and the modulation of diverse redox-sensitive signaling pathways in endothelial cells, which influence gene and protein expression (83). The redox-sensitive signaling pathways include nuclear factor (NF) κB and hypoxia-inducible factor 1. NF-κB activates proinflammatory cytokines (TNF-α, IL-6), chemokines (MCP-1 and IL-8), and adhesion molecules (ICAM, VCAM, selectin) (84). There is increasing evidence that such vascular wall inflammation plays a key role in the pathogenesis of vascular disease and that endothelial dysfunction is a precursor of the atherosclerotic process (85).

The endothelium plays a crucial role in the maintenance of vascular tone and structure. Normal endothelial tone and function is maintained through vasoactive mediators that include NO, endothelin-1 (ET-1), RAAS and xanthine oxidase (XO), and thromboxane. Alterations in the vascular milieu in which an imbalance occurs between the vasoconstrictive and vasorelaxant factors will alter endothelium-dependent vasorelaxation.

The pathophysiological effects of SDB including hypoxia, sympathetic activation, systemic inflammation, production of reactive oxygen species, endothelial dysfunction, and negative intrathoracic pressures provide the basis for a cascade of events that could initiate atherogenesis (86). Evidence suggests that OSA is an independent predictor of endothelial dysfunction (87) and that an imbalance occurs between the vasoconstrictive and vasorelaxant factors with improvement following treatment with continuous positive airway pressure (CPAP) therapy (88,89). More recently, direct evidence of endothelial dysfunction and inflammation has been demonstrated in vivo in vascular endothelium of patients with OSA (90) along with increased carotid intima-media thickness (91).

The role of hypoxia is supported by Savransky and colleagues who demonstrated induction of atherosclerosis in mice exposed to intermittent hypoxia (92). Treatment of OSA with CPAP has been found to reverse early atherosclerotic lesions in humans, supporting a causal relationship (93). OSA may also contribute to atherosclerosis indirectly by causing systolic hypertension, insulin resistance, and impaired lipid metabolism (94,95).

The vasculature in the human body serves not only as a conduit to deliver blood to the body's organs and tissues but is also an important modulator of the entire cardiovascular system. Aortic elastic properties are important determinants of blood pressure and LV function. By virtue of these elastic properties the aorta influences LV function and structure and coronary blood flow (96–98). Therefore, atherosclerosis, particularly in the aorta, may alter both mechanical and electrical cardiac function. The increased arterial stiffness observed in OSA may in turn contribute to increased LV afterload, diastolic dysfunction, and ultimately to LV hypertrophy (87,99). Furthermore, atherosclerosis involving the coronary arteries may cause coronary occlusion and ischemia with resultant myocardial damage and fibrosis. Therefore, by accelerating atherosclerosis, SDB can increase the tendency to cardiac arrhythmias either through direct alterations in the cellular substrate or indirectly by causing global cardiac remodeling.

B. Cardiac Remodeling

Cardiac remodeling changes the cardiac substrate and predisposes to arrhythmias. In athletes, cardiac remodeling may be beneficial, leading to more efficient myocyte and ventricular contraction. However, structural remodeling as occurs in hypertension and other medical conditions is maladaptive and referred to as LV hypertrophy. LV hypertrophy may be classified as eccentric or concentric hypertrophy (100). Concentric hypertrophy is characterized by both increased LV mass and relative wall thickness and is usually due to volume overload, whereas eccentric hypertrophy features an isolated LV mass increase, usually attributed to pressure overload. LV hypertrophy causes anatomic, cellular, and phenotypic changes in myocytes. The anatomic changes include an accumulation of type 1 collagen, extracellular fibrosis, and increased thickness of coronary artery walls. Cellular changes include cardiomyocyte hypertrophy, hyperplasia, and hypertrophy of the nonmuscular cells as a result of sarcomeric reorganization that causes myocyte lengthening (101). Phenotypic changes in myocytes are the result of complex changes in gene reprogramming (102), including the reexpression of immature fetal cardiac genes that are responsible for energy metabolism, motor unit modification, and encoding of hormonal pathways. Phenotypic changes may also result from blunted expression in genes that modify intracellular ion homeostasis (e.g., downregulation of sarcoplasmic reticulum calcium ATPase) and downregulation of parasympathetic and sympathetic receptors. Alterations in intracellular calcium handling lead to activation of transient inward current medicated by either Na^+/Ca^{2+} exchange, a nonspecific cationic current, or a calcium-activated chloride current (103). This new cardiocyte phenotype favors both automaticity and triggered activity (104). These changes culminate in the interference with normal myocyte contraction and relaxation and predispose to cardiac arrhythmias (105).

In patients with CSA and HF, LV remodeling is usually present as it is an early pathogenic marker of HF (106–108). However, there is evidence that OSA also promotes LV remodeling and dysfunction. Animal models of chronic intermittent hypoxia induce LV hypertrophy and global LV dysfunction independent of elevations in blood pressure (109,110). In the canine model of chronic OSA, acute sleep-related obstructive events were associated with increased LV afterload and decreases in fractional shortening, which chronically lead to sustained decreases in LV systolic performance (111). In these animal models the LV dysfunction is attributable to cardiomyocyte hypertrophy, apoptosis, and altered gene profile expression (109,110,112,113). Furthermore, oxidative stress and cytokines are implicated in the pathophysiology of intermittent hypoxia-induced LV remodeling (114,115).

Although animal models of intermittent hypoxia have demonstrated cardiac remodeling, the demonstration of changes in cardiac structures in human studies of OSA is somewhat more difficult due to confounding factors. Furthermore, variability in the severity of the disease and its development over many years may alter the cardiac effects. Most of the studies performed are small cross-sectional studies. Results and interpretation of these studies must be approached with caution as the presence of cardiac medications, hypertension, or other diseases that could affect diastolic function, incomplete or varying methodology in assessment of echocardiographic parameters (116–119), and lack of or an inadequately matched control group (116,120,121) may confound the results. However, both hemodynamic load and neurohormonal activation are known mechanisms that predispose to cardiac remodeling (122,123) and these are present in SDB. In general the majority of the studies have favored a higher prevalence of LV hypertrophy in OSA patients, especially in those with higher apnea-hypopnea index (AHI) (124,125). In non-obese children with OSA, there was an 11-fold increased risk for LV hypertrophy and 83% had eccentric hypertrophy. Those with OSA were also more likely to have RV dysfunction (126). In contrast, two studies did not find any relationship between LV hypertrophy and OSA, although differences in the calculation of the LV mass may account for some of these differences (117,127).

The association between LV hypertrophy and both atrial and ventricular arrhythmias is well documented (128,129). Moreover, a reduction in arrhythmogenesis is demonstrated upon reversal of LV hypertrophy (130,131). Furthermore, excessive hypertrophy has been associated with the development of LV dysfunction (132), which is a well-known independent predictor of sudden arrhythmic death (133). With the appearance of overt HF, there is a further decline in LV ejection fraction and a further increase in the incidence of complex ventricular arrhythmias.

Studies examining systolic and diastolic dysfunction in OSA and the effect of CPAP therapy are also conflicting. Most of these studies are uncontrolled and small cross-sectional analyses. A prospective cohort study of 169 patients found systolic dysfunction in 7.7% of OSA patients as assessed by radionuclide imaging. Ischemic cardiac disease was unlikely as there were no segmental LV wall motion abnormalities. However, 69% of these individuals were obese and 54% had hypertension. Despite this normalization of dysfunction was seen in all of the patients who had imaging following CPAP. Furthermore, compared with an untreated control group, subjects with OSA had reduced cardiac output during exercise suggested early systolic dysfunction, which improved on treatment with CPAP (135).

The evidence for OSA contributing to diastolic dysfunction is more robust. Diastolic dysfunction has been associated with moderate to severe OSA in a number of studies (116,118–120). In two studies, OSA independent of obesity was associated with increased LA size as well as impaired LV diastolic function (119,136). The authors propose that chronic diastolic dysfunction may cause increased LA size and predispose to atrial fibrillation (137). The most frequent abnormality observed in these studies is impaired isovolumic relaxation time and mitral deceleration time with a tendency to a higher LV mass, posterior wall, and interventricular septal thickness in OSA subjects. That diastolic dysfunction is associated independently with OSA is suggested by the reversal of some of these changes on application of CPAP (118–121).

C. Neurohormonal Dysfunction

OSA and CSA are associated with chronic abnormalities of cardiovascular autonomic regulation. It is important to recognize that these abnormalities are not limited to sleep but carry over into the daytime. Patients with OSA have higher daytime MSNA compared to controls matched for age, sex, and body mass index (138,139). This elevation of MSNA is a consistent finding, regardless of whether patients are hypertensive or not (139). Treatment of OSA either by tracheostomy (140) or by CPAP therapy leads to a reduction in overnight urinary catecholamine levels and daytime MSNA. However, in keeping with the concept that OSA fundamentally alters normal autonomic regulation, reversal of its autonomic effects by CPAP is not immediate. Only after several months of CPAP therapy does lowering of MSNA occur, and the effect is most pronounced in patients with the greatest number of hours of CPAP usage (141–143).

Cardiovascular autonomic regulation in OSA has also been assessed by examination of heart rate variability (HRV). It has been known for more than two decades that diminished overall HRV in the setting of cardiac disease is a harbinger of a worse prognosis (144,145). Conversely, higher overall HRV is though to denote better health. HRV can be further divided into specific frequency bands with differing physiological interpretation: high-frequency (0.15–0.4 Hz) HRV is modulated primarily by cardiac vagal activity and occurs at respiratory frequencies. HRV at low frequency (0.05–0.15 Hz) is thought to be modulated by sympathetic activity, although there is a controversy on this point (146) and very low frequency (0.01–0.05 Hz) variability is even less well understood.

In general, patients with OSA have been found to have HRV profiles consistent with poorer health, diminished parasympathetic, and increased sympathetic modulation of HR (139,147,148): total HRV and high-frequency power are reduced, whereas low-frequency power is increased. Furthermore, the severity of sleep apnea as quantified by the AHI has been observed to correlate with sympathetic activity, as assessed by low-frequency HRV (139). Treatment of OSA with CPAP has been shown to restore HRV indices toward normal, both acutely (149) and chronically (150), extending into wakefulness.

OSA and CSA may have particular importance in the setting of CHF. Patients with the combination of CHF and OSA have higher daytime MSNA than controls matched for age and ejection fraction (151). There is intriguing evidence that the HF state may actually alter the sympathetic response to obstructive apneas: patients with CHF have a higher MSNA response to simulated obstructive apneas (Mueller maneuvers) than to simple breath holds, whereas healthy controls have similar MSNA responses to both maneuvers (152). If so, OSA and CHF may act synergistically to undermine normal autonomic regulation. Treatment of OSA for one month with CPAP has been reported in a randomized controlled trial to reduce both daytime MSNA and BP, compared to an untreated group (153).

Surprisingly, given the consistency of the studies using MSNA, urinary norepinephrine has not been found to be elevated in CHF patients with OSA compared with those without (154), and although norepinephrine spillover rates are exceedingly high in patients with CHF and CSA, this appears to be a consequence of HF severity and not the severity of CSA (155). Nonetheless, treatment of OSA with CPAP for three months in the setting of HF significantly reduced norepinophrine spillover rate compared with untreated controls (156).

Studies of HRV in patients with CHF and sleep apnea have largely focused on CSA and have consistently shown overall diminished HRV, particularly in the high-frequency (parasympathetic) band (157,158). Interestingly, many groups report relatively preserved very low frequency power due to a discrete cyclical oscillation in heart rate associated with Cheyne–Stokes respiration itself (158,159). Again, it is important to note that these abnormalities are found not only during sleep, coincident with the abnormal respiratory patterns, but also during wakefulness (158,159). These findings have been extended to patients with CSA and asymptomatic LV dysfunction (19). Treatment of OSA with CPAP in the setting of HF has been reported to increase spectral parameters of parasympathetic modulation (high-frequency HRV) and restore sympathovagal balance (low frequency:high frequency ratio) (160).

Sympathetic overactivity leads to a number of metabolic and structural changes to the heart that are ultimately pro-arrhythmic, among them β-adrenoreceptor down-regulation and desensitization, enhanced G_i protein and G-protein receptor kinases (GRK) (161), and increased activity and amount of Na^+/H^+ exchanger NHE1 (162). In animal studies, NE has been demonstrated to result in hypertrophy of the myocardium (163,164). There is a correlation between increased SNA and LV hypertrophy in subjects with hypertension, suggesting that increased SNA may contribute to myocardial remodeling in humans (165). Therefore, while acute increases in SNA contribute to myocardial performance and maintain homeostasis, chronic elevations are maladaptive and result in myocardial damage, remodeling, contractile dysfunction, and cardiac arrhythmias. These changes may be mediated via chronic activation of NHE1, inducing intracellular Ca^{2+} overload and promoting repolarization (162,166). Evidence for the role of elevated SNA in arrhythmogenesis is demonstrated in both the heritable disorder catecholaminergic polymorphic ventricular tachycardia (CPVT) and HF. In CPVT abnormal calcium handling leads to abnormalities of repolarization called delayed after depolarization (DAD) and subsequent ventricular arrhythmias (167). In HF DAD-triggered ventricular arrhythmias are exhibited in association with elevated SNA and altered calcium handling (168–170). Persistent SNA activation may also cause insulin resistance indirectly via oxidative stress–induced inflammatory response and cause hypertension (171). In those with HF, SNA overactivity may also activate the RAAS.

V. Sleep Apnea and Cardiac Arrhythmias

Cardiac arrhythmias that have been described in association with OSA include sinus pauses, heart block, atrial fibrillation, and ventricular tachycardia (9). Such arrhythmias have been implicated as a cause of sudden nocturnal death in patients with OSA, although definitive proof of a causal relationship remains elusive. Still, given the prevalence of OSA, if even a minority of the arrhythmic events coinciding with its presence could be prevented through therapy directed toward its treatment, the clinical implications would be immense. The true extent of the problem remains uncertain because of the lack of well-designed prospective studies and widely varying prevalences of arrhythmias reported in different studies of OSA patients. Much of the variation probably relates to different referral patterns for OSA in different centers (9,10,172–176).

A. Bradycardia and Heart Block

A frequently noted feature of OSA is cyclic variation in HR: most typically, HR rises during hyperpneas and falls during apneas (75). In some cases, bradycardia during apnea can lead to sinus arrest and second- and third-degree heart block, a phenomenon thought to be vagally mediated. For many years, it was believed that episodes of nocturnal heart block frequently accompany OSA, and early studies reported a prevalence of 18% to 50% (9,177). However, a subsequent study comparing OSA patients with controls found a much lower prevalence of serious bradyarrhythmias (1–5%) that was no greater than in subjects without OSA (174). Recently, the Sleep Hearth Health Study (10) found a higher prevalence of first- and second-degree heart block among subjects with SDB than in those without (1.8% vs. 0.3% and 2.2% vs. 0.9%, respectively) but these differences did not reach statistical significance. The most likely explanation for these discordant results is the changing referral patterns of OSA as the disease becomes more widely recognized and diagnosed. Earlier studies tended to comprise patients with more severe OSA, more frequent and longer apneas, and worse apnea-related hypoxia, factors that are known to be associated with a higher risk of bradyarrhythmia and heart block (9,178,179).

The HR response to apneas varies greatly among individuals and only a minority of those with even severe OSA develop significant bradyarrhythmias. Hypoxia is known to influence HR differently depending on the presence or absence of ventilation and the balance of its parasympathetic and sympathetic stimulatory effects. In the absence of ventilation (e.g., during apnea), hypoxic stimulation of the carotid body is vagotonic and tends to cause bradycardia (71,72). Indeed, the bradycardia occurring during obstructive apneas can be attenuated by the administration of supplemental O_2 or atropine (180). In the presence of ventilation (e.g., hypoxic rebreathing), the situation is quite different: hypoxia causes tachycardia due to a lung inflation reflex that inhibits vagal outflow to the heart and permits unopposed cardiac sympathetic discharge. Not surprisingly, the HR responses to obstructive apneas can be quite different in different individuals despite similar burdens of OSA: HR can decrease, increase, or remain stable. This variability is probably due to individual differences in the severity of hypoxia, intrinsic hypoxic chemosensitivity and on the relative influence of hypoxia on vagal and sympathetic input to the sinoatrial node (181,182). Where parasympathetic influence predominates, HR slows, where sympathetic influence predominates, HR rises, and where vagal and sympathetic influences are relatively equal, HR may remain largely unchanged (43). The HR response to the resumption of airflow at apnea termination is much more consistent: HR invariably rises owing to disengagement of hypoxia-mediated cardiac vagal outflow and unopposed cardiac sympathetic discharge (58,68,183).

Even severe bradyarrhythmias during OSA are not primarily the result of fixed structural disease of the conduction system, but are rather a consequence of an increased vagal tone during apnea. Electrophysiological studies of 15 OSA patients with prolonged ventricular asystoles during obstructive apneas revealed that sinus node and atrioventricular conduction was normal or only slightly abnormal during wakefulness (184). In general, severe bradyarrhythmias occur in association with more frequent apneas and more severe degrees of apnea-related hypoxia (9,178,179). Abolition of OSA by tracheostomy or CPAP generally eliminates these bradyarrhythmias (9) and should be considered the therapy of choice, obviating the need for electrical pacing.

B. Ventricular Arrhythmias

Nocturnal ventricular arrhythmias occurring in association with OSA have been described by many groups. Guilleminault et al. (9) in a series of 400 patients, reported frequent (>2/min) ventricular ectopic beats during sleep in 20%. Although this study did not employ a control group comprising non-apneics, the ectopic beats were clearly sleep related, since their frequency diminished when they awoke, in contrast to the usual diurnal pattern observed in subjects known not to have sleep apnea (185,186). Several patients also had episodes of nonsustained ventricular tachycardia that occurred exclusively during sleep. Ventricular ectopy and tachycardia tend to occur in concert with relatively severe O_2 desaturation, suggesting that OSA triggers ventricular ectopy primarily by causing hypoxia (9,49). Shepard (49) reported almost no events observed above oxyhemoglobin saturation of 80%. The arrhythmogenic effects of hypoxia are many and include directly lowering the fibrillation threshold and reducing myocardial O_2 supply at the time of increased O_2 demand due to increases in sympathetic activity, BP, and HR. These effects would be magnified in the presence of coronary artery disease, possibly provoking frank ischemia (187) and arrhythmias. With these factors in mind, the most likely explanation of the lower prevalences of ventricular ectopy reported in some series of OSA patients may be related to less severe degrees of apnea-related hypoxia in those patients (173,174). In keeping with this concept, mild degrees of sleep apnea do not seem to result in ventricular ectopy that is more frequent than controls, even in the setting of preexisting coronary artery disease (176).

It must be emphasized that even if ventricular arrhythmias are confined to that subset of sleep apneics with the most severe OSA and apnea-related hypoxia, a very large number of patients may still be at risk of arrhythmias and nocturnal sudden death owing to the high prevalence of OSA in the general population. Three recent studies underscore this possibility. Firstly, patients with severe untreated OSA (AHI > 30) in a large prospective cohort study have been reported to suffer a higher incidence of fatal and nonfatal cardiovascular events compared to patients without sleep apnea (6). The incidence of cardiac events was not significantly higher in the cohort with mild-moderate sleep apnea (AHI = 5 to 30), a finding that again supports the notion that it may only be the group with severe OSA that is at risk.

Secondly, the Sleep Heart Health Study (10), a large multicenter community-based study, reported in a cross-sectional analysis a significantly higher prevalence of nonsustained ventricular tachycardia and complex ventricular ectopy in subjects with SDB compared with those without (4.8% vs. 0.9%). After matching for age, sex, body mass index, and prevalent coronary artery disease, individuals with SDB were found to have three times the odds of nonsustained ventricular tachycardia and twice the risk of complex ventricular ectopy. Finally, Gami and coworkers reported the intriguing observation that patients with OSA exhibit an altered circadian pattern of cardiac sudden death than those without SDB. Examining the death certificates of 112 Minnesota residents who had undergone diagnostic polysomnography and subsequently died suddenly from a cardiac cause, death was found to occur during the six hours between midnight and 6 a.m. in 46% of those with OSA compared with the 25% expected by chance (17) (Fig. 2). From the preceding discussion regarding the autonomic milieu of normal sleep, it follows that sudden cardiac death should be less common during sleep than wakefulness, and this is indeed what was found by these authors among subjects without OSA and in the general population (21% and 16% of sudden deaths between midnight and 6 a.m., respectively). While the question of whether OSA confers an increased risk of sudden death irrespective of time of day was left unanswered by this report, it is much more in keeping with the findings of the other studies (6,10) to suppose that OSA changes the circadian pattern of death by increasing the risk during sleep, rather than by somehow exerting a protective effect during the day.

OSA is very common in the general population, whereas CSA is rare. However, both CSA and OSA are common among patients with CHF. Moreover, the clinical impact of any pro-arrhythmic effect of SDB is magnified in the setting of HF due to the high mortality associated with CHF and the fact that about half of patients with CHF die of sudden cardiac death (188). CHF patients with hypocapnia ($PaCO_2 < 35$ mmHg) have

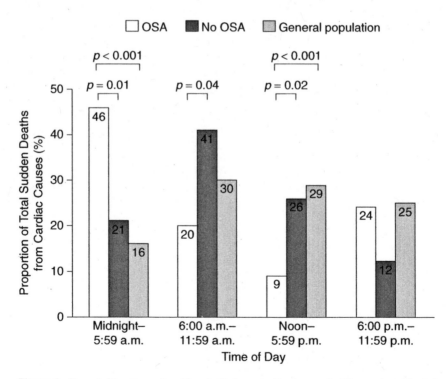

Figure 2 Day-night pattern of sudden death from cardiac causes in 78 persons with obstructive sleep apnea and 34 persons without and in the general population. *Abbreviation*: OSA, obstructive sleep apnea. *Source*: From Ref. 17.

been reported to have both a higher prevalence of CSA and a higher rate of ventricular ectopic beats than eucapnic patients (11). Similarly, severe CSA has been associated with a higher incidence of ventricular arrhythmias among patients with HF (19).

There is reason to believe that CSA is not merely associated with ventricular arrhythmias, both being sequela of underlying heart disease, but that CSA actually provokes arrhythmic events. Firstly, at least two groups have reported a reduction in the frequency of VPBs in association with treatment of CSA, either with CPAP (189) or inhaled carbon dioxide (41).

Secondly, there is often a stunning temporal relationship between CSA and ventricular ectopic events during sleep. Findley et al. (190) described in 1984 a patient experiencing ventricular ectopy in timing with the CSA cycle. VPBs were preferentially clustered during the hyperpneic phase of CSA and were largely absent during apnea. These findings were replicated in a series of 10 patients with CHF and CSA two decades later, in whom it was found that VPBs were more likely to occur during periods of the night when CSA was present than during normal breathing and that ectopic beats were again found to cluster during hyperpnea. Furthermore, eradication of CSA by administering inhaled CO_2 sufficient to raise $PaCO_2$ above the apneic threshold resulted in a reduction in the frequency of ectopy (Fig. 3) (41). Significantly, eradication of the hypoxic dips with supplemental oxygen was not sufficient to reduce ectopy as long as CSA itself persisted, suggesting that CSA-associated surges in respiratory drive and motor activity are pro-arrhythmic even in the absence of hypoxia.

These observations are consonant with what is known about the timing of acute physiological disturbances associated with CSA: it is during the hyperpneic phase of CSA that respiratory drive, HR, and BP are most elevated (76). Even nadir oxygen

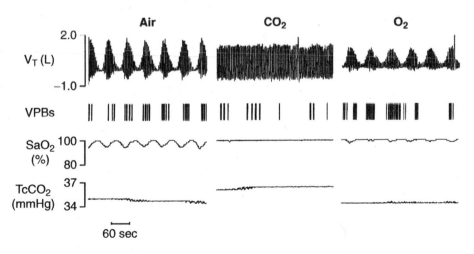

Figure 3 The effects of breathing room air, inhaled CO_2, and O_2 on the frequency of VPBs in one subject. Note VPBs (*vertical lines*) during the hyperneic phases of CSA while breathing room air, inhaled CO_2 (middle panel), and supplemental oxygen (*right panel*). *Abbreviations*: V_T, tidal volume; VPBs, ventricular premature beats; SaO_2, oxyhemoglobin saturation; $PtcCO_2$, transcutaneous PCO_2. *Source*: From Ref. 41.

saturation in CSA tends to occur during hyperpnea due to the effects of circulatory delay. In the case of OSA, however, it is during the apneic phase that increased respiratory drive, intrathoracic pressure changes, and blood gas alterations are at their most extreme. Accordingly, it is during apnea that one might expect ventricular irritability to be greatest. Indeed, this is the case: the phase relationship between ventricular ectopic beats and the breathing cycle was found to be reversed in patients with OSA; in those patients, VPBs were found to occur preferentially during apnea rather than hyperpnea (40).

C. Supraventricular Arrhythmias

The same mechanisms that predispose to ventricular arrhythmias (i.e., hypoxia, increased SNA, and myocardial stretch) might also trigger atrial arrhythmias, and, in particular, there has been a substantial amount of investigation into the link between OSA and atrial fibrillation.

The initial description of the association between atrial arrhythmias and sleep apnea was in the 1980s (9,173,191). Guilleminault observed atrial arrhythmias in 11% (3% with atrial fibrillation) of the 400 patients studied with severe OSA (mean RDI = 42). Twenty years intervened before the relationship between atrial fibrillation and sleep apnea underwent further scrutiny.

This resurgence of interest in the relationship between atrial fibrillation and OSA was ignited by Kanagala and coworkers who demonstrated prospectively that in a group of patients undergoing electrical cardioversion for atrial fibrillation there was an increased recurrence rate in those with either untreated OSA or noncompliant with OSA therapy (82%) compared with those compliant (42%, $p = 0.013$) and those without OSA (53%, $p = 0.009$) (137). The same group later reported that 49% of patients with atrial fibrillation had OSA compared with 32% of the general cardiology population ($p = 0.0004$). The relationship between OSA and atrial fibrillation was significant both without (OR 1.89; 1.28–2.82, $p = 0.002$) and with adjustment (OR 2.19; 1.4–3.42, $p = 0.0006$) for potential confounders (BMI, DM, NC, HTN) (192). In patients without cardiac disease, the prevalence of atrial arrhythmias in 247 patients with OSA (defined as AHI > 5/hr) was 6.1% with less than 1% with atrial fibrillation (193).

In the Sleep Heart Health Study, there was a fourfold risk of atrial fibrillation in patients with SDB compared with those without it after adjustment for potential confounders including BMI, age sex, and prevalent coronary heart disease [OR = 4.02 (1.03–15.74)] (10). 4.8% of the patients with SDB had atrial fibrillation and of those one-third had paroxysmal atrial fibrillation. A prospective postoperative study in patients following cardiac bypass grafting demonstrated the occurrence of atrial fibrillation in 32% of those with SDB versus 18% without (194). More recently, a Japanese study demonstrated an association between the severity of OSA as defined by the 3% oxygen desaturation index (ODI) and atrial fibrillation: the adjusted odds ratio for mild (ODI 5–15/hr) was 2.47, and for moderate to severe SDB was 5.66 (ODI $\geq$ 15) (195). Perhaps the strongest evidence to date in favor of a causal relationship between OSA and atrial fibrillation comes from Gami and coworkers, who retrospectively examined 3542 subjects for the occurrence of incident atrial fibrillation. OSA was present in 74% of the subjects and there was a mean follow-up of 4.7 years. The presence of OSA (AHI > 5) was a strong predictor of incident atrial fibrillation (HR 2.181–3.54, $p = 0.002$). Atrial fibrillation occurred in 4.3% with OSA and 2.1% without OSA (196).

It should be noted, however, that not all investigators have found evidence supporting the association: using a case-control design, Porthan reported a similar prevalence of SDB in a group of patients with atrial fibrillation without other cardiac disease compared with controls (32% versus 29%, $p = 0.22$) (197). Results from studies involving patients with pacemakers have also been discordant. Ambulatory sleep monitoring in 192 patients with pacemaker insertion did not demonstrate any significant relationship between atrial fibrillation and SDB. However, 47.4% of these patients had an RDI > 10/hr (198). The high prevalence of sleep apnea (59%) has been confirmed in a subsequent study of consecutive patients with pacemakers (199). In another group of patients with pacemakers, those at high or low risk of OSA did not seem to be at significantly different risk for recurrence of atrial fibrillation (200). Interestingly, however, OSA is a reported risk factor for the return of pulmonary vein conduction following ablation for atrial fibrillation (201).

The association between atrial fibrillation and sleep apnea is not restricted to OSA, but also extends to CSA. However, there are few studies. In the largest retrospective study, atrial fibrillation was found to be a significant independent risk factor for CSA in patients with congestive HF following adjustments for both BMI and LV ejection fraction (OR 4.13; 95% CI 1.53–11.14, $p < 0.05$) (8). The increased prevalence of atrial fibrillation in patients with CSA and HF was later confirmed in a prospective study (202). Idiopathic CSA is also strongly associated with atrial fibrillation, suggesting that the presence of LV dysfunction is not part of the causal pathway linking these disorders (203).

D. Treatment

There are very few studies in which the effect of treating SDB on cardiac arrythmias has been tested. One of the earliest and still most impressive remains an uncontrolled study from the pre-CPAP era in which treatment of OSA by tracheostomy was associated with elimination of bradyarrhythmias in all 50 patients and alleviation of ventricular ectopic activity in 14 of 18 patients (9). As is the case with most of the early studies, the severity of OSA among these 50 patients was extremely high. Similar results have been reported, however, using nasal CPAP in more moderate cases (178,184,204).

In one of the few randomized trials to date, Ryan (205) reported a 58% reduction in the frequency of VPBs in patients with OSA and CHF who were randomized to CPAP treatment for one month. Left unanswered is the question of whether treatment of OSA with CPAP reduces the incidence of more malignant arrhythmias such as ventricular tachycardia or sudden death. However, it may be worth emphasizing that a general principle of arrhythmia management is to first correct any underlying physiological derangements such as electrolyte disturbances or hypoxia that are known to increase ventricular irritability and lower fibrillation threshold. Treatment of OSA would seem to be a logical extension of this principle.

Abolition of CSA in the setting of HF has also been reported to reduce ventricular ectopy, whether by application of CPAP (189) or through administration of inhaled CO_2 (41). Disappointingly, a recent randomized controlled trial of CPAP for the treatment of CSA in the setting of HF did not show survival benefit in an intention to treat analysis (206). However, the lack of survival benefit in this trial may very well have been due to the failure of CPAP to abolish CSA in many subjects. Since a subsequent post hoc analysis did show improved survival in the subgroup of patients in whom AHI fell below

15 (207), the question as to whether a more effective means of eliminating CSA might improve survival overall remains unsettled. In this regard, adaptive servoventilation, a novel mode of positive pressure therapy specifically designed to treat CSA (208) may be promising.

VI. Conclusion

OSA is a very common disease in the general population and CSA, while less common, is very prevalent in patients with CHF who are already at high risk for lethal arrhythmias and sudden cardiac death. Both OSA and CSA exert physiological effects that acutely subject the myocardium to pro-arrhythmic triggering stimuli such as hypoxia and surges in sympathetic activity. Over time, there is mounting evidence that these disturbances may also alter the very cardiac substrate, rendering it more susceptible to arrhythmias as well—a potentially lethal combination of acute and chronic effects acting in synergy.

Further elucidation of the relevant signaling pathways is essential. While there is strong evidence that sleep apnea causes cardiac injury and remodeling through a variety of mechanisms, it is not known which are most important or confer the most risk. A better understanding of the relevant physiology might lead to better risk stratification of patients with sleep apnea, and targeted therapies, such as correcting hypoxia or suppressing arousals. Indeed, with knowledge of the signaling pathways leading from SDB to athe-rosclerosis, LV hypertrophy, and cardiac arrhythmias, pharmacological agents directed toward specific adverse effects of OSA might play a significant role in the future.

Until that time, eradication of OSA itself must remain the primary therapeutic goal and the mainstay of treatment. With successful administration of CPAP or other therapy, OSA and all its accompanying "downstream" deleterious effects can in theory be eradicated. This approach is not without its drawbacks: CPAP is not always well tolerated or accepted by many patients. Still, with the mounting evidence that untreated sleep apnea can lead to serious and even fatal consequences, clinicians must screen for and treat SDB as best they can.

References

1. Young T, Palta M, Dempsey J, et al. The occurrence of sleep-disordered breathing among middle-aged adults. N Engl J Med 1993; 328:1230–1235.
2. Leung RS, Bradley TD. Sleep apnea and cardiovascular disease. Am J Respir Crit Care Med 2001; 164:2147–2165.
3. Shahar E, Whitney CW, Redline S, et al. Sleep-disordered breathing and cardiovascular disease: cross-sectional results of the Sleep Heart Health Study. Am J Respir Crit Care Med 2001; 163:19–25.
4. Peppard PE, Young T, Palta M, et al. Prospective study of the association between sleep-disordered breathing and hypertension. N Engl J Med 2000; 342:1378–1384.
5. Arzt M, Young T, Finn L, et al. Association of sleep-disordered breathing and the occurrence of stroke. Am J Respir Crit Care Med 2005; 172:1447–1451.
6. Marin JM, Carrizo SJ, Vicente E, et al. Long-term cardiovascular outcomes in men with obstructive sleep apnoea-hypopnoea with or without treatment with continuous positive airway pressure: an observational study. Lancet 2005; 365:1046–1053.
7. Javaheri S, Parker TJ, Liming JD, et al. Sleep apnea in 81 ambulatory male patients with stable heart failure. Types and their prevalences, consequences, and presentations. Circulation 1998; 97:2154–2159.

8. Sin DD, Fitzgerald F, Parker JD, et al. Risk factors for central and obstructive sleep apnea in 450 men and women with congestive heart failure. Am J Respir Crit Care Med 1999; 160:1101–1106.

9. Guilleminault C, Connolly SJ, Winkle RA. Cardiac arrhythmia and conduction disturbances during sleep in 400 patients with sleep apnea syndrome. Am J Cardiol 1983; 52:490–494.

10. Mehra R, Benjamin EJ, Shahar E, et al. Association of nocturnal arrhythmias with sleep-disordered breathing: The Sleep Heart Health Study. Am J Respir Crit Care Med 2006; 173:910–916.

11. Javaheri S, Corbett WS. Association of low $PaCO_2$ with central sleep apnea and ventricular arrhythmias in ambulatory patients with stable heart failure. Ann Intern Med 1998; 128:204–207.

12. Shah M, Akar FG, Tomaselli GF. Molecular basis of arrhythmias. Circulation 2005; 112: 2517–2529.

13. Singh BN. Significance and control of cardiac arrhythmias in patients with congestive cardiac failure. Heart Fail Rev 2002; 7:285–300.

14. Kahan T, Bergfeldt L. Left ventricular hypertrophy in hypertension: its arrhythmogenic potential. Heart 2005; 91:250–256.

15. Knollmann BC, Roden DM. A genetic framework for improving arrhythmia therapy. Nature 2008; 451:929–936.

16. Zheng ZJ, Croft JB, Giles WH, et al. Sudden cardiac death in the United States, 1989 to 1998. Circulation 2001; 104:2158–2163.

17. Gami AS, Howard DE, Olson EJ, et al. Day-night pattern of sudden death in obstructive sleep apnea. N Engl J Med 2005; 352:1206–1214.

18. AHA. Heart Disease and Stroke Statistics—Update. Dallas, Texas: American Heart Association, 2008.

19. Lanfranchi PA, Somers VK, Braghiroli A, et al. Central sleep apnea in left ventricular dysfunction: prevalence and implications for arrhythmic risk. Circulation 2003; 107:727–732.

20. Hanly PJ, Zuberi-Khokhar NS. Increased mortality associated with Cheyne-Stokes respiration in patients with congestive heart failure. Am J Respir Crit Care Med 1996; 153:272–276.

21. McGinty D, Szymusiak R. Neurobiology of sleep. In: Saunders NA, Sullivan CE, eds. Sleep and breathing: second edition. New York: Marcel Dekker, 1994:1–26.

22. Phillipson EA, Bowes G. Control of breathing during sleep. In: Cherniack NS, Widdicombe JG, eds. Handbook of Physiology: Vol 2, Control of breathing. Bethesda, MD: Williams and Wilkins, 1986:649–689.

23. Trinder J. Respiratory and cardiac activity during sleep onset. In: Bradley TD, Floras JS, eds. Sleep apnea: implications in cardiovascular and cerebrovascular disease. New York: Marcel Dekker, 2000:337–354.

24. Phillipson EA. Control of breathing during sleep. Am Rev Respir Dis. 1978; 118:909–939.

25. Orem J, Osorio I, Brooks E, et al. Activity of respiratory neurons during NREM sleep. J Neurophysiol 1985; 54:1144–1156.

26. White DP, Weil JV, Zwillich CW. Metabolic rate and breathing during sleep. J Appl Physiol 1985; 59:384–391.

27. Somers VK, Dyken ME, Mark AL, et al. Sympathetic-nerve activity during sleep in normal subjects. N Engl J Med 1993; 328:303–307.

28. Shepard JW Jr. Gas exchange and hemodynamics during sleep. Med Clin North Am 1985; 69:1243–1264.

29. Hornyak M, Cejnar M, Elam M, et al. Sympathetic muscle nerve activity during sleep in man. Brain 1991; 114:1281–1295.

30. Okada H, Iwase S, Mano T, et al. Changes in muscle sympathetic nerve activity during sleep in humans. Neurology 1991; 41:1961–1966.

31. Mancia G. Autonomic modulation of the cardiovascular system during sleep. N Engl J Med 1993; 328:347–349.
32. Kong TQ Jr., Goldberger JJ, Parker M, et al. Circadian variation in human ventricular refractoriness. Circulation 1995; 92:1507–1516.
33. Lown B, Tykocinski M, Garfein A, et al. Sleep and ventricular premature beats. Circulation 1973; 48:691–701.
34. Orem J. Neuronal mechanisms of respiration in REM sleep. Sleep 1980; 3:251–267.
35. Chandler SH, Chase MH, Nakamura Y. Intracellular analysis of synaptic mechanisms controlling trigeminal motoneuron activity during sleep and wakefulness. J Neurophysiol 1980; 44:359–371.
36. Snyder F, Hobson JA, Morrison DF, et al. Changes in respiration, heart rate, and systolic blood pressure in human sleep. J Appl Physiol 1964; 19:417–22.
37. Tilkian AG, Guilleminault C, Schroeder JS, et al. Hemodynamics in sleep-induced apnea. Studies during wakefulness and sleep. Ann Intern Med 1976; 85:714–719.
38. Ringler J, Basner RC, Shannon R, et al. Hypoxemia alone does not explain blood pressure elevations after obstructive apneas. J Appl Physiol 1990; 69:2143–2148.
39. Leung RS, Lorenzi-Filho G, Floras JS, et al. Entrainment of blood pressure and heart rate by Cheyne-Stokes respiration in patients with congestive heart failure. Am J Respir Crit Care Med 2000; 161:A865.
40. Ryan CM, Juvet S, Leung R, et al. Timing of nocturnal ventricular ectopy in heart failure patients with sleep apnea. Chest 2008; 133(4):934–940 [Epub February 8, 2008].
41. Leung RS, Diep TM, Bowman ME, et al. Provocation of ventricular ectopy by Cheyne-Stokes respiration in patients with heart failure. Sleep 2004; 27:1337–1343.
42. Serizawa T, Vogel WM, Apstein CS, et al. Comparison of acute alterations in left ventricular relaxation and diastolic chamber stiffness induced by hypoxia and ischemia. Role of myocardial oxygen supply-demand imbalance. J Clin Invest 1981; 68:91–102.
43. Bonsignore MR, Romano S, Marrone O, et al. Different heart rate patterns in obstructive apneas during NREM sleep. Sleep 1997; 20:1167–1174.
44. Nakao K, Ohgushi M, Yoshimura M, et al. Hyperventilation as a specific test for diagnosis of coronary artery spasm. Am J Cardiol 1997; 80:545–549.
45. Barrabes JA, Garcia-Dorado D, Padilla F, et al. Ventricular fibrillation during acute coronary occlusion is related to the dilation of the ischemic region. Basic Res Cardiol 2002; 97:445–451.
46. Coronel R, Wilms-Schopman FJ, deGroot JR. Origin of ischemia-induced phase 1b ventricular arrhythmias in pig hearts. J Am Coll Cardiol 2002; 39:166–176.
47. Beardslee MA, Lerner DL, Tadros PN, et al. Dephosphorylation and intracellular redistribution of ventricular connexin43 during electrical uncoupling induced by ischemia. Circ Res 2000; 87:656–662.
48. Wu J, McHowat J, Saffitz JE, et al. Inhibition of gap junctional conductance by long-chain acylcarnitines and their preferential accumulation in junctional sarcolemma during hypoxia. Circ Res 1993; 72:879–889.
49. Shepard JW Jr., Garrison MW, Grither DA, et al. Relationship of ventricular ectopy to oxyhemoglobin desaturation in patients with obstructive sleep apnea. Chest 1985; 88:335–340.
50. Willich SN, Goldberg RJ, Maclure M, et al. Increased onset of sudden cardiac death in the first three hours after awakening. Am J Cardiol 1992; 70:65–68.
51. Tofler GH, Gebara OC, Mittleman MA, et al. Morning peak in ventricular tachyarrhythmias detected by time of implantable cardioverter/defibrillator therapy. The CPI Investigators. Circulation 1995; 92:1203–1208.
52. Naughton M, Benard D, Tam A, et al. Role of hyperventilation in the pathogenesis of central sleep apneas in patients with congestive heart failure. Am Rev Respir Dis 1993; 148:330–338.

53. Xie A, Wong B, Phillipson EA, et al. Interaction of hyperventilation and arousal in the pathogenesis of idiopathic central sleep apnea. Am J Respir Crit Care Med 1994; 150:489–495.
54. Horner RL, Rivera MP, Kozar LF, et al. The ventilatory response to arousal from sleep is not fully explained by differences in CO(2) levels between sleep and wakefulness. J Physiol 2001; 534:881–890.
55. O'Donnell CP, Ayuse T, King ED, et al. Airway obstruction during sleep increases blood pressure without arousal. J Appl Physiol 1996; 80:773–781.
56. Trinder J, Merson R, Rosenberg JI, et al. Pathophysiological interactions of ventilation, arousals, and blood pressure oscillations during cheyne-stokes respiration in patients with heart failure. Am J Respir Crit Care Med 2000; 162:808–813.
57. Naughton MT, Benard DC, Liu PP, et al. Effects of nasal CPAP on sympathetic activity in patients with heart failure and central sleep apnea. Am J Respir Crit Care Med 1995; 152:473–479.
58. Horner RL, Brooks D, Kozar LF, et al. Immediate effects of arousal from sleep on cardiac autonomic outflow in the absence of breathing in dogs. J Appl Physiol 1995; 79:151–162.
59. Suzuki M, Ogawa H, Okabe S, et al. Digital recording and analysis of esophageal pressure for patients with obstructive sleep apnea-hypopnea syndrome. Sleep Breath 2005; 9:64–72.
60. White SG, Fletcher EC, Miller CC III. Acute systemic blood pressure elevation in obstructive and nonobstructive breath hold in primates. J Appl Physiol 1995; 79:324–330.
61. Chen L, Scharf SM. Comparative hemodynamic effects of periodic obstructive and simulated central apneas in sedated pigs. J Appl Physiol 1997; 83:485–494.
62. Bradley TD, Hall MJ, Ando S, et al. Hemodynamic effects of simulated obstructive apneas in humans with and without heart failure. Chest 2001; 119:1827–1835.
63. Franz MR. Mechano-electrical feedback in ventricular myocardium. Cardiovasc Res 1996; 32:15–24.
64. Somers VK, Dyken ME, Clary MP, et al. Sympathetic neural mechanisms in obstructive sleep apnea. J Clin Invest 1995; 96:1897–1904.
65. Hedner J, Ejnell H, Sellgren J, et al. Is high and fluctuating muscle nerve sympathetic activity in the sleep apnoea syndrome of pathogenetic importance for the development of hypertension? J Hypertens Suppl 1988; 6:S529–S531.
66. Leuenberger U, Jacob E, Sweet L, et al. Surges of muscle sympathetic nerve activity during obstructive apnea are linked to hypoxemia. J Appl Physiol 1995; 79:581–588.
67. Portaluppi F, Provini F, Cortelli P, et al. Undiagnosed sleep-disordered breathing among male nondippers with essential hypertension. J Hypertens 1997; 15:1227–1233.
68. Somers VK, Mark AL, Zavala DC, et al. Contrasting effects of hypoxia and hypercapnia on ventilation and sympathetic activity in humans. J Appl Physiol 1989; 67:2101–2106.
69. Lugliani R, Whipp BJ, Wasserman K. A role for the carotid body in cardiovascular control in man. Chest 1973; 63:744–750.
70. Bernthal T, Green W Jr., Revzin AM. Role of the carotid body chemoreceptors in hypoxic cardiac acceleration. Proc Soc Exp Biol Med 1951; 143:361–372.
71. Daly MdB, Scott MJ. The cardiovascular responses to stimulation of the carotid chemoreceptors in the dog. J Physiol 1963; 165:179–197.
72. Daly MdB, Scott MJ. The effects of stimulation of the carotid body chemoreceptors on heart rate in the dog. J Physiol 1958; 144:148–166.
73. Ponikowski P, Anker SD, Chua TP, et al. Oscillatory breathing patterns during wakefulness in patients with chronic heart failure: clinical implications and role of augmented peripheral chemosensitivity. Circulation 1999; 100:2418–2424.
74. Solin P, Roebuck T, Johns DP, et al. Peripheral and central ventilatory responses in central sleep apnea with and without congestive heart failure. Am J Respir Crit Care Med 2000; 162:2194–2200.

75. Guilleminault C, Connolly S, Winkle R, et al. Cyclical variation of the heart rate in sleep apnoea syndrome. Mechanisms, and usefulness of 24 h electrocardiography as a screening technique. Lancet 1984; 1:126–131.
76. Leung RS, Floras JS, Lorenzi-Filho G, et al. Influence of Cheyne-Stokes respiration on cardiovascular oscillations in heart failure. Am J Respir Crit Care Med 2003; 167:1534–1539.
77. Richardson DW, Wasserman AJ, Patterson JL Jr. General and regional circulatory responses to change in blood pH and carbon dioxide tension. J Clin Invest 1961; 40:31–43.
78. Wilcox I, McNamara SG, Dodd MJ, et al. Ventilatory control in patients with sleep apnoea and left ventricular dysfunction: comparison of obstructive and central sleep apnoea. Eur Respir J 1998; 11:7–13.
79. Javaheri S. A mechanism of central sleep apnea in patients with heart failure. N Engl J Med 1999; 341:949–954.
80. Narkiewicz K, Pesek CA, van de Borne PJ, et al. Enhanced sympathetic and ventilatory responses to central chemoreflex activation in heart failure. Circulation 1999; 100:262–267.
81. Enson Y, Giuntini C, Lewis ML, et al. The influence of hydrogen ion concentration and hypoxia on the pulmonary circulation. J Clin Invest 1964; 43:1146–1162.
82. De Caterina R, Libby P, Peng HB, et al. Nitric oxide decreases cytokine-induced endothelial activation. Nitric oxide selectively reduces endothelial expression of adhesion molecules and proinflammatory cytokines. J Clin Invest 1995; 96:60–68.
83. Dworakowski R, Alom-Ruiz SP, Shah AM. NADPH oxidase-derived reactive oxygen species in the regulation of endothelial phenotype. Pharmacol Rep 2008; 60:21–28.
84. Barnes PJ, Karin M. Nuclear factor-kappaB: a pivotal transcription factor in chronic inflammatory diseases. N Engl J Med 1997; 336:1066–1071.
85. Ross R. Atherosclerosis—an inflammatory disease. N Engl J Med 1999; 340:115–126.
86. Wolk R, Kara T, Somers VK. Sleep-disordered breathing and cardiovascular disease. Circulation 2003; 108:9–12.
87. Kato M, Roberts-Thomson P, Phillips BG, et al. Impairment of endothelium-dependent vasodilation of resistance vessels in patients with obstructive sleep apnea. Circulation 2000; 102:2607–2610.
88. Ip MS, Lam B, Chan LY, et al. Circulating nitric oxide is suppressed in obstructive sleep apnea and is reversed by nasal continuous positive airway pressure. Am J Respir Crit Care Med 2000; 162:2166–2171.
89. Schulz R, Schmidt D, Blum A, et al. Decreased plasma levels of nitric oxide derivatives in obstructive sleep apnoea: response to CPAP therapy. Thorax 2000; 55:1046–1051.
90. Jelic S, Padeletti M, Kawut SM, et al. Inflammation, oxidative stress, and repair capacity of the vascular endothelium in obstructive sleep apnea. Circulation 2008; 117:2270–2278.
91. Lorenz MW, Markus HS, Bots ML, et al. Prediction of clinical cardiovascular events with carotid intima-media thickness: a systematic review and meta-analysis. Circulation 2007; 115:459–467.
92. Savransky V, Nanayakkara A, Li J, et al. Chronic intermittent hypoxia induces atherosclerosis. Am J Respir Crit Care Med 2007; 175:1290–1297.
93. Drager LF, Bortolotto LA, Figueiredo AC, et al. Effects of continuous positive airway pressure on early signs of atherosclerosis in obstructive sleep apnea. Am J Respir Crit Care Med 2007; 176:706–712.
94. Libby P. Changing concepts of atherogenesis. J Intern Med 2000; 247:349–358.
95. Punjabi NM, Polotsky VY. Disorders of glucose metabolism in sleep apnea. J Appl Physiol 2005; 99:1998–2007.
96. Kelly RP, Tunin R, Kass DA. Effect of reduced aortic compliance on cardiac efficiency and contractile function of in situ canine left ventricle. Circ Res 1992; 71:490–502.
97. Urschel CW, Covell JW, Sonnenblick EH, et al. Effects of decreased aortic compliance on performance of the left ventricle. Am J Physiol 1968; 214:298–304.

98. Wilcken DE, Charlier AA, Hoffman JI, et al. Effects of alterations in aortic impedance on the performance of the ventricles. Circ Res 1964; 14:283–293.
99. Drager LF, Bortolotto LA, Figueiredo AC, et al. Obstructive sleep apnea, hypertension, and their interaction on arterial stiffness and heart remodeling. Chest 2007; 131:1379–1386.
100. Ganau A, Devereux RB, Roman MJ, et al. Patterns of left ventricular hypertrophy and geometric remodeling in essential hypertension. J Am Coll Cardiol 1992; 19:1550–1558.
101. Gerdes AM, Capasso JM. Structural remodeling and mechanical dysfunction of cardiac myocytes in heart failure. J Mol Cell Cardiol 1995; 27:849–856.
102. Swynghedauw B. Molecular mechanisms of myocardial remodeling. Physiol Rev 1999; 79:215–262.
103. Pogwizd SM, Schlotthauer K, Li L, et al. Arrhythmogenesis and contractile dysfunction in heart failure: roles of sodium-calcium exchange, inward rectifier potassium current, and residual beta-adrenergic responsiveness. Circ Res 2001; 88:1159–1167.
104. Lorell BH, Carabello BA. Left ventricular hypertrophy: pathogenesis, detection, and prognosis. Circulation 2000; 102:470–479.
105. Krauser DG, Devereux RB. Ventricular hypertrophy and hypertension: prognostic elements and implications for management. Herz 2006; 31:305–316.
106. Levy D, Garrison RJ, Savage DD, et al. Prognostic implications of echocardiographically determined left ventricular mass in the Framingham Heart Study. N Engl J Med 1990; 322:1561–1566.
107. Pfeffer MA, Braunwald E. Ventricular remodeling after myocardial infarction. Experimental observations and clinical implications. Circulation 1990; 81:1161–1172.
108. Verdecchia P, Schillaci G, Borgioni C, et al. Adverse prognostic significance of concentric remodeling of the left ventricle in hypertensive patients with normal left ventricular mass. J Am Coll Cardiol 1995; 25:871–878.
109. Fletcher EC, Bao G. The rat as a model of chronic recurrent episodic hypoxia and effect upon systemic blood pressure. Sleep 1996; 19:S210–S212.
110. Fletcher EC, Lesske J, Behm R, et al. Carotid chemoreceptors, systemic blood pressure, and chronic episodic hypoxia mimicking sleep apnea. J Appl Physiol 1992; 72;1978–1984.
111. Parker JD, Brooks D, Kozar LF, et al. Acute and chronic effects of airway obstruction on canine left ventricular performance. Am J Respir Crit Care Med 1999; 160:1888–1896.
112. Chen L, Einbinder E, Zhang Q, et al. Oxidative stress and left ventricular function with chronic intermittent hypoxia in rats. Am J Respir Crit Care Med 2005; 172:915–920.
113. Chen L, Zhang J, Gan TX, et al. Left ventricular dysfunction and associated cellular injury in rats exposed to chronic intermittent hypoxia. J Appl Physiol 2008; 104:218–223.
114. Hayashi T, Yamashita C, Matsumoto C, et al. Role of gp91phox-containing NADPH oxidase in left ventricular remodeling induced by intermittent hypoxic stress. Am J Physiol Heart Circ Physiol 2008; 294:H2197–H2203.
115. Barth W, Deten A, Bauer M, et al. Differential remodeling of the left and right heart after norepinephrine treatment in rats: studies on cytokines and collagen. J Mol Cell Cardiol 2000; 32:273–284.
116. Fung JW, Li TS, Choy DK, et al. Severe obstructive sleep apnea is associated with left ventricular diastolic dysfunction. Chest 2002; 121:422–429.
117. Niroumand M, Kuperstein R, Sasson Z, et al. Impact of obstructive sleep apnea on left ventricular mass and diastolic function. Am J Respir Crit Care Med 2001; 163:1632–1636.
118. Arias MA, Garcia-Rio F, Alonso-Fernandez A, et al. Obstructive sleep apnea syndrome affects left ventricular diastolic function: effects of nasal continuous positive airway pressure in men. Circulation 2005; 112:375–383.
119. Otto ME, Belohlavek M, Romero-Corral A, et al. Comparison of cardiac structural and functional changes in obese otherwise healthy adults with versus without obstructive sleep apnea. Am J Cardiol 2007; 99:1298–1302.

120. Dursunoglu N, Dursunoglu D, Ozkurt S, et al. Effects of CPAP on left ventricular structure and myocardial performance index in male patients with obstructive sleep apnoea. Sleep Med 2007; 8:51–59.

121. Shivalkar B, Van de Heyning C, Kerremans M, et al. Obstructive sleep apnea syndrome: more insights on structural and functional cardiac alterations, and the effects of treatment with continuous positive airway pressure. J Am Coll Cardiol 2006; 47:1433–1439.

122. Cohn JN, Ferrari R, Sharpe N. Cardiac remodeling—concepts and clinical implications: a consensus paper from an international forum on cardiac remodeling. Behalf of an International Forum on Cardiac Remodeling. J Am Coll Cardiol 2000; 35:569–582.

123. Opie LH, Commerford PJ, Gersh BJ, et al. Controversies in ventricular remodelling. Lancet 2006; 367:356–367.

124. Hedner J, Ejnell H, Caidahl K. Left ventricular hypertrophy independent of hypertension in patients with obstructive sleep apnoea. J Hypertens 1990; 8:941–946.

125. Noda A, Okada T, Yasuma F, et al. Cardiac hypertrophy in obstructive sleep apnea syndrome. Chest 1995; 107:1538–1544.

126. Amin RS, Kimball TR, Bean JA, et al. Left ventricular hypertrophy and abnormal ventricular geometry in children and adolescents with obstructive sleep apnea. Am J Respir Crit Care Med 2002; 165:1395–1399.

127. Davies RJ, Crosby J, Prothero A, et al. Ambulatory blood pressure and left ventricular hypertrophy in subjects with untreated obstructive sleep apnoea and snoring, compared with matched control subjects, and their response to treatment. Clin Sci (Colch) 1994; 86:417–424.

128. Haider AW, Larson MG, Benjamin EJ, et al. Increased left ventricular mass and hypertrophy are associated with increased risk for sudden death. J Am Coll Cardiol 1998; 32:1454–1459.

129. McLenachan JM, Henderson E, Morris KI, et al. Ventricular arrhythmias in patients with hypertensive left ventricular hypertrophy. N Engl J Med 1987; 317:787–792.

130. Okin PM, Devereux RB, Jern S, et al. Regression of electrocardiographic left ventricular hypertrophy during antihypertensive treatment and the prediction of major cardiovascular events. JAMA 2004; 292:2343–2349.

131. Rials SJ, Wu Y, Xu X, et al. Regression of left ventricular hypertrophy with captopril restores normal ventricular action potential duration, dispersion of refractoriness, and vulnerability to inducible ventricular fibrillation. Circulation 1997; 96:1330–1336.

132. Quinones MA, Greenberg BH, Kopelen HA, et al. Echocardiographic predictors of clinical outcome in patients with left ventricular dysfunction enrolled in the SOLVD registry and trials: significance of left ventricular hypertrophy. Studies of Left Ventricular Dysfunction. J Am Coll Cardiol 2000; 35:1237–1244.

133. Cohn JN. Structural basis for heart failure. Ventricular remodeling and its pharmacological inhibition. Circulation 1995; 91:2504–2507.

134. Laaban JP, Pascal-Sebaoun S, Bloch E, et al. Left ventricular systolic dysfunction in patients with obstructive sleep apnea syndrome. Chest 2002; 122:1133–1138.

135. Alonso-Fernandez A, Garcia-Rio F, Arias MA, et al. Obstructive sleep apnoea-hypoapnoea syndrome reversibly depresses cardiac response to exercise. Eur Heart J 2006; 27:207–215.

136. Romero-Corral A, Somers VK, Pellikka PA, et al. Decreased right and left ventricular myocardial performance in obstructive sleep apnea. Chest 2007; 132:1863–1870.

137. Kanagala R, Murali NS, Friedman PA, et al. Obstructive sleep apnea and the recurrence of atrial fibrillation. Circulation 2003; 107:2589–2594.

138. Carlson JT, Hedner J, Elam M, et al. Augmented resting sympathetic activity in awake patients with obstructive sleep apnea. Chest 1993; 103:1763–1768.

139. Narkiewicz K, Montano N, Cogliati C, et al. Altered cardiovascular variability in obstructive sleep apnea. Circulation 1998; 98:1071–1077.

140. Fletcher EC, Miller J, Schaaf JW, et al. Urinary catecholamines before and after tracheostomy in patients with obstructive sleep apnea and hypertension. Sleep 1987; 10:35–44.
141. Hedner J, Darpo B, Ejnell H, et al. Reduction in sympathetic activity after long-term CPAP treatment in sleep apnoea: cardiovascular implications. Eur Respir J 1995; 8:222–229.
142. Narkiewicz K, Kato M, Phillips BG, et al. Nocturnal continuous positive airway pressure decreases daytime sympathetic traffic in obstructive sleep apnea. Circulation 1999; 100:2332–2335.
143. Waradekar NV, Sinoway LI, Zwillich CW, et al. Influence of treatment on muscle sympathetic nerve activity in sleep apnea. Am J Respir Crit Care Med 1996; 153:1333–1338.
144. Kleiger RE, Miller JP, Bigger JT Jr., et al. Decreased heart rate variability and its association with increased mortality after acute myocardial infarction. Am J Cardiol 1987; 59:256–262.
145. Ponikowski P, Anker SD, Chua TP, et al. Depressed heart rate variability as an independent predictor of death in chronic congestive heart failure secondary to ischemic or idiopathic dilated cardiomyopathy. Am J Cardiol 1997; 79:1645–1650.
146. Task. Heart rate variability: standards of measurement, physiological interpretation and clinical use. Task Force of the European Society of Cardiology and the North American Society of Pacing and Electrophysiology. Circulation 1996; 93:1043–1065.
147. Noda A, Yasuma F, Okada T, et al. Circadian rhythm of autonomic activity in patients with obstructive sleep apnea syndrome. Clin Cardiol 1998; 21:271–276.
148. Wiklund U, Olofsson BO, Franklin K, et al. Autonomic cardiovascular regulation in patients with obstructive sleep apnoea: a study based on spectral analysis of heart rate variability. Clin Physiol 2000; 20:234–241.
149. Khoo MC, Kim TS, Berry RB. Spectral indices of cardiac autonomic function in obstructive sleep apnea. Sleep 1999; 22:443–451.
150. Roche F, Court-Fortune I, Pichot V, et al. Reduced cardiac sympathetic autonomic tone after long-term nasal continuous positive airway pressure in obstructive sleep apnoea syndrome. Clin Physiol 1999; 19:127–134.
151. Spaak J, Egri ZJ, Kubo T, et al. Muscle sympathetic nerve activity during wakefulness in heart failure patients with and without sleep apnea. Hypertension 2005; 46:1327–1332.
152. Bradley TD, Tkacova R, Hall MJ, et al. Augmented sympathetic neural response to simulated obstructive apnoea in human heart failure. Clin Sci (Lond).2003; 104:231–238.
153. Usui K, Bradley TD, Spaak J, et al. Inhibition of awake sympathetic nerve activity of heart failure patients with obstructive sleep apnea by nocturnal continuous positive airway pressure. J Am Coll Cardiol 2005; 45:2008–2011.
154. Solin P, Kaye DM, Little PJ, et al. Impact of sleep apnea on sympathetic nervous system activity in heart failure. Chest 2003; 123:1119–1126.
155. Mansfield D, Kaye DM, Brunner La Rocca H, et al. Raised sympathetic nerve activity in heart failure and central sleep apnea is due to heart failure severity. Circulation 2003; 107:1396–1400.
156. Mansfield DR, Gollogly NC, Kaye DM, et al. Controlled trial of continuous positive airway pressure in obstructive sleep apnea and heart failure. Am J Respir Crit Care Med 2004; 169:361–366.
157. Saul JP, Arai Y, Berger RD, et al. Assessment of autonomic regulation in chronic congestive heart failure by heart rate spectral analysis. Am J Cardiol 1988; 61:1292–1299.
158. Lanfranchi PA, Braghiroli A, Bosimini E, et al. Prognostic value of nocturnal Cheyne-Stokes respiration in chronic heart failure. Circulation 1999; 99:1435–1440.
159. Mortara A, Sleight P, Pinna GD, et al. Abnormal awake respiratory patterns are common in chronic heart failure and may prevent evaluation of autonomic tone by measures of heart rate variability. Circulation 1997; 96:246–252.

160. Gilman MP, Floras JS, Usui K, et al. Continuous positive airway pressure increases heart rate variability in heart failure patients with obstructive sleep apnoea. Clin Sci (Lond) 2008; 114:243–249.

161. Brodde OE, Bruck H, Leineweber K. Cardiac adrenoceptors: physiological and pathophysiological relevance. J Pharmacol Sci 2006; 100:323–337.

162. Leineweber K, Heusch G, Schulz R. Regulation and role of the presynaptic and myocardial Na$^+$/H$^+$ exchanger NHE1: effects on the sympathetic nervous system in heart failure. Cardiovasc Drug Rev 2007; 25:123–131.

163. Patel MB, Stewart JM, Loud AV, et al. Altered function and structure of the heart in dogs with chronic elevation in plasma norepinephrine. Circulation 1991; 84:2091–2100.

164. Simpson P. Norepinephrine-stimulated hypertrophy of cultured rat myocardial cells is an alpha 1 adrenergic response. J Clin Invest 1983; 72:732–738.

165. Schlaich MP, Kaye DM, Lambert E, et al. Relation between cardiac sympathetic activity and hypertensive left ventricular hypertrophy. Circulation 2003; 108:560–565.

166. Reiken S, Gaburjakova M, Gaburjakova J, et al. Beta-adrenergic receptor blockers restore cardiac calcium release channel (ryanodine receptor) structure and function in heart failure. Circulation 2001; 104:2843–2848.

167. Wehrens XH, Lehnart SE, Huang F, et al. FKBP12.6 deficiency and defective calcium release channel (ryanodine receptor) function linked to exercise-induced sudden cardiac death. Cell 2003; 113:829–840.

168. Marx SO, Reiken S, Hisamatsu Y, et al. PKA phosphorylation dissociates FKBP12.6 from the calcium release channel (ryanodine receptor): defective regulation in failing hearts. Cell 2000; 101:365–376.

169. Cohn JN, Levine TB, Olivari MT, et al. Plasma norepinephrine as a guide to prognosis in patients with chronic congestive heart failure. N Engl J Med 1984; 311:819–823.

170. Kaye DM, Lefkovits J, Jennings GL, et al. Adverse consequences of high sympathetic nervous activity in the failing human heart. J Am Coll Cardiol 1995; 26:1257–1263.

171. Pliquett RU, Fasshauer M, Bluher M, et al. Neurohumoral stimulation in type-2-diabetes as an emerging disease concept. Cardiovasc Diabetol 2004; 3:4.

172. Hoffstein V, Mateika S. Cardiac arrhythmias, snoring, and sleep apnea. Chest 1994; 106: 466–471.

173. Miller WP. Cardiac arrhythmias and conduction disturbances in the sleep apnea syndrome. Prevalence and significance. Am J Med 1982; 73:317–321.

174. Flemons WW, Remmers JE, Gillis AM. Sleep apnea and cardiac arrhythmias. Is there a relationship? Am Rev Respir Dis 1993; 148:618–621.

175. Laaban JP, Cassuto D, Orvoen-Frija E, et al. Cardiorespiratory consequences of sleep apnoea syndrome in patients with massive obesity. Eur Respir J 1998; 11:20–27.

176. Koehler U, Schafer H. Is obstructive sleep apnea (OSA) a risk factor for myocardial infarction and cardiac arrhythmias in patients with coronary heart disease (CHD)? Sleep 1996; 19:283–286.

177. Tilkian AG, Guilleminault C, Schroeder JS, et al. Sleep-induced apnea syndrome. Prevalence of cardiac arrhythmias and their reversal after tracheostomy. Am J Med 1977; 63:348–358.

178. Becker H, Brandenburg U, Peter JH, et al. Reversal of sinus arrest and atrioventricular conduction block in patients with sleep apnea during nasal continuous positive airway pressure. Am J Respir Crit Care Med 1995; 151:215–218.

179. Koehler U, Becker HF, Grimm W, et al. Relations among hypoxemia, sleep stage, and bradyarrhythmia during obstructive sleep apnea. Am Heart J 2000; 139:142–148.

180. Zwillich C, Devlin T, White D, et al. Bradycardia during sleep apnea. Characteristics and mechanism. J Clin Invest 1982; 69:1286–1292.

181. Douglas NJ, White DP, Weil JV, et al. Hypoxic ventilatory response decreases during sleep in normal men. Am Rev Respir Dis 1982; 125:286–289.

182. Sato F, Nishimura M, Shinano H, et al. Heart rate during obstructive sleep apnea depends on individual hypoxic chemosensitivity of the carotid body. Circulation 1997; 96:274–281.
183. Kato H, Menon AS, Slutsky AS. Mechanisms mediating the heart rate response to hypoxemia. Circulation 1988; 77:407–414.
184. Grimm W, Hoffmann J, Menz V, et al. Electrophysiologic evaluation of sinus node function and atrioventricular conduction in patients with prolonged ventricular asystole during obstructive sleep apnea. Am J Cardiol 1996; 77:1310–1314.
185. Hinkle LE Jr., Carver ST, Stevens M. The frequency of asymptomatic disturbances of cardiac rhythm and conduction in middle-aged men. Am J Cardiol 1969; 24(5):629–650.
186. Canada WB, Woodward W, Lee G, et al. Circadian rhythm of hourly ventricular arrhythmia frequency in man. Angiology 1983; 34:274–282.
187. Franklin KA, Nilsson JB, Sahlin C, et al. Sleep apnoea and nocturnal angina. Lancet 1995; 345:1085–1087.
188. Cleland JG, Chattopadhyay S, Khand A, et al. Prevalence and incidence of arrhythmias and sudden death in heart failure. Heart Fail Rev 2002; 7:229–242.
189. Javaheri S. Effects of continuous positive airway pressure on sleep apnea and ventricular irritability in patients with heart failure. Circulation 2000; 101:392–397.
190. Findley LJ, Blackburn MR, Goldberger AL, et al. Apneas and oscillation of cardiac ectopy in Cheyne-Stokes breathing during sleep. Am Rev Respir Dis 1984; 130:937–939.
191. Bartall HZ, Tye KH, Roper P, et al. Atrial flutter associated with obstructive sleep apnea syndrome. A case report. Arch Intern Med 1980; 140:121–122.
192. Gami AS, Pressman G, Caples SM, et al. Association of atrial fibrillation and obstructive sleep apnea. Circulation 2004; 110:364–367.
193. Olmetti F, La Rovere MT, Robbi E, et al. Nocturnal cardiac arrhythmia in patients with obstructive sleep apnea. Sleep Med 2008; 9:475–480.
194. Mooe T, Gullsby S, Rabben T, et al. Sleep-disordered breathing: a novel predictor of atrial fibrillation after coronary artery bypass surgery. Coron Artery Dis 1996; 7:475–478.
195. Tanigawa T, Yamagishi K, Sakurai S, et al. Arterial oxygen desaturation during sleep and atrial fibrillation. Heart 2006; 92:1854–1855.
196. Gami AS, Hodge DO, Herges RM, et al. Obstructive sleep apnea, obesity, and the risk of incident atrial fibrillation. J Am Coll Cardiol 2007; 49:565–571.
197. Porthan KM, Melin JH, Kupila JT, et al. Prevalence of sleep apnea syndrome in lone atrial fibrillation: a case-control study. Chest 2004; 125:879–885.
198. Fietze I, Rottig J, Quispe-Bravo S, et al. Sleep apnea syndrome in patients with cardiac pacemaker. Respiration 2000; 67:268–271.
199. Geigel EJ, Chediak AD. Theophylline therapy for near-fatal Cheyne-Stokes respiration. Ann Intern Med 1999; 131:713–714.
200. Padeletti L, Gensini GF, Pieragnoli P, et al. The risk profile for obstructive sleep apnea does not affect the recurrence of atrial fibrillation. Pacing Clin Electrophysiol 2006; 29:727–732.
201. Sauer WH, McKernan ML, Lin D, et al. Clinical predictors and outcomes associated with acute return of pulmonary vein conduction during pulmonary vein isolation for treatment of atrial fibrillation. Heart Rhythm 2006; 3:1024–1028.
202. Javaheri S. Sleep disorders in systolic heart failure: a prospective study of 100 male patients. The final report. Int J Cardiol 2006; 106:21–28.
203. Leung RS, Huber MA, Rogge T, et al. Association between atrial fibrillation and central sleep apnea. Sleep 2005; 28:1543–1546.
204. Harbison J, O'Reilly P, McNicholas WT. Cardiac rhythm disturbances in the obstructive sleep apnea syndrome: effects of nasal continuous positive airway pressure therapy. Chest 2000; 118:591–595.

205. Ryan CM, Usui K, Floras JS, et al. Effect of continuous positive airway pressure on ventricular ectopy in heart failure patients with obstructive sleep apnoea. Thorax 2005; 60:781–785.
206. Bradley TD, Logan AG, Kimoff RJ, et al. Continuous positive airway pressure for central sleep apnea and heart failure. N Engl J Med 2005; 353:2025–2033.
207. Arzt M, Floras JS, Logan AG, et al. Suppression of central sleep apnea by continuous positive airway pressure and transplant-free survival in heart failure: a post hoc analysis of the Canadian Continuous Positive Airway Pressure for Patients with Central Sleep Apnea and Heart Failure trial (CANPAP). Circulation 2007; 115:3173–3180.
208. Teschler H, Dohring J, Wang YM, et al. Adaptive pressure support servo-ventilation. A novel treatment for Cheyne-Stokes respiration in heart failure. Am J Respir Crit Care Med 2001; 164:614–619.

13
Obstructive Sleep Apnea and Atherosclerosis

GERALDO LORENZI-FILHO and LUCIANO F. DRAGER
University of São Paulo, São Paulo, Brazil

I. Introduction

There is now evidence that obstructive sleep apnea (OSA) is associated with increased risk of myocardial infarction and stroke, independent of confounding factors (1–3). Atherosclerosis is a common pathological factor underlying all types of cardiovascular diseases and is the leading cause of coronary heart disease, stroke, and peripheral vascular disease (4). Therefore, atherosclerosis is an attractive intermediate mechanism to explain the link between OSA and cardiovascular morbidity and mortality (5). The mechanisms whereby OSA may contribute to atherosclerosis, however, are under investigation and not completely understood. Patients with OSA frequently present with one or several features of metabolic syndrome, including hypertension, central obesity, insulin resistance, and dyslipidemia. These are well-known risk factors for atherosclerosis (5). This observation raises the question of whether OSA is simply a marker that clusters with previously recognized and well-established risk factors for atherosclerosis. In this chapter, we shall explore the evidence that OSA is not simply an innocent bystander but may directly contribute to atherosclerosis.

There is now mounting evidence that OSA is not simply associated with but may trigger or contribute to hypertension (6), diabetes (7), and insulin resistance (8). These powerful mechanisms by which OSA may contribute to atherosclerosis are also discussed in other chapters of this book. In addition to this indirect link, this chapter will particularly explore the evidence that supports a direct causal link between OSA and atherosclerosis. The evidence of a causal link between OSA and atherosclerosis will be explored based on the criteria established by Koch in the 19th century to attribute an etiological agent to a disease. Although Koch's postulates were developed to test the causal relationship between infectious organism and a given disease, the rationale required to prove causality can be adapted and applied to other diseases such as OSA and atherosclerosis (9).

Following this line, the first question becomes, is there biological plausibility to support the hypothesis that OSA contributes to atherosclerosis? To answer this question, we will briefly review the knowledge about vascular biology, pathology, and risk factors for atherosclerosis. Compared with other well-known risk factors for atherosclerosis, such as smoking, hypertension, and hyperlipidemia (9), the studies on the association between OSA and atherosclerosis are in their infancy. Although the vast literature about atherosclerosis ignores OSA, this approach will provide a framework that may help shed light on the link between OSA and atherosclerosis. Second, according to an adaptation of Koch's postulate, a causal relationship between OSA and atherosclerosis will be explored in animal and in vitro studies. Third, small and well-controlled human studies as well as epidemiological studies will be presented to prove independent associations between OSA and atherosclerosis. As commented earlier, the perennial limitation of human studies is that the typical patient with OSA carries several risk factors for cardiovascular disease, including increasing age, obesity, hypertension, diabetes, and hyperlipidemia. One possibility to overcome this limitation is to focus on a small and well-selected group of OSA patients free of comorbidities and medications. Alternatively, epidemiological studies that include a large number of patients attempt to control for these confounding variables by statistical modeling. Another important tool is the use of continuous positive airway pressure (CPAP), a treatment that is well standardized and is able to virtually abolish OSA without major changes in confounding variables. Therefore, well-controlled treatment studies may provide further evidence for the independent cause-and-effect association between OSA and atherosclerosis. Collectively, studies using different models are very consistent and support the concept of a direct link between OSA and atherosclerosis by showing that it is biologically plausible and that OSA is independently associated with atherosclerosis in animal models and humans. There is good evidence that OSA may trigger a cascade of key factors involved in the genesis of atherosclerosis, including systemic inflammation, oxidative stress, vascular smooth cell activation, increased adhesion molecule expression, lymphocyte activation, increased lipid lowering in macrophages, lipid peroxidation, high-density lipoprotein dysfunction, and endothelial dysfunction (5). One major limitation in this area is that, in contrast to other cardiovascular outcomes that are easy to measure (for instance, hypertension), atherosclerosis is primarily a pathological alteration at the level of arteries. Human studies must therefore rely on surrogate markers of atherosclerosis. Finally, we shall critically review the large OSA treatment studies that, according to Koch's postulate, should show a reduction in cardiovascular events (9). The major limitation is that hard endpoints associated with atherosclerosis, such as myocardial infarction and stroke, are relatively rare events and bring the necessity of large randomized treatment studies that are not available to date. Therefore, we shall end up by discussing future areas of research.

II. Pathophysiology of Atherosclerosis

Atherosclerosis has traditionally been viewed to simply result from chronic deposition of lipids within the vessel wall of the medium-sized and large arteries. However, this concept has dramatically changed over the last two decades. The three key concepts that must be taken into account are (*i*) inflammation, occurring at the wall of the arteries, plays a major role in the genesis of atherosclerosis; (*ii*) the endothelial layer of the arteries and veins is not passive but may be regarded as an active organ that modulates vessel tone and inflammation; and (*iii*) atherosclerosis is a slow process that starts early in life and is the end result of multiple mechanisms (9,10).

In addition to the deposition of elevated and modified low-density lipoprotein (LDL) in the endothelium, several mechanisms and pathways are important in this process, including free radicals, infectious microorganisms, hypertension, shear stress, and toxins associated with smoking. Frequently, the combination of these and other factors leads to a compensatory inflammatory response at the endothelial level (11,12).

Endothelial dysfunction, once established, causes greater retention of LDL in the sub-endothelial space and further activates intracellular signaling molecules involved in gene expression (13). Upregulation of cell adhesion molecules on the endothelial surface facilitates the attraction of monocytes and lymphocytes to the arterial wall (14). Once the blood cells have attached, chemokines produced in the underlying intima stimulate them to migrate through the interendothelial junctions and into the sub-endothelial space (12). A cytokine or growth factor produced in the inflamed intima, macrophage colony-stimulating factor, induces monocytes entering the plaque to differentiate into macrophages (12). Macrophages that have been modified by oxidized LDL release a variety of inflammatory substances, cytokines, and growth factors. Uptake of strongly oxidized lipoproteins via scavenger receptors is known to promote foam cell formation in vitro and is thought to play a central role in atherogenesis. Among the many molecules that have been implicated in this process are monocyte chemotactic protein 1 (MCP-1) (15–17); intercellular adhesion molecule 1 (ICAM-1) (16); macrophage and granulocyte-macrophage colony-stimulating factors (17,18); soluble CD40 ligand (19); interleukin-1 (IL-1), IL-3, IL-8, and IL-18 (20–23); and tumor necrosis factor alpha (24,25). The key events involved in the genesis of atherosclerosis are summarized in Figure 1.

Cytokines play a pivotal role in the pathogenesis of atherosclerosis (27). The release of proinflammatory cytokines is stimulated by LDL modification, free-radical formation, hemodynamic stress, hypertension, and infection. These cytokines, especially IL-1 and tumor necrosis factor alpha, have a multitude of atherogenic effects. They enhance the expression of cell surface molecules such as ICAM-1, vascular cell adhesion molecule 1 (VCAM-1), CD40, CD40L, and selectins on endothelial cells, smooth muscle cells, and macrophages. Proinflammatory cytokines can also induce cell proliferation, contribute to the production of reactive oxygen species, stimulate matrix metalloproteinases, and induce tissue factor expression. Other cytokines, such as IL-4 and IL-10, are antiatherogenic.

A. The Antiatherosclerotic Effects of High-Density Lipoprotein

The high-density lipoprotein (HDL) particle consists of an outer hydrophobic layer of free cholesterol, phospholipid, and several apolipoproteins (apo A-I, AII, C, E, AIV, J, and D) on the surface. Apolipoprotein A-1 is the principal protein of HDL. Plasma HDL levels bear a strong independent inverse relationship with atherosclerotic cardiovascular disease. Although HDL has antioxidant, anti-inflammatory, vasodilating, and antithrombotic properties, the major hypothesis to explain the antiatherogenic properties of HDL is that HDL promotes a process of reverse cholesterol transport from arteries to the liver (28). The specific process involving efflux of cholesterol from macrophage foam cells in the artery wall has been termed macrophage reverse cholesterol transport (29) and is thought to be central to the antiatherogenic properties of HDL. The principal molecules involved in efflux of cholesterol from macrophage foam cells are adenosine triphosphate (ATP)-binding cassette transporter A1 (ABCA1) and ATP-binding cassette transporter gene G1 (ABCG1). ABCA1 is primarily responsible for the initiation of HDL formation, principally in the liver, and stimulates cholesterol efflux to lipid-poor apolipoproteins, while ABCG1 promotes efflux of cholesterol and oxysterols to HDL (30). An important lipid transfer protein, lecithin:cholesterol acyltransferase (LCAT), esterifies cholesterol on HDL particles, and this activity may help drive cholesterol efflux via passive efflux or the ABCG1 pathway. Another lipid transfer protein, cholesteryl ester transfer protein

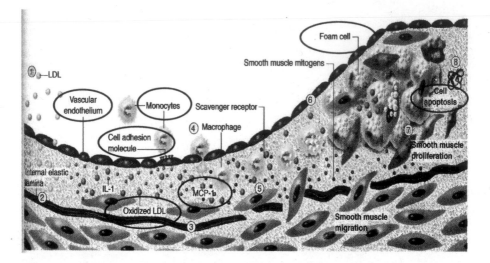

Figure 1 Pathogenesis of atherosclerosis. Schematic of the evolution of the atherosclerosis plaque. (**1**) Accumulation and modification of lipoprotein particles in the intima. Modifications include oxidation and glycation. (**2**) Oxidative stress, including products found in modified lipoproteins, can induce cytokine elaboration. (**3**) The cytokines thus induced increase expression of adhesion molecules for leukocytes that cause their attachment and chemoattractant molecules that direct their migration into the intima. (**4**) Blood monocytes, upon entering the artery wall in response to chemoattractant cytokines such as MCP-1. (**5**) Scavenger receptors mediate the uptake of modified lipoprotein particles and promote the development of foam cells (an important source of further cytokines). (**6**) Smooth muscle cells in the intima divide other smooth muscle cells that migrate into the intima from the media. (**7**) Smooth muscle cells can then divide and elaborate extracellular matrix, promoting extracellular matrix accumulation in the growing atherosclerotic plaque. (**8**) In the later stages, calcification can occur and fibrosis continues, sometimes accompanied by cell apoptosis. Circled text represent current evidences in OSA. *Abbreviations*: MCP-1, monocyte chemoattractant protein 1; IL-1, interleukin-1; LDL, low-density lipoprotein; OSA, obstructive sleep apnea. *Source*: Reproduced from Ref. 26.

(CETP), transfers cholesteryl ester from HDL to triglyceride-rich lipoproteins and to LDL as well as triglyceride from triglyceride-rich lipoproteins to HDL (31). In addition, HDLs have also been shown to increase endothelial nitric oxide synthase (eNOS) activity and protein levels in cultured endothelial cells (32) and to reverse the oxidized LDL-mediated decrease in nitric oxide (NO) production in endothelial cells (33). In humans, elevated HDL levels are less likely to be associated with abnormal vasoconstrictor responses in response to acetylcholine over diseased segments of coronary arteries (34).

B. Histological Changes

The first phase in atherosclerosis histologically presents as focal thickening of the intima with an increase in smooth muscle cells and extracellular matrix (35). These smooth muscle cells, which are possibly derived from hematopoietic stem cells (36), migrate and proliferate within the intima. This is followed by accumulation of intracellular lipid deposits or extracellular lipids or both, which produce the fatty streak. As these lesions expand, more smooth muscle cells migrate into the intima. The smooth muscle cells within the deep layer of the fatty streak are susceptible to apoptosis, which is associated with further macrophage infiltration, perhaps contributing to the transition of fatty streaks into atherosclerotic plaques (37). As atherosclerotic plaques develop and expand, they acquire their own microvascular network (*vasa vasorum*) extending from the adventitia through the media and into the thickened intima. These thin-walled vessels are prone to disruption, leading to hemorrhage within the substance of the plaque (38). Another phenomenon commonly observed in the progression of atherosclerosis is positive artery remodeling, a condition defined as a positive correlation between plaque and the external elastic membrane area due to a compensatory increase in a local vessel size in response to increasing plaque burden (39). This condition has been felt to be a compensatory mechanism in early artery disease, preventing luminal loss despite plaque accumulation.

C. Atherosclerosis and Cardiovascular Events

Atherosclerosis is generally asymptomatic. Plaque stenosis that exceeds 70% or 80% can produce a critical reduction in flow. These large lesions can, for instance, produce typical symptoms of angina pectoris. However, acute coronary and cerebrovascular syndromes (unstable angina, myocardial infarction, sudden death, and stroke) are typically due to rupture of plaques with less than 50% stenosis (40,41). Activated macrophages, T cells, and mast cells at sites of plaque rupture produce several types of molecules—inflammatory cytokines, proteases, coagulation factors, radicals, and vasoactive molecules that can destabilize lesions (11). All these factors inhibit the formation of stable fibrous caps, attack collagen in the cap, and initiate thrombus formation. These reactions can conceivably induce the activation and rupture of plaque, thrombosis, and ischemia. However, despite the significant advances in the pathogenesis of atherosclerosis, our present capacity to prevent plaque instability is poor.

D. Risk Factors for Atherosclerosis

Several well-established risk factors could be involved in the initiation, progression, and instability of the atherosclerosis process (Table 1). As a complex disease, multiple genetic and environmental factors frequently interact in the same individual to determine

Table 1 Traditional and Novel Atherosclerotic Risk Factors

Traditional risk factors	Novel risk factors[a]
Aging	C-reactive protein
Family history of coronary heart disease	Homocysteine
Family history of stroke	Fibrinogen
Hypertension	Fibrin D-dimer
Diabetes	Lipoprotein (a)
Hyperlipidemia	Tissue palsminogen activator and plasminogen activator inhibitor 1
Smoking	
Mental stress/depression	
Obesity	
Physical inactivity	

[a]Some of them there is no definitive consensus.
Source: Adapted from Ref. 9.

a particular clinical presentation. There is compelling evidence that atherosclerosis is likely to be caused by genetic variation in multiple cardiovascular candidate genes that individually exert a small effect on the development of peripheral arterial disease. Some risk factors, such as aging, are nonmodifiable. However, the majority of the risk factors for atherosclerosis can be modified with lifestyle changes and therapeutic opportunities. Recent discoveries of novel factors (Table 1) should improve risk estimation.

III. The Causal Link between Obstructive Sleep Apnea and Atherosclerosis

OSA is associated with three key acute mechanisms that may be deleterious to the cardiovascular system: recurrent asphyxia, arousals from sleep, and generation of negative intrathoracic pressure during futile efforts to breathe. Most animal models duplicate some but not all of these key features of OSA. On the other hand, the evidence in humans is usually hampered by the fact that the typical OSA patient presents with multiple risk factors for atherosclerosis, including dyslipidemia, hypertension, diabetes, smoking, and obesity.

IV. Experimental Studies

Animal studies are able to isolate one single mechanism associated with OSA and explore its cardiovascular effects. The most studied mechanism and the one that is thought to play the key role in the genesis of cardiovascular effects of OSA is intermittent hypoxia.

A. Animal Models

Interest in evaluating the link between hypoxia and atherosclerosis is not new. Several hypoxic models have been investigated. Studies on the impact of sustained hypoxia on atherosclerosis development are not new (42–45). In 1969, Kjeldsen et al. showed that hyperoxia reversed the atheromatosis in aorta of rabbits and suggested that hypoxia was atherogenic (46).

Helin et al. described for the first time the impact of intermittent hypoxia in the development of atherosclerosis in rabbits (47). These authors studied male albino rabbits exposed to intermittent nitrogen breathing every 30 seconds for 5 seconds, 15 minutes daily, over a period of three weeks, and every 30 seconds for 5 seconds over a period of 10 hours. A third group of animals was exposed continuously to 8% oxygen breathing for two weeks. The authors found that neither intermittent nor continuous hypoxia induced gross or microscopic alteration in the aorta. In contrast, the exposure to intermittent hypoxia for longer periods (>2 weeks) promoted significant reduction in the synthesis of glycosaminoglycans. Reductions of glycosaminoglycans compromise the mechanical properties of the aorta and lead to impaired healing of vascular injury (47). Despite this evidence, the model adopted by the pivotal study of Helin et al. was not designed to mimic the intermittent hypoxia commonly observed in patients with OSA.

Studies employing suitable models of sleep apnea have been developed only recently. The best evidences regarding the impact of intermittent hypoxia and atherosclerosis has been provided by Polotsky's group in Baltimore. Using adult male C57BL/6J mice, a murine model with low susceptibility to diet-induced atherosclerosis, this group described several pathways that predispose this strain to atherosclerosis after intermittent hypoxia. The protocol applied intermittent hypoxia capable of reducing FiO_2 to 5% around 60 times per hour, simulating what is frequently observed in patients with severe OSA (48). Two main pathways seem to be involved in the atherogenesis promoted by intermittent hypoxia: dyslipidemia and lipid peroxidation. In the first study by the Polotsky's group (49), an acute exposure (5 days) to intermittent hypoxia induced hyperlipidemia in lean mice, characterized by increases in total cholesterol, HDL, phospholipids, tryglycerides, and liver tryglycerides content. In lean mice, hyper-cholesterolemia during intermittent hypoxia was attributed to the hypoxia-inducible factor 1 in the liver, which activates sterol regulatory element–binding protein 1 (SREBP-1) and stearoyl-coenzyme A desaturase 1 (SCD-1), an important gene of try-glycerides and phospholipids biosynthesis controlled by SREBP-1. Others key genes involved in cholesterol biosynthesis, including SREBP-2 and 3-hydroxy-3-methyl-glutaryl-CoA (HMG CoA) reductase, were unaffected by intermittent hypoxia (49). In another study, the same group described that intermittent hypoxia over 12 weeks pro-moted an upregulation of genes involved with lipid biosynthesis in obese mice (50). Two years later, Li et al. described that in lean C57BL/6J mice a protocol of severe inter-mittent hypoxia (FiO_2 was reduced from 21% to 5%) for four weeks promoted a sig-nificant increase in fasting levels of total cholesterol and LDL in conjunction with an increase in lipoprotein secretion via upregulation of SCD-1 (51). Severe intermittent hypoxia also increased markedly lipid peroxidation in the liver. In contrast, moderate intermittent hypoxia (FiO_2 was reduced from 21% to 10%) did not induce hyper-lipidemia or change hepatic levels of SCD-1 but did cause lipid peroxidation in the liver at a reduced level relative to severe intermittent hypoxia, suggesting a severity dependence of intermittent hypoxia to induce hyperlipidemia and lipid peroxidation.

More recently, Savransky et al. (52) provided convincing evidence about the impact of intermittent hypoxia in atherosclerosis. The authors studied 40 male C57BL/6J mice, 8 weeks of age, fed either a high-cholesterol diet or a regular chow diet and subjected either to intermittent hypoxia or to intermittent air (control conditions) for 12 weeks. These animals are particularly resistant to atherosclerosis. However, 9 out of 10 mice exposed simultaneously to intermittent hypoxia and a high-cholesterol diet developed atherosclerotic lesions in the aortic origin and descending aorta. In contrast, atherosclerosis was not observed in mice exposed to intermittent air and a high-cho-lesterol diet or in mice exposed to intermittent hypoxia and a regular diet (Fig. 2). Although a high-cholesterol diet resulted in significant increases in serum total and LDL cholesterol levels and a decrease in HDL cholesterol, combined exposure to intermittent hypoxia and a high-cholesterol diet resulted in further increases in serum total choles-terol and LDL, with an additive impact on serum lipid peroxidation, and upregulation of SDC-1. The relative importance of SDC-1 on dyslipidemia and atherosclerosis induced by intermittent hypoxia was recently reinforced by an elegant study showing that SDC-1 deficiency attenuated intermittent hypoxia–induced dyslipidemia and atherosclerosis in mice (53). These results suggested that preexistent or coexisting dyslipidemia due to either genetic or environmental factors are necessary for expression of atherogenic properties of chronic intermittent hypoxia in this resistant model of atherosclerosis.

Another key mechanism by which chronic intermittent hypoxia may cause athe-rosclerosis is oxidative stress. The repetitive cycles of hypoxia and reoxygenation leads to excessive production of reactive oxygen species and oxidative stress in various organs

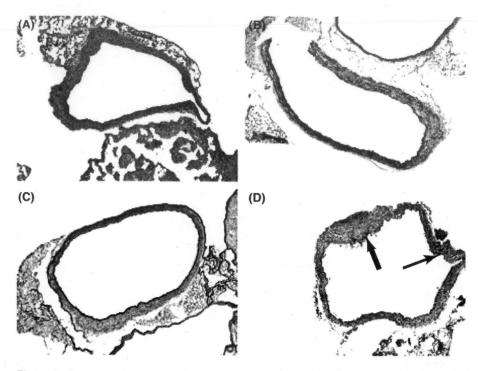

Figure 2 Representative cross sections of the ascending aorta (sinus of Valsalva) in C57BL/6J mice exposed to (**A**) intermittent air control conditions and regular diet, (**B**) chronic intermittent hypoxia and regular diet, (**C**) intermittent air and a high-cholesterol diet, or (**D**) chronic intermittent hypoxia and a high-cholesterol diet. Original magnification: 100×. The thick arrow points at the atherosclerotic plaque with a necrotic core. The thin arrow points at the fatty streak. *Source*: From Ref. 52.

and tissues (54). Chronic intermittent hypoxia also depletes antioxidant defenses and induces systemic oxidative stress with increased lipid peroxidation in serum, myocardium, and vasculature, which can predispose to vascular inflammation and atherosclerosis. However, there is no evidence to date in humans, linking markers of oxidative stress with markers of atherosclerosis in OSA.

B. In Vitro Studies

A number of in vitro studies have investigated the effects of hypoxia on monocyte adhesion to endothelial cells using either cell cultures or ex vivo arteries. The effects of hypoxia vary dramatically depending on experimental models. Adhesion molecule expression is altered by changes in temperature, pH, and shear stress. More importantly, the results are extremely dependent on the hypoxic regimen imposed on the system that varies from sustained hypoxia, long cycles of hypoxia mimicking models of ischemia, and reperfusion or repetitive hypoxia in short cycles, created to mimic the conditions experienced by OSA patients. Sustained hypoxia seems to have no effect or even confers a protective effect in such models. For instance, Ali et al. found no change in human umbilical vein endothelial cell (HUVEC) levels of E-selectin or ICAM-1 expression with 24 hours of 1% oxygen (55). Willian et al. found a downregulation of ICAM-1 and VCAM-1 in human microvascular endothelial cells and HUVECs exposed to sustained hypoxia (56). In contrast, long cycles of hypoxia-reoxygenation, an ischemia-reperfusion model, promoted endothelial cell adhesion. The exact mechanism by which hypoxia-reoxygenation promotes cell adhesion is controversial. Willian et al. found an increased expression of both adhesion molecules in HUVECs exposed to hypoxia for 4 hours followed by 16 to 28 hours at 21% oxygen (56). Ichikawa et al. demonstrated an increased expression of ICAM-1 and P-selectin, using HUVECs exposed to one hour of hypoxia, followed by one hour of reoxygenation (57). The increased adhesion in the latter study was not explained by increase in ICAM-1 or E-selectin, but it was due to increased CD11a/CD 18 and CD 11b/CD 18 interactions with ICAM-1. Interestingly enough, one cycle of hypoxia may precondition the system and be actually protective. Preconditioning of rat aortic endothelial cells with one hour of hypoxia and one hour of reoxygenation prevented an increase in adhesion molecule expression on subsequent exposure to anoxia-reoxygenation (58).

Like the studies in animals previously described, studies investigating the effects of short hypoxic cycles trying to mimic OSA were recently reported. Lattimore et al. did not find an increase in human monocyte adhesion to endothelial cells or adhesion molecule expression with short (4 hours) or prolonged (48 hours) repetitive intermittent hypoxia, even at levels of hypoxia as low as 5% oxygen or lower (2% oxygen) that are likely to be encountered at the level of the arterial endothelium of patients with OSA (59). The same study found that intermittent hypoxia enhanced lipid uptake into human macrophages and human cell formation from macrophages (59). Macrophage lipid loading is a key event in atherosclerosis that occurs within the arterial wall. In another relevant study, Dyugovskaya et al. found that in vitro intermittent hypoxia delayed neutrophil apoptosis of healthy subjects (60). Neutrophils possess the ability to produce large quantities of reactive oxygen species, which can cause DNA protein and lipid peroxidation. In addition, neutrophils release inflammatory leukotrienes and proteolytic enzymes, which may directly induce vascular damage. Therefore, apoptosis is thought to be a fundamental injury-limiting mechanism that is impaired after exposure to intermittent hypoxia in vitro. Using an in vitro model of intermittent hypoxia with HeLa cells transfected with reporter constructs and DNA-binding assays for the master transcriptional regulators of the inflammatory and adaptive pathways (NF-κB and HIF-1), Ryan et al. (61) found that intermittent hypoxia selectively activates NF-κB-dependent transcription over HIF-1-dependent transcription. It is possible that this selective inflammatory activation could be implicated in the genesis of atherosclerosis induced by intermittent hypoxia. On the other hand, the selective inflammatory activation by intermittent hypoxia could be an attractive strategy for future alternative therapy to patients with OSA.

V. Snoring—a Mechanical Force

Recently, it has been postulated that snoring is an atherogenic factor both in rabbits (62) and in humans (63). The rationale is that the vibration during snoring, transmitted though the surrounding tissues to the carotid artery wall, triggers an inflammatory cascade leading to early changes of atherosclerosis. Interestingly, opposite to intermittent hypoxia, snoring seems to promote atherosclerosis only in the carotid artery but not in other vascular beds (63). However, all these evidences points to an association more than a definitive cause-and-effect relationship between snoring and atherosclerosis (64). Future studies in this important area should be performed to clarify the relative role of snoring in the pathogenesis of carotid atherosclerosis.

VI. Clinical Studies

Several risk factors for atherosclerosis described in Table 1 are also closely associated with OSA. All these factors are clearly confounding factors. Increasing age, for instance, is an independent risk factor for OSA, hypertension, and atherosclerosis. Obesity is a risk factor for OSA, hypertension, and atherosclerosis. These interrelated conditions, frequently present in patients with OSA, obviously make the determination of an independent association between OSA and atherosclerosis more difficult.

OSA is now recognized as a cause of secondary hypertension, which in turn is one of the most important causes of atherosclerosis. This indirect link per se is relevant and is further explored in chapter 11. It must be stressed that vascular dysfunction associated with hypertension may occur in patients with OSA even without the overt diagnosis of hypertension. From the clinical perspective, several OSA patients who may be considered normotensive on the basis of office blood pressure (BP) measurements may actually turn out to be hypertensive when 24-hour BP is monitored (65). Another caveat is that the respiratory events associated with OSA are associated with cyclic BP surges at the end of each apnea or hypopnea. These events occur hundreds of times in patients with moderate to severe OSA and may not be fully depicted by 24-hour BP monitoring. It is therefore conceivable that BP oscillations associated with OSA promote cyclic shear stress oscillations in the aorta and large arteries that may in turn independently contribute to artery remodeling and poor cardiovascular outcome even in the absence of overt hypertension. There is also evidence that more subtle vasomotor perturbations, which may be measured indirectly by arterial stiffness, do occur within each obstructive event independent of BP oscillations. Arterial stiffness, a measure of arterial vessel resistance to deformation, is determined functionally by neurohumoral components, including endothelial relaxation factors, and by structural components, including collagen and elastin. Increased arterial stiffness is associated with increased pulse wave velocity and subsequent early wave reflection in systole. Increased vascular stiffness and the associated augmented sympathetic milieu may actually precede the onset of elevated BP. Jelic et al. measured arterial stiffness noninvasively during apneas and hypopneas in patients with OSA by determining the arterial augmentation index. The arterial augmentation index is derived from arterial wave reflection analysis and is defined as the ratio of augmented systolic pressure (due to the late systolic peak in the pressure waveform) to pulse pressure (66). The authors found that arterial stiffness increases acutely and transiently during obstructive events in both normotensive and hypertensive patients with OSA. These changes in arterial stiffness occurred in the late phase of the apnea, prior to any discernible alteration in BP or electroencephalogram arousal. These acute surges in arterial stiffness were transient and reversible and most likely reflect acutely impaired vascular endothelial relaxation and may be one of the first mechanisms by which OSA contributes to vascular dysfunction (66).

Several proinflammatory cytokines involved in the genesis of atherothrombosis can travel from local sites of inflammation to the liver, where they trigger protein synthesis characteristic of the acute phase response. C-reactive protein (CRP) is an acute phase reactant that is recognized as a major cardiovascular risk factor, independent of classic atherosclerotic risk factors such as blood lipids. More than simply a marker of inflammation, CRP may influence directly vascular vulnerability through several mechanisms, including enhanced expression of local adhesion molecules, increased expression of endothelial PAI-s, reduced endothelial NO bioactivity, altered LDL uptake by macrophages, and co-localization with complement within atherosclerotic lesions. Several prospective epidemiological studies have demonstrated that CRP, when measured with new high-sensitivity assays (hsCRP), strongly and independently predicts risk of myocardial infarction, stroke, peripheral arterial disease, and sudden cardiac death. HsCRP is also associated with pulse wave velocity in apparently healthy individuals (9). Having this background as a context, several studies but not all showed that OSA is independently associated with CRP. Moreover, there is also evidence that CRP may be reduced by treatment of OSA with CPAP (67). Yokoe et al. showed that levels of CRP, IL-6, and spontaneous production of IL-6 by monocytes are elevated in patients with OSA and are decreased by treatment with CPAP (68). One of the initial events in the development of atherosclerosis is the adhesion of monocytes to endothelial cells with subsequent transmigration into the vascular intima. Leukocyte and VCAMs, such as selectins, integrins, VCAM-1, and ICAM-1, affect this process. Levels of soluble cell adhesion molecules may serve as surrogate markers of the cellular expression of cell adhesion molecules. Chin et al. showed that soluble ICAM-1 levels and soluble E-selectin levels are increased in patients with OSA compared to controls and decrease after CPAP (69).

Several atherosclerotic markers or intermediate pathways, including reactive oxygen species, coagulation factors, systemic inflammation, and endothelial dysfunction, have been shown to be altered and to ameliorate or normalize after OSA treatment with CPAP (70–73). Dyugovskaya et al. found that neutrophil apoptosis is decreased and expression of selectins is increased in patients with OSA. Moreover, treatment with CPAP reversed both measures (60). Using freshly harvested venous endothelial cells and vascular reactivity (flow-mediated dilation) before and after four weeks of CPAP therapy, Jelic et al. found that OSA directly affects the vascular endothelium by promoting inflammation and oxidative stress while decreasing NO availability and repair capacity. Interestingly, effective CPAP therapy was associated with the reversal of these alterations (74).

Increased sympathetic activity is one of the most recognized features of OSA and is present not only during the night but also during the day. In turn, increased sympathetic activity may also play a major role in vascular remodeling. For instance, there is evidence that femoral artery wall thickness is associated with the level of sympathetic nerve activity in healthy men (75). In addition, CRP was also associated with arterial stiffness in apparently healthy individuals (76), suggesting that these mechanisms may interrelate closely in patients with OSA.

In the last two decades, several studies demonstrated an independent association between coronary and carotid atherosclerosis in OSA patients. However, most studies included patients with comorbidities (77–83). To avoid the typical confounding factors associated with OSA, Drager et al. (84) studied a group of relatively young male OSA

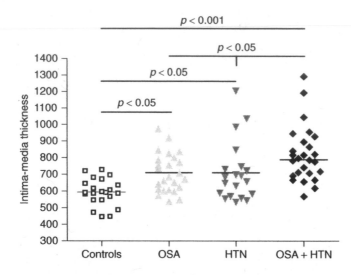

Figure 3 Carotid IMT in controls, patients with OSA, patients with HTN without OSA, and patients with OSA and HTN. Compared with the control group, carotid IMT and carotid diameter increased by 19.4% and 8.2% in the OSA group, 19.5% and 9.4% in the HTN group, and 40.3% and 20.6% in the OSA + HTN group, respectively. *Abbreviations*: OSA, obstructive sleep apnea; HTN, hypertension; IMT, intima-media thickness. *Source*: Modified from Ref. 86.

patients who were otherwise apparently healthy and free of comorbidities, including hypertension, diabetes, and smoking. Compared to appropriate controls with no OSA, patients with OSA presented early signs of atherosclerosis, including increased pulse wave velocity, carotid intima-media thickness, and carotid diameter. In addition, all vascular abnormalities were associated with the severity of OSA, as determined by their apnea-hypopnea index and minimal oxygen saturation. However, even in this highly selected group, the average body mass index was 29 kg/m^2 in both patients and controls and LDLs were borderline high in both groups. Therefore, as in the rodent model, these OSA patients may have been exposed to both OSA and dyslipidemia. More recently, Drager et al. (85) showed that patients in whom OSA and hypertension coexist exhibit significantly more vascular stiffness and heart remodeling than patients who suffer from only hypertension or OSA. Similar results were obtained in the carotid bed, suggesting an additive, harmful effect when the frequent combination of OSA and hypertension is present in the same individual (Fig. 3) (86). Thus, the harmful effects of OSA on the cardiovascular system may be multiplied in the presence of a second cardiovascular risk factor, such as dyslipidemia or hypertension.

To evaluate the hypothesis that OSA is an independent risk factor for athero-sclerosis, Drager et al. (87) performed a randomized study that evaluated the effects of four months of CPAP therapy on early markers of atherosclerosis, 24-hour BP monitoring, plasma CRP, and catecholamines in apparently healthy patients with severe OSA. Vascular properties, blood samples, and 24-hour BP monitoring were performed at study entry and after four months. Out of approximately 400 patients with established severe OSA, only a minority fulfilled the entry criteria, mainly due to the presence of

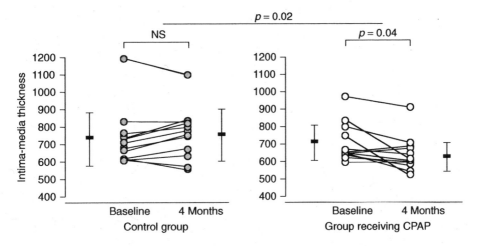

Figure 4 Individual values for the IMT. In the control group, IMT from baseline to four months [from 732 ± 164 to 740 ± 150 µm; 95% CI (−20.69 36.86)] was similar. In contrast, IMT significantly decreased in the group randomized to CPAP therapy [from 707 ± 105 to 645 ± 95 µm; 95% CI (−110.2 −14.07), $p = 0.04$]. The differences between groups remained significant ($p = 0.02$). Short horizontal lines and bars are mean ± SD. *Abbreviations*: IMT, intima-media thickness; CI, confidence interval; CPAP, continuous positive airway pressure; NS, not significant; SD, standard deviation. *Source*: Reproduced from Ref. 87.

comorbidities, including hypertension, diabetes, smoking, and chronic use of medications. The 24 patients studied were predominantly middle-aged and overweight. Four months of effective treatment with CPAP improved significantly validated markers of atherosclerosis in these normotensive middle-aged men with severe OSA. In addition, improvements in these early vascular markers were associated with reductions in markers of inflammation and sympathetic activation, as evaluated by plasma CRP and catecholamines, respectively. These effects occurred without concurrent changes in weight or lipids. In patients assigned to CPAP therapy, intima-media thickness (Fig. 4) and pulse wave velocity reverted to values similar to those reported previously in appropriate controls. Taken together, the results from this study provide evidence that OSA is an independent risk factor for atherosclerosis. The clinical importance of such findings is based on evidence that early detection of atherosclerotic disease processes and subsequent therapeutic interventions can alter significantly the natural course of cardiovascular disease.

VII. Conclusions

The clinical implication of atherosclerosis relies on the fact that this is a unifying mechanism linking OSA with several cardiovascular diseases, in particular coronary and cerebrovascular diseases. OSA, however, is not yet considered an established cause of atherosclerosis, especially by national or international cardiovascular societies. On the other hand, there is progressively more convincing evidence in support of a link between OSA and atherosclerosis. The biological plausibility, the dose-effect relationship between exposure to respiratory events and markers of atherosclerosis, the consistency of the results among different groups, and recent evidence that the treatment with CPAP reverses early signs of atherosclerosis suggest that OSA is an independent risk factor for atherosclerosis.

The impact of OSA can be evidenced when we compare the impact of the treatment of OSA with CPAP on vascular parameters with traditional forms of treatments for important risk factors to acute myocardial infraction and stroke, such as hypertension and dyslipidemia. Long-term studies showed that statins reduced carotid intima-media thickness after six months of therapy. Therefore, the observation in one study of a significant reduction on carotid intima-media thickness after only four months of effective CPAP is remarkable. However, further and larger studies are necessary to confirm these findings.

Therefore, there is an emergent necessity to advance in this important area through experimental and clinical research focused on advancing our current understanding of pathways involved with atherosclerosis, including lipid metabolism, inflammatory and immunologic regulation, endothelial repair and apoptosis, composition of plaque, angiogenesis, etc., and on exploring potential cross talk between mechanisms involved in the pathogenesis of atherosclerosis, such as sympathetic activity and renin-angiotensin-aldosterone system–mediated inflammatory gene expression (88). Recent advances in imaging technology (89) (magnetic resonance imaging, positron-emission tomography, intravascular ultrasound) offer many enticing prospects, including detecting atherosclerosis early, grouping individuals by the probability that they will develop symptoms of atherosclerosis, assessing the results of treatment of OSA, and improving the current understanding of the biology of atherosclerosis in this important sleep-disordered breathing. Finally, the observation of associations between OSA and poor cardiovascular outcome and mortality is based on observational studies. Prospective randomized studies will be necessary to fully establish OSA as a risk factor for atherosclerosis and poor cardiovascular outcome.

Acknowledgments

We are very grateful to Tatiana F. G. Galvão, MD, PhD, for her suggestions and critical review of the chapter and A. Falcetti Júnior for assistance on the figures in this chapter.

References

1. Marin JM, Carrizo SJ, Vicente E, et al. Long-term cardiovascular outcomes in men with obstructive sleep apnoea-hypopnoea with or without treatment with continuous positive airway pressure: an observational study. Lancet 2005; 365(9464):1046–1053.
2. Yaggi HK, Concato J, Kernan WN, et al. Obstructive sleep apnea as a risk factor for stroke and death. N Engl J Med 2005; 353(19):2034–2041.
3. Arzt M, Young T, Finn L, et al. Association of sleep-disordered breathing and the occurrence of stroke. Am J Respir Crit Care Med 2005; 172(11):1447–1451.
4. Pasterkamp G, de Klejin DP, Borst C. Arterial remodeling in atherosclerosis, restenosis and after alteration of blood flow: Potential mechanisms and clinical implications. Cardiovasc Res 2000; 45:843.
5. Lorenzi-Filho G, Drager LF. Obstructive sleep apnea and atherosclerosis: a new paradigm. Am J Respir Crit Care Med 2007; 175(12):1219–1221.

6. Peppard PE, Young T, Palta M, et al. Prospective study of the association between sleep-disordered breathing and hypertension. N Engl J Med 2000; 342(19):1378–1384.
7. Reichmuth KJ, Austin D, Skatrud JB, et al. Association of sleep apnea and type II diabetes: a population-based study. Am J Respir Crit Care Med 2005; 172(12):1590–1595.
8. Ip MS, Lam B, Ng MM. Obstructive sleep apnea is independently associated with insulin resistance. Am J Respir Crit Care Med 2002; 165:670–676.
9. Ridker PM, Libby P. Risk factors for atherothrombotic disease. In: Zipes D, Libby P, Bonow RO, et al., eds. Braunwald's Heart Disease. 7th ed. Elsevier Saunders, 2005:939–958.
10. Libby P. Changing concepts of atherogenesis. J Intern Med 2000; 247(3):349–358.
11. Ross R. Atherosclerosis–an inflammatory disease. N Engl J Med 1999; 340(2):115–126.
12. Hansson GK. Inflammation, atherosclerosis, and coronary artery disease. N. Engl J Med 2005; 352:1685–1695.
13. Fuster V, Moreno PR, Fayad ZA, et al. Atherothrombosis and high-risk plaque: part I: evolving concepts. J Am Coll Cardiol 2005; 46(6):937–954.
14. Mora R, Lupu F, Simionescu N. Prelesional events in atherogenesis. Colocalization of apolipoprotein B, unesterified cholesterol and extracellular phospholipid liposomes in the aorta of hyperlipidemic rabbit. Atherosclerosis 1987; 67(2–3):143–154.
15. Berliner JA, Navab M, Fogelman AM, et al. Atherosclerosis: basic mechanisms. Oxidation, inflammation, and genetics. Circulation 1995; 91(9):2488–2496.
16. Gawaz M, Neumann FJ, Dickfeld T, et al. Activated platelets induce monocyte chemotactic protein-1 secretion and surface expression of intercellular adhesion molecule-1 on endothelial cells. Circulation 1998; 98(12):1164–1171.
17. Tsao PS, Wang B, Buitrago R, et al. Nitric oxide regulates monocyte chemotactic protein-1. Circulation 1997; 96(3):934–940.
18. Takahashi M, Kitagawa S, Masuyama JI, et al. Human monocyte-endothelial cell interaction induces synthesis of granulocyte-macrophage colony-stimulating factor. Circulation 1996; 93 (6):1185–1193.
19. Mach F, Schönbeck U, Sukhova GK, et al. Functional CD40 ligand is expressed on human vascular endothelial cells, smooth muscle cells, and macrophages: implications for CD40-CD40 ligand signaling in atherosclerosis. Proc Natl Acad Sci U S A 1997; 94(5):1931–1936.
20. Rectenwald JE, Moldawer LL, Huber TS, et al. Direct evidence for cytokine involvement in neointimal hyperplasia. Circulation 2000; 102(14):1697–1702.
21. Brizzi MF, Formato L, Dentelli P, et al. Interleukin-3 stimulates migration and proliferation of vascular smooth muscle cells: a potential role in atherogenesis. Circulation 2001; 103(4): 549–554.
22. Simonini A, Moscucci M, Muller DW, et al. IL-8 is an angiogenic factor in human coronary atherectomy tissue. Circulation 2000; 101(13):1519–1526.
23. Tenger C, Sundborger A, Jawien J, et al. IL-18 accelerates atherosclerosis accompanied by elevation of IFN-gamma and CXCL16 expression independently of T cells. Arterioscler Thromb Vasc Biol 2005; 25(4):791–796.
24. Dixit VM, Green S, Sarma V, et al. Tumor necrosis factor-alpha induction of novel gene products in human endothelial cells including a macrophage-specific chemotaxin. J Biol Chem 1990; 265(5):2973–2978.
25. Tintut Y, Patel J, Parhami F, et al. Tumor necrosis factor-alpha promotes in vitro calcification of vascular cells via the cAMP pathway. Circulation 2000; 102(21):2636–2642.
26. Libby P. The vascular biology of atherosclerosis. In: Zipes DP, Libby P, Bonow RO, Braunwald E, eds. Braunwald's Heart Disease. A Textbook of Cardiovascular Medicine. 7th ed. Elsevier Saunders 2005: 925.
27. Young JL, Libby P, Schönbeck U. Cytokines in the pathogenesis of atherosclerosis. Thromb Haemost 2002; 88(4):554–567.

28. Glomset JA, Norum KR. The metabolic role of lecithin: cholesterol acyltransferase: per-
     spectives form pathology. Adv Lipid Res 1973; 11:1–65.
29. Cuchel M, Rader DJ. Macrophage reverse cholesterol transport: key to the regression of
     atherosclerosis? Circulation 2006; 113:2548–2555.
30. Tall AR. Cholesterol efflux pathways and other potential mechanisms involved in the athero-
     protective effect of high density lipoproteins. J Intern Med 2008; 263(3):256–273.
31. Stein O, Stein Y. Lipid transfer proteins (LTP) and atherosclerosis. Atherosclerosis 2005; 178
     (2):217–230.
32. Mineo C, Deguchi H, Griffin JH, et al. Endothelial and antithrombotic actions of HDL. Circ
     Res 2006; 98:1352–1364.
33. Uittenbogaard A, Shaul PW, Yuhanna IS, et al. High density lipoprotein prevents oxidized
     low density lipoprotein-induced inhibition of endothelial nitric-oxide synthase localization
     and activation in caveolae. J Biol Chem 2000; 275:11278–11283.
34. Zeiher AM, Schachlinger V, Hohnloser SH, et al. Coronary atherosclerotic wall thickening
     and vascular reactivity in humans. Elevated high-density lipoprotein levels ameliorate
     abnormal vasoconstriction in early atherosclerosis. Circulation 1994; 89:2525–2532.
35. Davies MJ, Woolf N, Rowles PM, et al. Morphology of the endothelium over atherosclerotic
     plaques in human coronary arteries. Br Heart J 1988; 60(6):459–464.
36. Sata M, Saiura A, Kunisato A, et al. Hematopoietic stem cells differentiate into vascular cells
     that participate in the pathogenesis of atherosclerosis. Nat Med 2002; 8(4):403–409.
37. Kockx MM, De Meyer GR, Muhring J, et al. Apoptosis and related proteins in different
     stages of human atherosclerotic plaques. Circulation 1998; 97(23):2307–2315.
38. Virmani R, Narula J, Farb A. When neoangiogenesis ricochets. Am Heart J 1998; 136(6):
     937–939.
39. Schoenhagen P, Ziada KM, Vince DG, et al. Arterial remodeling and coronary artery disease:
     the concept of "dilated" versus "obstructive" coronary atherosclerosis. J Am Coll Cardiol
     2001; 38(2):297–306.
40. Falk E, Shah PK, Fuster V. Coronary plaque disruption. Circulation 1995; 92(3):657–671.
41. Ambrose JA, Tannenbaum MA, Alexopoulos D, et al. Angiographic progression of coronary
     artery disease and the development of myocardial infarction. J Am Coll Cardiol 1988; 12(1):
     56–62.
42. Kipshidze NN. Effect of anoxia on the development of experimental coronary athero-
     sclerosis. Biull Eksp Biol Med 1959; 47(4):54–60.
43. Astrup P. Effects of hypoxia and of carbon monoxide exposures on experimental athero-
     sclerosis. Ann Intern Med 1969; 71(2):426–427.
44. Kjeldsen K, Wanstrup J, Astrup P. Enhancing influence of arterial hypoxia on the devel-
     opment of atheromatosis in cholesterol-fed rabbits. J Atheroscler Res 1968; 8:835–845.
45. Helin G, Helin P, Lorenzen I. The aortic glycosaminoglycans in arteriosclerosis induced by
     systemic hypoxia. Atherosclerosis 1970; 12:235–240.
46. Kjeldsen K, Astrup P, Wanstrup J. Reversal of rabbit atheromatosis by hyperoxia. J Athe-
     roscler Res 1969; 10:173–178.
47. Helin P, Garbarsch C, Lorenzen I. Effects of intermittent and continuous hypoxia on the
     aortic wall in rabbits. Atherosclerosis 1975; 21:325–335.
48. Tagaito Y, Polotsky VY, Campen MJ, et al. A model of sleep-disordered breathing in the
     C57BL/6J mouse. J Appl Physiol 2001; 91(6):2758–2766.
49. Li J, Thorne LN, Punjabi NM, et al. Intermittent hypoxia induces hyperlipidemia in lean
     mice. Circ Res 2005; 97(7):698–706.
50. Li J, Grigoryev DN, Ye SQ, et al. Chronic intermittent hypoxia upregulates genes of lipid
     biosynthesis in obese mice. J Appl Physiol 2005; 99(5):1643–1648.
51. Li J, Savransky V, Nanayakkara A, et al. Hyperlipidemia and lipid peroxidation are dependent
     on the severity of chronic intermittent hypoxia. J Appl Physiol 2007; 102(2):557–563.

52. Savransky V, Nanayakkara A, Li J, et al. Chronic Intermittent Hypoxia Induces Athero-sclerosis. Am J Respir Crit Care Med 2007; 175:1290–1297.

53. Savransky V, Jun J, Li J, et al. Dyslipidemia and atherosclerosis induced by chronic inter-mittent hypoxia are attenuated by deficiency of stearoyl coenzyme A desaturase. Circ Res 2008; 103(10):1173–1180.

54. Lavie L. Obstructive sleep apnoea syndrome - an oxidative stress disorder. Sleep Med Rev 2003; 7:35–51.

55. Ali MH, Schlidt SA, Hynes KL, et al. Prolonged hypoxia alters endothelial barrier function. Surgery 1998; 124(3):491–497.

56. Willian C, Schindler R, Frei U, et al. Increases in oxygen tension stimulate expression of ICAM-1 and VCAM-1 on human endothelial cells. Am J Physiol 1999; 276(6 Pt2): H2044–H2052.

57. Ichikawa H, Flores S, Kvietys PR, et al. Molecular mechanisms of anoxia-reoxygenation induced neutrhphil adherence to cultured endothelial cells. Circ Res 1997; 81(6):922–931.

58. Beauchamp P, Richard V, Tamion F, et al. Protective effects of preconditioning in cultured rat endothelial cells: effects on neutrophil adhesion and expression of ICAM-1 after anoxia and reoxygenation. Circulation 1999; 100(5):541–546.

59. Lattimore JD, Wilcox I, Nakhla S, et al. Repetitive hypoxia increases lipid loading in human macrophages-a potentially atherogenic effect. Atherosclerosis 2005; 179(2):255–259.

60. Dyugovskaya L, Polyakov A, Lavie P, et al. Delayed neutrophil apoptosis in patients with sleep apnea. Am J Respir Crit Care Med 2008; 17:544–554.

61. Ryan S, Taylor CT, McNicholas WT. Selective activation of inflammatory pathways by inter-mittent hypoxia in obstructive sleep apnea syndrome. Circulation 2005; 112(17):2660–2667.

62. Amatoury J, Howitt L, Wheatley JR, et al. Snoring-related energy transmission to the carotid artery in rabbits. J Appl Physiol 2006; 100(5):1547–1553.

63. Lee SA, Amis TC, Byth K, et al. Heavy snoring as a cause of carotid artery atherosclerosis. Sleep 2008; 31(9):1207–1213.

64. Drager LF, Lorenzi-Filho G. Heavy snoring and carotid atherosclerosis: is there more than an association? Sleep 2008; 31(10):1335.

65. Baguet JP, Lévy P, Barone-Rochette G, et al. Masked hypertension in obstructive sleep apnea syndrome. J Hypertens 2008; 26(5):885–892.

66. Jelic S, Bartels MN, Mateika JH, et al. Arterial stiffness increases during obstructive sleep apneas. Sleep 2002; 25(8):850–855.

67. Shamsuzzaman AS, Winnicki M, Lanfranchi P, et al. Elevated C-reactive protein in patients with obstructive sleep apnea. Circulation 2002; 105(21):2462–2464.

68. Yokoc T, Minoguchi K, Matsuo H, et al. Elevated levels of C-reactive protein and inter-leukin-6 in patients with obstructive sleep apnea syndrome are decreased by nasal continuous positive airway pressure. Circulation 2003; 107(8):1129–1134.

69. Chin K, Nakamura T, Shimizu K, et al. Effects of nasal continuous positive airway pressure on soluble cell adhesion molecules in patients with obstructive sleep apnea syndrome. Am J Med 2000; 109:562–567.

70. Kato M, Roberts-Thomson P, Phillips BG, et al. Impairment of endothelium-dependent vasodilation of resistance vessels in patients with obstructive sleep apnea. Circulation 2000; 102(21):2607–2610.

71. Ip MS, Tse HF, Lam B, et al. Endothelial function in obstructive sleep apnea and response to treatment. Am J Respir Crit Care Med 2004; 169(3):348–353.

72. Dyugovskaya L, Lavie P, Lavie L. Lymphocyte activation as a possible measure of athe-rosclerotic risk in patients with sleep apnea. Ann N Y Acad Sci 2005; 1051:340–350.

73. von Känel R, Loredo JS, Ancoli-Israel S, et al. Association between sleep apnea severity and blood coagulability: treatment effects of nasal continuous positive airway pressure. Sleep Breath 2006; 10(3):139–146.

74. Jelic S, Padeletti M, Kawut SM, et al. Inflammation, oxidative stress, and repair capacity of the vascular endothelium in obstructive sleep apnea. Circulation 2008; 117(17):2270–2278.
75. Dinenno FA, Jones PP, Seals DR, et al. Age-associated arterial wall thickening is related to elevations in sympathetic activity in healthy humans. Am J Physiol Heart Circ Physiol 2000; 278(4):H1205–H1210.
76. Yasmin, McEniery CM, Wallace S, et al. C-reactive protein is associated with arterial stiffness in apparently healthy individuals. Arterioscler Thromb Vasc Biol 2004; 24(5):969–674.
77. Peker Y, Kraiczi H, Hedner J, et al. An independent association between obstructive sleep apnoea and coronary artery disease. Eur Respir J 1999; 14(1):179–184.
78. Mooe T, Rabben T, Wiklund U, et al. Sleep-disordered breathing in men with coronary artery disease. Chest 1996; 109(3):659–663.
79. Hayashi M, Fujimoto K, Urushibata K, et al. Nocturnal oxygen desaturation correlates with the severity of coronary atherosclerosis in coronary artery disease. Chest 2003; 124(3):936–941.
80. Sorajja D, Gami AS, Somers VK, et al. Independent association between obstructive sleep apnea and subclinical coronary artery disease. Chest 2008; 133(4):927–933.
81. Silvestrini M, Rizzato B, Placidi F, et al. Carotid artery wall thickness in patients with obstructive sleep apnea syndrome. Stroke 2002; 33(7):1782–1785.
82. Suzuki T, Nakano H, Maekawa J, et al. Obstructive sleep apnea and carotid-artery intima-media thickness. Sleep 2004; 27(1):129–133.
83. Altin R, Ozdemir H, Mahmutyazicioğlu K, et al. Evaluation of carotid artery wall thickness with high-resolution sonography in obstructive sleep apnea syndrome. J Clin Ultrasound 2005; 33(2):80–86.
84. Drager LF, Bortolotto LA, Lorenzi MC, et al. Early signs of atherosclerosis in obstructive sleep apnea. Am J Respir Crit Care Med 2005; 172:613–618.
85. Drager LF, Bortolotto LA, Figueiredo AC, et al. Obstructive sleep apnea, hypertension, and their interaction on arterial stiffness and heart remodeling. Chest 2007; 131(5):1379–1386.
86. Drager LF, Bortolotto LA, Krieger EM, et al. Additive effects of obstructive sleep apnea and hypertension on early markers of carotid atherosclerosis. Hypertension 2009; 53(1):64–69.
87. Drager LF, Bortolotto LA, Figueiredo AC, et al. Effects of continuous positive airway pressure on early signs of atherosclerosis in obstructive sleep apnea. Am J Respir Crit Care Med 2007; 176(7):706–712.
88. Sahar S, Dwarakanath RS, Reddy MA, et al. Angiotensin II enhances interleukin-18 mediated inflammatory gene expression in vascular smooth muscle cells: a novel cross-talk in the pathogenesis of atherosclerosis. Circ Res 2005; 96(10):1064–1071.
89. Sanz J, Fayad ZA. Imaging of atherosclerotic cardiovascular disease. Nature 2008; 451(7181):953–957.

14
Sleep Apnea and Stroke

MASSIMILIANO M. SICCOLI and CLAUDIO L. BASSETTI
Department of Neurology, University Hospital of Zurich, Zurich, Switzerland

I. Introduction

The link between sleep apnea (SA) and cerebrovascular disease has been increasingly studied over the last 15 years. The interactions existing between SA and stroke are manifold: (*i*) SA of the obstructive type has been recognized as a possible independent risk factor for cardiovascular morbidity and mortality (1,2), including arterial hypertension (3–5), ischemic heart disease/heart failure/atrial fibrillation (5–10), sudden death (11), and stroke (7,9,12); (*ii*) ischemic brain damage and its consequences/complications [e.g., hypoxia, blood pressure (BP) elevation, immobilization, pain, cognitive and mood changes) may affect the regulation of sleep-wake and breathing control; (*iii*) hemodynamic changes secondary to SA may have a detrimental effect on the ischemic brain, eventually affecting the outcome of stroke; and (*iv*) disrupted night sleep and excessive daytime sleepiness related to SA may adversely affect neurological, cognitive, and psychiatric functions and consequently the rehabilitation outcome as well. Considering that SA is frequent in patients with stroke and transient ischemic attacks (TIAs) compared to the general population (13–15), this link has potentially major practical implications.

II. Clinical Features of Sleep Apnea in Acute Stroke

SA is highly prevalent in patients with ischemic stroke or TIA, with 50% to 70% of patients exhibiting an apnea-hypopnea index (AHI) $\geq$ 10/hr in the acute phase (13–17). The most common type of SA observed in acute stroke is the obstructive one, which has been reported in 36% to 90% (13–16,18,19) of patients. Obstructive SA (OSA) in acute ischemic stroke often reflects a preexisting situation in patients with high-risk cardiovascular profile and is therefore frequently associated with arterial hypertension, obesity, and diabetes. This type of SA may, but usually does not, exacerbate after stroke and improves less or does not improve at all on follow-up (15).

The second type observed in patients with acute stroke is central SA and central periodic breathing (or Cheyne–Stokes breathing), which is common as well and has been described in up to 40% of patients (13–20). Central SA and central periodic breathing in the acute phase of stroke often represents a new-onset stroke-related phenomenon. In such cases, a spontaneous recovery after stroke (15,17,21,22) is often observed (Figs. 1 and 2). Overall, patients with central SA seem to have a better outcome than those with obstructive SA (23). However, severe central SA persisting over weeks after stroke can be seen in patients with large hemispheric ischemic lesions and cardiac dysfunction (24). In this subgroup of patients, central SA is associated with a poor functional outcome (25).

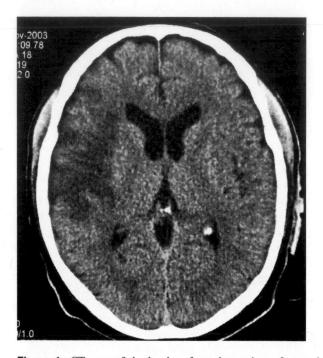

Figure 1 CT scan of the head performed two days after stroke onset, showing a right-sided ischemic infarction in the territory of the middle cerebral artery with involvement of the insula. *Case description*: A 52-year-old man was referred with acute weakness of the left arm and the left-sided face muscles, speech disturbances, and gait unsteadiness. In the clinical examination a slight left-sided palsy of the face, arm, and leg and a left hemisensory loss were found. The National Institutes of Health Stroke Scale was 5. BP at admission was 175/110 mmHg; heart rate was 88/ min. Respiration during the day was unremarkable, but frequent central apneas as well as irregular breathing were observed during sleep. Transesophageal echocardiography showed an ejection fraction <50%, plaques of the fourth degree in the aortic arch, and an aneurysm of the left ventricle (possibly residual, after myocardial infarction) but no patent foramen ovale. *Abbreviations*: CT, computed tomography; BP, blood pressure. *Source*: Courtesy of the Institute of Neuroradiology, University Hospital, Zurich, Switzerland.

More rarely (9–18%) (13–16), obstructive and central SA occur together. Obstructive events tend to predominate in the rapid eye movement (REM) sleep and central apneas/central periodic breathing in non-REM sleep (13,15,19). The different prevalence of obstructive and central SA reported in previous studies is in part due to (*i*) different assessment methods (i.e., full polysomnography versus portable devices) and (*ii*) different intervals between stroke and assessment of nocturnal breathing. The details of the studies exploring the prevalence of SA in the acute/subacute phase of stroke are summarized in Table 1.

No major differences have been reported, so far, in the frequency of SA regarding topography, subtype (ischemic versus hemorrhagic stroke or TIA), and etiology of

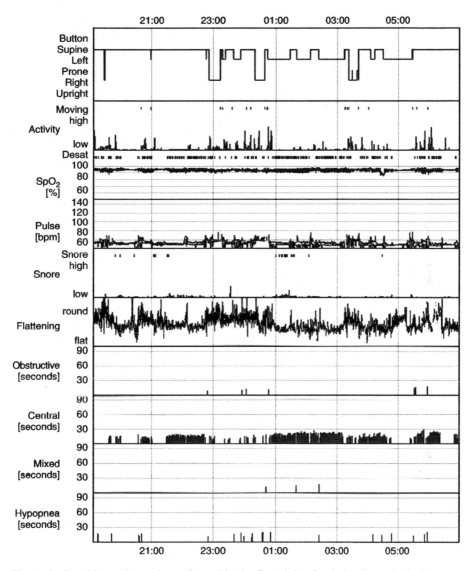

Figure 2 Portable respirography performed in the first night after ischemic stroke in the same patient as shown in Figure 1, showing severe central SA. *Respirographic data*: Apnea-hypopnea index 47/hr, apnea index 44/hr, obstructive apnea index 0/hr, central apnea index 44/hr, central periodic breathing during 50% of recording time, oxygen desaturation index 49/hr, minimal oxygen saturation 85%. Respirography performed three months after acute stroke showed normal findings; the apnea-hypopnea index was 1/hr.

Table 1 Detailed Representation of Studies Exploring the Prevalence of SA in the Acute/Subacute Phase of Stroke

Reference	N	Age	BMI	Time[a]	Type[b]	AHI	Obstructive apneas[c]	Central apneas[d]	CPB (%)
Bassetti[13]	59	62 ± 11	27.4 ± 5.0	12 (1–71) day	PSG	27 ± 29 ≥10/hr in 69%	90%	10%	37%[e]
Dyken[18]	24	65 ± 10	M, 27.8 ± 1.2 F, 32.9 ± 1.7	2–5 wk	PSG	M, 21.5 ± 4.2 W, 31.6 ± 8.8	M, 77% F, 64%		28%
Bassetti[19]	39	57 ± 15	≥29.0 in 38%	10 (1–49) day	PSG	≥10/hr in 69%	54%		
Bassetti[14]	80	60 ± 14	29.2 ± 8.4	9 (1–71) day	PSG	28 (0–140) ≥10/hr in 62.5%	94%	6%	
Parra[15]	161	72 ± 9	26.6 ± 3.9	48–72 hr	PR	21.2 ± 15.7 ≥10/hr in 71%	52%	38%	26%[e]
Iranzo[16]	50	67 ± 9	26.4 ± 3.2	11.6 ± 5.6 hr	PSG	27.7 ± 26.6 ≥10/hr in 62%	OAI = 4.5 ± 8.4 48%	CAI = 5.6 ± 10.1 6.5%	29%
Turkington[27]	120	79 ± 10	23.6 ± 4.0	Up to 24 hr	PR	≥10/hr in 61%	91%	9%	38% 12%[e]
Selic/Siccoli[107]	41	63 ± 13	27 ± 4	37 ± 25 hr	PR	23 ± 22	OAI = 2 ± 3	CAI = 8 ± 15	
Siccoli[17]	74	63 ± 13	28 ± 4	45 ± 26 hr	PR	20 ± 20 ≥10/hr in 68%	OAI = 3 ± 7	CAI = 7 ± 12	41%[e]

Data are expressed as mean and standard deviations, means and ranges, or percentages according to the corresponding original paper.
[a]Time, the interval between stroke onset and assessment of nocturnal breathing.
[b]Type of nocturnal breathing assessment.
[c]Obstructive apneas, percentage of patients with predominantly obstructive apneas.
[d]Central apneas, percentage of patients with predominantly central apneas.
[e]Percentage of patients with CPB during ≥10% of recording time.

Abbreviations: BMI, body mass index; PSG, full polysomnography; PR, portable respirography; M, male; F, female; AHI, apnea-hypopnea index (expressed as number of events per hour or as percentage of patients with AHI ≥10/hr); OAI, obstructive apnea index (number of obstructive apneas per hour); CAI, central apnea index (number of central apneas per hour); CPB (%), percentage of patients with central periodic breathing.

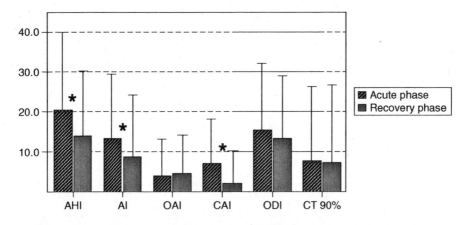

Figure 3 Evolution of respiratory parameters in 42 patients with acute ischemic stroke from the acute phase (1.5 ± 1.1 days) to the recovery phase (3.9 ± 1.1 months) after stroke. Data are means $\pm$ 1 standard deviation. * indicates $p < 0.05$, calculated for comparison between acute and recovery phase after stroke. *Abbreviations:* AHI, apnea-hypopnea index; AI, apnea-index; OAI, obstructive apnea index; CAI, central apnea index; ODI, oxygen desaturation index; CT90%, percent of registration time with oxygen saturation <90%. *Source*: From Ref. 29.

stroke (13–15,26,27). Bassetti et al. first reported an association of SA with macro-angiopathy (21). Furthermore, recent data suggest that stroke in distinct brain areas participating in autonomic/respiratory control (17,19,20,22) might be associated with a new-onset central SA or central periodic breathing after stroke.

SA improves in most patients from the acute to the recovery phase after stroke, with more than 50% of patients still exhibiting an AHI $\geq$ 10/hr three months after the acute event (15,21,28). This improvement is mainly due to a decrease of central apneas (15,29), whereas the obstructive component improves substantially less than the central one or, in most patients, remains unchanged (Fig. 3).

SA can present with a wide variety of sleep-wake and autonomic abnormalities/symptoms/signs, which are sometimes misinterpreted as consequences of the underlying brain damage. Nighttime symptoms of SA include sleep onset insomnia; respiratory noises (snoring, stridor); irregular or periodic respiration; apneas; agitated sleep with increased motor activity and frequent awakenings; sudden awakenings with or without choking sensations; shortness of breath, palpitations, and fear (panic attacks); orthopnea and increased sweating; and even sudden death during sleep. Daytime symptoms of SA are headaches, fatigue, and excessive daytime sleepiness; altered cognition with concentration and memory difficulties; irritability; and depression (30,31). Some stroke patients may exhibit breathing abnormalities during wakefulness as well, including dyspnea, apneas, inspiratory breath holding (apneustic breathing), irregular breathing, rapid shallow breathing (hyperpnea and central hyperventilation), or hiccups. In some patients with ischemic lesions involving the brainstem breathing control centers (32–34), an overlap of sleep-disordered breathing with sleep-wake disorder and/or autonomic abnormalities may be observed.

III. Sleep Apnea as a Cause of Stroke
A. Sleep Apnea and Increased Stroke Risk

It has been estimated that about 4% to 5% of men and 2% of women (35,36) in Western countries suffer from clinically significant obstructive apnea. SA, mainly of the obstructive type, is increasingly recognized as a possible independent risk factor for cardiovascular morbidity and mortality (1,2,37,38), including arterial hypertension (3–5), ischemic heart disease/heart failure/atrial fibrillation (5–10), sudden death during sleep (11), and, recently described, ventricular arrhythmias without heart failure (39). The condition of clinically significant obstructive apnea is even becoming more prevalent as the average population body weight rises. Severe obstructive SA is associated with a very high cardiovascular risk: over 10 years, 14% of this group is predicted to experience a stroke and 23% a myocardial infarction (36% combined risk) (40).

Sleep Apnea and Increased Risk of Hypertension

Part of this link is also due to the association between SA and arterial hypertension, which was found in several studies, independent of age, gender, smoking, alcohol, educational state, use of antihypertensive medication, and body mass index (BMI) (3–5,41–45).

An analysis of 709 patients from the Wisconsin Sleep Cohort (3) showed that an AHI > 15/hr was correlated to a threefold increased relative risk to develop new-onset arterial hypertension within four years. In the Sleep Heart Health Study (5), an association between SA and hypertension was found independent of age, gender, race, BMI, and neck circumference. This association was stronger in patients with a higher AHI (>30/hr); in this subgroup, 60% of patients were hypertensive (relative risk 1.5) compared to 40% in the group without SA (AHI < 5/hr). These studies provide a strong evidence of an association between SA and arterial hypertension, with a dose-response relationship depending on the severity of SA. However, the magnitude of this association remains modest in terms of increased absolute risk. The prevalence of OSA in patients with arterial hypertension is also higher compared with the normal population (46), and treatment with nasal continuous positive airway pressure (CPAP) reduces BP in hypertensive SA patients (47,48). Such an effect, which was found for both systolic and diastolic BP during sleep and wakefulness, is expected to be associated with a stroke risk reduction of about 20%.

History of Snoring and Increased Risk of Stroke

Whether obstructive SA may be considered an independent risk factor for stroke is still a matter of debate. The first evidence of a link between obstructive SA and an increased risk of prevalent and incident stroke was reported in epidemiological studies on habitual snoring as a surrogate marker of obstructive SA. These studies, which were performed with a case-control (49–53) or cross-sectional longitudinal (54–56) design, reported an increased risk of prevalent and incident stroke ranging from 1.26 to 10.3 (mean 1.66) (57) in patients with snoring, after adjusting for cardiovascular risk factors such as age, gender, obesity, arterial hypertension, diabetes, smoking, hypercholesterinemia, and alcohol consumption. The two largest cohort studies included, respectively, 4388 patients with a follow-up of three years (54) and 71,779 patients with a follow-up of eight years (56); habitual snoring was assessed in both studies with a mailed questionnaire; and outcome measures were incident fatal/nonfatal stroke and fatal/nonfatal coronary events. The adjusted risk for stroke in patients with habitual snoring was 2.08 [95% confidence interval (CI,) 1.5–3.77] and 1.33 (95% CI, 1.06–1.67). A cross-sectional longitudinal analysis of the Caerphilly cohort showed a high risk for stroke over a 10-year follow-up in males reporting more than one of the following symptoms assessed by questionnaires: snoring, witnessed apneas, daytime sleepiness, insomnia, and restless legs (58).

Documented Obstructive Sleep Apnea and Increased Risk of Stroke

A further evidence of a link between obstructive SA and increased stroke risk came from an analysis of the Sleep Hearth Health Study cohort (7). In this cross-sectional study, the association between sleep-disordered breathing assessed by unattended portable polysomnography at home and self-reported cardiovascular events including stroke were examined in 6242 free-living individuals. A total of 1023 individuals had mild to moderate SA (median AHI = 4.4/hr, interquartile range 1.3–11.0). For individuals in the upper quartile (AHI > 11/hr), the multivariable-adjusted odds ratio of prevalent cardiovascular events was 1.42 (95% CI, 1.13–1.78), and the relative odds of prevalent stroke compared with individuals in the lower quartile was 1.58 (95% CI, 1.02–2.46).

A second cross-sectional and longitudinal study performed with polysomnography in 1475 individuals of the Wisconsin Sleep Cohort (59) found that moderate to severe SA defined as AHI > 20/hr was linked to increased odds for prevalent (odds ratio adjusted for age, sex, BMI, alcohol, and smoking 4.33, 95% CI, 1.32–14.24, $p = 0.02$) and incident (unadjusted odds ratio 4.31, 95% CI, 1.31–14.15, $p = 0.02$; odds ratio adjusted for age, sex, and BMI 3.08, 95% CI, 0.74–12.81, $p = 0.12$) stroke over the next four years.

A prospective North American observational cohort study (12) performed in 697 individuals with obstructive SA (defined as AHI $\geq$ 5/hr with respiratory events predominantly of the obstructive type) and in 325 controls with a mean follow-up time of 3.4 years reported that obstructive SA was associated with an increased relative risk of stroke or death from any cause (unadjusted model: hazard ratio 2.24, 95% CI, 1.30–3.86, $p = 0.0004$; adjusted model: hazard ratio 1.97, 95% CI, 1.12–3.48, $p = 0.01$). This risk rose to 3.3 (95% CI, 1.74–6.26, $p = 0.005$) in patients with severe disease (AHI > 36/hr). More importantly, the increased risk was still present after adjustment for age, sex, race, smoking status, alcohol consumption, BMI, and the presence or absence of diabetes mellitus, hyperlipidemia, atrial fibrillation, and arterial hypertension. A drawback of this study was the fact that CPAP-treated and CPAP-untreated patients were included in the same analysis.

A large Spanish prospective observational cohort study (9) performed in 264 controls, 377 snorers, 403 patients with mild (AHI 5–30/hr) untreated obstructive SA, 235 patients with severe (AHI, 30/hr) untreated obstructive SA, and 372 patients with treated (CPAP) OSA with a 10-year follow-up showed that patients with severe untreated disease had a higher incidence of fatal (1.06 per 100 person-years) and non-fatal (2.13 per 100 person-years) cardiovascular events, including stroke, compared with the other groups; the adjusted odds ratio for fatal and nonfatal cardiovascular events in the group of patients with severe untreated disease compared to healthy individuals was 2.87 (95% CI, 1.17–7.51) and 3.17 (95% CI, 1.12–7.51), respectively. An obvious, major drawback of this study was the fact that decisions for treatment were not randomized.

A recent Swedish prospective study (60) performed on 392 patients with coronary artery disease showed that patients with SA (defined as AHI $\geq$ 5/hr) were associated with an increased risk of stroke [hazard ratio adjusted for age, BMI, left ventricular function, diabetes mellitus, gender, coronary intervention, hypertension, atrial fibrillation, a previous stroke or TIA, and smoking, 2.89 (95% CI, 1.37–6.09, $p = 0.005$)] over a follow-up time of 10 years. Patients with AHI $\geq$ 15/hr had a 3.56 (95% CI, 1.56–8.16) times increased risk of stroke than patients without SA, independent of confounders.

Case-control studies have tested the association between obstructive SA and silent vascular white matter lesions, with contrasting results (61,62). One recent study showed a higher percentage of silent brain lesions in patients with moderate to severe OSA (25.0%) compared to obese control subjects (6.7%) or patients with mild OSA (7.7%) (63). In one large population-based longitudinal study from the Sleep Heart Health Study cohort, the number of ischemic lesions correlated with the arousal frequency but not with the severity of obstructive SA. The clinical significance of these findings remains unclear (64).

B. Mechanisms
Chronic Effects
Several factors may contribute chronically to the increased risk of stroke in patients with obstructive SA. Whereas the link existing between obstructive SA and other cardiovascular risk factors (such as arterial hypertension, obesity, diabetes, hypercholesterinemia) may contribute to an increased stroke risk in these patients, there is also growing evidence that changes related to SA may contribute to increased atherosclerosis/atherogenesis in terms of a direct causative link. The potential underlying mechanisms are manifold and include vascular/endothelial, coagulatory, metabolic, and inflammatory/oxidative changes.

Vascular/Endothelial Factors
Endothelial function, particularly the activity of nitric oxide synthetase and circulating nitric oxide, which plays a role in the regulation of vascular tone and was shown to be impaired in hypertension and atherosclerosis (65,66), is impaired in obstructive SA (67), and treatment with CPAP was shown to promptly restore these changes (68–70). Levels of endothelin-1, which has potent vasoconstrictor and mitogenic effects, are increased in SA and significantly decrease after CPAP treatment (71). Hypoxemia-related endothelin release was shown to be associated with a sustained increase of BP also during daytime (71,72).

Coagulatory Factors
Prothrombotic changes with increased factor VII clotting activity, which is a marker of the extrinsic coagulation pathway, increased platelet activation and aggregation, and increased erythrocyte adhesiveness and aggregation (73) were documented in association with obstructive SA (74–76), both in vivo and in vitro.

Metabolic Factors
An increased prevalence of insulin resistance and diabetes mellitus has been shown in patients with obstructive SA, independent of body weight (77,78), and the extent of the impaired glucose tolerance was reduced after CPAP treatment (78,79). Sympathetic activation may be a possible mechanism playing a role in these changes. Levels of

leptin, an adipocyte-derived protein, which plays a role as an appetite suppressant in the central nervous system, were also shown to be increased in patients with obstructive SA (80,81). A decrease of leptin levels and intra-abdominal visceral fat was documented after CPAP treatment (82).

Inflammatory/Oxidative Factors

Increased serum levels of circulating inflammatory markers, particularly fibrinogen (83), C-reactive protein (84–86), serum amyloid A (87), inflammatory cytokines [interleukin-6 (IL-6) and IL-18] (85,88), and adhesion molecules (81,89,90) were documented in patients with OSA in previous studies. An increased level of circulating cell-derived microparticles was recently documented in patients with minimally symptomatic OSA compared to matched control subjects without OSA (91). Moreover, oxidative stress related to intermittent hypoxia and normoxia is increased in OSA (81,89). These factors may play a role in the development and progression of atherosclerosis in OSA. Accordingly, a significant increase of carotid intima-media thickness, percentage of carotid plaques, and serum levels of C-reactive protein, IL-6, and IL-18 in patients with OSA may place them at greater risk for stroke (88,92,93).

Acute Effects

Blood Pressure

Considering the strong association between arterial hypertension and obstructive SA, the presence of SA in the first days after stroke may have an impact on BP and, subsequently, on clinical evolution and the outcome. The evolution of BP in acute stroke and its impact on the outcome has been investigated in several studies. Up to 80% of patients with acute stroke are hypertensive after stroke onset, and elevated BP spontaneously declines over the following days (94,95). Both increased and decreased BP levels in acute stroke are linked to an unfavorable prognosis, suggesting a J-/U-shaped relationship between BP and stroke outcome (96–99). In addition, an alteration of circadian BP rhythms with loss of physiological nocturnal BP lowering (the so-called nondipping state) has been documented in the first days after stroke (100–103). However, despite the evidence of a strong association between SA and both hypertension and stroke, and considering the impact of elevated BP levels on the stroke outcome (102,104,105), the relationship between BP, SA, and stroke remains poorly investigated. In one study (106), an increased BP variability (as defined by number of 15 mmHg dips/hr) was documented in seven stroke patients with SA when compared with five patients without SA. A prospective study on 41 patients with acute ischemic stroke (107) showed an association between SA severity and higher 24-hour BP values (Fig. 4). In the same study, nondipping was linked to more severe strokes and to a worse short-term outcome. Preliminary data suggest that the presence of moderate to severe obstructive SA in the acute phase of stroke may be associated with sustained higher nocturnal BP levels in the recovery phase (29). The possible role of a sustained increased sympathetic activity related to obstructive SA needs to be tested in these patients. Further studies with larger numbers of patients are needed to better understand the impact of obstructive SA on BP evolution and their implication for stroke evolution/outcome and to identify subgroups of high-risk patients requiring a closer monitoring and more aggressive management of BP after stroke.

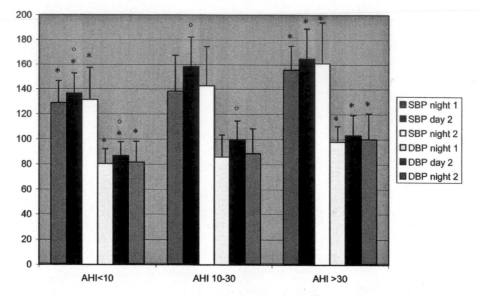

Figure 4 Mean systolic and diastolic blood pressure during the first night, the second day and the second night in 41 patients with acute ischemic stroke according to the severity of sleep apnea. AHI <10/hr indicates no sleep apnea, AHI between 10/hr and 30/hr indicates a mild to moderate sleep apnea, and AHI >30/hr indicates a moderate to severe sleep apnea. Data are means ± 1 standard deviation. * indicates statistical significance ($p < 0.05$) between patients without sleep apnea (AHI < 10) and those with moderate to severe sleep apnea (AHI > 30); ° indicates statistical significance ($p < 0.05$) between patients without sleep apnea (AHI < 10) and those with mild to moderate sleep apnea (AHI, 10–30). *Abbreviations*: AHI, apnea-hypopnea index; SBP, systolic blood pressure; DBP, diastolic blood pressure; night 1, first night after stroke onset; day 2, second day after stroke onset; night 2, second night after stroke onset. *Source*: From Ref. 107.

Cerebral Hemodynamics and Tissue Oxygenation

SA has been documented to adversely affect short-term evolution (16), duration of hospitalization (108), functional outcome, and mortality after stroke (18,21,106,109,110). Part of this association is possibly due to the detrimental effect of apneic events on not yet irreversibly damaged ischemic brain areas [the so-called penumbra (111)] in acute stroke. Apneic events were shown in several studies to be associated with a reduction of cerebral oxygenation (hypoxia) and with fluctuations in cerebral hemodynamics (112–116), whereas this effect is more pronounced for apneas of the obstructive type than for those of the central type. One study (114) found a significant decline in cerebral blood flow of the cerebri media occurring during apneas, especially of the obstructive type, associated with falls in oxygen saturation. Moreover, an abnormal cerebral vascular response to hypoxia/hypercapnia (117–119) and a close correlation between changes in cerebral blood flow and fluctuations in arterial BP (113,117,120) have been observed in patients with SA, indicating impaired cerebral autoregulation (121–123) and increased susceptibility to brain ischemia, which is particularly evident in the early morning. These abnormalities were shown to be corrected with CPAP treatment (115). In addition, OSA patients with a simultaneous monitoring of intracranial pressure showed a marked increase in intracranial pressure, which is in part related to negative intrathoracic pressure during apneas and to increased central venous volume (124), resulting in a decrease in cerebral perfusion pressure, especially during obstructive apneas (125). The magnitude of the increase in intracranial pressure correlated with the duration of apneas. Recently, near-infrared spectrophotometry, which allows measurements of cerebral tissue oxy- and deoxy-hemoglobin concentration, as well as brain tissue oxygenation, has been shown to be a useful noninvasive tool for assessment and monitoring of cerebral tissue oxygenation during apneic phases (126–128).

These observations support the evidence of a tight link between apneic events (particularly of the obstructive type) and cerebral hemodynamics, particularly brain oxygenation. The clinical implications of these changes, as well as their impact on stroke outcome, morbidity, and mortality, remain at the present time still unclear.

Sympathetic Nervous System

Obstructive SA has been shown to be associated with sustained increased sympathetic activity (81). Apneic events accompanying SA, mainly of the obstructive type, are associated with hypoxemia, arousal from sleep, intrathoracic pressure changes, and sympathetic activation (81,129). These responses are related to acute changes in cardiovascular function. Hypoxemia and hypercapnia result in chemoreflex activation with consequent sustained increase in sympathetic vasoconstrictor activity to peripheral blood vessels (81,130). This reflex response results in increased BP as well as increased levels of circulating catecholamines. The sympathetic activity and increase in BP are shown to be reduced after treatment with CPAP (131,132). Moreover, the association between SA and elevated cardiovascular risk, as well as early signs of atherosclerosis [i.e., carotid intima-media thickness (88,92)], is likely to be, in part, mediated by increased sympathetic activity.

In acute stroke, elevated BP levels, increased BP/heart rate variability (106), and altered physiological 24-hour BP pattern (nondipping state) are frequently observed (103,133). This is partly due to an increased stroke-related catecholamine and cortisol release, possibly reflecting the cerebral response to decreased perfusion in the ischemic penumbra, but also due to changes in the sleep-wake cycle and the acute stress of hospitalization (100,101,103). A relationship with stroke topography (cortical versus noncortical) and stroke etiology (hemorrhagic versus ischemic) has also been suggested (100–102). In addition, ischemic strokes in distinct cortical brain areas involved in central cardiovascular control (e.g., insula) were shown to be associated with profound alterations in cardiac function and BP, which may be linked to acute changes in central autonomic control (134–138).

IV. Sleep Apnea as a Consequence of Stroke

A. Breathing Disorder in Wakefulness as a Consequence of Stroke

In patients with stroke, disordered breathing is often the result of different factors overlapping: the brain damage per se, the preexisting cardiorespiratory conditions (obstructive SA or heart failure), and the indirect complications of brain damage (aspiration, lung edema, pain, immobility, respiratory infection, autonomic changes).

Brain damage affects breathing during wakefulness and/or sleep in different ways according to the type, extension, and topography of the lesion (139): (*i*) Involvement of afferent inputs to the medullary respiratory neurons (e.g., posterior spinal cord) (140) may lead to apneas of obstructive or central type; (*ii*) dysfunction of medullary respiratory neurons (e.g., in medullary stroke) may trigger central apneas, irregular breathing (Biot's or ataxic breathing), and failure of automatic breathing (Ondine's curse) during wakefulness and/or sleep; (*iii*) involvement of the efferent respiratory control at the level of respiratory neurons (e.g., in anterior medullary or spinal stroke) (141) may lead to central or obstructive apneas; and (*iv*) dysfunction of supramedullary (cortical, corticobulbar, or corticospinal) breathing control mechanisms can present with various forms of disordered breathing, mainly in the form of complex abnormalities of voluntary or automatic breathing (142–144). Lesions of different topographies involving the cortex, the corticobulbar tracts, or the corticospinal tracts may affect voluntary breathing either partially (respiratory apraxia) or completely (failure of voluntary breathing) (145,146).

Bilateral lesions in the ventrotegmental pons may be associated with inspiratory breath holding (apneustic breathing) or regular and rapid breathing (central neurogenic hyperventilation), whereas in pontomedullary lesions, complex abnormalities of voluntary and automatic breathing may be observed. These patients may exhibit irregular breathing (cluster breathing), central apneas, hiccups, and stridor during wakefulness and sleep.

B. Breathing Disorder in Sleep (Sleep Apnea) as a Consequence of Stroke

An acute ischemic brain lesion may cause a new-onset SA or worsen a preexisting SA, especially of the central type. Breathing disorders of the central type, such as central apneas or central periodic breathing, were traditionally reported both during wakefulness and sleep in patients with brainstem or bilateral/extensive hemispheric stroke with impaired level of consciousness (19,144,147) and in association with heart failure (24,148–151). Central SA or central periodic breathing occurring exclusively during sleep has been linked to large hemispheric ischemic lesions and poor functional outcome (17,25,152). Recent studies (14–16,19) suggest that this type of disordered breathing may also occur in the very acute phase in patients with unilateral lesions of variable topography involving autonomic (e.g., insula) or volitional (e.g., prefrontal region, capsula interna, thalamus) brain areas participating in respiratory control, even without a disturbed level of consciousness or heart failure (17,19,20,22). The pathogenetic mechanism underlying new-onset respiratory changes in acute stroke remains poorly understood. Distinct brainstem lesions may lead to a reduced CO_2 sensitivity (153), contributing to the disorder. The potential role of dysfunction in central autonomic control, in analogy to cardiovascular changes observed in patients with stroke in definite brain areas (e.g., insula) (137,138), remains to be investigated in these patients. This breathing pattern spontaneously recovers within weeks or months after stroke in most patients (15,21,22). Persisting central SA has been linked, on the other hand, with chronic heart failure (24,154,155).

Rarely, preexisting obstructive SA may worsen by a disturbed coordination of upper airway, intercostal, and diaphragmatic muscles due to brainstem or hemispheric lesions. In addition, both central SA and obstructive SA may potentiate each other (14).

V. Clinical Relevance of Sleep Apnea in Stroke Patients
A. Very Acute/Acute Phase after Ischemic Stroke

Little is known about the clinical implications of SA in the acute phase of ischemic stroke. Iranzo et al. (16) assessed 50 patients by polysomnography in the first night after brain infarction, showing that SA (defined as AHI ≥ 10/hr) was associated with early neurological worsening independent of other cardiovascular risk factors but not with unfavorable longer-term outcome. In the same study, moderate to severe SA (defined as AHI ≥ 25/hr) was significantly linked to stroke onset during sleep. Selic et al. (107) assessed 41 patients by portable respirography within the first four days after stroke onset, finding that SA severity was significantly associated with stroke severity and with worse short-term stroke outcome at hospital discharge. In the same study, SA severity was also associated with higher 24-hour BP levels in terms of a linear dose-response relationship. In a recent study assessing with questionnaires (however, without any objective measurement of nocturnal breathing) the risk of OSA in 190 patients, no association between the likelihood of OSA and stroke severity or early neurological worsening was observed (156). An association between the severity of SA and the duration of hospital stay has been observed in two studies (107,108). In one recent study, SA assessed within 24 hours after stroke onset defined as AHI ≥ 10/hr was independently associated with increased levels of C-reactive protein (157).

Whether SA, especially of the obstructive type, adversely affects the evolution of the ischemic penumbra in the acute stroke phase remains unclear. Preliminary data suggest that SA may be linked to a smaller regression of the perfusion deficit (measured by perfusion-weighted magnetic resonance imaging) in the ischemic brain area (158).

B. Subacute Chronic Phase after Ischemic Stroke

SA was shown to be associated with increased mortality (18,21,23,109,159) and poor functional outcome (30,109,159,160). Dyken et al. (18) reported a four-year mortality of 21% in 24 stroke patients with obstructive SA assessed by polysomnography within five weeks after stroke onset. Parra et al. (109) assessed SA severity with a portable device in a group of 161 patients within 72 hours after stroke onset, showing that AHI was an independent predictor of two-year mortality. In this study, 50% of follow-up deaths were cerebrovascular deaths, and 10 patients had a recurrent fatal stroke; each additional unit of AHI was associated with a 5% increased relative risk of death; and age, involvement of the middle cerebral artery, and coronary heart disease were reported as further independent predictors of mortality. Turkington et al. (159) reported that death after stroke was independently associated with stroke severity [measured by the Scandinavian Stroke Scale (161)] and severity of obstructive SA (estimated by the AHI) at six months follow-up, whereas longer apneic events were associated with higher mortality. The severity of OSA assessed in 113 patients during the subacute phase (weeks) after stroke has also been reported to be associated with higher fibrinogen levels that correlated with the duration of apneas and the minimal oxygen desaturation (83). Bassetti et al. (21) showed that AHI assessed with a portable device in a group of 131 patients with acute ischemic stroke within nine days after stroke onset was significantly higher among nonsurvivors after a follow-up of five years. One recent Swedish study performed on 151 patients with acute/subacute ischemic stroke showed that OSA detected 23 ± 8 days after stroke was associated with a higher risk of death in a 10-year follow-up compared to controls without OSA (adjusted hazard ratio 1.76,

95% CI, 1.05–2.95; $p = 0.03$), independent of age, gender, BMI, smoking, hypertension, diabetes mellitus, atrial fibrillation, the Mini-Mental State Examination score, and the Barthel index. In contrast, there was no difference in mortality between patients with central SA and controls (23).

Fewer data exist on SA severity and the long-term functional outcome or recurrence after the first stroke or TIA. Good et al. (30) studied 47 patients with pulse oximetry and 19 of them by polysomnography after a median time of 15 days following stroke and found that several oximetry variables (mean oxygen saturation, time spent less than 90% saturation, number of desaturations, and desaturation index) correlated with functional disability [measured by the Barthel index (162)] at discharge, with the functional improvement from admission to discharge, and with the ability to return home after discharge. Mean oxygen saturation and time spent with less than 90% saturation correlated with the ability to live at home at 3 months and with the risk of death at 12 months after stroke. Turkington et al. (159) reported that functional disability (measured by the Barthel index) was independently predicted by the minimum oxygen saturation measured in the acute stroke phase; the Barthel index was higher in the group of patients with OSA, but the difference compared to patients without SA did not reach statistical significance. In a recent study, SA detected 6.5 ± 3.2 days after stroke onset in the acute phase was associated with a worse functional outcome and to an increasing likelihood of dependency three months after stroke (110).

In terms of event recurrence after the first stroke or TIA, Martinez-Garcia et al. (160) observed that patients with moderate to severe (AHI $\geq$ 20/hr) SA assessed within two months after stroke who did not receive CPAP treatment had a fivefold-increased relative risk (adjusted odds ratio 5.09, 95% CI, 1.54–40.7) of recurrent stroke or TIA at an 18-month follow-up compared with treated SA patients.

Preliminary data suggest that the presence of witnessed apneas assessed by questionnaires in patients with first-ever stroke or TIA may independently be associated with a higher risk of event recurrence (Siccoli MM et al., unpublished data).

VI. Treatment of Sleep Apnea in Stroke Patients

Treatment of OSA in stroke patients represents a challenge. General treatment strategies should always include prevention and early treatment of secondary complications (e.g., aspiration, respiratory infections, pain) and cautious use or avoidance of sedative-hypnotic drugs, which may all negatively affect breathing control during sleep. It is usually recommended to place patients on their nonparetic side, since wrong positioning in the acute phase may also adversely affect oxygen saturation (163) and favor the occurrence of apneas (164). Weight loss may also help to improve obstructive SA after stroke.

In terms of long-term prevention after ischemic stroke, CPAP remains the treatment of choice for patients with OSA. Particularly, the benefit of CPAP treatment in patients with moderate to severe disease and (*i*) high cardiovascular risk profile, in terms of primary and secondary long-term prevention of incident cardiovascular events, including stroke (7,9,12,37,38,59,60), and (*ii*) excessive daytime sleepiness and/or impaired quality of life (165–170) have been clearly documented.

In contrast, the question about the benefit of CPAP treatment in patients with moderate to severe OSA during the first days to weeks after ischemic stroke remains controversial. A few publications suggest that early CPAP treatment may have favorable effects in stroke patients. In one prospective study (171), CPAP administered in the first weeks after stroke has been shown to significantly improve nocturnal BP and subjective well-being measured by a visual analogue scale after 10 days of treatment. In another randomized study with 63 patients (172), CPAP was shown to improve depressive symptoms in patients with severe stroke and SA after one week and one month of follow-up. Another study performed on 51 patients (160) showed an 80% reduction in the risk of stroke recurrence after 18 months of follow-up in patients started and maintained on CPAP within 2 months after stroke compared to those who did not tolerate CPAP treatment. Moreover, the cost-effectiveness of CPAP treatment has been proven in stroke patients (173). Only one randomized controlled CPAP treatment trial has been performed to date in stroke patients. Hsu et al. (174) assessed 66 patients with polysomnography within 14 to 18 days after ischemic stroke, randomizing 15 patients with severe OSA (AHI $\geq$ 30/hr) to CPAP and 15 to conventional treatment. At a follow-up of eight weeks and six months, no significant differences were observed between the two groups regarding the quality of life, neurological function, or excessive sleepiness; however, the CPAP use was poor (1.4 hr/night).

Two further factors need to be taken into account considering CPAP treatment in stroke patients. First, SA spontaneously improves in most patients from the acute to the recovery phase after stroke (15,21,28), and this improvement may occur early (within one week) in some patients. A follow-up respirography should therefore be considered before initiating treatment to confirm if the severity of obstructive apneas is severe enough to justify CPAP treatment. Secondly, long-term CPAP compliance is low in stroke patients. Previous studies report a variable CPAP compliance ranging from 22% to 70% at two to eight weeks after stroke (21,171,175,176). One study performed in 34 stroke patients reported a CPAP compliance of 11% at three months (175); in another study carried out by Bassetti et al. (21) in 66 patients, a compliance of 16% was observed at a five-year follow-up. In contrast, one recent pilot study performed in 12 patients within 48 hours after stroke onset showed CPAP acceptance of 84% in the first night of treatment, with a mean use of CPAP of 5.2 $\pm$ 4.0 hours (177).

Thus, CPAP treatment of patients with OSA in the first days/weeks after stroke remains a difficult and controversial issue, although the results of clinical studies on the impact of SA on stroke evolution and outcome would support early CPAP use. Early CPAP treatment may therefore be individually considered, mainly in younger (<70 years) patients with (*i*) mild to moderate neurological deficits without aphasia/facial weakness/neglect/dementia or severe coincidental illness, (*ii*) moderate to severe OSA (AHI $\geq$ 30/hr), and (*iii*) either a high cardiovascular risk profile, excessive daytime sleepiness, or both.

A prospective study with a large number of patients and adequate follow-up is needed to assess the acceptance and benefit of long-term CPAP treatment in stroke patients with OSA. In patients presenting predominantly with central apneas or central periodic breathing, oxygen may be beneficial (20). The benefit of CPAP treatment in stroke patients with central apneas or central periodic breathing has not been proven until now. In contrast, the efficacy of CPAP treatment in patients with central apnea or central periodic breathing and heart failure has been extensively investigated. A large randomized trial showed that CPAP treatment in patients with heart failure improved nocturnal oxygenation, increased the ejection fraction, lowered norepinephrine levels, and increased the distance walked in six minutes, but it did not affect survival (151). A further post hoc analysis revealed that a reduction of central apneas below the threshold of 15 events/hr was linked to a significant improvement in transplant-free survival (178). Other methods of ventilator support, such as adaptive servoventilation, were shown to prevent central apneas in stroke patients with heart failure more efficiently than CPAP or oxygen (179). Acetazolamide administered before sleep has been shown to improve central SA and related daytime symptoms in patients with heart failure (180) and may be considered in stroke patients as well.

References

1. He J, Kryger MH, Zorick FJ, et al. Mortality and apnea index in obstructive sleep apnea. Experience in 385 male patients. Chest 1988; 94:9–14.
2. Partinen M, Jamieson A, Guilleminault C. Long-term outcome for obstructive sleep apnea syndrome patients. Mortality. Chest 1988; 94:1200–1204.
3. Young T, Peppard P, Palta M, et al. Population-based study of sleep-disordered breathing as a risk factor for hypertension. Arch Intern Med 1997; 157:1746–1752.
4. Peppard PE, Young T, Palta M, et al. Prospective study of the association between sleep-disordered breathing and hypertension. N Engl J Med 2000; 342:1378–1384.
5. Nieto FJ, Young TB, Lind BK, et al. Association of sleep-disordered breathing, sleep apnea, and hypertension in a large community-based study. Sleep Heart Health Study. JAMA 2000; 283:1829–1836.
6. Hung J, Whitford EG, Parsons RW, et al. Association of sleep apnoea with myocardial infarction in men. Lancet 1990; 336:261–264.
7. Shahar E, Whitney CW, Redline S, et al. Sleep-disordered breathing and cardiovascular disease: cross-sectional results of the Sleep Heart Health Study. Am J Respir Crit Care Med 2001; 163:19–25.
8. Gami AS, Pressman G, Caples SM, et al. Association of atrial fibrillation and obstructive sleep apnea. Circulation 2004; 110:364–367.
9. Marin JM, Carrizo SJ, Vicente E, et al. Long-term cardiovascular outcomes in men with obstructive sleep apnoea-hypopnoea with or without treatment with continuous positive airway pressure: an observational study. Lancet 2005; 365:1046–1053.
10. Kanagala R, Murali NS, Friedman PA, et al. Obstructive sleep apnea and the recurrence of atrial fibrillation. Circulation 2003; 107:2589–2594.
11. Gami AS, Howard DE, Olson EJ, et al. Day-night pattern of sudden death in obstructive sleep apnea. N Engl J Med 2005; 352:1206–1214.
12. Yaggi HK, Concato J, Kernan WN, et al. Obstructive sleep apnea as a risk factor for stroke and death. N Engl J Med 2005; 353:2034–2041.
13. Bassetti C, Aldrich MS, Chervin RD, et al. Sleep apnea in patients with transient ischemic attack and stroke: a prospective study of 59 patients. Neurology 1996; 47:1167–1173.
14. Bassetti C, Aldrich MS. Sleep apnea in acute cerebrovascular diseases: final report on 128 patients. Sleep 1999; 22:217–223.
15. Parra O, Arboix A, Bechich S, et al. Time course of sleep-related breathing disorders in first-ever stroke or transient ischemic attack. Am J Respir Crit Care Med 2000; 161:375–380.
16. Iranzo A, Santamaria J, Berenguer J, et al. Prevalence and clinical importance of sleep apnea in the first night after cerebral infarction. Neurology 2002; 58:911–916.
17. Siccoli MM, Valko PO, Hermann DM, et al. Central periodic breathing during sleep in 74 patients with acute ischemic stroke—neurogenic and cardiogenic factors. J Neurol 2008; 255:1687–1692.
18. Dyken ME, Somers VK, Yamada T, et al. Investigating the relationship between stroke and obstructive sleep apnea. Stroke 1996; 27:401–407.

19. Bassetti C, Aldrich MS, Quint D. Sleep-disordered breathing in patients with acute supra- and infratentorial strokes. A prospective study of 39 patients. Stroke 1997; 28:1765–1772.

20. Nachtmann A, Siebler M, Rose G, et al. Cheyne-Stokes respiration in ischemic stroke. Neurology 1995; 45:820–821.

21. Bassetti CL, Milanova M, Gugger M. Sleep disordered breathing and acute stroke: diagnosis, risk factors, treatment, evolution and outcome. Stroke 2006; 37:967–972.

22. Hermann DM, Siccoli M, Kirov P, et al. Central periodic breathing during sleep in acute ischemic stroke. Stroke 2007; 38:1082–1084.

23. Sahlin C, Sandberg O, Gustafson Y, et al. Obstructive sleep apnea is a risk factor for death in patients with stroke: a 10-year follow-up. Arch Intern Med 2008; 168:297–301.

24. Nopmaneejumruslers C, Kaneko Y, Hajek V, et al. Cheyne-Stokes respiration in stroke: relationship to hypocapnia and occult cardiac dysfunction. Am J Respir Crit Care Med 2005; 171:1048–1052.

25. Rowat AM, Dennis MS, Wardlaw JM. Central periodic breathing observed on hospital admission is associated with an adverse prognosis in conscious acute stroke patients. Cerebrovasc Dis 2006; 21:340–347.

26. Wessendorf TE, Teschler H, Wang YM, et al. Sleep-disordered breathing among patients with first-ever stroke. J Neurol 2000; 247:41–47.

27. Turkington PM, Bamford J, Wanklyn P, et al. Prevalence and predictors of upper airway obstruction in the first 24 hours after acute stroke. Stroke 2002; 33:2037–2042.

28. Harbison J, Ford GA, James OFW, et al. Sleep-disordered breathing following acute stroke. QJM 2002; 95:741–747.

29. Siccoli MM, Birkmann S, Valko PO, et al. Effect of obstructive sleep apnea in acute ischemic stroke on blood pressure evolution and functional outcome. Abstract of the 20th Annual meeting of the Associated Professional Sleep Societies, June 2006, Salt Lake City, Utah, USA.

30. Good DC, Henkle JQ, Gelber D, et al. Sleep-disordered breathing and poor functional outcome after stroke. Stroke 1996; 27:252–259.

31. van der Werf SP, van den Broek HL, Anten HW, et al. Experience of severe fatigue long after stroke and its relation to depressive symptoms and disease characteristics. Eur Neurol 2001; 45:28–33.

32. Bogousslavsky J, Khurana R, Deruaz JP, et al. Respiratory failure and unilateral caudal brainstem infarction. Ann Neurol 1990; 28:668–673.

33. Rousseaux M, Hurtevent JF, Benaim C, et al. Late contralateral hyperhidrosis in lateral medullary infarcts. Stroke 1996; 27:991–995.

34. Kim BS, Kim YI, Lee KS. Contralateral hyperhidrosis after cerebral infarction. Clinicoanatomic correlations in five cases. Stroke 1995; 26:896–899.

35. Young T, Palta M, Dempsey J, et al. The occurrence of sleep-disordered breathing among middle-aged adults. N Engl J Med 1993; 328:1230–1235.

36. Stradling JR, Crosby JH. Predictors and prevalence of obstructive sleep apnoea and snoring in 1001 middle aged men. Thorax 1991; 46:85–90.

37. Young T, Finn L, Peppard PE, et al. Sleep disordered breathing and mortality: eighteen-year follow-up of the Wisconsin sleep cohort. Sleep 2008; 31:1071–1078.

38. Marshall NS, Wong KK, Liu PY, et al. Sleep apnea as an independent risk factor for all-cause mortality: the Busselton health study. Sleep 2008; 31:1079–1085.

39. Koshino Y, Satoh M, Katayose Y, et al. Association of sleep-disordered breathing and ventricular arrhythmias in patients without heart failure. Am J Cardiol 2008; 101:882–886.

40. Peker Y, Hedner J, Norum J, et al. Increased incidence of cardiovascular disease in middle-aged men with obstructive sleep apnea: a 7-year follow-up. Am J Respir Crit Care Med 2002; 166:159–165.

41. Kales A, Bixler EO, Cadieux RJ, et al. Sleep apnoea in a hypertensive population. Lancet 1984; 2:1005–1008.

42. Carlson JT, Hedner JA, Ejnell H, et al. High prevalence of hypertension in sleep apnea patients independent of obesity. Am J Respir Crit Care Med 1994; 150:72–77.
43. Hla KM, Young TB, Bidwell T, et al. Sleep apnea and hypertension. A population-based study. Ann Intern Med 1994; 120:382–388.
44. Worsnop CJ, Naughton MT, Barter CE, et al. The prevalence of obstructive sleep apnea in hypertensives. Am J Respir Crit Care Med 1998; 157:111–115.
45. Lavie P, Herer P, Hoffstein V. Obstructive sleep apnoea syndrome as a risk factor for hypertension: population study. BMJ 2000; 320:479–482.
46. Sjostrom C, Lindberg E, Elmasry A, et al. Prevalence of sleep apnoea and snoring in hypertensive men: a population based study. Thorax 2002; 57:602–607.
47. Faccenda JF, Mackay TW, Boon NA, et al. Randomized placebo-controlled trial of continuous positive airway pressure on blood pressure in the sleep apnea-hypopnea syndrome. Am J Respir Crit Care Med 2001; 163:344–348.
48. Pepperell JC, Ramdassingh-Dow S, Crosthwaite N, et al. Ambulatory blood pressure after therapeutic and subtherapeutic nasal continuous positive airway pressure for obstructive sleep apnoea: a randomised parallel trial. Lancet 2002; 359:204–210.
49. Spriggs DA, French JM, Murdy JM, et al. Snoring increases the risk of stroke and adversely affects prognosis. Q J Med 1992; 83:555–562.
50. Partinen M, Palomaki H. Snoring and cerebral infarction. Lancet 1985; 2:1325–1326.
51. Palomaki H. Snoring and the risk of ischemic brain infarction. Stroke 1991; 22:1021–1025.
52. Smirne S, Palazzi S, Zucconi M, et al. Habitual snoring as a risk factor for acute vascular disease. Eur Respir J 1993; 6:1357–1361.
53. Neau JP, Meurice JC, Paquereau J, et al. Habitual snoring as a risk factor for brain infarction. Acta Neurol Scand 1995; 92:63–68.
54. Koskenvuo M, Kaprio J, Partinen M, et al. Snoring as a risk factor for hypertension and angina pectoris. Lancet 1985; 1:893–896.
55. Jennum P, Sjol A. Snoring, sleep apnoea and cardiovascular risk factors: the MONICA II Study. Int J Epidemiol 1993; 22:439–444.
56. Hu FB, Willett WC, Manson JE, et al. Snoring and risk of cardiovascular disease in women. J Am Coll Cardiol 2000; 35:308–313.
57. Yaggi H, Mohsenin V. Obstructive sleep apnoea and stroke. Lancet Neurol 2004; 3:333–342.
58. Elwood P, Hack M, Pickering J, et al. Sleep disturbance, stroke, and heart disease events: evidence from the Caerphilly cohort. J Epidemiol Community Health 2006; 60:69–73.
59. Arzt M, Young T, Finn L, et al. Association of sleep-disordered breathing and the occurrence of stroke. Am J Respir Crit Care Med 2005; 172:1447–1451.
60. Valham F, Mooe T, Rabben T, et al. Increased risk of stroke in patients with coronary artery disease and sleep apnea: a 10-year follow-up. Circulation 2008; 118:955–960.
61. Harbison J, Gibson GJ, Birchall D, et al. White matter disease and sleep-disordered breathing after acute stroke. Neurology 2003; 61:959–963.
62. Davies CW, Crosby JH, Mullins RL, et al. Case control study of cerebrovascular damage defined by magnetic resonance imaging in patients with OSA and normal matched control subjects. Sleep 2001; 24:715–720.
63. Minoguchi K, Yokoe T, Tazaki T, et al. Silent brain infarction and platelet activation in obstructive sleep apnea. Am J Respir Crit Care Med 2007; 175:612–617.
64. Ding J, Nieto FJ, Beauchamp NJ Jr., et al. Sleep-disordered breathing and white matter disease in the brainstem in older adults. Sleep 2004; 27:474–479.
65. Panza JA, Quyyumi AA, Brush JE Jr., et al. Abnormal endothelium-dependent vascular relaxation in patients with essential hypertension. N Engl J Med 1990; 323:22–27.
66. Celermajer DS, Sorensen KE, Gooch VM, et al. Non-invasive detection of endothelial dysfunction in children and adults at risk of atherosclerosis. Lancet 1992; 340:1111–1115.

67. Kohler M, Craig S, Nicoll D, et al. Endothelial function and arterial stiffness in minimally symptomatic obstructive sleep apnea. Am J Respir Crit Care Med 2008; 178:984–988.
68. Ip MS, Lam B, Chan LY, et al. Circulating nitric oxide is suppressed in obstructive sleep apnea and is reversed by nasal continuous positive airway pressure. Am J Respir Crit Care Med 2000; 162:2166–2171.
69. Schulz R, Schmidt D, Blum A, et al. Decreased plasma levels of nitric oxide derivatives in obstructive sleep apnoea: response to CPAP therapy. Thorax 2000; 55:1046–1051.
70. Imadojemu VA, Gleeson K, Quraishi SA, et al. Impaired vasodilator responses in obstructive sleep apnea are improved with continuous positive airway pressure therapy. Am J Respir Crit Care Med 2002; 165:950–953.
71. Phillips BG, Narkiewicz K, Pesek CA, et al. Effects of obstructive sleep apnea on endothelin-1 and blood pressure. J Hypertens 1999; 17:61–66.
72. Allahdadi KJ, Walker BR, Kanagy NL. Augmented endothelin vasoconstriction in intermittent hypoxia-induced hypertension. Hypertension 2005; 45:705–709.
73. Peled N, Kassirer M, Kramer MR, et al. Increased erythrocyte adhesiveness and aggregation in obstructive sleep apnea syndrome. Thromb Res 2008; 121:631–636.
74. Bokinsky G, Miller M, Ault K, et al. Spontaneous platelet activation and aggregation during obstructive sleep apnea and its response to therapy with nasal continuous positive airway pressure. A preliminary investigation. Chest 1995; 108:625–630.
75. Eisensehr I, Ehrenberg BL, Noachtar S, et al. Platelet activation, epinephrine, and blood pressure in obstructive sleep apnea syndrome. Neurology 1998; 51:188–195.
76. Geiser T, Buck F, Meyer BJ, et al. In vivo platelet activation is increased during sleep in patients with obstructive sleep apnea syndrome. Respiration; international review of thoracic diseases. Respiration 2002; 69:229–234.
77. Brooks B, Cistulli PA, Borkman M, et al. Obstructive sleep apnea in obese noninsulin-dependent diabetic patients: effect of continuous positive airway pressure treatment on insulin responsiveness. J Clin Endocrinol Metab 1994; 79:1681–1685.
78. Punjabi NM, Sorkin JD, Katzel LI, et al. Sleep-disordered breathing and insulin resistance in middle-aged and overweight men. Am J Respir Crit Care Med 2002; 165:677–682.
79. Harsch IA, Schahin SP, Radespiel-Troger M, et al. Continuous positive airway pressure treatment rapidly improves insulin sensitivity in patients with obstructive sleep apnea syndrome. Am J Respir Crit Care Med 2004; 169:156–162.
80. Phillips BG, Kato M, Narkiewicz K, et al. Increases in leptin levels, sympathetic drive, and weight gain in obstructive sleep apnea. Am J Physiol Heart Circ Physiol 2000; 279: H234–H237.
81. Shamsuzzaman AS, Gersh BJ, Somers VK. Obstructive sleep apnea: implications for cardiac and vascular disease. JAMA 2003; 290:1906–1914.
82. Chin K, Shimizu K, Nakamura T, et al. Changes in intra-abdominal visceral fat and serum leptin levels in patients with obstructive sleep apnea syndrome following nasal continuous positive airway pressure therapy. Circulation 1999; 100:706–712.
83. Wessendorf TE, Thilmann AF, Wang YM, et al. Fibrinogen levels and obstructive sleep apnea in ischemic stroke. Am J Respir Crit Care Med 2000; 162:2039–2042.
84. Shamsuzzaman AS, Winnicki M, Lanfranchi P, et al. Elevated C-reactive protein in patients with obstructive sleep apnea. Circulation 2002; 105:2462–2464.
85. Yokoe T, Minoguchi K, Matsuo H, et al. Elevated levels of C-reactive protein and interleukin-6 in patients with obstructive sleep apnea syndrome are decreased by nasal continuous positive airway pressure. Circulation 2003; 107:1129–1134.
86. Ridker PM. Clinical application of C-reactive protein for cardiovascular disease detection and prevention. Circulation 2003; 107:363–369.
87. Svatikova A, Wolk R, Shamsuzzaman AS, et al. Serum amyloid a in obstructive sleep apnea. Circulation 2003; 108:1451–1454.

88. Minoguchi K, Yokoe T, Tazaki T, et al. Increased carotid intima-media thickness and serum inflammatory markers in obstructive sleep apnea. Am J Respir Crit Care Med 2005; 172:625–630.
89. Dyugovskaya L, Lavie P, Lavie L. Increased adhesion molecules expression and production of reactive oxygen species in leukocytes of sleep apnea patients. Am J Respir Crit Care Med 2002; 165:934–939.
90. El-Solh AA, Mador MJ, Sikka P, et al. Adhesion molecules in patients with coronary artery disease and moderate-to-severe obstructive sleep apnea. Chest 2002; 121:1541–1547.
91. Ayers L, Ferry B, Craig S, et al. Circulating cell-derived microparticles in patients with minimally-symptomatic obstructive sleep apnoea. Eur Respir J 2009; 33:574–580.
92. Silvestrini M, Rizzato B, Placidi F, et al. Carotid artery wall thickness in patients with obstructive sleep apnea syndrome. Stroke 2002; 33:1782–1785.
93. Drager LF, Bortolotto LA, Krieger EM, et al. Additive effects of obstructive sleep apnea and hypertension on early markers of carotid atherosclerosis. Hypertension 2009; 53:64–69.
94. Britton M, Carlsson A, de Faire U. Blood pressure course in patients with acute stroke and matched controls. Stroke 1986; 17:861–864.
95. Jorgensen HS, Nakayama H, Christensen HR, et al. Blood pressure in acute stroke. The Copenhagen Stroke Study. Cerebrovasc Dis 2002; 13:204–209.
96. Farnett L, Mulrow CD, Linn WD, et al. The J-curve phenomenon and the treatment of hypertension. Is there a point beyond which pressure reduction is dangerous? JAMA 1991; 265:489–495.
97. Kario K, Pickering TG, Matsuo T, et al. Stroke prognosis and abnormal nocturnal blood pressure falls in older hypertensives. Hypertension 2001; 38:852–857.
98. Castillo J, Leira R, Garcia MM, et al. Blood pressure decrease during the acute phase of ischemic stroke is associated with brain injury and poor stroke outcome. Stroke 2004; 35: 520–526.
99. Vemmos KN, Tsivgoulis G, Spengos K, et al. U-shaped relationship between mortality and admission blood pressure in patients with acute stroke. J Intern Med 2004; 255:257–265.
100. Lip GY, Zarifis J, Farooqi IS, et al. Ambulatory blood pressure monitoring in acute stroke. The West Birmingham Stroke Project. Stroke 1997; 28:31–35.
101. Morfis L, Schwartz RS, Poulos R, et al. Blood pressure changes in acute cerebral infarction and hemorrhage. Stroke 1997; 28:1401–1405.
102. Bhalla A, Wolfe CDA, Rudd AG. The effect of 24 h blood pressure levels on early neurological recovery after stroke. J Intern Med 2001; 250:121–130.
103. Jain S, Namboodri KK, Kumari S, et al. Loss of circadian rhythm of blood pressure following acute stroke. BMC Neurol 2004; 4:1.
104. Ahmed N, Wahlgren G. High initial blood pressure after acute stroke is associated with poor functional outcome. J Intern Med 2001; 249:467–473.
105. Aslanyan S, Weir CJ, Lees KR; for the GAIN International Steering Committee and Investigators. Elevated pulse pressure during the acute period of ischemic stroke is associated with poor stroke outcome. Stroke 2004; 35:e153–e155.
106. Turkington PM, Bamford J, Wanklyn P, et al. Effect of upper airway obstruction on blood pressure variability after stroke. Clin Sci (Lond) 2004; 107:75–79.
107. Selic C, Siccoli MM, Hermann DM, et al. Blood pressure evolution after acute ischemic stroke in patients with and without sleep apnea. Stroke 2005; 36:2614–2618.
108. Kaneko Y, Hajek VE, Zivanovic V, et al. Relationship of sleep apnea to functional capacity and length of hospitalization following stroke. Sleep 2003; 26:293–297.
109. Parra O, Arboix A, Montserrat JM, et al. Sleep-related breathing disorders: impact on mortality of cerebrovascular disease. Eur Respir J 2004; 24:267–272.
110. Yan-Fang S, Yu-Ping W. Sleep-disordered breathing: impact on functional outcome of ischemic stroke patients. Sleep Med 2009; 10(7):717–719.

111. Schlaug G, Benfield A, Baird AE, et al. The ischemic penumbra: operationally defined by diffusion and perfusion MRI. Neurology 1999; 53:1528–1537.

112. Siebler M, Nachtmann A. Cerebral hemodynamics in obstructive sleep apnea. Chest 1993; 103:1118–1119.

113. Hayakawa T, Terashima M, Kayukawa Y, et al. Changes in cerebral oxygenation and hemodynamics during obstructive sleep apneas. Chest 1996; 109:916–921.

114. Netzer N, Werner P, Jochums I, et al. Blood flow of the middle cerebral artery with sleep-disordered breathing : correlation with obstructive hypopneas. Stroke 1998; 29:87–93.

115. Diomedi M, Placidi F, Cupini L, et al. Cerebral hemodynamic changes in sleep apnea syndrome and effect of continuous positive airway pressure treatment. Neurology 1998; 51:1051–1056.

116. Leslie WD, Wali S, Kryger M, et al. Blood flow of the middle cerebral artery with sleep-disordered breathing: correlation with obstructive hypopneas response. Stroke 1999; 30: 188a–190a.

117. Loeppky JA, Voyles WF, Eldridge MW, et al. Sleep apnea and autonomic cerebrovascular dysfunction. Sleep 1987; 10:25–34.

118. Foster GE, Hanly PJ, Ostrowski M, et al. Effects of continuous positive airway pressure on cerebral vascular response to hypoxia in patients with obstructive sleep apnea. Am J Respir Crit Care Med 2007; 175:720–725.

119. Foster GE, Poulin MJ, Hanly PJ. Intermittent hypoxia and vascular function: implications for obstructive sleep apnoea. Exp Physiol 2007; 92:51–65.

120. Balfors EM, Franklin KA. Impairment of cerebral perfusion during obstructive sleep apneas. Am J Respir Crit Care Med 1994; 150:1587–1591.

121. Furtner M, Staudacher M, Frauscher B, et al. Cerebral vasoreactivity decreases overnight in severe obstructive sleep apnea syndrome: a study of cerebral hemodynamics. Sleep Med 2009; 10(7):717–719.

122. Nasr N, Traon AP, Czosnyka M, et al. Cerebral autoregulation in patients with obstructive sleep apnea syndrome during wakefulness. Eur J Neurol 2009; 16:386–391.

123. Urbano F, Roux F, Schindler J, et al. Impaired cerebral autoregulation in obstructive sleep apnea. J Appl Physiol 2008; 105:1852–1857.

124. Shiomi T, Guilleminault C, Stoohs R, et al. Leftward shift of the interventricular septum and pulsus paradoxus in obstructive sleep apnea syndrome. Chest 1991; 100:894–902.

125. Jennum P, Borgesen SE. Intracranial pressure and obstructive sleep apnea. Chest 1989; 95:279–283.

126. Al-Rawi PG, Smielewski P, Kirkpatrick PJ. Evaluation of a near-infrared spectrometer (NIRO 300) for the detection of intracranial oxygenation changes in the adult head. Stroke 2001; 32:2492–500.

127. Wolf M, Weber O, Keel M, et al. Comparison of cerebral blood volume measured by near infrared spectroscopy and contrast enhanced magnetic resonance imaging. Adv Exp Med Biol 1999; 471:767–773.

128. Toronov V, Webb A, Choi JH, et al. Investigation of human brain hemodynamics by simultaneous near-infrared spectroscopy and functional magnetic resonance imaging. Med Phys 2001; 28:521–527.

129. Lanfranchi P, Somers VK. Obstructive sleep apnea and vascular disease. Respir Res 2001; 2:315–319.

130. Somers VK, Dyken ME, Clary MP, et al. Sympathetic neural mechanisms in obstructive sleep apnea. J Clin Invest 1995; 96:1897–1904.

131. Narkiewicz K, Kato M, Phillips BG, et al. Nocturnal continuous positive airway pressure decreases daytime sympathetic traffic in obstructive sleep apnea. Circulation 1999; 100: 2332–2335.

132. Kohler M, Pepperell JC, Casadei B, et al. CPAP and measures of cardiovascular risk in males with OSAS. Eur Respir J 2008; 32:1488–1496.
133. Verdecchia P, Porcellati C, Schillaci G. Ambulatory blood pressure. An independent predictor of prognosis in essential hypertension. Hypertension 1994; 24:790–801.
134. Oppenheimer SM, Kedem G, Martin WM. Left-insular cortex lesions perturb cardiac autonomic tone in humans. Clin Auton Res 1996; 6:131–140.
135. Christensen H, Boysen G, Christensen AF, et al. Insular lesions, ECG abnormalities, and outcome in acute stroke. J Neurol Neurosurg Psychiatry 2005; 76:269–271.
136. Oppenheimer S. Cerebrogenic cardiac arrhythmias: cortical lateralization and clinical significance. Clin Auton Res 2006; 16:6–11.
137. Laowattana S, Zeger SL, Lima JA, et al. Left insular stroke is associated with adverse cardiac outcome. Neurology 2006; 66:477–483.
138. Ay H, Koroshetz WJ, Benner T, et al. Neuroanatomic correlates of stroke-related myocardial injury. Neurology 2006; 66:1325–1329.
139. Bassetti CL, Gugger M. Sleep disordered breathing in neurologic disorders. Swiss Med Wkly 2002; 132:109–115.
140. Lahuerta J, Buxton P, Lipton S, et al. The location and function of respiratory fibres in the second cervical spinal cord segment: respiratory dysfunction syndrome after cervical cordotomy. J Neurol Neurosurg Psychiatry 1992; 55:1142–1145.
141. Howard RS, Thorpe J, Barker R, et al. Respiratory insufficiency due to high anterior cervical cord infarction. J Neurol Neurosurg Psychiatry 1998; 64:358–361.
142. Plum F. Hyperpnea, hyperventilation, and brain dysfunction. Ann Intern Med 1972; 76:328.
143. Plum F, Brown HW. Neurogenic factors in periodic breathing. Trans Am Neurol Assoc 1961; 86:39–42.
144. Plum F, Swanson AG. Central neurogenic hyperventilation in man. AMA Arch Neurol Psychiatry 1959; 81:535–549.
145. Munschauer FE, Mador MJ, Ahuja A, et al. Selective paralysis of voluntary but not limbically influenced automatic respiration. Arch Neurol 1991; 48:1190–1192.
146. Davis JN. Autonomous breathing. Report of a case. Arch Neurol 1974; 30:480–483.
147. Lee MC, Klassen AC, Resch JA. Respiratory pattern disturbances in ischemic cerebral vascular disease. Stroke 1974; 5:612–616.
148. Sin DD, Fitzgerald F, Parker JD, et al. Risk factors for central and obstructive sleep apnea in 450 men and women with congestive heart failure. Am J Respir Crit Care Med 1999; 160:1101–1106.
149. Bradley TD, Floras JS. Sleep apnea and heart failure: part II: central sleep apnea. Circulation 2003; 107:1822–1826.
150. Leung RS, Huber MA, Rogge T, et al. Association between atrial fibrillation and central sleep apnea. Sleep 2005; 28:1543–1546.
151. Bradley TD, Logan AG, Kimoff RJ, et al. Continuous positive airway pressure for central sleep apnea and heart failure. N Engl J Med 2005; 353:2025–2033.
152. Rowat AM, Wardlaw JM, Dennis MS. Abnormal breathing patterns in stroke: relationship with location of acute stroke lesion and prior cerebrovascular disease. J Neurol Neurosurg Psychiatry 2007; 78:277–279.
153. Morrell MJ, Heywood P, Moosavi SH, et al. Unilateral focal lesions in the rostrolateral medulla influence chemosensitivity and breathing measured during wakefulness, sleep, and exercise. J Neurol Neurosurg Psychiatry 1999; 67:637–645.
154. Solin P, Roebuck T, Johns DP, et al. Peripheral and central ventilatory responses in central sleep apnea with and without congestive heart failure. Am J Respir Crit Care Med 2000; 162:2194–2200.
155. Javaheri S. A mechanism of central sleep apnea in patients with heart failure. N Engl J Med 1999; 341:949–954.

156. Koch S, Zuniga S, Rabinstein AA, et al. Signs and symptoms of sleep apnea and acute stroke severity: is sleep apnea neuroprotective? J Stroke Cerebrovasc Dis 2007; 16:114–118.
157. Dziewas R, Ritter M, Kruger L, et al. C-reactive protein and fibrinogen in acute stroke patients with and without sleep apnea. Cerebrovasc Dis 2007; 24:412–417.
158. Siccoli MM, Tettenborn B, Kollias SS, et al. Acute ischemic stroke and sleep apnea: evolution of clinical and radiological parameters within three days after stroke onset. Abstracts of the 8th World Congress on Sleep Apnea, September 2006, Montréal, Canada.
159. Turkington PM, Allgar V, Bamford J, et al. Effect of upper airway obstruction in acute stroke on functional outcome at 6 months. Thorax 2004; 59:367–371.
160. Martinez-Garcia MA, Galiano-Blancart R, Roman-Sanchez P, et al. Continuous positive airway pressure treatment in sleep apnea prevents new vascular events after ischemic stroke. Chest 2005; 128:2123–2129.
161. Multicenter trial of hemodilution in ischemic stroke—background and study protocol. Scandinavian Stroke Study Group. Stroke 1985; 16:885–890.
162. Granger CV, Dewis LS, Peters NC, et al. Stroke rehabilitation: analysis of repeated Barthel index measures. Arch Phys Med Rehabil 1979; 60:14–17.
163. Rowat AM, Wardlaw JM, Dennis MS, et al. Patient positioning influences oxygen saturation in the acute phase of stroke. Cerebrovasc Dis 2001; 12:66–72.
164. Dziewas R, Hopmann B, Humpert M, et al. Positional sleep apnea in patients with ischemic stroke. Neurol Res 2008; 30:645–648.
165. Jenkinson C, Davies RJ, Mullins R, et al. Comparison of therapeutic and subtherapeutic nasal continuous positive airway pressure for obstructive sleep apnoea: a randomised prospective parallel trial. Lancet 1999; 353:2100–2105.
166. Jenkinson C, Stradling J, Petersen S. Comparison of three measures of quality of life outcome in the evaluation of continuous positive airways pressure therapy for sleep apnoea. J Sleep Res 1997; 6:199–204.
167. Jenkinson C, Davies RJ, Mullins R, et al. Long-term benefits in self-reported health status of nasal continuous positive airway pressure therapy for obstructive sleep apnoea. Q J Med 2001; 94:95–99.
168. Engleman HM, Kingshott RN, Wraith PK, et al. Randomized placebo-controlled crossover trial of continuous positive airway pressure for mild sleep apnea/hypopnea syndrome. Am J Respir Crit Care Med 1999; 159:461–467.
169. Engleman HM, Martin SE, Kingshott RN, et al. Randomised placebo controlled trial of daytime function after continuous positive airway pressure (CPAP) therapy for the sleep apnoea/hypopnoea syndrome. Thorax 1998; 53:341–345.
170. Giles TL, Lasserson TJ, Smith BH, et al. Continuous positive airways pressure for obstructive sleep apnoea in adults. Cochrane Database Syst Rev 2006; (1):CD001106.
171. Wessendorf TE, Wang YM, Thilmann AF, et al. Treatment of obstructive sleep apnoea with nasal continuous positive airway pressure in stroke. Eur Respir J 2001; 18:623–629.
172. Sandberg O, Franklin KA, Bucht G, et al. Nasal continuous positive airway pressure in stroke patients with sleep apnoea: a randomized treatment study. Eur Respir J 2001; 18: 630–634.
173. Brown DL, Chervin RD, Hickenbottom SL, et al. Screening for obstructive sleep apnea in stroke patients: a cost-effectiveness analysis. Stroke 2005; 36:1291–1293.
174. Hsu CY, Vennelle M, Li HY, et al. Sleep-disordered breathing after stroke: a randomised controlled trial of continuous positive airway pressure. J Neurol Neurosurg Psychiatry 2006; 77:1143–1149.
175. Hui DSC, Choy DKL, Wong LKS, et al. Prevalence of sleep-disordered breathing and continuous positive airway pressure compliance*: results in Chinese patients with first-ever ischemic stroke. Chest 2002; 122:852–860.

176. Palombini L, Guilleminault C. Stroke and treatment with nasal CPAP. Eur J Neurol 2006; 13:198–200.
177. Scala R, Turkington PM, Wanklyn P, et al. Acceptance, effectiveness and safety of continuous positive airway pressure in acute stroke: a pilot study. Respir Med 2009; 103:59–66.
178. Arzt M, Floras JS, Logan AG, et al. Suppression of central sleep apnea by continuous positive airway pressure and transplant-free survival in heart failure: a post hoc analysis of the Canadian continuous positive airway pressure for patients with central sleep apnea and heart failure trial (CANPAP). Circulation 2007; 115:3173–3180.
179. Teschler H, Dohring J, Wang YM, et al. Adaptive pressure support servo-ventilation: a novel treatment for Cheyne-Stokes respiration in heart failure. Am J Respir Crit Care Med 2001; 164:614–619.
180. Javaheri S. Acetazolamide improves central sleep apnea in heart failure: a double-blind, prospective study. Am J Respir Crit Care Med 2006; 173:234–237.

15
Circadian Rhythm of Cardiac and Cerebrovascular Ischemic Events

DAN SORAJJA
Mayo Clinic, Scottsdale, Arizona, U.S.A.

APOOR S. GAMI
Midwest Heart Specialists, Elmhurst, Illinois, U.S.A.

I. Myocardial Infarction and Sudden Cardiac Death

Heart disease remains the leading cause of morbidity and mortality in developed countries (1). Abundant data from both retrospective and prospective observational studies and trials have consistently demonstrated a diurnal variation to the occurrence of cardiac ischemic events, including myocardial infarction and sudden cardiac death. These diurnal patterns of disease incidence may reflect the circadian variation and environmental day-night pattern of various pathophysiological cardiovascular disease mechanisms. Sleep-disordered breathing, due to its own unique nocturnal pathophysiology, may play an important role in the diurnal variation of these cardiovascular events.

The incidence of myocardial infarction peaks in the late morning hours or soon after awakening. Strategies that have been used to identify the time of onset of myocardial infarction in these analyses included assessments of the timing of cardiac biomarker elevations and the onset of patient symptoms. Reproducible findings from several population-based studies and trials have shown a three- to fourfold increase in the frequency of myocardial infarction between 6 a.m. and noon, with a peak between 8 a.m. and 9 a.m. and a trough beginning at 6 p.m. and a nadir between 11 p.m. and 1 a.m. (2–11). In a meta-analysis of data for 66,635 patients, nonfatal, acute myocardial infarction occurred in 31.5% of the patients between 6 a.m. and 12 p.m., with a relative risk of 1.38 during this time period (Fig. 1) (12). Notably, in many studies, the morning peak in myocardial infarctions was not observed in patients taking β-adrenergic receptor antagonists (β-blockers) (2,3,5). An important correlative observation was that myocardial infarctions were more frequent, not just in these morning hours, but more specifically in the three hours after waking and in relation to stress or emotional upset (Fig. 2) (13–19). Some data suggest a bimodal peak in myocardial infarction incidence, with a second peak in events during the evening (6 p.m. to midnight). Subgroup analyses from these studies suggest that an additional evening peak is more likely in patients with preexisting heart or vascular disease, in working rather than retired patients, and in Mediterranean Caucasians rather than British Caucasians (10,14,20–23).

Sudden cardiac death is the most common cause of heart disease–related death in the United States (24–26). It is usually due to ventricular dysrhythmias in the setting of acute myocardial infarction (27). It follows, then, that the diurnal variation in the

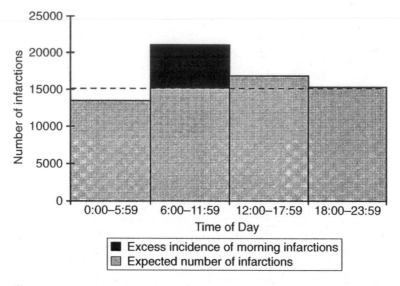

Figure 1 Circadian pattern of nonfatal myocardial infarction ($n = 66,635$). *Source*: From Ref. 12.

incidence of sudden cardiac death parallels that of myocardial infarction. Strategies used to identify the time of sudden cardiac death included evaluation of death certificate data and review of emergency medical system calls for out-of-hospital cardiac arrests. As for myocardial infarction, data from several population-based studies have reproducibly shown a peak incidence of sudden cardiac death in the late morning, between 6 a.m. and noon (8,27–31). A meta-analysis including 19,390 patients from 19 studies confirmed that 30.1% of sudden cardiac deaths occurred during this time period, with a relative risk of 1.29 compared to the rest of the day (Fig. 3) (12). In a few studies, the use of β-blockers and calcium channel blockers, but not amiodarone, was shown to attenuate the diurnal variation of sudden cardiac death (32–35). Some studies describe a second nocturnal peak in sudden cardiac death (36–40), and there are conflicting data regarding the presence of a diurnal variation of sudden cardiac death in heart failure patients (41–43).

Data from implantable cardioverter-defibrillators have provided insights into the diurnal variation of ventricular dysrhythmias in patients at risk for sudden cardiac death due to structural heart disease. Studies have generally shown that ventricular dys-rhythmias diagnosed and treated by the devices had a peak incidence between 6 a.m. and noon, a second evening peak, and an attenuation of diurnal variation in patients taking β-blockers or with marked ventricular dysfunction (44–48).

II. Ischemic Stroke

Stroke is the leading cause of long-term disability in developed countries (1). Epi-demiological data have demonstrated a diurnal variation to the incidence of stroke. As for cardiac ischemic events, these patterns likely reflect the circadian variation of pathophysiological cardiovascular disease mechanisms, which may be modified by sleep-disordered breathing.

The incidence of stroke peaks in the late morning hours, between 6 a.m. and noon, and it is at its lowest between midnight and 6 a.m. (9,49–61). Multiple population-based

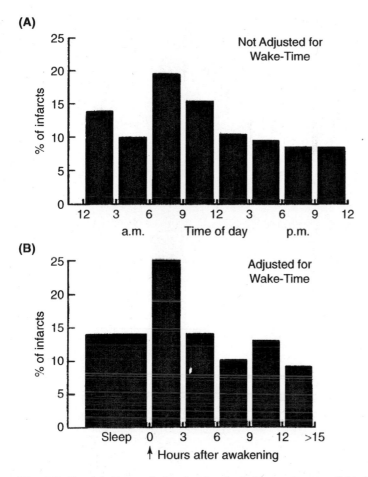

(A)

(B)

Figure 2 Panel A: Bar graph showing that the incidence of myocardial infarction in the TRIMM pilot study ($n = 224$) exhibited a significant ($p < 0.01$) circadian variation with a peak incidence from 6 a.m. to 9 a.m. The relative risk of myocardial infarction during this three-hour interval compared with other times of day was 1.8 (95% CI, 1.3–2.4). Panel B: Bar graph showing that, after adjustment for the individual patients' wake times, the morning peak was more pronounced compared with the baseline circadian variation. The relative risk of myocardial infarction during the initial three-hour interval after awakening was 2.4 (95% CI, 1.8–3.1) compared with other times of day. *Abbreviations*: TRIMM, triggers and mechanisms of myocardial infarction; CI, confidence interval. *Source*: From Ref. 4.

studies from varying regions have consistently demonstrated that over 50% of all ischemic strokes occur during the late morning hours (50,56,59). It was noted that about a quarter of them occur within the first hour after awakening (56). This diurnal pattern existed, regardless of age, sex, and ethnicity; however, it was not present in smokers (62). Insufficient data exist regarding the effect of medications and other disease conditions on the circadian variation of ischemic stroke.

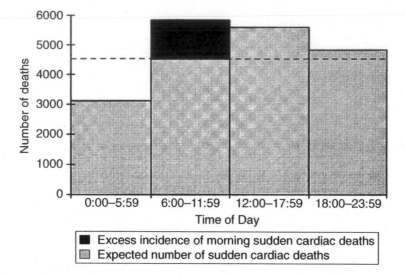

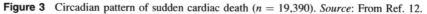

Figure 3 Circadian pattern of sudden cardiac death ($n = 19,390$). *Source*: From Ref. 12.

III. Pathophysiology

The diurnal variation of cardiac and cerebrovascular ischemic events may be related to the circadian rhythm of various physiological processes as well as day-night patterns of environmental stimuli (Fig. 4). An additional important role is played by behavioral and environmental triggering events (Fig. 2).

Cardiac autonomic balance likely plays a critical role in increasing the late morning incidence of both cardiac and cerebral events. Increased heart rate and decreased heart rate variability, both reflections of increased sympathetic tone, correspond to ischemic burden and are risk markers for sudden cardiac death (63–67). Plasma epinephrine concentration is selectively increased by awakening, and plasma norepinephrine concentration increases with standing (68,69). Indirect evidence of the role of the autonomic nervous system was observed in multiple studies by the attenuation of the morning increase in myocardial infarctions and sudden cardiac deaths in patients taking β-blockers (2,3,5,34,70). The loss of the circadian variation of cardiovascular events in patients with advanced heart failure may be due to their chronic increase in sympathetic tone, with persistently elevated plasma norepinephrine concentrations (71,72). Smokers have also been shown to lack this diurnal variation, and this also may be due to their persistently elevated sympathetic tone, reflected by high plasma epinephrine concentrations throughout the day (73,74).

There is a relationship between diurnal blood pressure variability and the risk of stroke. Even treated hypertensive patients with normal blood pressure during clinic visits have early morning blood pressure surges (73–76). Patients with blood pressure surges of 55 mmHg or more are more likely to have ischemic brain lesions than patients without them (77). Individuals who lack the usual nocturnal decrease in blood pressure ("nondippers") have a substantially increased risk of stroke, which can be lowered in

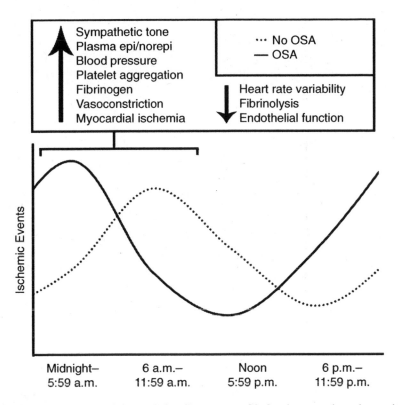

Figure 4 Pathophysiology of circadian pattern of ischemic events in patients with and without OSA. *Abbreviation*: OSA, obstructive sleep apnea.

some patients by converting them to "dippers" by countering sympathetic overactivity with β-adrenergic blockers (78,79).

The circadian variation in the function of platelets and coagulation proteins also is likely to play an important role in the incidence of morning ischemic events. Platelet aggregation increases between 6 a.m. and 9 a.m. compared to the remainder of the day (80–83), and this also correlates with the assumption of an upright posture (80). Patients with ST-elevation myocardial infarction treated with coronary intervention were found to have the highest degree of platelet aggregability between 4 a.m. and 8 a.m. (84). Indirect support of the clinical relevance of the circadian variability in platelet aggregation comes from the observation that aspirin reduces morning myocardial infarctions by 59% but myocardial infarctions during other times of the day by only 34% (11).

Other critical mechanisms of thrombosis follow a circadian pattern. Peak plasma fibrinogen levels occur at noon (82). Tissue-type plasminogen activator concentrations are the lowest at night, until 6 a.m. Concurrent with this, plasminogen activator inhibitor activity peaks during the same hours (85). Together, these processes decrease fibrinolytic potential during the morning hours. This has been substantiated during clinical cardiac ischemic events (86). Among patients with acute myocardial infarction treated with thrombolytic agents, thrombolysis resistance was greater during the morning and thrombolysis success was greater at night (87,88).

Vascular function also follows a circadian pattern, which has implications for both cardiac and cerebrovascular events. Flow-mediated endothelium-dependent vasodilation decreases in the morning after waking, and α-adrenergic vasoconstriction increases during the morning (89,90). Also, coronary artery segments with abnormal endothelial function show accentuated measures of dysfunction during the late morning hours (between 6 a.m. and 1 p.m.) (91). The myocardial ischemic threshold is lower in the morning, suggesting an increased coronary vascular resistance (92). ST-segment monitoring shows that asymptomatic myocardial ischemia peaks in the morning, except in patients who are treated with β-blockers (93), and it does not necessarily correlate with physical activity or stress (94).

Environmental stimuli and behavioral patterns have an impact on the diurnal variation of ischemic events. It can be difficult to distinguish the true biological circadian variation of various pathophysiological processes versus the day-night variation of these processes caused by patterned environmental events. For example, while an abundance of data demonstrates the peak incidence of sudden cardiac death between 6 a.m. and noon, a careful study that assessed the time of patients' awakening demonstrated that sudden cardiac death correlated strongest with the three-hour time period after waking (Fig. 2) (95). Some of the mechanisms of ischemic events correlate better with individuals' activities that are usually associated with the late morning (such as waking) rather than the actual time of day in which they occur. For example, night shift workers have higher sympathetic tone and higher systolic blood pressure during the night (96), populations that practice siesta have a late afternoon peak of ischemic events (97), and plasma tissue plasminogen and plasminogen activator inhibitor concentrations are altered in shift workers (98). The performance of exercise and other strenuous activity in the hours after waking may contribute to the day-night pattern that has been observed. The risk of acute myocardial infarction is significantly higher in the hour after heavy exertion, particularly in individuals who perform exercise infrequently (15,17,99,100). This holds true for sudden cardiac death, with a significant increase in risk during and in the 30 minutes after strenuous exercise (101). The contribution of emotional stress has been established, as well. The incidence of *tako-tsubo* cardiomyopathy, also known as "stress cardiomyopathy" due to its occurrence during dramatic psychosocial stresses, peaks between 6 a.m. and noon (102). Anger and occupational stress both have been linked to a significantly increased risk of myocardial infarction (14,16,18,19).

IV. Effects of Obstructive Sleep Apnea

Obstructive sleep apnea (OSA) not only increases the risk of both ischemic cardiac and cerebrovascular diseases but also alters the usual circadian variation of these events. Acute nocturnal pathophysiological mechanisms related to obstructive apneas may lead to coronary, aortic, or cerebrovascular plaque rupture, with arterial thrombosis and resultant myocardial infarction, sudden cardiac death, transient ischemic attack, or stroke (103). Repetitive collapse of the airway during obstructive apneic sleep leads to hypoxemia, sometimes severe and prolonged, which can result in acute myocardial ischemia and ventricular arrhythmias (104–106). Also, this hypoxemia and hypercapnia activate the chemoreflex, which augments sympathetic nerve activity (107–109). The resultant decrease in heart rate variability and alteration in ventricular repolarization characteristics increase the risk of sudden cardiac death (63,66,67,110). The increased sympathetic tone also produces an elevated blood pressure, and each apnea can be associated with a significant blood pressure surge (111–113). These blood pressure elevations can increase myocardial oxygen demand and promote ischemia, especially in the setting of hypoxemia (106). Furthermore, the obstructive apneic events create marked fluctuations in intrathoracic and cardiac transmural pressures, which can increase cardiac afterload, increase myocardial oxygen demand, and promote ischemia and dysrhythmias (106,114–117). OSA also modifies the circadian variation of factors affecting arterial thrombosis. In contrast to patients without OSA, in whom platelet activation and thrombotic factors favor morning ischemic events, patients with OSA exhibit increased platelet activation, higher fibrinogen concentrations, and decreased fibrinolytic activity during the night (118–122).

Epidemiological data have demonstrated a striking change in the day-night patterns of myocardial infarction and sudden cardiac death in patients with OSA, but data are lacking for cerebrovascular diseases. Patients with OSA were much more likely to experience an acute myocardial infarction between midnight and 6 a.m. compared to patients without OSA, in whom the frequency of acute myocardial infarction was highest between 6 a.m. and noon (Fig. 5) (123). In fact, over 90% of the patients having an acute myocardial infarction during the night and early morning hours had OSA (123). Similarly, sudden cardiac death occurred more frequently during the night in patients with OSA, with nearly half of sudden cardiac deaths in OSA patients occurring between midnight and 6 a.m. The relative risk of sudden cardiac death for OSA patients during the night was 2.33 compared to other times of the day (Fig. 6) (124).

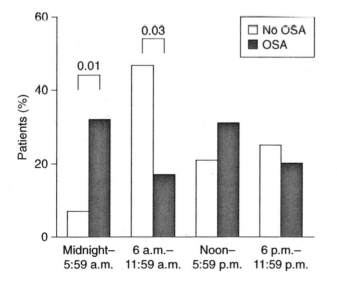

Figure 5 Day-night pattern of myocardial infarction in persons with ($n = 64$) and without ($n = 28$) OSA. *Abbreviation*: OSA, obstructive sleep apnea. *Source*: From Ref. 123.

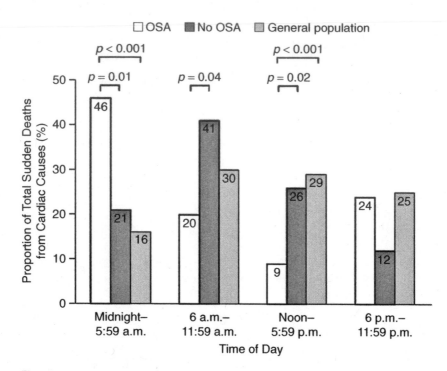

Figure 6 Day-night pattern of sudden death from cardiac causes in persons with ($n = 78$) and without ($n = 34$) OSA and the general population. *Abbreviation*: OSA, obstructive sleep apnea. *Source*: From Ref. 124.

V. Conclusions

Cardiac and cerebrovascular ischemic events in the general population occur with an established day-night pattern. This pattern can be explained by various pathophysiological mechanisms that follow a biological circadian rhythm or by a diurnal variation based on environmental and behavioral events. These patterns are modified by relatively few factors, including certain medications and diseases (i.e., β-adrenergic blockers and heart failure), as well as the unique and striking effects of OSA. A better understanding of the expected and altered diurnal rhythms of cardiac and cerebrovascular ischemic events may lead to novel and focused interventions to prevent and treat these conditions.

References

1. American Heart Association and American Stroke Association. Heart Disease and Stroke Statistics: 2008 Update At-a-Glance. Dallas, TX: American Heart Association and American Stroke Association, 2008:1–43.
2. Muller JE, Stone PH, Turi ZG, et al. Circadian variation in the frequency of onset of acute myocardial infarction. N Engl J Med 1985; 313:1315–1322.

3. Willich SN, Linderer T, Wegscheider K, et al. Increased morning incidence of myocardial infarction in the ISAM Study: absence with prior beta-adrenergic blockade. ISAM Study Group. Circulation 1989; 80:853–858.

4. Willich SN, Lowel H, Lewis M, et al. Association of wake time and the onset of myocardial infarction. Triggers and mechanisms of myocardial infarction (TRIMM) pilot study. TRIMM Study Group. Circulation 1991; 84:VI62–V167.

5. Tofler GH, Muller JE, Stone PH, et al. Modifiers of timing and possible triggers of acute myocardial infarction in the Thrombolysis in Myocardial Infarction Phase II (TIMI II) Study Group. J Am Coll Cardiol 1992; 20:1049–1055.

6. Morning peak in the incidence of myocardial infarction: experience in the ISIS-2 trial. ISIS-2 (Second International Study of Infarct Survival) Collaborative Group. Eur Heart J 1992; 13:594–598.

7. Gnecchi-Ruscone T, Piccaluga E, Guzzetti S, et al. Morning and Monday: critical periods for the onset of acute myocardial infarction. The GISSI 2 Study experience. Eur Heart J 1994; 15:882–887.

8. van der Palen J, Doggen CJ, Beaglehole R. Variation in the time and day of onset of myocardial infarction and sudden death. N Z Med J 1995; 108:332–334.

9. Wang H, Kingsland R, Zhao H, et al. Time of symptom onset of eight common medical emergencies. J Emerg Med 1995; 13:461–469.

10. Hjalmarson A, Gilpin EA, Nicod P, et al. Differing circadian patterns of symptom onset in subgroups of patients with acute myocardial infarction. Circulation 1989; 80:267–275.

11. Ridker PM, Manson JE, Buring JE, et al. Circadian variation of acute myocardial infarction and the effect of low-dose aspirin in a randomized trial of physicians. Circulation 1990; 82:897–902.

12. Cohen MC, Rohtla KM, Lavery CE, et al. Meta-analysis of the morning excess of acute myocardial infarction and sudden cardiac death. Am J Cardiol 1997; 79:1512–1516.

13. Goldberg RJ, Brady P, Muller JE, et al. Time of onset of symptoms of acute myocardial infarction. Am J Cardiol 1990; 66:140–144.

14. Behar S, Halabi M, Reicher-Reiss H, et al. Circadian variation and possible external triggers of onset of myocardial infarction. SPRINT Study Group. Am J Med 1993; 94:395–400.

15. Mittleman MA, Maclure M, Tofler GH, et al. Triggering of acute myocardial infarction by heavy physical exertion. Protection against triggering by regular exertion. Determinants of myocardial infarction onset study investigators. N Engl J Med 1993; 329:1677–1683.

16. Mittleman MA, Maclure M, Sherwood JB, et al. Triggering of acute myocardial infarction onset by episodes of anger. Determinants of Myocardial Infarction Onset Study Investigators. Circulation 1995; 92:1720–1725.

17. Willich SN, Lewis M, Lowel H, et al. Physical exertion as a trigger of acute myocardial infarction. Triggers and Mechanisms of Myocardial Infarction Study Group. N Engl J Med 1993; 329:1684–1690.

18. Moller J, Hallqvist J, Diderichsen F, et al. Do episodes of anger trigger myocardial infarction? A case-crossover analysis in the Stockholm Heart Epidemiology Program (SHEEP). Psychosom Med 1999; 61:842–849.

19. Moller J, Theorell T, de Faire U, et al. Work related stressful life events and the risk of myocardial infarction. Case-control and case-crossover analyses within the Stockholm Heart Epidemiology Programme (SHEEP). J Epidemiol Community Health 2005; 59:23–30.

20. Peters RW, Zoble RG, Liebson PR, et al. Identification of a secondary peak in myocardial infarction onset 11 to 12 hours after awakening: the Cardiac Arrhythmia Suppression Trial (CAST) experience. J Am Coll Cardiol 1993; 22:998–1003.

21. Thompson DR, Blandford RL, Sutton TW, et al. Time of onset of chest pain in acute myocardial infarction. Int J Cardiol 1985; 7:139–148.

22. Hansen O, Johansson BW, Gullberg B. Circadian distribution of onset of acute myocardial infarction in subgroups from analysis of 10,791 patients treated in a single center. Am J Cardiol 1992; 69:1003–1008.
23. Spielberg C, Falkenhahn D, Willich SN, et al. Circadian, day-of-week, and seasonal variability in myocardial infarction: comparison between working and retired patients. Am Heart J 1996; 132:579–585.
24. Zheng ZJ, Croft JB, Giles WH, et al. Sudden cardiac death in the United States, 1989 to 1998. Circulation 2001; 104:2158–2163.
25. Rea TD, Pearce RM, Raghunathan TE, et al. Incidence of out-of-hospital cardiac arrest. Am J Cardiol 2004; 93:1455–1460.
26. Kannel WB, Wilson PW, D'Agostino RB, et al. Sudden coronary death in women. Am Heart J 1998; 136:205–212.
27. Muller JE, Ludmer PL, Willich SN, et al. Circadian variation in the frequency of sudden cardiac death. Circulation 1987; 75:131–138.
28. Willich SN, Levy D, Rocco MB, et al. Circadian variation in the incidence of sudden cardiac death in the Framingham Heart Study population. Am J Cardiol 1987; 60:801–806.
29. Levine RL, Pepe PE, Fromm RE, Jr., et al. Prospective evidence of a circadian rhythm for out-of-hospital cardiac arrests. JAMA 1992; 267:2935–2937.
30. Willich SN, Lowel H, Lewis M, et al. Weekly variation of acute myocardial infarction. Increased Monday risk in the working population. Circulation 1994; 90:87–93.
31. Martens P, Calle P, Hubloue I, et al. Does age have an effect on the time of occurrence of cardiac arrest of presumed cardiac etiology? Belgian Cardiopulmonary-Cerebral Resuscitation Study Group. Cardiology 1995; 86:197–201.
32. Behrens S, Ney G, Fisher SG, et al. Effects of amiodarone on the circadian pattern of sudden cardiac death (Department of Veterans Affairs Congestive Heart Failure-Survival Trial of Antiarrhythmic Therapy). Am J Cardiol 1997; 80:45–48.
33. Peters RW, Mitchell LB, Brooks MM, et al. Circadian pattern of arrhythmic death in patients receiving encainide, flecainide or moricizine in the Cardiac Arrhythmia Suppression Trial (CAST). Am Coll Cardiol 1994; 23:283–289.
34. Peters RW, Muller JE, Goldstein S, et al. Propranolol and the morning increase in the frequency of sudden cardiac death (BHAT Study). Am J Cardiol 1989; 63:1518–1520.
35. Andersen L, Sigurd B, Hansen J. Verapamil and circadian variation of sudden cardiac death. Am Heart J 1996; 131:409–410.
36. Savopoulos C, Ziakas A, Hatzitolios A, et al. Circadian rhythm in sudden cardiac death: a retrospective study of 2,665 cases. Angiology 2006; 57:197–204.
37. Cho JG, Park HW, Rhew JY, et al. Clinical characteristics of unexplained sudden cardiac death in Korea. Jpn Circ J 2001; 65:18–22.
38. Kirschner RH, Eckner FA, Baron RC. The cardiac pathology of sudden, unexplained nocturnal death in Southeast Asian refugees. JAMA 1986; 256:2700–2705.
39. Nademanee K, Veerakul G, Nimmannit S, et al. Arrhythmogenic marker for the sudden unexplained death syndrome in Thai men. Circulation 1997; 96:2595–2600.
40. Munger RG, Booton EA. Bangungut in Manila: sudden and unexplained death in sleep of adult Filipinos. Int J Epidemiol 1998; 27:677–684.
41. Moser DK, Stevenson WG, Woo MA, et al. Timing of sudden death in patients with heart failure. J Am Coll Cardiol 1994; 24:963–967.
42. Casaleggio A, Maestri R, La Rovere MT, et al. Prediction of sudden death in heart failure patients: a novel perspective from the assessment of the peak ectopy rate. Europace 2007; 9:385–390.
43. Carson PA, O'Connor CM, Miller AB, et al. Circadian rhythm and sudden death in heart failure: results from Prospective Randomized Amlodipine Survival Trial. J Am Coll Cardiol 2000; 36:541–546.

44. Behrens S, Ehlers C, Bruggemann T, et al. Modification of the circadian pattern of ventricular tachyarrhythmias by beta-blocker therapy. Clin Cardiol 1997; 20:253–257.
45. Tofler GH, Gebara OC, Mittleman MA, et al. Morning peak in ventricular tachyarrhythmias detected by time of implantable cardioverter/defibrillator therapy. The CPI Investigators. Circulation 1995; 92:1203–1208.
46. Grimm W, Walter M, Menz V, et al. Circadian variation and onset mechanisms of ventricular tachyarrhythmias in patients with coronary disease versus idiopathic dilated cardiomyopathy. Pacing Clin Electrophysiol 2000; 23:1939–1943.
47. Englund A, Behrens S, Wegscheider K, et al. Circadian variation of malignant ventricular arrhythmias in patients with ischemic and nonischemic heart disease after cardioverter defibrillator implantation. European 7219 Jewel Investigators. J Am Coll Cardiol 1999; 34:1560–1568.
48. Kozak M, Krivan L, Semrad B. Circadian variations in the occurrence of ventricular tachyarrhythmias in patients with implantable cardioverter defibrillators. Pacing Clin Electrophysiol 2003; 26:731–735.
49. Marler JR, Price TR, Clark GL, et al. Morning increase in onset of ischemic stroke. Stroke 1989; 20:473–476.
50. Argentino C, Toni D, Rasura M, et al. Circadian variation in the frequency of ischemic stroke. Stroke 1990; 21:387–389.
51. Pasqualetti P, Natali G, Casale R, et al. Epidemiological chronorisk of stroke. Acta Neurol Scand 1990; 81:71–74.
52. Ricci S, Celani MG, Vitali R, et al. Diurnal and seasonal variations in the occurrence of stroke: a community-based study. Neuroepidemiology 1992; 11:59–64.
53. Wroe SJ, Sandercock P, Bamford J, et al. Diurnal variation in incidence of stroke: Oxfordshire community stroke project. BMJ 1992; 304:155–157.
54. Gallerani M, Manfredini R, Ricci L, et al. Chronobiological aspects of acute cerebrovascular diseases. Acta Neurol Scand 1993; 87:482–487.
55. Tsementzis SA, Gill JS, Hitchcock ER, et al. Diurnal variation of and activity during the onset of stroke. Neurosurgery 1985; 17:901–904.
56. Marsh EE 3rd, Biller J, Adams HP Jr., et al. Circadian variation in onset of acute ischemic stroke. Arch Neurol 1990; 47:1178–1180.
57. Moulin T, Tatu L, Crepin-Leblond T, et al. The Besancon Stroke Registry: an acute stroke registry of 2,500 consecutive patients. Eur Neurol 1997; 38:10–20.
58. Stergiou GS, Vemmos KN, Pliarchopoulou KM, et al. Parallel morning and evening surge in stroke onset, blood pressure, and physical activity. Stroke 2002; 33:1480–1486.
59. Elliott WJ. Circadian variation in the timing of stroke onset: a meta-analysis. Stroke 1998; 29:992–996.
60. Agnoli A, Manfredi M, Mossuto L, et al. [Relationship between circadian rhythms and blood pressure and the pathogenesis of cerebrovascular insufficiency.] Rev Neurol (Paris) 1975; 131:597–606.
61. Hayashi S, Toyoshima H, Tanabe N, et al. Daily peaks in the incidence of sudden cardiac death and fatal stroke in Niigata Prefecture. Jpn Circ J 1996; 60:193–200.
62. Haapaniemi H, Hillbom M, Juvela S. Weekend and holiday increase in the onset of ischemic stroke in young women. Stroke 1996; 27:1023–1027.
63. Priori SG, Aliot E, Blomstrom-Lundqvist C, et al. Task Force on Sudden Cardiac Death of the European Society of Cardiology. Eur Heart J 2001; 22:1374–1450.
64. Wannamethee G, Shaper AG, Macfarlane PW, et al. Risk factors for sudden cardiac death in middle-aged British men. Circulation 1995; 91:1749–1756.
65. Shaper AG, Wannamethee G, Macfarlane PW, et al. Heart rate, ischaemic heart disease, and sudden cardiac death in middle-aged British men. Br Heart J 1993; 70:49–55.

66. Algra A, Tijssen JG, Roelandt JR, et al. Heart rate variability from 24-hour electrocardiography and the 2-year risk for sudden death. Circulation 1993; 88:180–185.

67. Kiviniemi AM, Tulppo MP, Wichterle D, et al. Novel spectral indexes of heart rate variability as predictors of sudden and non-sudden cardiac death after an acute myocardial infarction. Ann Med 2007; 39:54–62.

68. Dodt C, Breckling U, Derad I, et al. Plasma epinephrine and norepinephrine concentrations of healthy humans associated with nighttime sleep and morning arousal. Hypertension 1997; 30:71–76.

69. Andrews NP, Gralnick HR, Merryman P, et al. Mechanisms underlying the morning increase in platelet aggregation: a flow cytometry study. J Am Coll Cardiol 1996; 28:1789–1795.

70. Peters RW. Circadian patterns and triggers of sudden cardiac death. Cardiol Clin 1996; 14:185–194.

71. Cohn JN, Johnson GR, Shabetai R, et al. Ejection fraction, peak exercise oxygen consumption, cardiothoracic ratio, ventricular arrhythmias, and plasma norepinephrine as determinants of prognosis in heart failure. The V-HeFT VA Cooperative Studies Group. Circulation 1993; 87:VI5–V16.

72. Porter TR, Eckberg DL, Fritsch JM, et al. Autonomic pathophysiology in heart failure patients. Sympathetic-cholinergic interrelations. J Clin Invest 1990; 85:1362–1371.

73. Hayano J, Yamada M, Sakakibara Y, et al. Short- and long-term effects of cigarette smoking on heart rate variability. Am J Cardiol 1990; 65:84–88.

74. Siess W, Lorenz R, Roth P, et al. Plasma catecholamines, platelet aggregation and associated thromboxane formation after physical exercise, smoking or norepinephrine infusion. Circulation 1982; 66:44–48.

75. Ishikawa J, Kario K, Hoshide S, et al. Determinants of exaggerated difference in morning and evening blood pressure measured by self-measured blood pressure monitoring in medicated hypertensive patients: Jichi Morning Hypertension Research (J-MORE) Study. Am J Hypertens 2005; 18:958–965.

76. Redon J, Roca-Cusachs A, Mora-Macia J. Uncontrolled early morning blood pressure in medicated patients: the ACAMPA study. Analysis of the Control of Blood Pressure using Abulatory Blood Pressure Monitoring. Blood Press Monit 2002; 7:111–116.

77. Kario K, Pickering TG, Umeda Y, et al. Morning surge in blood pressure as a predictor of silent and clinical cerebrovascular disease in elderly hypertensives: a prospective study. Circulation 2003; 107:1401–1406.

78. Zakopoulos N, Stamatelopoulos S, Moulopoulos S. Effect of hypotensive drugs on the circadian blood pressure pattern in essential hypertension: a comparative study. Cardiovasc Drugs Ther 1997; 11:795–799.

79. O'Brien E, Sheridan J, O'Malley K. Dippers and non-dippers. Lancet 1988; 2:397.

80. Brezinski DA, Tofler GH, Muller JE, et al. Morning increase in platelet aggregability. Association with assumption of the upright posture. Circulation 1988; 78:35–40.

81. Tofler GH, Brezinski D, Schafer AI, et al. Concurrent morning increase in platelet aggregability and the risk of myocardial infarction and sudden cardiac death. N Engl J Med 1987; 316:1514–1518.

82. Petralito A, Mangiafico RA, Gibiino S, et al. Daily modifications of plasma fibrinogen platelets aggregation, Howell's time, PTT, TT, and antithrombin II in normal subjects and in patients with vascular disease. Chronobiologia 1982; 9:195–201.

83. Jafri SM, VanRollins M, Ozawa T, et al. Circadian variation in platelet function in healthy volunteers. Am J Cardiol 1992; 69:951–954.

84. De Luca G, Suryapranata H, Ottervanger JP, et al. Circadian variation in myocardial perfusion and mortality in patients with ST-segment elevation myocardial infarction treated by primary angioplasty. Am Heart J 2005; 150:1185–1189.

85. Andreotti F, Davies GJ, Hackett DR, et al. Major circadian fluctuations in fibrinolytic factors and possible relevance to time of onset of myocardial infarction, sudden cardiac death and stroke. Am J Cardiol 1988; 62:635–637.
86. Huber K, Rosc D, Resch I, et al. Circadian fluctuations of plasminogen activator inhibitor and tissue plasminogen activator levels in plasma of patients with unstable coronary artery disease and acute myocardial infarction. Thromb Haemost 1988; 60:372–376.
87. Kurnik PB. Circadian variation in the efficacy of tissue-type plasminogen activator. Circulation 1995; 91:1341–1346.
88. Kono T, Morita H, Nishina T, et al. Circadian variations of onset of acute myocardial infarction and efficacy of thrombolytic therapy. J Am Coll Cardiol 1996; 27:774–778.
89. Panza JA, Epstein SE, Quyyumi AA. Circadian variation in vascular tone and its relation to alpha-sympathetic vasoconstrictor activity. N Engl J Med 1991; 325:986–990.
90. Otto ME, Svatikova A, Barretto RB, et al. Early morning attenuation of endothelial function in healthy humans. Circulation 2004; 109:2507–2510.
91. el-Tamimi H, Mansour M, Pepine CJ, et al. Circadian variation in coronary tone in patients with stable angina. Protective role of the endothelium. Circulation 1995; 92:3201–3205.
92. Quyyumi AA, Panza JA, Diodati JG, et al. Circadian variation in ischemic threshold. A mechanism underlying the circadian variation in ischemic events. Circulation 1992; 86:22–28.
93. Mulcahy D, Keegan J, Cunningham D, et al. Circadian variation of total ischaemic burden and its alteration with anti-anginal agents. Lancet 1988; 2:755–759.
94. Rocco MB, Barry J, Campbell S, et al. Circadian variation of transient myocardial ischemia in patients with coronary artery disease. Circulation 1987; 75:395–400.
95. Willich SN, Goldberg RJ, Maclure M, et al. Increased onset of sudden cardiac death in the first three hours after awakening. Am J Cardiol 1992; 70:65–68.
96. Sternberg H, Rosenthal T, Shamiss A, et al. Altered circadian rhythm of blood pressure in shift workers. J Hum Hypertens 1995; 9:349–353.
97. Lopez F, Lee KW, Marin F, et al. Are there ethnic differences in the circadian variation in onset of acute myocardial infarction? A comparison of 3 ethnic groups in Birmingham, UK and Alicante, Spain. Int J Cardiol 2005; 100:151–154.
98. Andreotti F, Kluft C. Circadian variation of fibrinolytic activity in blood. Chronobiol Int 1991; 8:336–351.
99. Hallqvist J, Moller J, Ahlbom A, et al. Does heavy physical exertion trigger myocardial infarction? A case-crossover analysis nested in a population-based case-referent study. Am J Epidemiol 2000; 151:459–467.
100. Giri S, Thompson PD, Kiernan FJ, et al. Clinical and angiographic characteristics of exertion-related acute myocardial infarction. JAMA 1999; 282:1731–1736.
101. Albert CM, Mittleman MA, Chae CU, et al. Triggering of sudden death from cardiac causes by vigorous exertion. N Engl J Med 2000; 343:1355–1361.
102. Kurisu S, Inoue I, Kawagoe T, et al. Circadian variation in the occurrence of tako-tsubo cardiomyopathy: comparison with acute myocardial infarction. Int J Cardiol 2007; 115: 270–271.
103. Lopez-Jimenez F, Sert Kuniyoshi FH, Gami A, et al. Obstructive sleep apnea: implications for cardiac and vascular disease. Chest 2008; 133:793–804.
104. Hanly P, Sasson Z, Zuberi N, et al. ST-segment depression during sleep in obstructive sleep apnea. Am J Cardiol 1993; 71:1341–1345.
105. Philip P, Guilleminault C. ST segment abnormality, angina during sleep and obstructive sleep apnea. Sleep 1993; 16:558–559.
106. Gami AS, Somers VK. Implications of obstructive sleep apnea for atrial fibrillation and sudden cardiac death. J Cardiovasc Electrophysiol 2008; 19:997–1003.
107. Phillips BG, Kato M, Narkiewicz K, et al. Increases in leptin levels, sympathetic drive, and weight gain in obstructive sleep apnea. Am J Physiol 2000; 279:H234–H237.

108. Somers VK, Mark AL, Zavala DC, et al. Influence of ventilation and hypocapnia on sympathetic nerve responses to hypoxia in normal humans. J Appl Physiol 1989; 67:2095–2100.
109. Somers VK, Mark AL, Zavala DC, et al. Contrasting effects of hypoxia and hypercapnia on ventilation and sympathetic activity in humans. J Appl Physiol 1989; 67:2101–2106.
110. Roche F, Barthelemy JC, Garet M, et al. Continuous positive airway pressure treatment improves the QT rate dependence adaptation of obstructive sleep apnea patients. Pacing Clin Electrophysiol 2005; 28:819–825.
111. Kala R, Fyhrquist F, Eisalo A. Diurnal variation of plasma angiotensin II in man. Scand J Clin Lab Invest 1973; 31:363–365.
112. Millar-Craig MW, Bishop CN, Raftery EB. Circadian variation of blood-pressure. Lancet 1978; 1:795–797.
113. Portaluppi F, Bagni B, degli Uberti E, et al. Circadian rhythms of atrial natriuretic peptide, renin, aldosterone, cortisol, blood pressure and heart rate in normal and hypertensive subjects. J Hypertens 1990; 8:85–95.
114. Arias MA, Garcia-Rio F, Alonso-Fernandez A, et al. Obstructive sleep apnea syndrome affects left ventricular diastolic function: effects of nasal continuous positive airway pressure in men. Circulation 2005; 112:375–383.
115. Buda AJ, Pinsky MR, Ingels NB Jr., et al. Effect of intrathoracic pressure on left ventricular performance. N Engl J Med 1979; 301:453–459.
116. Fessler HE, Brower RG, Wise RA, et al. Mechanism of reduced LV afterload by systolic and diastolic positive pleural pressure. J Appl Physiol 1988; 65:1244–1250.
117. Otto ME, Belohlavek M, Romero-Corral A, et al. Comparison of cardiac structural and functional changes in obese otherwise healthy adults with versus without obstructive sleep apnea. Am J Cardiol 2007; 99:1298–1302.
118. Eisensehr I, Ehrenberg BL, Noachtar S, et al. Platelet activation, epinephrine, and blood pressure in obstructive sleep apnea syndrome. Neurology 1998; 51:188–195.
119. Rangemark C, Hedner JA, Carlson JT, et al. Platelet function and fibrinolytic activity in hypertensive and normotensive sleep apnea patients. Sleep 1995; 18:188–194.
120. Sanner BM, Konermann M, Tepel M, et al. Platelet function in patients with obstructive sleep apnoea syndrome. Eur Respir J 2000; 16:648–652.
121. Wessendorf TE, Thilmann AF, Wang YM, et al. Fibrinogen levels and obstructive sleep apnea in ischemic stroke. Am J Respir Crit Care Med 2000; 162:2039–2042.
122. Nobili L, Schiavi G, Bozano E, et al. Morning increase of whole blood viscosity in obstructive sleep apnea syndrome. Clin Hemorheol Microcirc 2000; 22:21–27.
123. Kuniyoshi FH, Garcia-Touchard A, Gami AS, et al. Day-night variation of acute myocardial infarction in obstructive sleep apnea. J Am Coll Cardiol 2008; 52:343–346.
124. Gami AS, Howard DE, Olson EJ, et al. Day-night pattern of sudden death in obstructive sleep apnea. N Engl J Med 2005; 352:1206–1214.

16

Quantitative Models of Periodic Breathing and Cheyne–Stokes Respiration

MICHAEL C. K. KHOO

University of Southern California, Los Angeles, California, U.S.A.

I. Introduction

Cheyne–Stokes respiration (CSR) is an exaggerated form of periodic breathing (PB) in which the ventilatory pattern displays a cyclic variation between periods of hyperpnea and periods of apnea or hypopnea. The classic pattern of CSR is one in which the apneic phase is followed by breaths that gradually wax and subsequently wane in amplitude until the next period of apnea occurs. CSR has long been associated with both congestive heart failure (CHF) and neurologic disease (1–3). As such, there has been a long-running controversy on whether the pathogenetic mechanisms underlying CSR are primarily neurological or cardiovascular in origin (3). Guyton et al. (4) induced CSR in anesthetized dogs by artificially lengthening the carotid arteries, thereby prolonging lung-to-brain circulation time (CT). Since it was known that patients with CHF commonly have prolonged CTs (5), these workers concluded that their results supported a cardiovascular mechanism for CSR. On the other hand, careful analysis of their results shows that only one-third of the experimental preparations developed CSR in spite of extremely long circulation times that ranged from two to five minutes. Furthermore, with such drastic interventions, neurological damage in some of the preparations could not be ruled out. In support of the neurological mechanism, Brown and Plum (6) found that 5 of the 28 patients with CSR that they studied were free of heart disease, although all had some kind of neurological lesion. On the other hand, numerous reports have indicated that PB can also appear in healthy subjects under a variety of circumstances. For instance, it is now well known that PB is a common occurrence in normal sojourners to high altitude, particularly when these subjects are asleep (7–11). This condition disappears when the subjects return to sea level. Douglas and Haldane (12) found that PB could be induced transiently following forced hyperventilation for about two minutes or during administration of a hypoxic gas mixture. PB is also commonly observed during sleep onset and in the light stages of sleep (13,14). Furthermore, PB frequently occurs in apparently healthy infants in the first few months of life but becomes uncommon thereafter (15,16).

The appearance of PB under relatively physiological circumstances as well as in highly pathological conditions, in the form of CSR, suggests that there might be some commonality to these apparently disparate entities. Douglas and Haldane (12) suggested that PB was simply a manifestation of the dynamics of an automatic control system constantly attempting to restore itself toward equilibrium as it responds to perturbations from the external. This "instability hypothesis" has been the basis of several theoretical models of PB that have been proposed over the past few decades (17,18). The primary goal of this chapter is to review the fundamental notions of control engineering that underlie the instability hypothesis and to determine whether the predictions of these quantitative models are consistent with empirical observations, with particular attention to CSR in the context of CHF. For details of many other aspects of CSR or PB, the reader is referred to many excellent reviews of the subject that exist in the literature (19–26). This chapter also addresses various issues related to ventilatory control stability that are often misunderstood or misinterpreted. Although obstructive or mixed apneas have been reported in subjects displaying CSR, the present work focuses primarily on the mechanisms that lead to central apnea.

II. Respiratory Control Instability: Theoretical Considerations

A. Basic Notions

The homeostatic control of most physiological processes, from basic cellular inter-actions up to the level of integrated multiorgan systems, is achieved through the use of negative feedback. In respiratory control, alterations in arterial blood gas tensions stimulate the chemoreflexes to produce ventilatory adjustments that act to restore Pa_{CO_2} and Pa_{O_2} toward their equilibrium levels. It is important to note that the feedback is "negative" because the corrective action taken by the respiratory controller is always opposite in sign to the original change in ventilation. Thus, a transient bout of hyperpnea would produce lower Pa_{CO_2} and higher Pa_{O_2}, which, acting through the chemoreflexes, would subsequently elicit a decrease in ventilation. Homeostatic regulation would work perfectly if the corrective change in ventilation (i.e., the decrease) were instantaneously produced, thereby canceling the effects of the original bout of hyperpnea. However, in reality, there are delays in the feedback process, and it is this physical and temporal separation of chemoreception from the lungs that constitutes the fundamental reason for respiratory instability.

Figure 1 illustrates more clearly how this kind of instability can come about. For the sake of simplicity, we consider a very rudimentary model of the chemical control of respiration in which there is only one chemoreflex pathway and the effects of any hypoxia can be ignored (Fig. 1A). We assume that the system is operating at some equilibrium level when it is perturbed by a disturbance (X) that transiently lowers ventilation: This disturbance may be a spontaneous occlusion of the upper airways, for instance. As shown in Figure 1B–D, the drop in ventilation produces an increase in Pa_{CO_2} in the lungs. If the chemosensors were located in the lungs, the increase in Pa_{CO_2} (ΔPa_{CO_2}) would translate rapidly into a compensatory increase in ventilation (ΔV_E), which would partially or completely offset the effect of the rest of the original hypopnea. However, the chemosensors are not located in the lungs, and time is needed for the blood with higher Pa_{CO_2} to reach these receptors. As a consequence, the respiratory controller does not respond to the original disturbance until most of it has already entered the system. Since there is now nothing to offset this mistimed corrective action, the net result is an overcompensation of the original disturbance, which produces an under-shooting in Pa_{CO_2} and subsequently a decrease in ventilation. This cascade of events leads to an oscillatory ventilatory response, which Haldane had referred to as "hunting." A crucial ingredient of this oscillatory response is the totality of delays and lags inherent

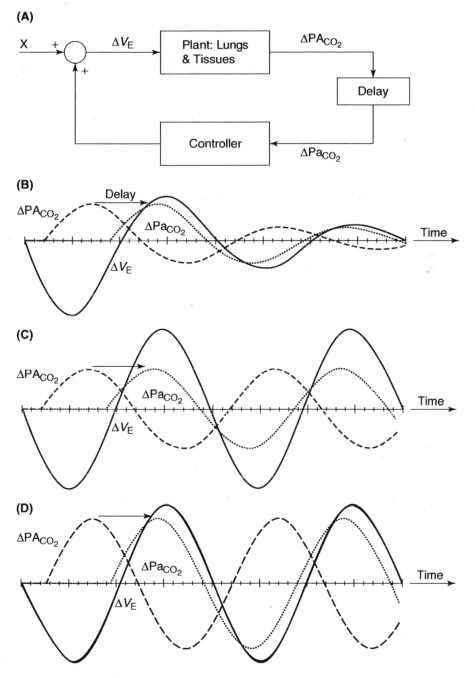

Figure 1 (A) Simplified schematic representation of the chemical control of respiration. (**B–D**) Illustration of how a sustained oscillation can come about (see accompanying text for details).

in the entire chemical control loop: If the corrective action by the controller is delayed to the extent that it becomes out of phase ($\varphi = 180°$) with the preceding disturbance, there will be a tendency for the oscillation to propagate. This antisynchronous timing is crucial, since otherwise there will be cancellative interference between the propagated disturbance and subsequent corrective changes.

Whether the closed-loop response to the initial hypopneic disturbance will be a brief oscillation that is quickly damped out (Fig. 1B) or a more sustained oscillation (Fig. 1C, D) depends on factors other than the circulatory delay. In Figure 1C, the initial hypopnea produces an increase in Pa_{CO_2} that is of the same magnitude as in Figure 1B. However, the increase in Pa_{CO_2} subsequently produces an overshooting in ventilation that is twice as large as that in Figure 1B. In this case, a doubling in "controller gain" or ventilatory response to CO_2 is the factor responsible for propagating the oscillation, which otherwise would have been damped out.

Figure 1D illustrates another way in which the initial hypopneic disturbance can produce a sustained oscillation. In this case, the controller gain is assumed to be the same as that in Figure 1B. Thus, the only way in which an oscillatory response can be sustained is for changes in ventilation to produce larger changes in Pa_{CO_2} compared to those in Figure 1B. The ratio of the magnitude of Pa_{CO_2} to the magnitude of ΔV_E is known as the "plant gain." In Figure 1D, the plant gain is doubled, leading to a sustained oscillatory response similar to that displayed in Figure 1C. The plant gain is inversely related to the amount of "damping" in the gas exchanger portion of the system. In a system that has large CO_2 and O_2 stores, there will be a large amount of damping in the system, since a given change in ventilation will lead to a smaller fluctuation in Pa_{CO_2} or Pa_{O_2}. This is equivalent to saying that the system in this case has a low plant gain.

In the situations depicted in Figure 1C and D, either controller gain or plant gain was doubled while the other was assumed constant. These cases reflect only two out of an infinite number of possible combinations that would produce a sustained oscillatory response. For instance, a 50% increase in both controller and plant gains can also lead to a self-sustained oscillation. Thus, the stability of the closed-loop response depends on the *combined* gains of the plant and controller, as well as the total lag inherent in the forward and feedback portions of the respiratory control system. In the parlance of control engineering, stability is dependent on the system property known as "loop gain" (LG). To take into account both magnitude and phase considerations, LG can be represented in the form of a complex variable:

$$LG = |LG|e^{-j\varphi} \tag{1a}$$

where

$$|LG| = G_{cont} \times G_{plant} \tag{1b}$$

and

$$\varphi = \varphi_{cont} + \varphi_{plant} + \varphi_{delay} \tag{1c}$$

In the above set of equations, j is the square root of -1, and G_{cont} and G_{plant} are the magnitudes of controller and plant gains, respectively, while φ represents the sum of the phase lags of all components that make up the plant (φ_{plant}) and controller (φ_{cont}) as well as the phase lag contribution (φ_{delay}) from the circulatory delay. An oscillation becomes self-sustaining when φ equals $180°$ and the product $G_{cont} \times G_{plant}$ attains the value of unity (27,28). These conditions constitute the Nyquist stability criterion (29), a fundamental theorem in classic control theory. Other theoretical models of respiratory control have employed different stability analysis techniques (30–32). A common limitation of all these analyses is the assumption of small perturbations, so that the nonlinear equations characterizing the system can be linearized around some equilibrium point. As such, the quantitative predictions that arise from these analyses must be interpreted as estimates of those system parameters in the period immediately following the initiation of oscillatory behavior.

When the magnitude of LG is larger than unity, the system becomes unstable, so any small perturbations due to noise entering the chemoreflex loop will be amplified, spawning an oscillation of rapidly increasing magnitude. Eventually, this growth will be limited by saturating nonlinearities in the controller and plant as these become progressively more dominant with increasing oscillation amplitude. However, the conversion of an initially low-amplitude ventilatory oscillation into a stable limit cycle with repetitive episodes of central apnea can occur very rapidly—in the time course of only a few breaths (33). In a sense, the term *respiratory instability* is a misnomer, since fully developed CSR patterns generally represent highly stable oscillations.

B. Analysis of Loop Gain

Although the preceding discussion is useful for describing in a general way how respiratory instability can come about, there are a number of important details that need to be highlighted. These details strongly affect the predictions that can be made, which, in turn, provide the means for validating or improving the model. The first important point is that controller gain and plant gain, as shown in equation (1b), are not constant values but are complex functions of frequency. Consider, for instance, plant gain. Plant gain encompasses all the influences that would affect the translation of a given change in ventilation into a change in Pa_{CO_2} or Pa_{O_2}. For simplicity, we limit the present discussion here to only CO_2, although similar considerations apply also to O_2. Lung and tissue gas stores of CO_2 affect the rapidity of the CO_2 exchange process and thus have a direct influence on system damping or, conversely, plant gain. When CO_2 stores are large, fluctuations in ventilation exert a smaller effect on alveolar and arterial Pa_{CO_2} changes. Thus, these stores act like a low-pass filter, attenuating the effects of rapid ventilatory fluctuations more than those of slow changes in ventilation. Further insight can be obtained by considering some of the mathematics behind this assertion. Assuming the simplest flow-through model of CO_2 exchange in the lungs, we have:

$$V_L \frac{dPa_{CO_2}}{dt} = (V_E - V_D)(PI_{CO_2} - Pa_{CO_2}) + MR_{CO_2} \tag{2}$$

where V_L represents the effective volume of CO_2 stored in the lungs, pulmonary blood, and lung tissue; PI_{CO_2} is the inspired CO_2 gas tension; and MR_{CO_2} is the metabolic production rate of CO_2. To deduce the magnitude of the plant gain for CO_2, $G_{plant}^{CO_2}$ (defined as $\Delta Pa_{CO_2}/\Delta V_E$), from this simplified gas exchange model, we assume small sinusoidal fluctuations in V_E (ΔV_E) and solve equation (2) to deduce how these translate into sinusoidal fluctuations in Pa_{CO_2} (ΔPa_{CO_2}). This can be done with the application of some calculus and the use of Laplace transforms (27–29). The resulting expression shows that $G_{\text{plant}}^{CO_2}$ depends strongly on the frequency f of the oscillations in V_E and Pa_{CO_2}:

$$G_{\text{plant}}^{CO_2}(f) = \frac{Pa_{CO_2} - PI_{CO_2}}{\sqrt{4\pi^2 f^2 V_L^2 + MR_{CO_2}^2/(Pa_{CO_2} - PI_{CO_2})^2}} \tag{3}$$

In the above equation, it can be seen that $G_{\text{plant}}^{CO_2}$ is largest when $f = 0$, that is, plant gain magnitude is maximized in the steady state. However, as f increases, the expression on the right-hand side of equation (3) decreases, since its denominator becomes progressively larger. The inherent response time of the gas exchange process also produces a lag in the phase of the resulting sinusoidal fluctuations in Pa_{CO_2} relative to those in V_E. This lag, φ_{plant}, contributes to the overall lag φ associated with LG. For the simple gas exchange model represented by equation (2), φ_{plant} takes the form:

$$\phi_{\text{plant}}(f) = \tan^{-1}\left(\frac{2\pi f V_L}{V_E - V_D}\right) \tag{4}$$

From the expression for $G_{\text{plant}}^{CO_2}$ in equation (3), it can be seen that administration of inhaled CO_2 raises PI_{CO_2} as well as Pa_{CO_2}. But since Pa_{CO_2}, does not increase as much as PI_{CO_2}, this reduces $G_{\text{plant}}^{CO_2}$ at all frequencies. Therefore, hypercapnia induced by exogenous means enhances system stability. On the other hand, equation (3) also predicts that endogenously induced hypercapnia (increasing Pa_{CO_2} without changing PI_{CO_2}), such as what occurs during sleep onset, raises $G_{\text{plant}}^{CO_2}$ over the whole range of frequencies and makes respiratory control less stable. A somewhat unexpected prediction is that $G_{\text{plant}}^{CO_2}$ is also increased when the metabolic rate is reduced. As discussed below, this is another factor that promotes instability during sleep.

Equations (3) and (4) provide the simplest possible mathematical descriptions of the plant gain for CO_2. The equivalent expression for the magnitude of plant gain for O_2 may be similarly derived, and this is given as:

$$G_{\text{plant}}^{O_2}(f) = \frac{PI_{O_2} - Pa_{O_2}}{\sqrt{4\pi^2 f^2 V_L^2 + MR_{O_2}^2/(PI_{O_2} - Pa_{O_2})^2}} \tag{5}$$

Much more complicated expressions arise when other important components, such as the influences of body CO_2 and O_2 stores and mixing in the vasculature, are taken into account. Detailed consideration of these factors may be found in Khoo et al. (27). However, the key point is that all these components contribute to the frequency dependence of plant gain magnitude and phase. Moreover, the respiratory controller is also frequency dependent, since both central and peripheral chemoreflexes have response times that span a range from 10 to 200 seconds (34–36). The net result is that LG magnitude and phase also vary with frequency. Figure 2 illustrates these considerations. Using the model of Khoo et al. (37), we have computed how LG would change with frequency under conditions simulating a normal subject during wakefulness. Only the range of frequencies from 0.01 to 0.05 Hz is shown, since this covers the range of periodicities (20–100 seconds) generally observed in PB. While LG magnitude falls with increasing frequency, the phase lag rises. To determine whether spontaneous oscillations can occur, we apply the criteria for stability that were outlined earlier. We begin by

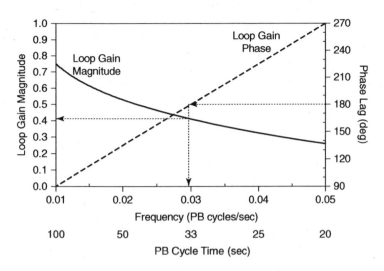

Figure 2 Loop gain magnitude and phase as functions of frequency (or, equivalently, periodic breathing cycle time) in a simulated "normal" subject during wakefulness.

searching for the frequency at which φ becomes 180°. In this case (as indicated by the dotted arrows), the corresponding oscillation cycle time is 34 seconds. Next, we determine the LG magnitude at this periodicity, which turns out to be slightly above 0.4. Thus, under the conditions simulated by the model, the system will tend to "resonate" with a frequency of ~0.03 Hz (corresponding to the 34-second periodicity) when perturbed by noise or other extraneous influences. However, these oscillations will be rapidly damped out, since the LG magnitude is substantially lower than unity.

The second important detail that is often not discussed is the *multifactorial* nature of LG. This arises because ventilatory fluctuations produce simultaneous changes in both Pa_{CO_2} and Pa_{O_2}. At the level of the controller, changes in Pa_{CO_2} and Pa_{O_2} and their interactions contribute to the total response in ventilatory output. This may be further decomposed into contributions arising from the central and peripheral chemoreceptors. Thus, from a functional viewpoint, there are multiple feedback loops. Consider the following steady state description of the ventilatory response to hypercapnia and hypoxia:

$$V_E = G_C(Pa_{CO_2} - I_C) + G_P(\lambda + e^{-0.05Pa_{O_2}})(Pa_{CO_2} - I_P) \qquad (6)$$

where G_C and G_P are the central and peripheral gain factors, and I_C and I_P are the corresponding apneic thresholds. The above controller model assumes that central chemoreflex drive is not affected by hypoxia and that all hypercapnic-hypoxic interaction exists at the peripheral chemoreflex level. It should be noted that equation (6) is essentially the same as the controller equation of Khoo et al. (37), with a small modification added to ensure that a residual peripheral chemoreflex drive λ exists during hyperoxia [review by Cunningham et al. (38)]. Using perturbation analysis, it can be shown that the response of the above controller (ΔV_E) to small changes in both $Pa_{CO_2}(\Delta Pa_{CO_2})$ and $Pa_{O_2}(\Delta Pa_{O_2})$ can be decomposed into three ventilatory drive contributions:

$$\Delta V_E = \Delta V_C + \Delta V_P^{CO_2} + V_P^{O_2} \tag{7}$$

where

$$\Delta V_C = G_C \Delta Pa_{CO_2} \tag{8}$$

$$\Delta V_P^{CO_2} = G_P(\lambda + e^{-0.05Pa_{O_2}})\Delta Pa_{CO_2} \tag{9}$$

and

$$\Delta V_P^{\dot{O}_2} = -0.05 G_P(Pa_{CO_2} - I_P)e^{-0.05Pa_{O_2}}\Delta Pa_{O_2} \tag{10}$$

ΔV_C represents the contribution from the central chemoreflex, which depends only on ΔPa_{CO_2}. $\Delta V_P^{CO_2}$ and $\Delta V_P^{CO_2}$ represent the responses of the peripheral chemoreflexes to ΔPa_{CO_2} and ΔPa_{O_2}, respectively. This delineation is important, since it highlights the fact that stability considerations now must be extended to incorporate the effects of at least three feedback loops, as depicted schematically in Figure 3A.

To determine LG for this multiple feedback loop model, we combine equations (8), (9), and (10) with the plant gain expressions in equations (3) and (5) to obtain the individual components that correspond to each of the feedback loops: LGc for the central chemoreflex loop, $LG_P^{CO_2}$ for the peripheral CO_2 loop, and $LG_P^{O_2}$ for the peripheral O_2 loop. Since each of these loops has its own dynamic characteristics, at any given frequency of stimulation, the responses from these different contribution sources will differ in both magnitude and phase. Thus, although V_E is assumed to be the sum of V_C, $V_P^{CO_2}$, and $V_P^{O_2}$, computation of the overall LG involves the vectorial addition of LG_C, $LG_P^{CO_2}$, and $LG_P^{O_2}$ so that the differences in magnitude and phase can be accounted for, that is:

$$|LG(f)| = \sqrt{|LG_C(f)|^2 + |LG_P^{CO_2}(f)|2 + |LG_P^{O_2}(f)|^2} \tag{11}$$

$$\phi(f) = \phi_C(f) + \phi_P^{CO_2}(f) + \phi_P^{O_2}(f) \tag{12}$$

To illustrate how these three components affect the overall LG, we present the results of this kind of computation performed for the example of the awake, normal subject discussed earlier (Fig. 2). The gain factors representing the central (G_C) and peripheral (G_P) chemoreflexes were assigned values so that, under normoxic conditions, peripheral CO_2 chemosensitivity would constitute roughly 28% of the combined steady state hypercapnic response slope. Figure 3B shows a vector diagram in which the overall LG is decomposed into its three components: LG_C, $LG_P^{CO_2}$, and $LG_P^{O_2}$. Using the right horizontal axis to represent $\varphi = 0°$, we adopt the convention that depicts an increase in φ as a clockwise rotation of any given vector. Consistent with our earlier results in Figure 2, at the frequency corresponding to a 34-second cycle time, LG is represented as a vector of length 0.4 that points horizontally to the left ($\varphi = 180°$). Because of vectorial summation, both the magnitude and the phase of each individual component play important roles in determining the magnitude of overall LG. For example, the central

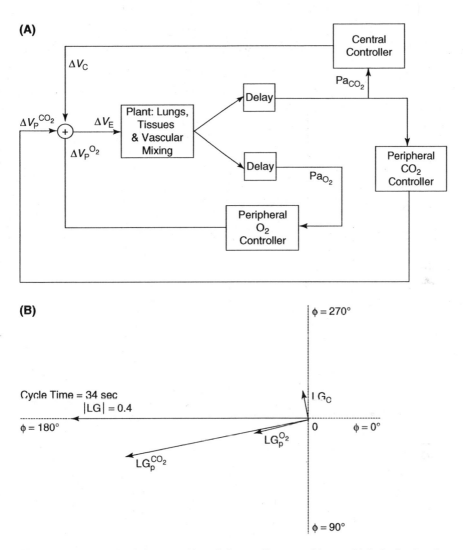

Figure 3 (A) Functional decomposition of chemoreflex control into multiple feedback pathways. (B) Vectorial decomposition of loop gain into its central, peripheral CO_2, and peripheral O_2 components.

chemoreflex component contribution is only about 2% due to the fact that the magnitude of LG_C is small and φ is 262° (almost perpendicular to the horizontal axis) at this oscillation frequency; this may be attributed to the sluggishness of the medullary chemoreflex response. At this periodicity, the peripheral CO_2 component contributes most (~77%) to the overall LG. However, it is interesting to note that the peripheral O_2 component, even under these relatively normoxic circumstances, remains significant, contributing substantially more (~21%) to the overall LG than the central component.

C. Nonlinear Models

It is important to recognize that a key assumption implicit in all that has been discussed thus far is linearity. This assumption is approximately valid when the fluctuations in V_E, Pa_{CO_2}, and Pa_{O_2} do not exceed certain limits. When larger changes occur, these computations of local stability must be repeated at new system "set points." For example, the expression for $G_{plant}^{CO_2}$ in equation (3) assumes that we are considering small changes in V_E and Pa_{CO_2} around a fixed average level of $Pa_{CO_2} - PI_{CO_2}$. Changes in the operating levels of PI_{CO_2}, Pa_{CO_2}, metabolic rate, and lung CO_2 stores will lead to changes in $G_{plant}^{CO_2}$ and φ_{plant} at all frequencies—that is, the curves shown in Figure 2 will shift with changes in these model parameters.

In the analysis summarized by equations (6) to (9), we underestimated the controller response to simultaneous changes in Pa_{CO_2} and Pa_{O_2}, since the calculations did not include the nonlinear term that reflects multiplicative interaction between hypercapnia and hypoxia. We have estimated that the linearity assumption would produce an error no higher than 25% in model predictions as long as the swings in blood gases do not exceed 10 Torr. However, the errors increase dramatically when the changes in blood gases or ventilation become larger or when the effects of a "hard nonlinearity," such as the occurrence of apnea, begin to dominate the dynamics of the system.

One analytical technique that can take into consideration certain types of nonlinearities is the "describing function" method (39), which may be viewed as an extension of Nyquist stability analysis. This method establishes the conditions necessary for the development of a "stable" limit cycle. The assumptions are (*i*) the closed-loop system in question can be partitioned in a linear dynamic component and a serially connected *static* nonlinearity; (*ii*) the linear dynamic component is low pass in nature; and (*iii*) because of assumption (*ii*), the oscillation that is sustained around the loop is sinusoidal in pattern. An extended LG is deduced from the product of the transfer function of the linear component and the gain function that relates the output of the static nonlinearity to its input (i.e., the "describing function"). Analogous to the Nyquist stability criterion, this extended LG can be shown to be equal to negative unity when a stable limit cycle exists. We have used this method to estimate the periodicity and amplitude of the limit cycle oscillation associated with CHF (29). However, because of the constraints posed by the assumptions on which it is based, the describing function method can be seen at best to provide an approximate analysis of closed-loop stability.

For the analysis of more complicated nonlinear models, it is necessary to resort to the use of computer simulation. The general procedure here is to model respiratory control as a system of coupled differential equations that are solved numerically by finite difference methods. A numerical solution allows stability characteristics to be explored over a wide range of parameter variations. Over the past several decades, many of these computer models have been proposed (37,40–44), each differing from the others in the level of complexity being represented and in the assumptions made about the physiological processes underlying various system components. The advantage of these models is that they allow the complexity of physiological reality to be better represented. This can lead to improved quantitative predictions. On the other hand, the increased complexity often leaves one with little physical insight into which factors are most responsible in initiating and propagating the ventilatory periodicities. As well, since these models are highly parameterized, selecting the combination of parameter values to be deployed in any given simulation can be problematic, since the values of many parameters are unknown.

D. Empirical Evidence of Respiratory Control Instability

A considerable body of evidence from human and animal studies has accumulated over the years to support the notion that, in most cases, PB is the result of unstable respiratory control. We have seen from the example illustrated in Figure 3B that, under normal physiological conditions, LG is derived predominantly from peripheral CO_2 and O_2 contributions, with the central chemoreflex contribution playing a minimal role. It follows that since hypoxia increases peripheral chemoreflex gain, PB should also become more prevalent. Indeed, various studies have demonstrated significant increases in the incidence and strength of ventilatory oscillations with growing severity of hypoxia (7–12,45,46). Taking into account the rise in cardiac output and the lowering of the lung washout time constant for O_2 (due to a steeper slope of the blood O_2 dissociation curve in hypoxia), our model also predicts a decrease in cycle time with increasing hypoxia (27). This prediction has been validated with the empirical finding that the intensity of ventilatory oscillations increases and cycle time decreases with ascent to high altitude (9). On the other hand, at more extreme altitudes, the decrease in cycle time appears to level off at ~ 20 seconds (8,10). This is predicted by the model if the assumption is made that there is no further increase in cardiac output and shortening of circulatory delay at these extremely hypoxic levels. In several studies involving animal preparations, interventions that enhance the relative importance of peripheral drive have also been found to increase the incidence of PB. Examples of such interventions are the administration of hypoxic inhalation mixtures (47), central drive depression by focal cooling of the medulla (48), and augmentation of carotid chemoreceptor sensitivity by blocking dopamine receptors (49).

The instability hypothesis predicts that inhalation of hypercapnic or hyperoxic mixtures depress plant gain and therefore should eliminate or attenuate PB. This is consistent with most experimental and clinical studies of PB (3,48,49), although some researchers have reported the persistence of PB despite O_2 administration (13,50,51). One possible explanation for this discrepancy is that O_2 inhalation tends to increase oscillation cycle time and thus lengthen the duration of apnea; this, in turn, could act to offset the reduction in plant gain.

As one can deduce from equation (3), a decrease in lung stores for CO_2 and O_2 increases plant gain, since smaller volumes would lead to reduced damping of fluctuations in alveolar and arterial blood gases. This explains the increased incidence of PB in subjects that are in the supine position relative to those that are seated, since the horizontal posture leads to a reduction in functional residual capacity (52). Several models have also predicted the transient appearance of PB following passive hyperventilation and the ensuing apnea (27,39,41). These predictions have been validated in anesthetized dogs (47) and humans during sleep (53).

Substantial differences in hypercapnic and hypoxic chemosensitivities exist between individuals. It follows from the instability hypothesis that the incidence of PB should be higher in subjects with larger chemosensitivities. A number of studies on humans have demonstrated strong statistical correlations between the incidence of PB and hypoxic or hypercapnic gains (8,11,54,55). Xie et al. (54) found that the central and peripheral chemosensitivities of patients with PB and idiopathic central sleep apnea are roughly twice as large as the corresponding measures of controller gain in normal controls. Data from the study of Chapman et al. (55) also suggest that a stronger degree of hypercapnic-hypoxic interaction may promote greater susceptibility to the development of periodic respiration.

According to the instability hypothesis, an initially small oscillation grows into a large-amplitude limit cycle, and repetitive episodes of apnea are produced when its hypoventilatory portions attain zero ventilation. Support for this mechanism of apnea production is evident in the study of Waggener et al. (56), who demonstrated, using a comb-filtering technique, that the vast majority of periodic apneas seen in premature infants coincide with the minimum phase of the dominant ventilatory oscillation.

Contrary to what is observed in adult humans and in many animal preparations, inhalation of hypoxic gas mixtures *suppresses* PB in newborn lambs and human infants (57,58). While this observation appears to contradict the instability hypothesis, closer examination of the components of LG resolves the discrepancy. In the adult human, we have shown that the increase in LG produced by hypoxia is derived primarily from a substantial increase in $LG_P^{CO_2}$, which in turn is due to the elevation of CO_2 controller gain in hypoxia (27). Counterintuitively, $LG_P^{O_2}$ remains unchanged or may even decrease, since a reduction in O_2 plant gain during hypoxia offsets the increase in O_2 controller gain. In newborn lambs and human preterm infants, it is also known that the ventilatory responses to hypercapnia and hypoxia are additive rather than multiplicative, that is, hypoxia does not increase CO_2 controller gain but merely shifts the CO_2 ventilatory response curve to the left. Wilkinson et al. (58) used the instability hypothesis to demonstrate that this results in an overall reduction in LG, since, in this case, $LG_P^{CO_2}$ is zero and LG is dominated by $LG_P^{O_2}$, which *decreases* in hypoxia due to the dominant effect of the reduction in O_2 plant gain (equation 5).

III. Respiratory Control Instability in Congestive Heart Failure

A. Relative Importance of Circulatory Delay Vs. Controller Gain

Several mathematical models of PB have shown that the prolongation of circulatory delay destabilizes chemoreflex control (27,31,32,40,41). However, close analysis of the behavior of these models indicates that the relationship between stability and circulatory delay is highly dependent on other key model parameters. Consequently, in some cases, CSR could only be produced under highly unrealistic conditions. For example, in Milhorn's study (40), the circulatory delay had to be increased to 3½ minutes before the model was able to oscillate spontaneously. We believe that this was probably due to the exclusion of the peripheral chemoreflex from their controller. The 1966 model of Longobardo et al. (41), assuming a more reasonable circulatory delay of 30 seconds for CHF and normal chemoreflex gain, was able to simulate CSR with a periodicity of about 2 minutes. However, the model did not oscillate spontaneously, and CSR occurred only after posthyperventilation apnea. This "inertia" may have resulted from the considerable amount of damping that was assumed by the inclusion of the entire volume of arterial blood (2.4 L) as a component of lung CO_2 and O_2 storage.

Applying the kind of analysis that was presented in section II.B, we have computed the LG for a hypothetical subject with CHF. The results of these calculations are

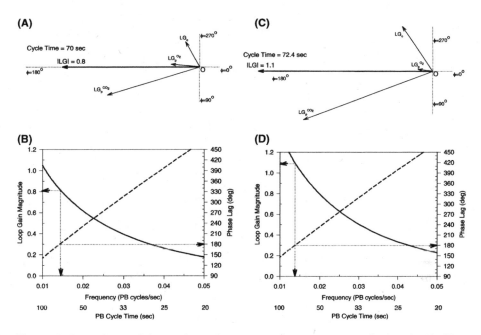

Figure 4 Dependence of loop gain on frequency and component contributions in (**A, B**) a simulated subject with prolonged circulatory delay and reduced cardiac output and (**C, D**) a simulated subject with prolonged circulatory delay, reduced cardiac output, and increased hypercapnic ventilatory response.

displayed in Figure 4A and B. All model parameters were assigned the same values as those employed for the normal subject (Figs. 2 and 3B), except that cardiac output was halved and the lung-to-ear circulation delay was doubled to 18 seconds. As Figure 4B clearly demonstrates, the longer delay is reflected in the much steeper rate of increase in phase lag ϕ with frequency relative to the normal case. LG magnitude is also increased over the whole range of frequencies displayed. The frequency at which ϕ becomes $180°$ now corresponds to a cycle time of 70 seconds. However, LG magnitude at this periodicity is 0.8, a value large enough to permit the occurrence of underdamped oscillations in ventilation but insufficient for engendering self-sustained periodic behavior. The vector diagram in Figure 4A shows the breakdown of LG into its three components at the periodicity of 70 seconds. The peripheral CO_2 component continues to dominate, accounting for $\sim 68\%$ of the overall LG. However, the central contribution now plays a significantly larger role ($>10\%$) in determining overall LG compared to 2% in the case for the normal subject. This example shows that a doubling of circulatory delay by itself promotes instability but may not be sufficient for the generation of self-sustained oscillation. Figure 4C and D illustrates the results of another simulation of CSR in CHF. Here, in addition to the assumption of a doubling in circulatory delay, we have also assumed a doubling of the hypercapnic sensitivities of both central and peripheral chemoreceptors; the hypoxic sensitivity in normocapnia was left unchanged (see below). The computations indicate that these alterations in model parameters elevate the LG magnitude (at $\varphi = 180°$) to a value exceeding unity, thus allowing self-sustained oscillation to occur at a periodicity of approximately 72 seconds.

The model calculations displayed in Figure 4 suggest that an increased controller gain or some other supplemental factor may be the distinguishing parameter that differentiates subjects with CSR from those without CSR in the population of patients with CHF. Indeed, while CSR is a common occurrence, it does not occur in all subjects with CHF (59). Both groups of CHF patients have been found to have similar left ventricular ejection fraction (60–62) and similar lung-to-ear circulatory delay (62). Wilcox et al. (63) found, in 34 CHF patients with CSR, hypercapnic ventilatory response slopes that were, on average, approximately twice the levels found in normals and patients with obstructive sleep apnea (OSA). Hypoxic sensitivities, however, were not different. In a more recent study, Solin et al. (64) measured both central and peripheral ventilatory responses to CO_2 using the rebreathing and single-breath CO_2 test, respectively. They found central CO_2 sensitivity to be almost three times and peripheral CO_2 sensitivity to be twice as large in CHF patients with CSR versus CHF patients without CSR. These findings are consistent with the assumptions we made in predicting LG in CHF-CSR (Fig. 4C and D).

We have also performed model computations using other circulatory delay times, ranging from 8 to 20 seconds. In each case, we determined the cycle duration of the sustained oscillation that would occur when the hypercapnic controller gains were increased to sufficiently high levels. We found a linear relationship between lung-to-ear delay (T_D) and circulation time (CT) that followed the regression equation:

$$CT = -2.91 + 4.14\,T_D \tag{13}$$

This result is remarkably consistent with experimental studies that have also examined the relationship between circulatory delay and cycle time (65,66).

B. Role of Hypocapnia

Patients with CHF and CSR have also been reported to be more hypocapnic than CHF controls without PB (62,66). Solin et al. (64) have argued that the hypocapnia and hyperventilation stem from the higher controller gain in these subjects. Comparison of subjects from these two groups with similar left ventricular ejection fractions and cardiac output have led to the finding that left ventricular diastolic volume is larger in the subjects with both CHF and CSR (67). Increased filling pressures can lead to pulmonary vascular congestion and consequently a decrease in pulmonary gas volume. The reduction in gas stores (V_L in equation 3) would certainly promote instability by elevating plant gain. Pulmonary congestion could also be partly responsible for the hyperventilation and hypocapnia generally found in this type of patient, through the stimulation of vagally mediated reflexes that effectively increase controller gain (67). The hypocapnia itself could be a destabilizing factor if it acts to silence the medullary chemoreceptors, leaving the regulation of breathing to the sole custody of the peripheral chemoreflex, which would subject the system to considerably greater volatility. Current models of PB have assumed that the CO_2 controller gain remains constant for a given Pa_{O_2} level above and below the eupneic point. On the other hand, experiments applying pressure support ventilation to produce quasi-steady hypocapnic conditions have found the apneic threshold during sleep to be at a higher level of PC_{O_2} than would have been expected from a simple extrapolation

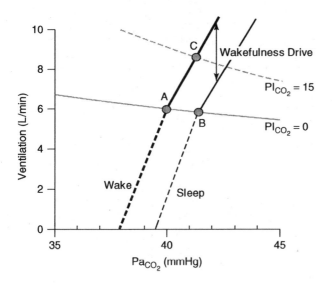

Figure 5 Schematic plots of the controller responses to CO_2 (*dark lines*) in wakefulness and sleep and the metabolic hyperbolac for CO_2 under eucapnic conditions (*solid gray curve*) and during inhalation of CO_2 (*broken gray curve*). The magnitude of the wakefulness drive is represented in this scheme as the vertical offset between the wake and sleep controller response lines. See text for further details.

of the hypercapnic ventilatory response line below the eupneic point (68). This suggests that the CO_2 ventilatory sensitivity may be higher below eupnea compared to hypercapnia, as illustrated in Figure 5 (broken lines compared to solid lines). Increased controller gain in hypocapnia is certainly a factor that would promote CSR.

C. Effects of Sleep: The Wakefulness Drive

While CSR can occur during wakefulness in CHF, the periodicities that are generally observed are patterns that include episodes of hypopneas or ventilatory oscillations that are barely visible unless analyzed by spectral analysis or comb-filtering techniques (69). Ventilatory periodicities that include apnea and the accompanying large fluctuations in blood gases generally occur during sleep. Reduction of Pa_{CO_2} by a few mmHg through passive hyperventilation can easily induce apnea in sleeping subjects, whereas the same intervention rarely leads to the cessation of breathing in wakefulness (53). These observations are due to some extent to the changeover in the behavioral control mode that so dominates wakefulness to the automatic chemoreflex-based control of ventilation that occurs during sleep. Thus, the removal of voluntary and nonspecific environmental influences may simply unmask the underlying oscillatory dynamics of a marginally stable system (70).

Fink suggested the existence of an input to the respiratory centers, a "wakefulness stimulus," that is dependent on the level of vigilance (71). The withdrawal of this supplemental drive to breathe during sleep onset is equivalent to a "downward" shift of the CO_2 ventilatory response line, which results in an increase in the CO_2 apneic threshold, as depicted in Figure 5. Assuming that the metabolic rate remains unchanged with sleep (in reality, of course, there is a small reduction), withdrawal of the wakefulness stimulus leads to a small increase inPa_{CO_2}, as indicated in Figure 5 by the shift in the steady state operating point from A to B. As one can deduce from equation (3), this endogenous increase in Pa_{CO_2} raises plant gain, which, in turn, increases LG, thereby making the chemoreflex control of ventilation less stable. This prediction is consistent with Bulow's observation that individuals with the largest increases in apneic threshold are also most likely to exhibit PB during sleep (13). On the other hand, the same level of elevated Pa_{CO_2} (as represented by Fig. 5C) can be attained in wakefulness through the inhalation of a CO_2-enriched mixture. But, in this case, plant gain is reduced (equation 3), and thus LG is also correspondingly decreased, resulting in a more stable system. Thus, plant gain can be increased or decreased for the same level of Pa_{CO_2} elevation, and thus hypercapnia can be destabilizing or stabilizing. The directionality of the change depends on whether the increase in Pa_{CO_2} is achieved endogenously (as in sleep) or through exogenous means (CO_2 inhalation). This explanation may be useful in clearing up some of the confusion as to whether hypercapnia promotes or suppresses PB (72).

We have also demonstrated in model simulations that for a given magnitude of wakefulness drive, the increase in Pa_{CO_2} that accompanies sleep onset is dependent on controller gain (37). For subjects with normal hypercapnic ventilatory response slopes, the model predicts the sleep-induced increase in Pa_{CO_2} to be on the order of 4 Torr. However, a doubling of controller gain can reduce this Pa_{CO_2} increase to <2 Torr. The form of this predicted dependence of Pa_{CO_2} increase on controller gain is consistent with experimental data (73). The explanation for this result becomes self-evident when the effect of sleep is conceptualized as a "downward" shift (equal to the magnitude of the wakefulness drive, as shown in Fig. 5) as opposed to a "rightward" shift of the CO_2 response line. For the same downward shift (i.e., the same magnitude of wakefulness drive withdrawal), a larger increase in the apneic threshold for CO_2 is produced with a low-gain controller compared to what would result for a controller with high gain. These results are consistent with the characteristics of a negative feedback system.

As alluded to earlier, equation (3) (sect. II.B) predicts that changes in two other factors that normally accompany sleep also predispose the system to elevated plant gain and consequently increased LG. First, as we have noted in the previous section, the change in posture from standing or sitting to the supine position leads to a decrease in functional residual capacity and lung CO_2 stores, which reduces system damping. Second, the reduction in the metabolic rate that accompanies sleep can also lead to an increase in plant gain. Furthermore, low metabolic rates tend to produce longer apneas, since Pa_{CO2} takes a longer time to recover to levels necessary to reinitiate breathing during apnea (43). This is consistent with the greater amounts of PB observed in patients with hypothyroidism (74) as well as in diabetics during hemodialysis using acetate-buffered dialysate (75).

On the other hand, it is known that the ventilatory responses to hypercapnia and hypoxia are depressed with increasing depth of sleep (76,77). This decreased controller gain would act to promote stability in respiratory control. However, we have demonstrated in a computer model that the elevation in plant gain that accompanies sleep onset is likely to more than offset any depression in controller gain during the light stages of quiet sleep, thus leading to a greater propensity for instability (78). As sleep depth increases, the progressive depression of chemoresponsiveness eventually becomes the more dominant factor, leading to decreased LG and greater stability during slow-wave sleep. This explanation is compatible with the well-known finding that PB occurs mostly in the light stages of quiet sleep and only rarely in stage 4 sleep (13,14,76,77). It has been shown that the closed-loop ventilatory response to dynamic changes in inhaled CO_2 (under hyperoxic conditions) is preserved during stage 2 sleep, while central controller gain is reduced significantly (79). As well, applying pseudorandom-binary forcing of inhaled CO_2, Khoo et al. (80) found no significant decrease in dynamic controller (central + peripheral) gain in normal subjects during normoxic sleep.

D. Respiratory Effects of Transient State Changes

The process of the wakefulness stimulus withdrawal in itself constitutes a large disturbance to the respiratory chemoreflexes. For individuals with normal levels of hypercapnic sensitivity, model calculations predict that the magnitude of the wakefulness drive has to be on the order of 6 to 7 L/min to achieve the increases in Pa_{CO_2} of 4 to 5 Torr that have been reported frequently in sleep studies (13,77). This implies that if Pa_{CO_2} could be maintained at waking levels during sleep onset [e.g., through passive hyperventilation (53)], most subjects would be apneic. Colrain and coworkers (81) have demonstrated that the reduction in ventilatory drive at sleep onset is not only substantial but that much of this loss can take effect in the course of a few breaths. Withdrawal of a large wakefulness drive with such a rapid time course could lead to a period of apnea, since there would not be sufficient time for the respiratory chemostat to compensate for the imposed disturbance. The large changes in arterial blood gases accompanying this initial period of apnea could subsequently push the system into oscillation if LG were sufficiently high. There have indeed been a number of reports of a greater tendency for PB to occur in subjects who fall asleep abruptly (13,77).

In cases where LG is greatly depressed due to substantial reduction in controller gain during sleep—e.g., in patients with primary alveolar hypoventilation syndrome—a different kind of "instability" may appear. Rapid withdrawal of wakefulness drive would lead to apnea. Since there is little or no controller gain, there is insufficient drive to terminate the apnea. Consequently, blood gases deteriorate to the point where an arousal is triggered, restoring the wakefulness drive to some extent. Breathing is reinitiated with large inspiratory drives in the initial breaths because of the poor blood gas levels. As blood gases return to normal, drowsiness may set in again and the next transition to sleep occurs. Recent model simulations show that this type of instability can lead to repetitive large fluctuations in ventilation and arterial blood gases with periodicities that are roughly double those reported in normals under high-LG conditions (37,78). In a situation of low LG, the respiratory control system is also more susceptible to being affected by external influences. Therefore, respiratory oscillations secondary to oscillations in other organ systems, such as primary fluctuations in arterial blood pressure (82), may appear.

It is most likely, however, that the CSR that occurs in patients with CHF involves both chemoreflex- and arousal-mediated instabilities, since hypercapnic chemosensitivity in this group of subjects is either normal or higher than normal (63,64). In our previous modeling study (37), we have shown that conditions of moderate-to-high controller gain can give rise to a variety of patterns in which the chemoreflex-mediated instability interacts with the arousal-driven instability. In some situations, arousal may

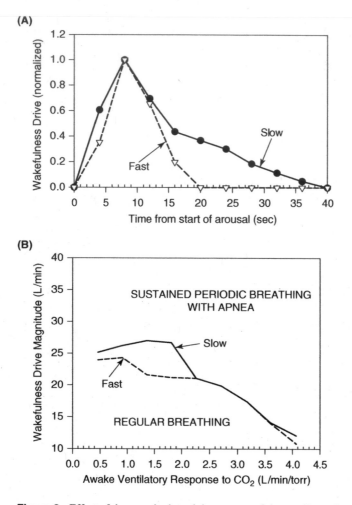

Figure 6 Effect of the magnitude and time course of the ventilatory increase induced by transient arousal on respiratory stability. (A) Time courses of the "fast" and "slow" types of arousal patterns; (B) Stability boundaries corresponding to the "fast" and "slow" arousals (see accompanying text for details). *Source*: Modified from Ref. 90.

accompany every hyperpneic episode in the PB cycle. In other situations, arousal may occur on every other cycle. Another simulation study has shown a similar wealth of complex oscillatory patterns under conditions of hypoxic sleep (83). A study by Hanly and Zuberi-Khokhar (84) has shown the frequency of arousals in CHF patients with CSR to be significantly higher than that in normal patients as well as CHF patients without CSR. This beneficial effect of oxygen therapy in reducing CSR and frequency of arousals has been demonstrated in both theoretical (37,83) and clinical studies (85,86).

The arousal that occurs during the hyperpneic phase of each CSR cycle contributes to the amplification of the hyperpnea that is already present, thereby promoting an even more potent level of hypocapnia that acts subsequently to prolong the apnea that follows. In an analysis of breathing patterns at extreme altitude (33), we found that ventilation was significantly higher in those hyperpneic phases of the PB cycle that were accompanied by arousal than in cycles not associated with arousal. Xie et al. (87) showed in patients with idiopathic central sleep apnea that apnea duration lengthened as the degree of hyperventilation in the preceding hyperpneic phase increased.

Work in our laboratory suggests that the time course of the transient bout of increased ventilatory drive that accompanies arousal may be as important as the magnitude of this hyperpnea in affecting subsequent respiratory stability (88,89). Using acoustic stimulation to provoke transient arousal, we measured the time course of the ventilatory increase accompanying the arousals. These experiments were conducted on normal subjects and patients with OSA breathing under continuous positive airway pressure to minimize the influence of changes in upper airway resistance. The measurements allowed us to incorporate into our original model (37) the time course of the wakefulness drive during arousal. The results obtained from computer simulations performed with the modified model are displayed in Figure 6. Stability of the model was assessed by determining the lowest value of the wakefulness drive accompanying arousal that would predict sustained oscillatory activity: Values above this "stability boundary" produced PB with apnea, while values below the boundary produced an inherently stable response to arousal. Figure 6A shows the two types of arousal-induced ventilatory profiles found in our subjects that were employed in the simulations: one depicting a very abrupt bout of hyperpnea lasting about 20 seconds (OSA subjects) and the other representing a somewhat more gradual time course lasting over 40 seconds (normal patients). The effects of the different arousal time courses on model stability are displayed in Figure 6B for a range of controller gains. Both cases show stability boundaries that are tilted to the right—i.e., it is easier for an arousal to lead to subsequent sustained PB when the controller gain is high. However, the "fast" arousal time course was substantially more destabilizing at low-to-moderate values of controller gain.

IV. Other Mechanisms Affecting Ventilatory Stability
A. Upper Airway Resistance

The loss of wakefulness stimulus that accompanies sleep also leads to a general reduction in tonic activity of the upper airway muscles (77). Thus, airway resistance is generally higher during sleep than in wakefulness. This may account for part of the apparent decrease in chemoresponsiveness that accompanies sleep (90). Although apneas are generally not of the obstructive variety in the PB of patients with CHF, it is likely that less dramatic fluctuations in upper airway resistance do occur. These can play a significant role in precipitating and amplifying periodic ventilation in the following way (19): If upper airway resistance were to increase with increasing ventilatory motor output, the resulting changes in inspiratory airflow would be attenuated. Conversely, changes in upper airway resistance that occur out of phase with ventilatory motor output would lead to an amplification of fluctuations in airflow, thereby exerting a destabilizing influence on respiratory control. The consequent fluctuations in blood gases, ventilatory pump activity, and upper airway muscle activity could eventually lead to events that include complete upper airway closure (91,92).

During hypoxia-induced PB in sleeping normal patients, Hudgel et al. (93) found in six of the nine subjects that upper airway resistance fluctuated between low values at the most hyperpneic breath and high values at the most hypopneic breath; in the remaining three subjects, there were no significant fluctuations. It is noteworthy that, in the first group of subjects, upper airway resistance increased substantially during the PB cycle only when the ratio of upper airway to chest wall inspiratory electromyographic activity decreased below 0.8; on the other hand, in the second group of subjects who did not show significant fluctuations in resistance, this ratio did not fall below 0.8. This finding suggests one of two possibilities for the development of obstructed breaths during PB. The first is that the electrical activities of the upper airways and chest may be related to the respective pressures in a highly nonlinear fashion, while the second is that the recruitment of the upper airway muscles may be slower than that of the inspiratory pump muscles. Warner et al. (94), who studied a group of snorers, showed that the tendency for resistance to fluctuate during hypoxia-induced PB was higher in those subjects who already had a high baseline airway resistance during sleep, whereas the subjects with close-to-normal baseline resistance exhibited little change.

B. Short-Term Potentiation
It has been demonstrated in anesthetized animals (95) and awake humans (96) that the abrupt removal of any drive that produces active hyperventilation leads not to apnea but to a more gradual decay in ventilation. Although this phenomenon was previously referred to as *ventilatory afterdischarge*, it is now generally known as *short-term potentiation* (STP), since it is believed to be the respiratory manifestation of a general form of central nervous system memory. Figure 7A depicts a functional representation of this kind of "signal processing" at the level of the respiratory centers. The classic STP response is illustrated in the top tracing of Figure 7B. In response to a step stimulus (dark bar in Fig. 7B), the phrenic output shows a virtually instantaneous response, but this is followed by a relatively slower rise to the maximum response. Following the removal of the stimulus, there is an abrupt partial reduction in response followed by the slower "afterdischarge." Previous studies (95,96) have shown that the "on" time constant to be smaller than the "off" time constant.

Following a period of ventilatory excitation, the STP response would be expected to exert a "braking" effect to the subsequent removal of the stimulus, thus counterbalancing any tendency toward hypopnea or apnea that might follow the loss of chemical drive. Thus, STP acts to improve the stability of respiratory control by providing additional damping to the system, in effect low-pass-filtering the neural output from the respiratory controller. As such, it has been suggested that the impairment of STP, either structural or functional, may be necessary for a given individual to develop PB with apnea (19). Some recent evidence suggests that this might be the case in CHF patients who have CSR. Ahmed et al. (97) measured the ventilatory responses to hyperoxia immediately following a brief exposure to hypoxia in awake CHF patients who exhibited CSR during sleep and age-matched normal patients. In the CHF-CSR group, posthypoxic-hyperoxic ventilation fell much more rapidly than in the normal patients, who showed the expected gradual decline characteristic of STP.

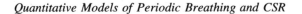

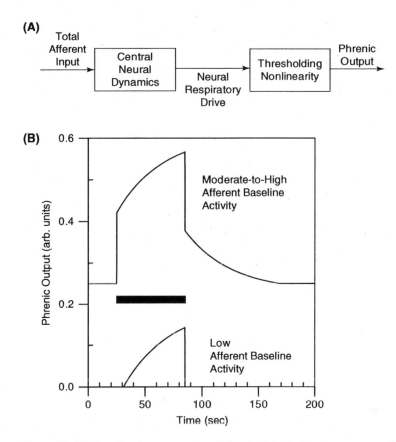

Figure 7 (**A**) Functional representation of the physiological processes responsible for short-term potentiation in ventilatory control; (**B**) Predicted response in phrenic discharge to a step increase in total afferent input (e.g., from carotid sinus stimulation), indicated by the *dark bar*, under conditions of moderate-to-high baseline drive (*upper tracing*) and low baseline drive (*lower tracing*).

Although the general consensus is that STP promotes ventilatory stability, inclusion of this factor into mathematical models of PB indicates only a modest stabilizing effect (18). Apart from the possible loss of this stabilizing mechanism through disease, several studies have demonstrated that STP appears to be highly sensitive to various factors that may be present under nonpathological conditions. STP has been shown to be attenuated by hypocapnia (95) and sustained hypoxia (98). Since CSR is generally associated with some hypoxia and repetitive phases of hypocapnia, it is conceivable that these conditions may interact to override the stabilizing mechanism after each period of hyperpnea, allowing the subsequent apnea to occur. Although it has been reasonably well established that the mechanism for STP remains intact during non–rapid eye movement sleep in normal patients (99), the study by Gleeson and Sweer (100) suggests that its damping effects on ventilatory changes are reduced in sleep relative to wakefulness. This, along with several other factors, may help to account for the greater prevalence of CSR during sleep. Studies in an anesthetized cat preparation demonstrated that, under baseline conditions of hypocapnia, the magnitude of the STP response to carotid sinus stimulation was substantially reduced (101). Below a certain level of P_{CO_2}, the direct effect of the STP response accompanying the start of stimulation disappeared, while the time constant of STP development became longer. Following cessation of the stimulus, however, the STP "off" response consisted only of the direct effect, with no afterdischarge component. This is illustrated in the lower tracing of Figure 7B. Eldridge and Gill-Kumar explained this observation by hypothesizing that activation of STP can exist at subthreshold levels of phrenic activity (101). This is certainly consistent with the processing scheme depicted in Figure 7A, in which a thresholding nonlinearity is placed downstream of the functional block representing central neural dynamics. The net effect of this kind of "subthreshold STP" on the ventilatory control system would be to dampen the effects of excitatory stimuli that increase ventilation but not have any "braking" effect on effects of inhibitory stimuli that act to promote apnea.

V. Conclusion

Quantitative models have played a major role in providing an improved understanding of the underlying mechanisms that give rise to CSR or PB. By using the unambiguous language of mathematics, models allow different researchers to use and test the same assumptions with minimal confusion. Since the equations employed in the model are based, at least in large part, on what is known about the physiological processes in question, they also serve the useful purpose of archiving past knowledge in compact form. The inherent self-consistency of the model derives from the operational rules of the mathematics employed, providing a logical accounting system for dealing with the multiple physiological variables and parameters, as well as their interactions with one another. Mathematical models have been particularly useful in demonstrating that most instances of CSR can be "explained" as a manifestation of disordered control, which may stem from the convergence of multiple factors, each of which influences the dynamics of the ventilatory control system. The early models of CSR were relatively simple closed-loop systems, but the incorporation of new empirical findings and the availability of improved computational tools have spurred the development of much more realistic and sophisticated models in recent years. Nevertheless, many questions remain to be resolved. An example is the effect of hypoxia-induced ventilatory depression on overall respiratory stability—a part of the effect on ventilation derives from the chemoresponsiveness of cerebral blood flow, which has been quantified (102). However, a less studied, and definitely much less quantified, part of this stems from the direct effects of hypoxia on the respiratory neurons. Another example is the interaction between the ventilatory responses of the central and peripheral chemoreceptors. In a recent model (43), Topor et al. showed that increased central chemosensitivity, in combination with a prolonged circulatory delay, can lead to CSR; in contrast, increased peripheral chemosensitivity alone could not produce CSR. As well, they found that their model was more easily destabilized by increasing central chemoreflex gain than by a combined increase in both central and peripheral gains. These findings require further investigation, since they appear to run counter to the predictions made by other PB models. Other unresolved issues in CSR modeling pertain to the interaction between the chemical control of ventilation and the respiratory pattern generator, as well as the interaction between the respiratory and cardiovascular control systems. As new empirical findings come to light, it is likely that our current models will become inadequate, and newer, more all-encompassing models would have to be developed to assimilate and "explain" the expanded array of observations.

Acknowledgment

The author's original work described herein and the preparation of this chapter were supported by NIH grants EB-001978, HL-090451, HL-02536, and HL-90451 and the American Lung Association.

References

1. Cheyne J. A case of apoplexy in which the fleshy part of the heart was converted into fat. Dublin Hosp Rep II 1818; 2:216–223.
2. Traube L. Zur theorie des Cheyne-Stokes 'schen atsmungsphanomen. Berl Klin Wochenschr 1874; 11:185–209.
3. Dowell AR, Buckley CE III, Cohen R, et al. Cheyne-Stokes respiration: a review of clinical manifestations and critique of physiological mechanisms. Arch Intern Med 1971: 127:712–726.
4. Guyton AC, Crowell JW, Moore JW. Basic oscillating mechanism of Cheyne-Stokes breathing. Am J Physiol 1956; 187:395–398.
5. Pryor WW. Cheyne-Stokes respiration in patients with cardiac enlargement and prolonged circulation time. Circulation 1951; 4:233–238.
6. Brown HW, Plum F. The neurological basis of Cheyne-Stokes respiration. Am J Med 1961; 30:849–861.
7. Mosso A. Life of Man on the High Alps. London: T Fisher Unwin, 1898.
8. Lahiri S, Maret K, Sherpa MG. Dependence of high altitude sleep apnea on ventilatory sensitivity to hypoxia. Respir Physiol 1983; 52:281–301.
9. Waggener TB, Brusil PJ, Kronauer RE, et al. Strength and cycle time of high-altitude ventilatory patterns in unacclimatized humans. J Appl Physiol 1984; 36:576–581.
10. West JB, Peters RM Jr., Aksnes G, et al. Nocturnal periodic breathing at altitudes of 6,300 and 8,050 m. J Appl Physiol 1986; 61:280–287.
11. White DP, Gleeson K, Pickett C, et al. Altitude acclimatization: influence on periodic breathing and chemoresponsiveness during sleep. J Appl Physiol 1987; 63:401–412.
12. Douglas CG, Haldane JS. The causes of periodic or Cheyne-Stokes breathing. J Physiol 1909; 38:401–419.
13. Bulow K. Respiration and wakefulness in man. Acta Physiol Scand 1963; 59(suppl 209): 1–110.
14. Webb P. Periodic breathing during sleep. J Appl Physiol 1974; 37:899–903.
15. Shannon DC, Carley DW, Kelly DH. Periodic breathing: quantitative analysis and clinical description. Pediatr Pulmonol 1988; 4:98–102.
16. Waggener TB. The relationship between abnormalities in respiratory control and apnea in infants. Respir Care 1986; 31:622–627.
17. Khoo MCK. Determinants of ventilatory instability and variability. Respir Physiol 2000; 122: 167–182.
18. Cherniack NS, Longobardo G. Mathematical models of periodic breathing and their usefulness in understanding cardiovascular and respiratory disorders. Exp Physiol 2006; 91: 295–305.
19. Younes M. The physiologic basis of central apnea and periodic breathing. Curr Pulmonol 1989; 10:265–326.

20. Bruce EN, Daubenspeck JA. Mechanisms and analysis of ventilatory stability. In: Dempsey JA, Pack AI, eds. Regulation of Breathing. 2nd ed. New York: Marcel Dekker, 1995:285–314.
21. Khoo MCK. Periodic breathing. In: Crystal RG, West JB, Barnes PJ, et al., eds. The Lung: Scientific Foundations. 2nd ed. NY: Raven Press, 1996:1851–1863.
22. Dempsey JA, Smith CA, Harms CA, et al. Sleep-induced breathing instability. Sleep 1996; 19:236–247.
23. Khoo MCK. Periodic breathing and central apnea. In: Altose M, Kawakami Y, eds. Control of Breathing in Health and Disease. New York: Marcel Dekker, 1998: 203–250.
24. Dempsey JA, Smith CA, Wilson CR, et al. Sleep-induced respiratory instabilities. In: Pack AI, ed. Pathogenesis, Diagnosis and Treatment of Sleep Apnea. New York: Marcel Dekker, 2002; 57–98.
25. Geraldo Lorenzi-Filho, Pedro R Genta, Adelaide C. Figueiredo, et al. Cheyne-Stokes respiration in patients with congestive heart failure: causes and consequences. Clinics 2005; 60 (4):333–344.
26. Bradley TD, Floras JS. Sleep apnea and heart failure. Part II: Central sleep apnea. Circulation 2003; 107:1822–1826.
27. Khoo MCK, Kronauer RE, Strohl KP, et al. Factors inducing periodic breathing in humans: a general model. J Appl Physiol 1982; 53:644–659.
28. Carley DW, Shannon DC. A minimal mathematical model of human periodic breathing. J Appl Physiol 1988; 65:1400–1409.
29. Khoo MCK. Physiological Control Systems: Analysis, Simulation and Estimation. Wiley/ IEEE Press, 2000.
30. Glass L, Mackey MC. Pathological conditions resulting from instabilities in physiological control systems. Ann NY Acad Sci 1979; 316:214–235.
31. Francis DP, Willson K, Davies C, et al. Quantitative general theory for periodic breathing in chronic heart failure and its clinical implications. Circulation 2000; 102:2214–2221.
32. Batzel JJ, Tran HT. Stability of the human respiratory control system. II. Analysis of a three-dimensional delay state-space model. J Math Biol 2000; 41:80–102.
33. Khoo MCK, Anholm JD, Ko SW, et al. Dynamics of periodic breathing and arousal during sleep at extreme altitude. Respir Physiol 1996; 103:33–43.
34. Bellville JW, Whipp BJ, Kaufmann RD, et al. Central and peripheral chemoreflex loop gain in normal and carotid body-resected subjects. J Appl Physiol 1979; 46:843–853.
35. Robbins PA. The ventilatory response of the human respiratory system to sine waves of alveolar carbon dioxide and hypoxia. J Physiol 1984; 350:461–474.
36. Berkenbosch A, Ward DS, Olievier CN, et al. Dynamics of ventilatory response to step changes in P_{CO2} of blood perfusing the brain stem. J Appl Physiol 1989; 66:2168–2173.
37. Khoo MCK, Gottschalk A, Pack AI. Sleep-induced periodic breathing and apnea: a theoretical study. J Appl Physiol 1991; 70:2014–2024.
38. Cunningham DJC, Robbins PA, Wolff CB. Integration of respiratory responses to changes in alveolar partial pressures of CO_2 and O, and in arterial pH. In: Fishman AP, ed. Handbook of Physiology: The Respiratory System. Bethesda, MD: American Physiological Society, 1987:475–528.
39. Atherton DP. Nonlinear Control Engineering. New York: Van Nostrand-Reinhold, 1982.
40. Milhorn HT Jr., Guyton AC. An analog computer analysis of Cheyne-Stokes breathing. J Appl Physiol 1965; 20:328–333.
41. Longobardo GS, Cherniack NS, Fishman AP. Cheyne-Stokes breathing produced by a model of the human respiratory system. J Appl Physiol 1966; 21:1839–1846.
42. Longobardo GS, Evangelisti CJ, Cherniack NS. Effects of neural drives on breathing in the awake state in humans. Respir Physiol 2002; 129:317–333.
43. Topor ZL, Vasilakos C, Younes M, et al. Model-based analysis of sleep-disordered breathing in congestive heart failure. Respir Physiol Neurobiol 2007; 155:82–92.

44. Ivanova OV, Khoo MCK. Simulation of cardiorespiratory variability using PNEUMA. Proceedings of the 26th Annual International Conference of the IEEE EMBS, 2004: 3901–3904.
45. Carley DW, Shannon DC. Relative stability of human respiration during progressive hypoxia. J Appl Physiol 1988; 65:1389–1399.
46. Anholm JD, Powles ACP, Downey R, et al. Operation Everest II: arterial oxygen saturation and sleep at extreme simulated altitude. Am Rev Respir Dis 1992; 145:817–826.
47. Cherniack NS, Longobardo GS, Levine OR, et al. Periodic breathing in dogs. J Appl Physiol 1966; 21:1847–1854.
48. Cherniack NS, von Euler C, Homma I, et al. Experimentally induced Cheyne-Stokes breathing. Respir Physiol 1979; 37:185–200.
49. Lahiri S, Hsiao C, Zhang R, et al. Peripheral chemoreceptors in respiratory oscillations. J Appl Physiol 1985; 58:1901–1908.
50. Greene AJ. Clinical studies of respiration IV: some observations on Cheyne-Stokes respiration. Arch Intern Med 1933; 52:454–463.
51. Motta J, Guilleminault C. Effects of oxygen administration on sleep-induced apneas. In: Guilleminault C, Dement WC, eds. Sleep Apnea Syndromes. New York: Alan R Liss, 1978.
52. Anthony AJ, Cohn AE, Steele JM. Studies on Cheyne-Stokes respiration. J Clin Invest 1932; 11:1321–1341.
53. Dempsey JA, Skatrud JB. A sleep-induced apneic threshold and its consequences. Am Rev Respir Dis 1986; 133:1163–1170.
54. Xie A, Rutherford R, Rankin F, et al. Hypocapnia and increased ventilatory responsiveness in patients with idiopathic sleep apnea. Am J Respir Crit Care 1995; 152:1950–1955.
55. Chapman KR, Bruce EN, Gothe B, et al. Possible mechanisms of periodic breathing during sleep. J Appl Physiol 1988; 64:1000–1008.
56. Waggener TB, Stark AR, Cohlan BA, et al. Apnea duration is related to ventilatory oscillation characteristics in newborn infants. J Appl Physiol 1984; 57:536–544.
57. Rigatto H, Brady JP, de la Torre Verduzco R. Chemoreceptor reflexes in preterm infants: 1. The effect of gestational and postnatal age on the ventilatory response to inhalation of 100% and 15% oxygen. Pediatrics 1975; 55:604–613.
58. Wilkinson MH, Sia K, Skuza EM, et al. Impact of changes in inspired oxygen and carbon dioxide on respiratory instability in the lamb. J Appl Physiol 2005; 98:437–446.
59. Quaranta AJ, D'Alonzo GE, Krachman SL. Cheyne-Stokes respiration during sleep in congestive heart failure. Chest 1997; 111:467–473.
60. Findley LJ, Zwillich CW, Ancoli-Israel S, et al. Cheyne-Stokes breathing during sleep in patients with congestive heart failure. South Med J 1985; 78:11–15.
61. Hanly PJ, Zuberi-Khokhar NS. Increased mortality associated with Cheyne-Stokes respiration in patients with congestive heart failure. Am J Respir Crit Care Med 1996; 153:272–276.
62. Naughton MT, Benard D, Tam A, et al. Role of hyperventilation in the pathogenesis of central apneas in patients with congestive heart failure. Am Rev Respir Dis 1993; 148:330–338.
63. Wilcox I, McNamara SG, Dodd MJ, et al. Ventilatory control in patients with sleep apnoea and left ventricular dysfunction: comparison of obstructive and central sleep apnoea. Eur Respir J 1998; 11:7–13.
64. Solin P, Roebuck T, Johns DP, et al. Peripheral and central ventilatory responses in central sleep apnea with and without congestive heart failure. Am J Respir Crit Care Med 2000; 162:2194–2200.
65. Millar TW, Hanly PJ, Hunt B, et al. The entrainment of low frequency breathing periodicity. Chest 1990; 98:1143–1148.
66. Hall MJ, Xie A, Rutherford R, et al. Cycle length of periodic breathing in patients with and without heart failure. Am J Respir Crit Care Med 1996; 154: 376–381.

67. Tkacova R, Hall MJ, Liu PP, et al. Left ventricular volume in patients with heart failure and Cheyne-Stokes respiration during sleep. Am J Respir Crit Care Med 1997; 156:1549–1555.

68. Dempsey JA. Crossing the apnoeic threshold: causes and consequences. Exp Physiol 2004; 90(1):13–24.

69. Brusil PJ, Waggener TB, Kronauer RE, et al. Methods for identifying respiratory oscillations disclose altitude effects. J Appl Physiol 1980; 48:545–556.

70. Cherniack NS. Sleep apnea and its causes. J Clin Invest 1984; 73:1501–1506.

71. Fink BR. Influence of cerebral activity in wakefulness on regulation of breathing. J Appl Physiol 1961; 16:15–20.

72. Manisty CH, Wilson K, Wensel R, et al. Development of respiratory control instability in heart failure: a novel approach to dissect the pathophysiological mechanisms. J Physiol 2006; 577:387–401.

73. Gothe B, Altose MD, Goldman MD, et al. Effect of quiet sleep on resting and CO_2-stimulated breathing in humans. J Appl Physiol 1981; 50:724–730.

74. Skatrud J, Iber C, Ewart R, et al. Disordered breathing during sleep in hypothyroidism. Am Rev Respir Dis 1981; 124:325–329.

75. DeBacker WA, Heyrman RM, Wittesaele WM, et al. Ventilation and breathing patterns during hemodialysis-induced carbon dioxide unloading. Am Rev Respir Dis 1987; 136:406–410.

76. Douglas NJ. Control of breathing during sleep. Clin Sci 1984; 67:465–471.

77. Phillipson EA, Bowes G. Control of breathing during sleep. In: Handbook of Physiology: The Respiratory System II. Bethesda, MD: American Physiological Society, 1987:649–690.

78. Khoo MCK. Modeling the effect of sleep state on respiratory stability. In: Khoo MCK, ed. Modeling and Parameter Estimation in Respiratory Control. New York: Plenum Press, 1989:193–204.

79. Modarreszadeh M, Bruce EN, Hamilton H, et al. Ventilatory stability to CO_2 disturbances in wakefulness and quiet sleep. J Appl Physiol 1995; 79:1071–1081.

80. Khoo MCK, Yang F, Shin JW, et al. Estimation of dynamic chemorefiex gain in wakefulness and NREM sleep. J Appl Physiol 1995; 78:1052–1064.

81. Colrain IM, Trinder J, Fraser G. Ventilation during sleep onset. J Appl Physiol 1987; 50:2067–2074.

82. Preiss G, Iscoe S, Polosa C. Analysis of a periodic breathing pattern associated with Mayer waves. Am J Physiol 1975; 228:768–774.

83. Saunders KB, Stradling J. Chemoreceptor drives and short sleep-wake cycles during hypoxia: a simulation study. Ann Biomed Eng 1993; 21:465–474.

84. Hanly P, Zuberi-Khokhar N. Daytime sleepiness in patients with congestive heart failure and Cheyne-Stokes respiration. Chest 1995; 107:952–958.

85. Hanly PJ, Millar TW, Steljes DG, et al. The effect of oxygen on respiration and sleep in congestive heart failure. Ann Intern Med 1989; 111:777–782.

86. Franklin KA, Eriksson P, Sahlin C, et al. Reversal of central sleep apnea with oxygen. Chest 1997; 111:163–169.

87. Xie A, Wong B, Phillipson EA, et al. Interaction of hyperventilation and arousal in the pathogenesis of idiopathic central sleep apnea. Am J Respir Crit Care Med 1994; 150:489–495.

88. Khoo MCK, Koh SSW, Shin JJW, et al. Ventilatory dynamics during transient arousal from NREM sleep: implications for respiratory control stability. J Appl Physiol 1996; 80:1475–1484.

89. Khoo MCK, Berry RB. Modeling the interaction between arousal and chemical drive in sleep-disordered breathing. Sleep 1996; 19:S167–S169.

90. Dempsey JA, Skatrud JB. Fundamental effects of sleep state on breathing. Curr Pulmonol 1988; 9:267–304.

91. Onal E, Lopata M. Periodic breathing and the pathogenesis of occlusive sleep apneas. Am Rev Respir Dis 1982; 126:676–680.

92. Alex CG, Onal E, Lopata M. Upper airway occlusion during sleep in patients with Cheyne-Stokes respiration. Am Rev Respir Dis 1986; 133:42–45.
93. Hudgel DW, Chapman KR, Faulks C, et al. Changes in inspiratory muscle electrical activity and upper airway resistance during periodic breathing induced by hypoxia during sleep. Am Rev Respir Dis 1987; 135:899–906.
94. Warner G, Skatrud JB, Dempsey JA. Effect of hypoxia-induced periodic breathing on upper airway obstruction during sleep. J Appl Physiol 1987; 62:2201–2211.
95. Eldridge FL. Maintenance of respiration by central neural feedback mechanisms. Fed Proc 1977; 36:2400–2404.
96. Tawadrous FD, Eldridge FL. Posthyperventilation breathing patterns after active hyperventilation in man. J Appl Physiol 1974; 37:353–356.
97. Ahmed M, Serrette C, Kryger MH, et al. Ventilatory instability in patients with congestive heart failure and nocturnal Cheyne-Stokes breathing. Sleep 1994; 17:527–534.
98. Holtby SG, Berezanski DJ, Anthonisen NR. The effect of 100% oxygen on hypoxic eucapnic ventilation. J Appl Physiol 1988; 65:1157–1162.
99. Badr MS, Skatrud JB, Dempsey JA. Determinants of poststimulus potentiation in humans during NREM sleep. J Appl Physiol 1992; 73:1958–1971.
100. Gleeson K, Sweer LW. Ventilatory pattern after hypoxic stimulation during wakefulness and NREM sleep. J Appl Physiol 1993; 75:397–404.
101. Eldridge FL, Gill-Kumar P. Central neural respiratory drive and after discharge. Respir Physiol 1980; 40:49–63.
102. Poulin MJ, Liang PJ, Robbins PA. Dynamics of the cerebral blood flow response to step changes in end-tidal P_{CO2} and P_{O2} in humans. J Appl Physiol 1996; 81:1084–1095.

17
Pathophysiological Interactions Between Sleep Apnea and Heart Failure

DAI YUMINO
Toronto Rehabilitation Institute, University of Toronto, Toronto, Ontario, Canada; Tokyo Women's Medical University, Tokyo, Japan

JOHN S. FLORAS
Mount Sinai Hospital and University Health Network, University of Toronto, Toronto, Ontario, Canada

T. DOUGLAS BRADLEY
Toronto Rehabilitation Institute, University Health Network and Mount Sinai Hospital, University of Toronto, Toronto, Ontario, Canada

I.   Introduction

In the United States, heart failure (HF), which affects approximately 5 million people, is the largest source of inpatient hospital costs for any single disease affecting patients over 65 years of age (1). As more patients survive acute myocardial infarction but are left with ventricular systolic dysfunction that may progress later in life (1), and as more elderly develop hypertension, its principal risk factor (2), the incidence and prevalence of HF, and as a consequence the number of deaths attributable to this condition have increased steadily. Despite better contemporary HF therapy, it has been estimated that the drug regimens introduced since 1985 have lengthened the life expectancy of the average HF patient by only 9 to 18 months (3), indicating an evident need and opportunity for new therapeutic strategies.

It is now appreciated that obstructive and central sleep apneas (OSA and CSA, respectively) are often present in patients with HF (4–7), in whom they reduce life expectancy independently of other known risk factors (8–12). Furthermore, their treatment by nasal continuous positive airway pressure (CPAP) can lead to improvements in objective measures of ventricular structure and function and in patients well-being (13–19).

Activation of the sympathetic nervous system is both a consequence and a fundamental marker of adverse prognosis in HF (20–23). During sleep, both obstructive and central apneas trigger repetitive bursts of sympathetic outflow (24), resulting in increased nocturnal urinary norepinephrine excretion (25). During wakefulness, such patients exhibit sustained increases in efferent muscle sympathetic nerve discharge and plasma norepinephrine concentrations relative to appropriate controls (24–26). These observations have advanced the hypothesis that these two conditions (HF and sleep apnea) summate to increase further central sympathetic outflow to the heart and peripheral vasculature. But augmented sympathetic nervous system activity (SNA) is only one of several consequences of sleep apnea with important adverse implications for ventricular systolic and diastolic function. Others are hemodynamic: increased left ventricular (LV) wall stress (27,28), attenuation of the normal fall in nocturnal blood pressure (BP) (24,29); chemical: intermittent hypoxia and oscillations in PCO_2 (30,31); inflammatory; and prothrombotic (32–36).

Findings such as these have stimulated intense investigation of three concepts: (*i*) sleep-related breathing disorders play an important role in the genesis, pathophysiology, and evolution of HF; (*ii*) their consideration within the differential diagnosis of conditions that could participate in such processes, their identification, and their quantification are important components of the evaluation of HF patients; and (*iii*) when sleep-related breathing disorders coexist with HF, specific treatment, such as CPAP or supplemental oxygen (13–19,37–39), should be considered and tested as adjunctive therapies. The rapidly growing body of evidence in support of these three concepts has been summarized in an American Heart Association and American College of Cardiology Foundation joint Scientific Statement on Sleep Apnea and Cardiovascular Disease (40) and two subsequent commentaries (41,42), and has been considered by writing committees developing clinical guidelines for HF investigation and management. The most recent American Heart Association statement on HF management (1) lists treatment of sleep apnea under "Drugs and Interventions Under Active Investigation" and states "It is hoped that such studies will provide information about the efficacy and safety of this approach (to treatment of sleep-related breathing disorders) and help identify patients most likely to benefit..."

At the outset it is important to recognize that the diagnosis and appropriate treatment of sleep-related breathing disorders in the setting of HF necessitates a novel and collaborative approach to the management of these patients, guided by specialized knowledge of sleep disorders medicine and access to specialized laboratory facilities and expertise in the use of respiratory devices. The diagnosis of OSA and CSA rests on the demonstration of recurrent apneas and hypopneas during polysomnography. When these sleep-related breathing disorders persist despite optimal medical therapy for HF, they may require treatment through nonpharmacological means, such as CPAP, that require particular expertise for their successful delivery (8,13–19).

In this chapter, we present evidence in support of the concept that coexistent sleep-related breathing disorders affect adversely the cardiovascular and autonomic nervous systems of patients with HF, and comment briefly on the impact of therapy targeted at sleep apnea on the HF state, a topic discussed in detail elsewhere in this volume (see chap. 19). Our specific goals are (*i*) to present the epidemiological evidence for a link between sleep-related breathing disorders and HF, (*ii*) to describe the pathophysiological consequences of OSA and CSA and their impact on the failing heart, and (*iii*) to identify gaps in knowledge in need of resolution regarding pathophysiological interactions between sleep apnea and HF. Unless stated otherwise, our discussion is specific to HF patients with impaired systolic function.

II. Epidemiology of Sleep-Related Breathing Disorders in Chronic Heart Failure

The epidemiology regarding sleep-related breathing disorders and its potential relationship to cardiovascular diseases in the general population is discussed elsewhere in this volume (see chap. 10). Consequently, herein, we confine our discussion to the epidemiology of sleep apnea, as it relates to HF. In this regard, an important observation from a cross-sectional analysis of the Sleep Heart Health Study was that the presence of OSA was associated with increased odds of having HF (43).

In otherwise healthy Americans, the prevalence of OSA, defined as an apnea-hypopnea index (AHI) exceeding 10 to 15, is approximately 7% to 10% (44), with a male:female ratio of approximately 2.5:1. However, CSA is rare with a prevalence of less than 1% (45,46). By contrast, two small prospective studies that employed full polysomnography, but studied only men, detected an AHI $\geq$15 in 49% of 100 patients (12% OSA and 37% CSA) (5) and in 53% of 55 patients (15% OSA and 38% CSA) (6). Recently, in a prospective epidemiological study involving 218 men and women with systolic HF treated with optimal medical therapy and evaluated by formal poly-somnography, Yumino et al. (7) found the prevalence of OSA and CSA (AHI $\geq$ 15) to be 47% (26% OSA and 21% CSA). As in the general population (44), the prevalence of OSA was approximately 2.5-fold higher in men than in women (30% vs. 12%). This was also the case for CSA (24% vs. 10%, respectively) (7). Multivariable analysis revealed that OSA was independently associated with older age, male sex, and greater BMI, whereas CSA was associated independently with older age, male sex, atrial fibrillation, lower awake PCO_2, and diuretic use. These prevalences and associations are similar to those identified earlier in our retrospective study of 450 HF patients (47). Although most OSA-related phenotypes are similar in subjects with and without HF, patients with HF have a lower BMI for a given AHI than the general population (48), indicating that factors other than obesity must be playing a relatively more important role in the pathogenesis of their upper airway obstruction. One factor that may be at play in patients with HF is daytime fluid retention, with its redistribution, when patients lie down at night, from edematous legs to peripharyngeal tissues rendering the pharynx more col-lapsible during sleep (49–52). A second mechanism that would facilitate CSA and exacerbate OSA, discussed in detail below, and elsewhere in this volume (see chap. 16), may be respiratory control system instability with increased loop gain resulting from low cardiac output, increased circulation time, and augmented peripheral and/or central chemosensitivity (53).

A noteworthy finding in an epidemiological study of patients with HF by Yumino et al. (7) was that over their seven-year enrollment period (1997–2004), the relative prevalence of OSA and CSA remained constant and similar to that observed in patients studied before the widespread introduction of β-blockers and spironolactone (47), despite the increased penetration of these drugs over this time period (7). These and contemporaneous data (54) suggest that the mortality benefits of these medications in clinical trials (55,56) cannot be attributed primarily to suppression of OSA or CSA.

III. Effects of Sleep on Cardiovascular Function in Healthy Subjects

Normally, metabolic rate, SNA, heart rate, stroke volume, cardiac output, and systemic BP all fall progressively from wakefulness through stages 1 to 4 of non–rapid eye movement (NREM) sleep (57–61), whereas vagal tone increases (59,62). The net effect of these changes is to reduce myocardial workload. Genes regulating carbohydrate utilization, fatty acid oxidation, and mitochondrial function exhibit circadian patterns of expression in anticipation of the normal diurnal variation in these several stimuli to myocardial oxygen demand (63). Although the deeper stages of NREM sleep are characterized by relative stability of the autonomic and circulatory systems, from time to time NREM sleep is punctuated by spontaneous K complexes and arousals from sleep followed by transient increases in muscle sympathetic nerve activity (MSNA), heart rate, and BP (61,64). These observations emphasize the important influence of subtle changes in sleep state on the autonomic and circulatory systems.

Sleep-related alterations in respiratory patterns parallel those of the autonomic and circulatory systems. As subjects proceed from stage 1 to stage 4 sleep, there are progressive reductions in central respiratory drive and minute ventilation and an increase in $PaCO_2$ (65). Respiratory rhythm and ventilatory output are also very stable in the deeper stages of NREM sleep. It is presumed that this is because ventilation is under purely chemical-metabolic control (65,66). Brief arousals into wakefulness are associated with transient increases in respiratory drive and ventilation (65,67) paralleled by increases in MSNA during NREM sleep (59,61). These observations should not be surprising. Hypercapnia and hypoxia stimulate both the respiratory chemoreceptors and the central sympathetic neurons, and the neural connections between the respiratory control and the central cardiovascular sympathetic centers in the nucleus tractus solitarius permit the modulation of central sympathetic outflow by respiratory drive and rhythm (68).

During rapid eye movement (REM) sleep, breathing becomes less dependent on metabolic drive and more so on non-metabolic and behavioral factors such as dream content (65,69). Patterns of breathing and SNA become irregular and begin to diverge: there is a further depression of respiratory drive with reductions in ventilation (65), but SNA and BP increase (59,61). The cause of this dissociation between central respiratory drive and central sympathetic outflow during REM sleep remains unclear. However, because adults spend approximately 80% to 85% of their total sleep time in NREM sleep, in general sleep relaxes the cardiovascular system. Disruption of this relative tranquility by recurrent apneas during sleep has adverse consequences for the heart and circulation.

IV. Pathophysiological Effects of OSA in HF

Upper airway occlusion during sleep is caused by a sleep-related withdrawal of upper airway inspiratory muscle tone superimposed on a narrow, highly compliant pharynx (70–72). As a result, the pharynx collapses during sleep, leading to obstructive apnea. The probability of obstructive apnea is increased if residual muscle tone is insufficient to counter peripharyngeal compressive forces, for example, increased neck circumference due to adipose tissue or edema. The latter may account for the higher relative prevalence of OSA in men and women with fluid retaining states, such as HF and renal failure (4,6,7,44), than in the general population.

Support for this concept comes from a recent study in which Redolfi and colleagues (52) quantified overnight changes in leg fluid volume, neck circumference, and the AHI in nonobese men referred for polysomnography because of suspicion of OSA. Remarkably, the AHI of these men was directly proportional to both the amount of fluid displaced and the increase in neck circumference overnight. In addition, the volume of fluid shifted was a function of time spent sitting over the course of the day. These novel data suggest that even otherwise healthy men accumulate fluid in their legs after sitting for prolonged periods. When they lie down, a proportion of this fluid moves rostrally into the neck and peripharyngeal tissues, increasing tissue pressure and augmenting any underlying predisposition to pharyngeal collapse (49–52).

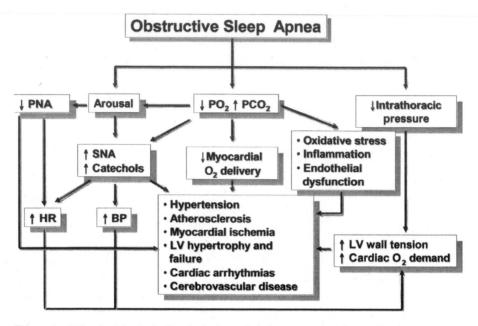

Figure 1 Pathophysiological effects of obstructive sleep apnea on the cardiovascular system. *Abbreviations*: PNA, parasympathetic nervous system activity; PO_2, partial pressure of oxygen; PCO_2, partial pressure of carbon dioxide; SNA, sympathetic nervous system activity; HR, heart rate; BP, blood pressure; LV, left ventricular. *Source*: From Ref. 41.

Upper airway occlusion triggers a cascade of mechanical, hemodynamic, autonomic, chemical, inflammatory, and metabolic consequences, plus chronic aftereffects, all capable of initiating or exacerbating cardiovascular disease (Fig. 1) (41). Four key pathophysiological features of OSA with adverse consequences for the cardiovascular system merit emphasis as a prelude to more detailed discussion in the context of HF: generation of exaggerated negative intrathoracic pressure (Pit) against the occluded airway, development of hypoxia during apnea, arousal from sleep at termination of apnea, and sympathoexcitation.

A. Negative Intrathoracic Pressure

The increase in LV afterload caused by the generation of negative Pit is a hemodynamic disturbance unique to OSA. During obstructive apnea, PaO_2 falls and $PaCO_2$ rises, causing an increase in respiratory drive. Exaggerated negative Pit is generated during each vigorous but futile inspiratory effort (Fig. 2). This struggle to breathe persists until an arousal terminates the apnea. This exaggerated negative Pit alters the loading conditions of the heart in several ways. First, the pressure gradient between intracavitary (LV) and extracavitary (i.e., intrathoracic or pericardial) pressure is augmented, thus increasing end-systolic LV transmural pressure (LVPtm) (27,28,73,74), a principal determinant of LV afterload. In some OSA patients with

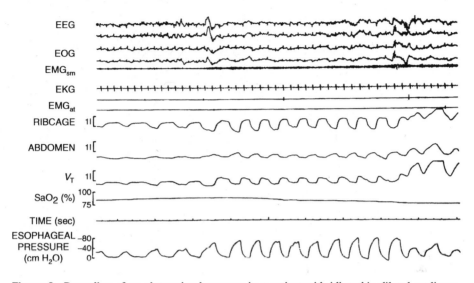

EEG

EOG

EMG$_{sm}$

EKG

EMG$_{at}$

RIBCAGE

ABDOMEN

V_T

SaO$_2$ (%)

TIME (sec)

ESOPHAGEAL
PRESSURE
(cm H$_2$O)

Figure 2 Recording of an obstructive hypopnea in a patient with idiopathic dilated cardiomy-opathy during stage 2 sleep. The three key features of obstructive sleep apnea are illustrated. First, paradoxical rib cage motion during hypopnea is accompanied by marked subatmospheric intra-thoracic pressure (i.e., esophageal pressure) swings during inspiratory efforts. This negative pressure is generated by the inspiratory muscles, which increases left ventricular afterload by increasing transmural pressure during systole (i.e., transmural pressure = systolic left ventricular pressure–esophageal pressure). Second, over the course of the hypopnea, a marked reduction in oxyhemoglobin saturation (SaO$_2$) occurs. Third, an arousal from sleep (EEG and EMG$_{sm}$ channels) terminates the hypopnea. *Abbreviations*: EEG, electroencephalogram; EKG, electrocardiogram; EMG$_{sm}$, submental electromyogram; EMG$_{at}$, anterior tibialis electromyogram; EOG, electro-oculogram; V_T, tidal volume. *Source*: From Ref. 18.

normal LV function, these increases in afterload, in conjunction with declining oxygen saturation, can trigger ischemic changes in the electrocardiogram (75). Second, the exaggerated negative intrathoracic pressure increases venous return to the right heart. This, combined with apnea-induced hypoxic pulmonary vasoconstriction, causes right ventricular (RV) distention that can shift the intraventricular septum leftward during diastole, thereby impeding LV filling (76–79). The higher LV afterload caused by this negative intrathoracic pressure can also reduce the rate of LV relaxation, thereby increasing the impedance to LV filling and increasing LV filling pressures (27,80). By one or more of these mechanisms, generation of exaggerated negative Pit during Mueller maneuvers or obstructive apneas can induce marked reductions in diastolic function, stroke volume, and cardiac output that are proportional to the degree of negative Pit (28,79–81). This combination could explain reports of OSA triggering nocturnal ischemia and acute pulmonary edema (82–85). The extent to which each of these factors contributes to reductions in cardiac output probably varies over the course of each apnea and may be further influenced by the underlying contractile state of the myocardium.

B. Hypoxia

Intermittent hypoxia during obstructive apneas can adversely affect cardiac performance through several mechanisms. Hypoxia causes pulmonary vasoconstriction and increases pulmonary artery pressures (81,86). The resultant increase in RV afterload may reduce right-sided cardiac output or cause RV distension and a leftward intraventricular septal shift during diastole (76–79,87). Several studies in animals have shown that intermittent hypoxia, as a model for the recurrent hypoxia of sleep apnea, causes acute and chronic histological and structural damage to the heart that can lead to remodeling (88–91). Hypoxia can also reduce cardiac output by depressing directly cardiac contractility (89–91) and by impairing the relaxation of both ventricles (92). It is also a potent stimulator of the sympathetic nervous system (88,93). Increasing $PaCO_2$ during apnea has an effect on MSNA additive to that of hypoxia (94).

Also, intermittent hypoxia can induce oxygen free radical production (32,33), activate inflammatory pathways that impair vascular endothelial function (34–36), and increase BP independently of activation of the sympathetic nervous system (95). Nonrandomized uncontrolled trials report that treatment of OSA with CPAP lowered C-reactive protein (34) and the nuclear factor-κB–dependent cytokines tumor necrosis factor α (TNF-α) and interleukin 6 (35,36). Individuals with OSA exhibit attenuated endothelium-dependent vasodilatation (96) and decreased circulating markers of nitric oxide. CPAP increases both (97). OSA can also promote lipoprotein oxidation, increase expression of adhesion molecules and monocyte adherence to endothelial cells, and provoke vascular smooth muscle proliferation (32,98–100). These adverse vascular effects, combined with increased sympathetic vasoconstrictor activity and inflammation, could contribute to the development or progression of hypertension and atherosclerosis (101,102).

C. Arousal

Obstructive apneas, whether spontaneously occurring or experimentally induced, are almost invariably terminated by a brief arousal in response to hypoxia, hypercapnia, and ineffectual inspiratory efforts (103–105). In this setting, arousal from sleep is a critical defense mechanism that stimulates the pharyngeal dilator muscles permitting restoration of upper airway patency and airflow (106). However, arousals from sleep, a form of alerting response, can also trigger increases in SNA and BP, and parasympathetic withdrawal with surges in heart rate (59,64). Also, by disrupting sleep, recurrent arousals can induce excessive daytime sleepiness and fatigue.

D. Sympathoexcitation

In obstructive apnea, the sympathetic nervous system is activated by at least five stimuli acting in concert: apnea, hypoxia, hypercapnia, reduced cardiac output, and arousal from sleep (20,59,94,107–109). During normal breathing, lung inflation stimulates pulmonary vagal afferents with inhibitory effects on tonic sympathetic outflow (20,107,110). During apnea, afferent nerve discharge ceases, removing this restraining influence on central sympathetic outflow. At the onset of a Mueller maneuver or an obstructive apnea, there is an initial increase in LV transmural pressure and inhibition of MSNA; the latter likely reflects the reflex response to stimulation of aortic arch and ventricular mechanoreceptors (108,111). However, the longer these disturbances are sustained, the greater the increase in MSNA. These could be due to chemical stimuli (108) or to reductions in cardiac output and BP, which unload the carotid baroreceptors (28,79,86,111). In two studies involving healthy humans, the magnitude of such sympathoexcitation was similar toward the end of breath-holds with and without superimposed negative Pit, indicating the predominance of chemoreceptor excitatory influence on sympathetic activity at this time point (108,111).

Shortly after resumption of breathing (rather than at the exact termination of apnea), MSNA peaks and BP surges to reach or exceed its baseline value (24,59,108,109,112). This slight but definite lag in the neural response to this stimulus may reflect the summation of circulatory delay between changes in arterial blood gas tension in the lung, their detection by peripheral and central chemoreceptors, central processing of afferent input and conduction velocity of the efferent reflex response, and the latency between cortical arousal and its maximum expression within efferent post-ganglionic muscle sympathetic nerve traffic. The neurally mediated surge in BP (29,113) will in turn inhibit MSNA reflexively by stimulating arterial and ventricular baroreceptors (23). Lung reinflation (24,110,114), and the resolution of hypoxia and hypercapnia will also cause MSNA to diminish.

These nocturnal events appear to have aftereffects that persist into wakefulness so that subjects with OSA but normal LV systolic function exhibit greater MSNA, plasma norepinephrine (NE) concentrations, and BP variability but less heart rate variability compared to subjects without OSA (24,109,115,116). In an observational study, daytime MSNA fell by 14% after six months of nightly use of CPAP (117). Several mechanisms may contribute to this sustained adrenergic activation. Acutely, exposure to brief episodes of intermittent hypoxia evokes long-lasting sympathetic activation and BP elevation that persist after termination of the hypoxic stimulus (118,119). Chronically, there may be central adaptation, with upward resetting of sympathetic outflow during wakefulness. In rats, altered dopamine and NE content of carotid bodies after intermittent hypoxia are accompanied by greater increases in sympathetic discharge and BP than induced by sustained hypoxia (120). In humans, chemoreceptor reflex deactivation by breathing 100% O_2 suppresses MSNA in OSA patients but not in healthy controls (121).

E. Implications for Patients at Risk for HF

Unless identified and treated, the exposure of the cardiovascular system to these repetitive insults over months or years could render individuals with OSA susceptible to nocturnal and daytime hypertension, myocardial ischemia, arrhythmias, impaired ventricular function, and ventricular septal hypertrophy (75,80–82,84,122–127). It is therefore not surprising that epidemiological studies report a significant association between OSA and HF (43) and OSA and premature cardiovascular mortality (128). Several pathological mechanisms might underpin these relationships.

Systemic hypertension during wakefulness, a key risk factor for HF, has been detected in approximately 50% to 60% of patients with OSA (37,79–81). Cross-sectional studies have shown increased odds of hypertension independent of obesity if OSA is present (129,130). In a prospective study the odds of developing hypertension over four to eight years was 2.89 (95% CI 1.46–5.64), independent of confounders, for an AHI >15 versus 0 events/hr (131). The degree to and the mechanism by which acute apnea–induced decreases in PaO_2 and elevations in $PaCO_2$ and sympathetic outflow might mediate long-term increases in BP in OSA remain to be determined.

Using a canine model, Brooks et al. (132) provided the first demonstration that several weeks of experimentally induced OSA could cause hypertension both during sleep apnea and wakefulness; BP returned to baseline levels a few weeks after removal of this noxious stimulus. Exposure during sleep to acoustic stimuli that provoked arousals and elevations in BP equal to those observed during OSA did not lead to sustained hypertension during wakefulness, indicating that additional stimuli, such as intermittent hypoxia during obstructive apneas, were necessary for its development. In rats, chronic intermittent exposure to hypoxia induced sustained arterial hypertension mediated by carotid chemoreflex stimulation of the sympathetic nervous system (102,133,134).

Studies in humans have yet to establish definitively the contribution of hypoxia to acute or chronic BP elevation. Acute administration of O_2 to patients with OSA does not prevent increases in BP at the termination of apnea (112). No relationship between the degree of nocturnal hypoxia and daytime systemic BP has been detected thus far in patients with OSA (135,136). However, the severity of hypoxia does relate to the frequency of arrhythmias such as sinus bradycardia, second-degree heart block, and supraventricular and ventricular ectopy and tachycardia (60,122,137,138).

The mechanical, neurohumoral, inflammatory, endothelial, and free radical–generating effects of OSA may act singularly or in concert to alter acutely and chronically LV structure and function. The pro-atherosclerotic consequences of OSA have been discussed in detail in elsewhere in this volume (chap. 13). Repetitive abrupt increases in LVPtm, over time, could induce ventricular remodeling, dilatation, and systolic dysfunction in subjects at risk, whether due to a genetic predisposition, prior occult myocarditis, or recent infarction (139). OSA can also cause LV diastolic dysfunction (140) that is at least partially reversible through treatment with CPAP (141). At the cellular level, acute pressure overload, which occurs upon generation of negative Pit, can decrease sarcoplasmic reticulum calcium ATPase pump activity and increase phospholamban (142). This slows the removal of calcium from the cytosol, resulting in impaired ventricular relaxation. Over time, such impairment would be exacerbated by afterload-stimulated myocyte hypertrophy and alterations in the collagen matrix. In addition, OSA appears to stress selectively the interventricular septum (143) through the combination of increased RV afterload secondary to hypoxic pulmonary vasoconstriction and increased LV afterload secondary to negative Pit generation and elevations in systemic BP. In one recent study of patients with OSA but without HF, interventricular septal thickness related directly to the AHI. After six months of CPAP therapy there was significant regression of interventricular septal but not posterior wall thickness and improved LV systolic function (144).

F. Implications for Patients with HF

OSA may be particularly deleterious when it coexists with HF. Sympathoadrenal activation is a major risk factor for premature death in patients with HF (21,22), and the contractile function of the failing left ventricle is more sensitive than the normal ventricle to acute or chronic increases in afterload.

In patients with HF, generation of negative intrathoracic pressure during Mueller maneuvers, mimicking obstructive apneas, causes an increase in LV and intrathoracic aortic transmural pressures that increase aortic arch baroreceptor stimulation. This leads to an initial suppression of MSNA. However, as the Mueller maneuver progresses, the increased LVPtm leads to a drop in stroke volume and BP that then augments sympathetic activity via unloading of the carotid sinus baroreceptors. At termination of Mueller maneuvers, MSNA increases more than during breath-holds of the same length without negative intrathoracic pressure in patients with HF, but not in healthy subjects (145). Thus, patient with HF may be more prone to sympathetic overactivation in response to obstructive apneas than subjects with normal ventricular function. Indeed, it appears that there is a summation of SNA arising from the influence of HF and sleep apnea as illustrated in Figures 3 and 4; MSNA is higher during wakefulness in HF patients with OSA than in those without it (26).

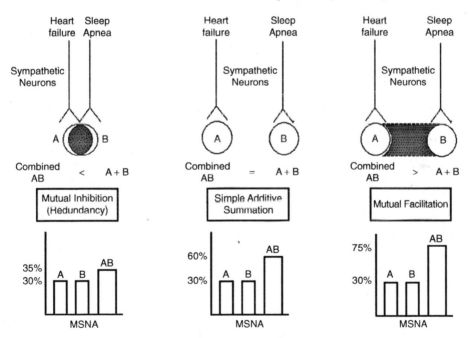

Figure 3 Possible interactions between heart failure and sleep apnea in activating the sympathetic nervous system. There may be mutual inhibition in which the total sympathetic nervous system activity is less than the sum of that due to HF and sleep apnea; an additive effect in which the total is equal to the sum of the HF and sleep apnea effects; or facilitation in which the total is greater than the sum of the HF and sleep apnea effects. *Abbreviation*: MSNA, muscle sympathetic nerve activity. *Source*: From Ref. 23.

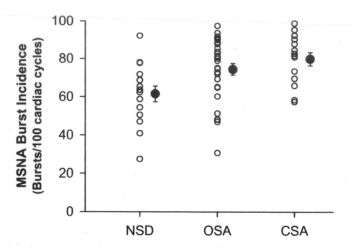

Figure 4 Scatter plots plus mean and SEM of muscle sympathetic nerve activity (MSNA) expressed as bursts per 100 heart beats from patients with heart failure (HF) measured during wakefulness. Compared with subjects with no sleep disordered breathing (NSD), MSNA was 11 bursts/100 cardiac cycles higher in those with coexisting obstructive sleep apnea (OSA) ($p = 0.032$) and 17 bursts/100 cardiac cycles higher in those with coexisting central sleep apnea (CSA) ($p = 0.006$). *Source*: Data from Ref. 26.

Because sympathetic activation during sleep arises as a result of apneas and arousals from sleep and not necessarily as a compensatory response to defend tissue perfusion, it may be particularly noxious to the diseased myocardium. Chronically elevated sympathetic nervous activity is linked to abnormal calcium cycling and calcium leakage in the failing myocardium, contributing to a decrease in myocardial contractility over time (146,147). In addition, increases in sympathetic nervous activity can enhance spontaneous inward currents through calcium channels, enhancing the likelihood of spontaneous repolarization, development of arrhythmias, and sudden death (148). Furthermore, chronic exposure of the myocardium to excess SNA and circulating catecholamines increases cardiac myocyte injury, apoptosis, and necrosis and contributes to hypertrophy and adverse remodeling (149).

The contractile function of the failing heart is highly sensitive to changes in afterload (150,151). Thus, it is of particular concern to note that the normal fall in BP during sleep is reversed in patients with HF and OSA (29). Some patients with treated HF may be normotensive during daytime clinic visits but hypertensive at night. In eight pharmacologically treated patients, studied during overnight polysomnography, average systolic BP increased from 120 mmHg during wakefulness to 132 mmHg during stage 2 sleep ($p < 0.05$) (Fig. 5 and Table 1) (29). The highest systolic BP was observed during the ventilatory period of stage 2 sleep. However, systolic arterial BP is not the only source of increased LV afterload in these patients. During paroxysms of apnea and hypopnea, patients abruptly generate levels of negative Pit reaching as much as -90 cmH$_2$O, (-65 mmHg) (Fig. 2). The effects of this increase in LVPtm on afterload are

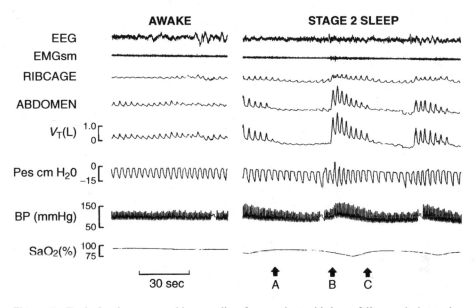

Figure 5 Typical polysomnographic recording from patient with heart failure and obstructive sleep apnea while awake and during stage 2 sleep: **A** to **B**, obstructive apnea; **B** to **C**, ventilatory period; and **A** to **C**, entire apnea-ventilatory cycle. Inspiratory esophageal pressure (Pes) swings during apnea indicate their obstructive nature. Blood pressure (BP) increases from wakefulness to stage 2 sleep and is higher during ventilatory period than during apnea. These increases in BP occurred even though the patient was normotensive while awake and on BP-lowering drugs. *Abbreviations*: EEG, electroencephalogram; EMG_{sm}, submental electromyogram; and V_T, tidal volume. *Source*: From Ref. 29.

functionally equivalent to those caused by sudden surges in systemic arterial BP of the same magnitude. It should therefore not be surprising that we (and others) have observed profound reductions in stroke volume and cardiac output from the onset of simulated obstructive apneas at more modest levels of negative Pit (74,152,153). These changes are greater in magnitude than those evoked by the same stimulus in matched control subjects with normal ventricular function (28,152). Moreover, these adverse effects on hemodynamics persist well into the recovery period after the termination of simulated obstructive apnea (28). These findings suggest that the contractile function of the myocardium is so impeded by this extra load that there may be a sustained impairment of contractility lasting beyond the stimulus exposure.

When one considers that the typical patient with OSA experiences between 10 and 60 obstructive events per hour of sleep, each lasting between 15 and 60 seconds, the implications of these repetitive and profound nocturnal changes in loading conditions become particularly significant for the patient with compromised ventricular function, regardless of etiology. But if flow-limiting coronary artery lesions are also present, these exaggerated negative Pit swings could precipitate myocardial ischemia even in the absence of hypoxia (77). Hypoxia can also directly impair myocardial contractility (91). These effects may be more pronounced in patients with associated coronary artery disease

Table 1 Effects of Obstructive Sleep Apnea on Cardiovascular and Respiratory Variables

Variable	Awake	Stage 2 sleep		
		Mean stage 2 sleep	Apnea	Ventilatory period
BP_{dias} (mmHg)	74.7 ± 4.1	79.3 ± 6.1	77.1 ± 5.6	80.6 ± 6.5[a]
BP_{sys} (mmHg)	120.4 ± 7.8	131.8 ± 10.6[b]	129.4 ± 10.6	133.9 ± 10.9[b,a]
Pes_{sys} (mmHg)	−4.2 ± 0.6	−5.4 ± 1.0	−4.6 ± 1.2	−6.1 ± 1.0[b,a]
$LVPtm_{sys}$ (mmHg)	124.4 ± 7.7	137.2 ± 10.8[b]	133.9 ± 10.0	140.2 ± 10.6[c,d]
HR (bpm)	83.3 ± 5.8	82.1 ± 5.8	80.1 ± 5.9[b]	83.9 ± 5.6[d]
Pes_{amp} (mmHg)	9.3 ± 1.4	12.2 ± 1.4	9.1 ± 1.3	15.2 ± 2.0[b,a]
RR (breaths/min)	19.9 ± 2.6	20.5 ± 1.7	19.1 ± 1.7	20.8 ± 1.8

These data demonstrate that in patients with heart failure, obstructive sleep apnea increases BP, negative Pes_{sys} swings, $LVPtm_{sys}$, HR, and inspiratory Pes_{amp} during stage 2 sleep compared with wakefulness.
[a]$p < 0.05$ versus apnea.
[b]$p < 0.05$ versus wakefulness.
[c]$p < 0.01$ versus wakefulness.
[d]$p < 0.01$ versus apnea.
Abbreviations: BP_{dias}, diastolic blood pressure; BP_{sys}, systolic blood pressure; HR, heart rate; $LVPtm_{sys}$, systolic LV transmural pressure; Pes_{amp}, amplitude of inspiratory esophageal pressure swings; Pes_{sys}, systolic esophageal pressure; RR, respiratory rate.
Source: From Ref. 29.

than in those without. Indeed, increased systolic LVPtm causes greater reductions in LV ejection fraction in patients with ischemic heart disease than in healthy subjects (152). Thus, the myocardial stresses induced by OSA could have more adverse effects on prognosis in patients with ischemic HF than in those with nonischemic HF (154).

Brady- and tachyarrhythmias are frequent causes of death in HF (155,156). The combination of increases in LV afterload, hypoxia, and increased SNA during OSA could all facilitate development of myocardial ischemia and arrhythmias during sleep, especially in patients with HF due to coronary artery disease (30,137,154,157). Indeed, Yumino et al. (154) recently reported that coexisting sleep apnea increased the risk of death, and in particular sudden death, in patients with ischemic HF but not in those with nonischemic HF.

In patients with preexisting ventricular dysfunction, abrupt and recurrent reductions in Pit, in conjunction with elevations in systemic arterial pressure and hypoxia, could trigger acute contractile impairment and nocturnal pulmonary edema, as has been reported in some patients with OSA (82,83,85,126). Over time, these repetitive increases in LV afterload may be sufficient to stimulate ventricular hypertrophy, blunt baroreflex sensitivity, or exacerbate preexisting HF (18,143,158–160). Apnea-associated hypertension and hypoxia-induced myocardial contractile impairment would further aggravate these processes (29). In our two-dimensional echocardiographic study of patients with HF due to nonischemic cardiomyopathy, subjects with coexisting OSA had a higher prevalence of LV hypertrophy (defined as LV thickness ≥12 mm) than those without OSA (48% vs. 15%, $p = 0.016$), even though both groups had similar body mass indices and daytime BP (143). This remodeling was greatest for the interventricular septum;

septal thickness was greater in those with OSA (10.9 vs. 9.3 mm, $p < 0.001$) and correlated with the AHI ($r = 0.59$, $p < 0.001$). In contrast, there was no difference in LV posterior wall thickness between the two groups. Of note, increased wall thickness for a given end-diastolic dimension places patients at increased risk of cardiovascular events (159). Although differences in right-heart function and morphology between HF patients with and without OSA were not assessed, the available data suggest that in patients with nonischemic cardiomyopathy the summation of the right- and left-sided stresses exerted by OSA provoke selective hypertrophy of the septum. These findings were replicated subsequently in a population of patients with OSA but without HF (144).

As HF advances, activation of the sympathoadrenal, renin-angiotensin-aldosterone, vasopressin, and endothelin systems could predispose to or exacerbate OSA by causing sodium and water retention and peripharyngeal edema (52). Another potential contributory factor that might also account for the higher prevalence of OSA in HF is respiratory control system instability consequent to low cardiac output, increased circulation time, and augmented peripheral and/or central chemosensitivity. This concept of increased loop gain (53), which predisposes the respiratory system to alternating episodes of hyperventilation (i.e., ventilatory overshoot) and apnea (i.e., ventilatory undershoot), is discussed in detail elsewhere in this volume (see chap. 16). However, it should be noted that if reduced central output to the respiratory muscles during the undershoot phase affects also the upper airway dilator muscles, the pharynx may narrow and collapse. In the non-HF population, high loop gain might explain a small proportion of the variability in AHI in a minority of those with OSA (53). However, cardiac output, LV filling pressure, and peripheral or central chemosensitivity to CO_2 do not differ between HF patients with OSA and those without sleep-related breathing disorders and there is as yet no firm evidence that such a mechanism plays a role in the pathogenesis of OSA in patients with HF. It is much more likely that these factors contribute to the pathogenesis of CSA as discussed below (161–166).

V. Central Sleep Apnea (Cheyne–Stokes Respiration) in HF

CSA in association with Cheyne–Stokes respiration (CSR) is a form of periodic breathing in which central apneas during sleep alternate regularly with hyperpneas to create a crescendo-decrescendo pattern of tidal volume (V_T) with a prolonged cycle length (161). The periodic breathing cycle length is directly related to the lung-peripheral chemoreceptor circulation time and inversely to cardiac output (162). Although CSA appears to arise secondary to HF, once initiated it may participate in a pathophysiological vicious cycle that contributes to deterioration in cardiovascular function, as illustrated in Figure 6. However, currently debated is whether CSA is simply a reflection of severely compromised cardiac function with elevated LV filling pressure (163), or whether CSA exerts unique and independent pathological effects on the failing myocardium. Many of the pathophysiological consequences of OSA are also manifested in CSA, increasing mortality risk of such patients (9,10). However, in contrast to OSA, HF acts as the initial stimulus to CSA, with respiratory control system instability required for its maintenance.

A. Respiratory Control System Instability

Ventilation during sleep is dependent mainly on the metabolic rather than the behavioral respiratory control system. The principal stimulus to ventilation during sleep is $PaCO_2$

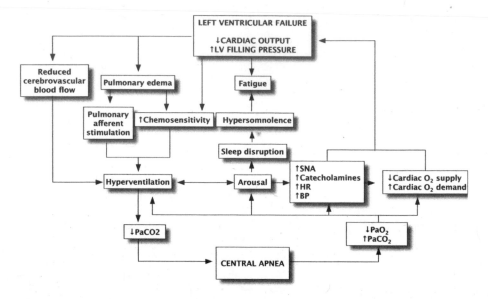

Figure 6 Pathophysiologic scheme of central sleep apnea (CSA) in heart failure (HF). Note that HF itself contributes to the development of CSA, which, in turn, has adverse effects on the myocardium including hypoxia and increased sympathetic nervous system activity (SNA). In addition, arousals disrupt sleep and may contribute to fatigue and sleepiness. *Abbreviations*: BP, blood pressure; HR, heart rate; LV, left ventricular. *Source*: From Ref. 161.

(164). A key factor predisposing to respiratory control system instability and CSA is chronic hyperventilation, setting eupneic $PaCO_2$ close to the apnea threshold. Compared with HF patients without CSA, those with CSA have increased peripheral and central chemoresponsiveness that promotes hyperventilation and hypocapnia (165,166) and exhibit lower $PaCO_2$ during wakefulness and sleep (167,168). Hyperventilation is triggered by lung congestion irritating pulmonary vagal afferent C fibers that stimulate central respiratory drive (163,169–171). Compared with HF patients without CSA, those with CSA have significantly higher pulmonary capillary wedge pressures and, presumably, more lung congestion (163). Indeed, in patients with HF, $PaCO_2$ is inversely proportional to pulmonary capillary wedge pressure (170), and lowering wedge pressure results in a rise in $PaCO_2$ and alleviation of CSA (163,170). During sleep, rostral fluid displacement (52) could increase the probability of hyperventilation by raising pulmonary venous pressure.

In NREM sleep, there is a reduction in central respiratory drive and loss of the nonchemical drive to breathe that maintain ventilation during wakefulness even when $PaCO_2$ falls below the apnea threshold. Ventilation decreases, and $PaCO_2$ and the apneic $PaCO_2$ threshold increase during the transition from wakefulness to NREM sleep. Consequently, CSR occurs more frequently during NREM sleep, when breathing becomes critically dependent on the metabolic control system, than during either wakefulness or REM sleep (164,168,172). As long as $PaCO_2$ remains greater than the apneic threshold, rhythmic breathing continues. However, in HF patients with CSA, $PaCO_2$ tends not to increase from wakefulness to sleep (4,173), but the apneic threshold does. The closer the prevailing $PaCO_2$ is to the apnea threshold the more likely it is that central apnea will occur in response to a given increase in ventilation. The critical role of hypocapnia in triggering central apneas is demonstrated by the observation that raising $PaCO_2$ by inhalation of a CO_2-enriched gas abolishes CSA immediately (Fig. 7) (31).

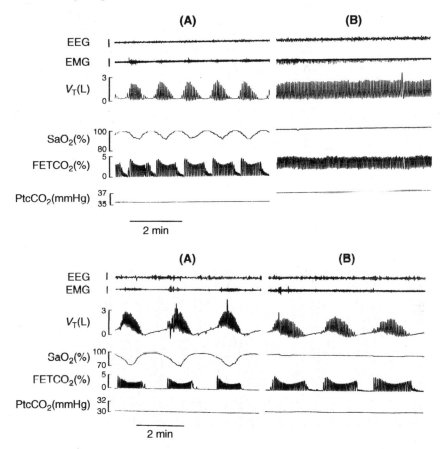

Figure 7 (Upper panel): Representative polysomnographic recordings from a patient during S2 sleep while breathing air (**A**) and CO_2 (**B**). Central apneas are abolished by CO_2 inhalation in association with an increase in the fraction of end-tidal CO_2 ($FETCO_2$) above the level during hyperpneas preceding apneas, and a 1.6-mmHg increase in transcutaneous PCO_2 ($PtcCO_2$). Abolition of Cheyne-Stokes respiration with central sleep apneas was also associated with elimination of dips in arterial oxygen saturation (SaO_2). (Lower panel) Recording from a different patient than shown in the upper panel during S2 sleep while breathing air (**A**) and O_2 (**B**). Although O_2 inhalation abolishes dips in Sa_{O2}, Cheyne–Stokes respiration with central sleep apneas persists. There were no significant effects of O_2 inhalation on either $FETCO_2$ or $PtcCO_2$. *Source*: From Ref. 31.

Abnormalities of cerebrovascular reactivity to CO_2 in patients with HF may also contribute to respiratory instability. Normal reflex changes in cerebrovascular blood flow provides an important counterregulatory mechanism that serves to minimize the change in hydrogen ion concentration [H^+] at the central chemoreceptor, thereby stabilizing the breathing pattern in the face of perturbations in $PaCO_2$. Compared with HF patients without CSA, those with CSA have impaired cerebral blood flow responses to CO_2 so that the fall in flow for a given decrease in arterial $PaCO_2$ is reduced. This permits a greater reduction in brain $PaCO_2$ and [H^+]. The chemoreceptors will then be exposed to a greater degree of alkalosis than normal, with a consequent greater tendency to develop ventilatory undershoot and hence central apnea (174).

Several additional factors such as metabolic alkalosis, low functional residual capacity, upper airway instability, and hypoxia may further contribute to respiratory instability and CSA. Metabolic alkalosis resulting from diuretic use in patients with HF could decrease the gap between the prevailing $PaCO_2$ and the apneic threshold (175). In sleeping dogs, metabolic alkalosis increases the apnea threshold to a greater degree than eupneic $PaCO_2$. As a result, dogs are more susceptible to periodic breathing during metabolic alkalosis (176). Indeed, we recently reported that use of diuretics, which can promote metabolic alkalosis, is an independent predictor of the presence of CSA in HF (7). Javaheri (177) also showed, in patients with HF, that CSA improved in response to induction of metabolic acidosis by the administration of acetazolamide even though this drug also reduced $PaCO_2$.

Patients with HF may have reduced functional residual capacity for several reasons including cardiomegaly, pleural effusion, and pulmonary edema. Large functional residual capacity acts as an O_2 and CO_2 reservoir that dampens oscillations in PaO_2 and $PaCO_2$, which occur during apneas (178,179), and therefore tends to stabilize respiration. However, Naughton et al. (168) reported that lung volume in stable ambulatory HF patients with CSR-CSA does not differ from that in patients without it. Thus, the role of reduced lung volume in the pathogenesis of CSA remains unclear.

Upper airway instability may also play a role in the pathogenesis of CSA. Alex et al. (180) described upper airway occlusion at the onset and end of some central apneas in selected HF patients. If upper airway resistance increases as ventilation decreases during the decrescendo phase of the hyperpneic segment of CSA, ventilatory undershoot is more likely to occur. The occasional occluded breath noted at the onset of central apnea during CSA is compatible with this concept (180). In addition, Tkacova et al. (181) observed that in a subset of HF patients with approximately equal numbers of obstructive and central respiratory events during sleep, obstructive events predominated at the beginning of the night, while central events predominated toward the end of the night in association with an increase in circulation time and fall in PCO_2. These observations suggest that pharyngeal obstruction may predispose to central events in association with an overnight deterioration in cardiovascular function, possibly related to the adverse effects of negative intrathoracic pressure and intermittent hypoxia on cardiac function, and increased tendency to hyperventilate.

Prolongation of circulation time secondary to reduced cardiac output with delayed transmission of altered arterial blood gas tensions from the lung to the peripheral and central chemoreceptors could theoretically promote CSR by facilitating ventilatory overshoot and undershoot. Guyton et al. (182) induced CSR in sedated dogs by inserting a length of tubing between the aorta and carotid artery to prolong the transit time from the lungs to the chemoreceptors. However, CSR was induced only when the lung-to-carotid body circulation time exceeded one minute, a delay far greater than described in patients with HF. In addition, several studies have shown that cardiac output, left ventricular ejection fraction (LVEF), and lung-to-chemoreceptor circulation time do not differ between HF patients with and without CSA (163,168). Consequently, prolonged circulation time appears not to play a key role in initiating CSA in most patients with HF. Rather, its major influence appears to be on the durations of the hyperpneic phase and of the total periodic breathing cycle (162).

Since the alterations in arterial blood gas tensions in the pulmonary circulation in response to changes in ventilation arrive via the systemic arterial circulation in a graded fashion, once $PaCO_2$ has risen above the apnea threshold, increases in tidal volumes and ventilation occur gradually, reaching a peak only several breaths after apnea termination. Similarly, as $PaCO_2$ falls in response to the gradual increase in the preceding ventilation, tidal volumes diminish gradually until apnea ensues once $PaCO_2$ has fallen below threshold. Thus, the prolonged transit time from the lungs to the peripheral chemoreceptors sculpts the classic crescendo-decrescendo pattern of tidal volumes during hyperpnea. However, apnea length appears not to be affected by prolonged circulation time but rather is proportional to the preceding decrease in $PaCO_2$ (162,183). Compared with patients with CSA but without HF, patients with HF and CSA have much longer hyperpnea with more gradual increases and decreases in tidal volume, but similar apnea duration (162,184). Thus, differences in the total cycle duration of periodic breathing between patients with and without HF are primarily modulated by differences in hyperpnea, but not apnea duration.

B. Arousals

Whereas in OSA arousals act as a defense mechanism to terminate apneas and activate pharyngeal muscles that allow resumption of airflow, in CSA, they appear to instigate central apneas by provoking ventilatory overshoot (185). There exists a strong correlation between the magnitude of arousal and both ventilation during hyperpnea and subsequent apnea duration (67,168,172). If there is an abnormally high sensitivity to $PaCO_2$, which is characteristic of HF patients with CSA, ventilatory overshoot occurs, which drives $PaCO_2$ down below the set point. If the patient then returns to NREM sleep, $PaCO_2$ lies below the higher apnea threshold, and central apnea occurs. Recurrent arousals during the ventilatory phase of CSA propagates CSA (113,168,172). However, if recurrent arousals do not occur during the ventilatory phase, ventilatory overshoot is dampened, respiration stabilizes, and CSA resolves. Whereas alleviation of OSA in HF by CPAP reduces the frequency of arousals (15), alleviation of CSA in HF by CPAP does not (185). These data reinforce the notion that arousals associated with CSA should be considered causal, rather than a consequence of this breathing disorder.

C. Negative Intrathoracic Pressure

In contrast to obstructive apneas, no inspiratory efforts are made during central apneas (Fig. 8). Consequently, any changes in LV afterload during the apneic phase would be mediated primarily by changes in systemic BP. In sedated animals, prolonged central apneas lower heart rate because of hypoxia but have no effect on stroke volume (186),

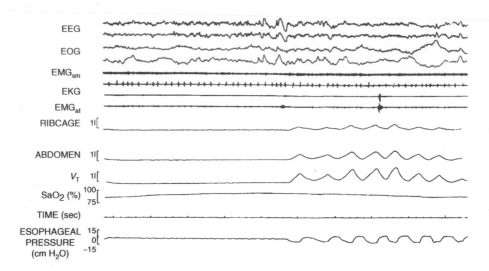

Figure 8 Central apnea during stage 2 sleep in a patient with heart failure (HF). It illustrates the absence of negative intrathoracic (i.e., esophageal) pressure swings during the apnea. *Abbreviations*: EEG, electroencephalogram; EKG, electrocardiogram; EMG$_{sm}$, submental electromyogram; EMG$_{at}$, anterior tibialis electromyogram; EOG, electrooculogram; SaO$_2$, oxyhemoglobin saturation; V_T, tidal volume.

whereas in conscious humans with HF, central apneas do not seem to cause significant alterations in heart rate, stroke volume, or cardiac output, probably because afterload is not increased and hypoxia is too mild to reduce heart rate or impair cardiac contractility (153).

By contrast, a substantial degree of negative Pit can be generated during hyperpnea. Thus, in some respects, the hyperpneic phase of these cycles replicates some of the adverse loading conditions of OSA. In addition, this inspiratory effort is probably one factor provoking arousal from sleep (103,187). It has been reported that paroxysmal nocturnal dyspnea in patients with HF can be related to the hyperpneic phase of CSA, probably through this mechanism (188).

D. Hypoxia

Hypoxia at high altitude initiates CSA by stimulating hyperventilation and lowering PaCO$_2$ below the apnea threshold (189). High-altitude periodic breathing can be abolished by administration of either supplemental O$_2$ or CO$_2$ (189). However, HF patients with CSA are generally not hypoxic so that hypoxia is unlikely to be a primary cause of CSR-CSA in most, but is more likely a consequence (113,167,168). Nevertheless, hypoxic dips during apneas could accentuate the tendency to hyperventilate upon termination of central apnea by amplifying the ventilatory overshoot in response to CO$_2$ when PaCO$_2$ increases above the ventilatory threshold (190). Ventilatory overshoot with propagation of CSA may therefore be facilitated by even mild apnea-related hypoxia.

Several studies investigated the effects of supplemental oxygen in patients with HF and CSR-CSA (37–39,191,192). These demonstrated inconsistent results; some showed a reduction in the AHI, while others did not (Fig. 7). These data support the hypothesis that hypoxia plays a role in aggravating CSA, but that it is not the major determinant of its development in most patients with HF.

E. Apnea and Hyperpnea

During central apnea, the absence of lung inflation deactivates pulmonary stretch receptors, and disinhibits central sympathetic nervous system outflow. This effect summates with apnea-related hypoxia and rises in $PaCO_2$ and with postapneic arousals to cause cyclical surges in SNA in synchrony with the ventilatory oscillations of CSA (193,194). These effects cause a generalized increase in SNA manifested as higher overnight urinary norepinephrine concentration in HF patients with CSA than in those without CSA (195). These data strongly suggest, first, that CSA can trigger sympathetic activation in certain patients with HF, and, second, that the increased SNA in these patients is not simply a compensatory response to low cardiac output but is directly related to the sleep apnea disorder. It may therefore represent excessive and pathological sympathoexcitation.

Oscillations in respiratory output that drive cyclic breathing also appear to entrain cardiovascular oscillations: during apneas heart rate and BP fall, while during hyperpneas they rise. These effects are complex and differ between normal rhythmic breathing and periodic breathing. For example, oscillations in heart rate and BP during normal breathing are entrained by respiration so that the spectral power of these oscillations is concentrated in the high-frequency range (0.15–0.5 Hz) at the respiratory frequency— the so-called respiratory sinus arrhythmia (113,196). The very low frequency (0.0049– 0.05 Hz) heart rate and BP oscillations normally observed during rhythmic breathing, however, are not related to respiration. The major effect of periodic breathing and CSA is to shift the majority of power in the heart rate variability and BP spectra from the high- and low-frequency (0.05–0.15 Hz) ranges into the very low frequency band at precisely the periodic breathing cycle frequency (113,196), even though respiratory sinus arrhythmia is still present. This shift of spectral power is a marker for poor prognosis in HF patients (197).

By applying spectral analysis and time-domain methods in subjects trained to perform simulated periodic breathing while awake, Lorenzi-Filho et al. (113) demonstrated that the periodic ventilatory pattern can amplify oscillations in BP and heart rate and entrain them at precisely the same very low frequency as the periodic breathing cycle (Fig. 9). This replicates the pattern of cardiovascular oscillations observed during CSA in HF patients (109,110). The implication of these data are that surges in BP and heart rate just after the termination of central and possibly obstructive apneas in patients with HF are related in part to increases in V_T and respiratory frequency (70). The concordance of heart rate and BP likely reflects synchronization of central respiratory and sympathetic neuronal output to the respiratory and cardiovascular systems, respectively. Importantly, such changes were observed in awake subjects with normal ventricular function in the absence of hypoxia and were not affected by inhalation of CO_2. They also occurred in the absence of arousals from sleep. HF patients with CSA would be anticipated to manifest even greater surges in BP, heart rate, and MSNA

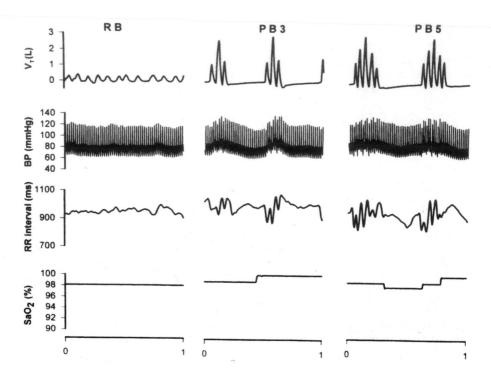

Figure 9 Recordings of tidal volume (V_T), blood pressure (BP), R-wave to R-wave interval from an electrocardiogram (RR interval), and oxyhemoglobin saturation (SaO_2) in one subject while awake during regular breathing (RB), voluntary periodic breathing with three-breath and five-breath hyperpneas (PB3 and PB5, respectively). Oscillations in BP and the RR interval were present during RB, but they became more prominent and regular, and were entrained at the periodic breathing cycle frequency during PB3 and PB5. SaO_2 did not decrease during PB3 or PB5 because overall, the subject hyperventilated. This figure also illustrates that oscillations in BP and RR interval can occur in the absence of hypoxia and arousals from sleep. *Source*: From Ref. 113.

during sleep in response to oscillations in ventilation, due to the additive effects of hypoxia, arousals from sleep, and ventricular dysfunction.

The magnitudes of these heart rate and BP fluctuations are proportional to the magnitude of fluctuations in ventilation (196,198). When CSR is spontaneously present during wakefulness in patients with HF, these cardiovascular oscillations continue in the absence of arousals from sleep, indicating that arousals are not the primary stimulus to augmentations of heart rate and BP during hyperpneas. During sleep, arousals have only a minor influence on these oscillations which is proportional to the augmentation in ventilation that accompanies them. Accordingly, it seems that as with respiratory sinus arrhythmia, such synchronous oscillations in ventilation, heart rate, and BP optimize ventilation/perfusion matching, so that an increase in heart rate during hyperpnea maintains perfusion of the lung at a time of maximum cardiac output and oxygen intake, while during apnea heart rate and perfusion decrease at a time when oxygen intake is reduced (196,199). Abolition of these very low frequency oscillations in heart rate and BP that accompany abolition of CSA indicates that these cardiovascular oscillations are caused by CSA (196).

Ventricular premature beats are also more frequent during periods of CSA than during periods of normal breathing. These are entrained to the ventilatory phase of CSA; ectopic beats occur more frequently during hyperpnea than apnea (200). Abolition of CSA by inhalation of a CO_2-enriched gas reduced the frequency of these ventricular ectopic beats. These observations suggest that in CSA, sympathetic activation during hyperpnea triggers ventricular ectopy (193). If so, this would contribute to the higher mortality of HF patients with CSA than in those without this breathing disorder (9,10).

Of equal interest is the observation that among patients with atrial fibrillation, in whom heart rate is generally chaotic and not influenced by normal breath-to-breath alterations in ventilation, the influence of CSA is so profound that it entrains heart rate oscillations at the very low frequency of periodic breathing even in the absence of breath-to-breath heart rate variability (201,202). In patients with atrial fibrillation, tachycardia during hyperpnea is associated with reduced atrioventricular nodal refractoriness and increased concealed conduction, whereas bradycardia during apnea is associated with increased atrioventricular nodal refractoriness and reduced concealed conduction. These observations indicate that fluctuations in respiratory drive and ventilation during CSA influence heart rate and BP variability through autonomic influences: increased sympathetic activation during hyperpnea likely reduces atrioventricular nodal refractoriness to increase the ventricular response to atrial fibrillation, whereas a relative increase in cardiac vagal activity during apnea likely increases the degree of concealed conduction and irregularity in heart rate.

F. Sympathoexcitation

The sympathetic stimulatory effects of CSA are not confined to sleep but also carry over into wakefulness. Daytime plasma norepinephrine concentrations are significantly higher in HF patients with CSA than in those without it, and are directly related to the frequency of arousals from sleep and to the degree of apnea-related hypoxia, but not to LVEF (195). MSNA is also significantly higher in HF patients with CSA than in HF patients without sleep apnea, and also unrelated to LVEF (26). Nevertheless, debate remains as to whether evidence for greater sympathetic activation in HF patients with CSA than without CSA reflects an independent consequence of this breathing disorder, or, is a manifestation of greater disease severity, as has been proposed by Mansfield et al. (203). However, the observations that treatment of CSA with either nocturnal oxygen or CPAP lowers SNA both during sleep and wakefulness (16,19,39,195) indicate that CSA contributes to sympathetic activation during wakefulness, as well as during sleep, with potential adverse consequences for myocardial performance and mortality (9,10) similar to those described earlier for patients with OSA and HF. Thus, CSA appears to participate in a vicious pathophysiological cycle involving the cardiovascular, respiratory, and autonomic nervous systems, as illustrated in Figure 6. It remains to be determined whether there is a direct cause-effect relationship between CSA and risk for morbidity and mortality in patients with HF.

VI. Treatment of Sleep Apnea in Patients with HF

Treatment of OSA and CSA in HF will be discussed only briefly, since this topic is the subject of another chapter in this volume (see chap. 19). Since most patients with HF who also have OSA or CSA do not complain of excessive daytime sleepiness (48), a primary objective of treating OSA and CSA is to improve cardiovascular function and clinical outcomes related to HF. However, there is still no consensus as to whether OSA and CSA should be treated in patients without symptoms of sleep apnea. In the case of CSA, the optimal therapeutic approach has yet to be established.

Conventional drug management of HF is unlikely to affect OSA and therefore would not be expected to attenuate or abolish its hemodynamic or sympathoneural consequences (7). Therefore, the maximum benefits to be derived from identifying OSA in HF patients would most likely accrue from its elimination by specific therapy. Indeed, the approach to OSA in the setting of HF should be similar to that for OSA in the absence of HF. The therapy of choice in most cases of OSA is CPAP. Short-term randomized controlled trials have demonstrated that treating OSA with CPAP in HF patients can improve LV systolic function; reduce SNA, BP, and frequency of ventricular ectopy; and improve vagal modulation of heart rate variability, baroreflex sensitivity and, in those with subjective daytime hypersomnolence, quality of life (13–15,19,160). The attenuation of MSNA during wakefulness is particularly interesting in that the treatment of OSA by CPAP reduced sympathetic firing rates to levels documented in HF patients without sleep apnea (19,26). This observation is consistent with the concept that sympathoexcitatory stimuli related to HF and OSA interact centrally through a process of additive summation (Fig. 3) (19). Furthermore, this reduction in sympathetic vasoconstrictor tone was accompanied by a parallel fall in systolic BP (19). In an observational study, Wang et al. also reported a trend, although not significant, for CPAP to reduce mortality in HF patients with OSA (8). However, no randomized trials have tested the effects of treating OSA on morbidity and mortality in HF patients.

A number of approaches to the therapy of CSA in patients with HF can be taken, depending on the weight one places on the pathophysiological significance of this breathing disorder. If one adopts the view that CSA itself is simply a reflection of the severity of cardiac failure, then pharmacological or device therapy of HF might alleviate this breathing disturbance. In a short-term study involving patients with mild CSA, atrial biventricular pacing reduced significantly the AHI; this change correlated with concurrent reductions in mitral regurgitation (204). This strategy has yet to be tested in longer-term randomized clinical trials. If, on the other hand, CSA is accompanied by symptoms of sleep disruption or sleep apnea such as restless sleep, insomnia, paroxysmal nocturnal dyspnea, or excessive daytime sleepiness, then specific treatment of CSA may be of additional and independent benefit. Finally, if one takes the approach that CSA plays a role in the progression of HF, then considerable attention should be directed toward the specific abolition of this condition. Nocturnal supplemental O_2 has been shown to attenuate CSA and cause modest short-term (1–4 weeks) reductions in nocturnal urinary norepinephrine concentrations and daytime exercise capacity (38,39). However, no direct benefits of O_2 therapy to the cardiovascular system have been demonstrated.

The most thoroughly tested treatment for CSA in the setting of HF—and the one so far shown to have the greatest clinical benefit is CPAP. The multicenter, long-term

Canadian Positive Airway Pressure (CANPAP) trial for central sleep apnea in heart failure demonstrated that CPAP improved nocturnal oxygenation, increased LVEF, lowered norepinephrine levels, and increased six-minute walking distance (16). However, despite excellent compliance with its use, CPAP proved to be relatively ineffective overall in suppressing CSA (the residual group mean AHI was 19 events/hr; i.e., greater than 15 events/hr, which was the trial entry criterion) and did not improve heart transplant–free survival (16). This finding raised the question as to how results of a clinical trial should be interpreted if the intervention applied does not demonstrate efficacy in the study population overall. Encouragingly, a post hoc secondary analysis based on efficacy revealed that if CSA was suppressed to below an AHI of 15 (CPAP-CSA-suppressed group), survival was improved significantly compared with the control group and the subgroup in whom CPAP did not suppress AHI <15 (CPAP-CSA-unsuppressed group) (205).

Of the 100 CPAP-treated patients in whom three-month polysomnographic data were available, CSA was suppressed in 57, from a mean of 34 events/hr to 6 events/hr, whereas mean AHI did not change over time in the 110 control patients (from 38 to 36 events/hr). At baseline, there was no significant difference in any clinical characteristic between CSA-suppressed and the control group. Compared with control subjects, increases in LVEF and heart transplantation–free survival were significantly greater ($p < 0.001$ and 0.043, respectively) in the CSA-suppressed group (205). Lack of suppression in patients randomly allocated CPAP was not due to nonadherence: the hours of CPAP use and the positive pressure applied were identical in patients with suppressed and unsuppressed CSA, yet the AHI on treatment in the latter group ($n = 43$) was 35 events/hr. These post hoc observations suggested that in HF patients, effective treatment of CSA might indeed improve heart transplant–free survival if CSA could be suppressed shortly after its initiation. Consequently, the question as to whether specific treatment of OSA and CSA will improve survival of patients with HF remains open. Large-scale randomized trials will be required to test this hypothesis.

VII. Conclusions and Future Directions

In the course of this chapter we have reviewed evidence that sleep apnea, whether primarily obstructive or central in nature, can have pathological effects in patients with HF that are known to worsen prognosis. Furthermore, sleep apnea may elicit symptoms of paroxysmal nocturnal dyspnea, restless sleep, daytime hypersomnolence, and fatigue. Another pathological consideration that warrants further investigation is the impact of sleep deprivation or disruption on the progression of HF. Patients with HF, whether or not they have coexisting sleep apnea, typically have fragmented sleep architecture as well as reduced sleep time; the total amount of sleep in such patients has been consistently reported to average only 4.5 hr/night, 70 minutes less than control subjects without HF (7,16,48). Indeed, these patients experience such frequent arousals and spend such little time in slow wave and REM sleep that the cardiovascular system may not enjoy the restorative effects of uninterrupted sleep.

These adverse cardiovascular effects of OSA and CSA are by and large not amenable to pharmacological therapy but may be specifically attenuated or eliminated by CPAP in the case of OSA or by CPAP, or possibly O_2 or other forms of positive airway pressure, such as adaptive servoventilation in the case of CSA (206,207). These findings highlight the need to consider OSA and CSA in the differential diagnosis of conditions that could contribute to the development and progression of LV dysfunction in patients with HF. Indeed, consideration of sleep apnea and polysomnography may become an important aspect of cardiac transplant evaluation. Recent epidemiological studies suggest that recognition of key clinical signs and a few laboratory tests may direct physicians toward considering the diagnosis and management of sleep-related breathing disorders in patients with HF. These studies also raise the question of whether sleep apnea is a primary cause of death during sleep in many patients with HF.

There are few well-controlled clinical trials of treatment of CSA and OSA in such patients, but those studies in which CPAP was used have reported favorable medium-term outcomes with respect to sleep apnea and sleep quality, LV function, SNA, respiratory muscle strength, and quality of life. These studies also demonstrate reductions in PNE and atrial natriuretic peptide concentrations, which are important markers of increased mortality in patients with HF. Such observations indicate the need for more research to fully elucidate mechanisms that contribute to the pathogenesis of OSA and CSA in HF. Once such mechanisms have been identified, better approaches to therapy of OSA and CSA may emerge for testing in large randomized trials with important morbidity and mortality endpoints. To be successful, such trials will require (*i*) greater involvement of respiratory physicians with expertise in sleep apnea in clinical and academic HF programs; (*ii*) efficient methods of identifying patients with moderate to severe apnea who might benefit from specific therapy; (*iii*) drug, pressure support, or electrophysiological device therapy to more effectively abolish CSA; and (*iv*) well-funded adequately powered tests of the hypothesis that effective treatment of sleep apnea, whether central or obstructive, will improve prognosis.

Acknowledgments

Some of the work described in this chapter was supported by operating grants MRC UI-14909 and MOP-82731 from the Canadian Institutes of Health Research, and by Grants in Aid T4050 and T4938 and Program Grant PRG 5276 from the Heart and Stroke Foundation of Ontario. D. Yumino was supported by an unrestricted research fellowship from Fuji-Respironics Inc., and J.S. Floras by a Canada Research Chair in Integrative Cardiovascular Biology and a Career Investigator Award from the Heart and Stroke Foundation of Ontario.

References

1. Hunt SA, Abraham WT, Chin MH, et al. ACC/AHA 2005 Guideline Update for the Diagnosis and Management of Chronic Heart Failure in the Adult: a report of the American College of Cardiology/American Heart Association Task Force on Practice Guidelines (Writing Committee to Update the 2001 Guidelines for the Evaluation and Management of Heart Failure): developed in collaboration with the American College of Chest Physicians and the International Society for Heart and Lung Transplantation: endorsed by the Heart Rhythm Society. Circulation 2005; 112:e154–e235.
2. Vasan RS, Beiser A, Seshadri S, et al. Residual lifetime risk for developing hypertension in middle-aged women and men: The Framingham Heart Study. JAMA 2002; 287:1003–1010.

3. Francis GS, Tang WH. Histamine, mast cells, and heart failure: is there a connection? J Am Coll Cardiol 2006; 48:1385–1386.
4. Ferrier K, Campbell A, Yee B, et al. Sleep-disordered breathing occurs frequently in stable outpatients with congestive heart failure. Chest 2005; 128:2116–2122.
5. Javaheri S. Sleep disorders in systolic heart failure: a prospective study of 100 male patients. The final report. Int J Cardiol 2006; 106:21–28.
6. Vazir A, Hastings PC, Dayer M, et al. A high prevalence of sleep disordered breathing in men with mild symptomatic chronic heart failure due to left ventricular systolic dysfunction. Eur J Heart Fail 2007; 9:243–250.
7. Yumino D, Wang H, Floras JS, et al. Prevalence and physiological predictors of sleep apnea in patients with heart failure and systolic dysfunction. J Card Fail 2009; 15:279–285.
8. Wang H, Parker JD, Newton GE, et al. Influence of obstructive sleep apnea on mortality in patients with heart failure. J Am Coll Cardiol 2007; 49:1625–1631.
9. Lanfranchi PA, Braghiroli A, Bosimini E, et al. Prognostic value of nocturnal Cheyne-Stokes respiration in chronic heart failure. Circulation 1999; 99:1435–1440.
10. Sin DD, Logan AG, Fitzgerald FS, et al. Effects of continuous positive airway pressure on cardiovascular outcomes in heart failure patients with and without Cheyne-Stokes respiration. Circulation 2000; 102:61–66.
11. Corra U, Pistono M, Mezzani A, et al. Sleep and exertional periodic breathing in chronic heart failure: prognostic importance and interdependence. Circulation 2006; 113:44–50.
12. Javaheri S, Shukla R, Zeigler H, et al. Central sleep apnea, right ventricular dysfunction, and low diastolic blood pressure are predictors of mortality in systolic heart failure. J Am Coll Cardiol 2007; 49:2028–2034.
13. Gilman MP, Floras JS, Usui K, et al. Continuous positive airway pressure increases heart rate variability in heart failure patients with obstructive sleep apnoea. Clin Sci (Lond) 2008; 114:243–249.
14. Ryan CM, Usui K, Floras JS, et al. Effect of continuous positive airway pressure on ventricular ectopy in heart failure patients with obstructive sleep apnoea. Thorax 2005; 60:781–785.
15. Kaneko Y, Floras JS, Usui K, et al. Cardiovascular effects of continuous positive airway pressure in patients with heart failure and obstructive sleep apnea. N Engl J Med 2003; 348:1233–1241.
16. Bradley TD, Logan AG, Kimoff RJ, et al. Continuous positive airway pressure for central sleep apnea and heart failure. N Engl J Med 2005; 353:2025–2033.
17. Mansfield DR, Gollogly NC, Kaye DM, et al. Controlled trial of continuous positive airway pressure in obstructive sleep apnea and heart failure. Am J Respir Crit Care Med 2004; 169:361–366.
18. Malone S, Liu PP, Holloway R, et al. Obstructive sleep apnoea in patients with dilated cardiomyopathy: effects of continuous positive airway pressure. Lancet 1991; 338:1480–1484.
19. Usui K, Bradley TD, Spaak J, et al. Inhibition of awake sympathetic nerve activity of heart failure patients with obstructive sleep apnea by nocturnal continuous positive airway pressure. J Am Coll Cardiol 2005; 45:2008–2011.
20. Floras JS. Clinical aspects of sympathetic activation and parasympathetic withdrawal in heart failure. J Am Coll Cardiol 1993; 22:72A–84A.
21. Kaye DM, Lambert GW, Lefkovits J, et al. Neurochemical evidence of cardiac sympathetic activation and increased central nervous system norepinephrine turnover in severe congestive heart failure. J Am Coll Cardiol 1994; 23:570–578.
22. Cohn JN, Levine TB, Olivari MT, et al. Plasma norepinephrine as a guide to prognosis in patients with chronic congestive heart failure. N Engl J Med 1984; 311:819–823.
23. Floras JS. Sympathetic nervous system activation in human heart failure: clinical implications of an updated model. J Am Coll Cardiol 2009; 54:375–385.

24. Somers VK, Dyken ME, Clary MP, et al. Sympathetic neural mechanisms in obstructive sleep apnea. J Clin Invest 1995; 96:1897–1904.

25. Naughton MT, Rahman MA, Hara K, et al. Effect of continuous positive airway pressure on intrathoracic and left ventricular transmural pressures in patients with congestive heart failure. Circulation 1995; 91:1725–1731.

26. Spaak J, Egri ZJ, Kubo T, et al. Muscle sympathetic nerve activity during wakefulness in heart failure patients with and without sleep apnea. Hypertension 2005; 46:1327–1332.

27. Virolainen J, Ventila M, Turto H, et al. Effect of negative intrathoracic pressure on left ventricular pressure dynamics and relaxation. J Appl Physiol 1995; 79:455–460.

28. Bradley TD, Hall MJ, Ando S, et al. Hemodynamic effects of simulated obstructive apneas in humans with and without heart failure. Chest 2001; 119:1827–1835.

29. Tkacova R, Rankin F, Fitzgerald FS, et al. Effects of continuous positive airway pressure on obstructive sleep apnea and left ventricular afterload in patients with heart failure. Circulation 1998; 98:2269–2275.

30. Shepard JW Jr., Garrison MW, Grither DA, et al. Relationship of ventricular ectopy to oxyhemoglobin desaturation in patients with obstructive sleep apnea. Chest 1985; 88:335–340.

31. Lorenzi-Filho G, Rankin F, Bies I, et al. Effects of inhaled carbon dioxide and oxygen on Cheyne-Stokes respiration in patients with heart failure. Am J Respir Crit Care Med 1999; 159:1490–1498.

32. Dyugovskaya L, Lavie P, Lavie L. Increased adhesion molecules expression and production of reactive oxygen species in leukocytes of sleep apnea patients. Am J Respir Crit Care Med 2002; 165:934–939.

33. Schulz R, Mahmoudi S, Hattar K, et al. Enhanced release of superoxide from polymorphonuclear neutrophils in obstructive sleep apnea. Impact of continuous positive airway pressure therapy. Am J Respir Crit Care Med 2000; 162:566–570.

34. Yokoe T, Minoguchi K, Matsuo H, et al. Elevated levels of C-reactive protein and interleukin-6 in patients with obstructive sleep apnea syndrome are decreased by nasal continuous positive airway pressure. Circulation 2003; 107:1129–1134.

35. Ryan S, Taylor CT, McNicholas WT. Selective activation of inflammatory pathways by intermittent hypoxia in obstructive sleep apnea syndrome. Circulation 2005; 112:2660–2667.

36. Ryan S, Taylor CT, McNicholas WT. Predictors of elevated nuclear factor-kappaB-dependent genes in obstructive sleep apnea syndrome. Am J Respir Crit Care Med 2006; 174:824–830.

37. Hanly PJ, Millar TW, Steljes DG, et al. The effect of oxygen on respiration and sleep in patients with congestive heart failure. Ann Intern Med 1989; 111:777–782.

38. Andreas S, Clemens C, Sandholzer H, et al. Improvement of exercise capacity with treatment of Cheyne-Stokes respiration in patients with congestive heart failure. J Am Coll Cardiol 1996; 27:1486–1490.

39. Staniforth AD, Kinnear WJ, Starling R, et al. Effect of oxygen on sleep quality, cognitive function and sympathetic activity in patients with chronic heart failure and Cheyne-Stokes respiration. Eur Heart J 1998; 19:922–928.

40. Somers VK, White DP, Amin R, et al. Sleep apnea and cardiovascular disease: an American Heart Association/american College Of Cardiology Foundation Scientific Statement from the American Heart Association Council for High Blood Pressure Research Professional Education Committee, Council on Clinical Cardiology, Stroke Council, and Council on Cardiovascular Nursing. In collaboration with the National Heart, Lung, and Blood Institute National Center on Sleep Disorders Research (National Institutes of Health). Circulation 2008; 118:1080–1111.

41. Bradley TD, Floras JS. Obstructive sleep apnoea and its cardiovascular consequences. Lancet 2009; 373:82–93.

42. Floras JS. Should sleep apnoea be a specific target of therapy in heart failure? Heart 2009; 95:1041–1046.

43. Shahar E, Whitney CW, Redline S, et al. Sleep-disordered breathing and cardiovascular disease: cross-sectional results of the Sleep Heart Health Study. Am J Respir Crit Care Med 2001; 163:19–25.

44. Young T, Palta M, Dempsey J, et al. The occurrence of sleep-disordered breathing among middle-aged adults. N Engl J Med 1993; 328:1230–1235.

45. Bixler EO, Vgontzas AN, Ten Have T, et al. Effects of age on sleep apnea in men. I. Prevalence and severity. Am J Respir Crit Care Med 1998; 157:144–148.

46. Bixler EO, Vgontzas AN, Lin HM, et al. Prevalence of sleep-disordered breathing in women: effects of gender. Am J Respir Crit Care Med 2001; 163:608–613.

47. Sin DD, Fitzgerald F, Parker JD, et al. Risk factors for central and obstructive sleep apnea in 450 men and women with congestive heart failure. Am J Respir Crit Care Med 1999; 160:1101–1106.

48. Arzt M, Young T, Finn L, et al. Sleepiness and sleep in patients with both systolic heart failure and obstructive sleep apnea. Arch Intern Med 2006; 166:1716–1722.

49. Chiu KL, Ryan CM, Shiota S, et al. Fluid shift by lower body positive pressure increases pharyngeal resistance in healthy subjects. Am J Respir Crit Care Med 2006; 174:1378–1383.

50. Shiota S, Ryan CM, Chiu KL, et al. Alterations in upper airway cross-sectional area in response to lower body positive pressure in healthy subjects. Thorax 2007; 62(10):868–872.

51. Su MC, Chiu KL, Ruttanaumpawan P, et al. Lower body positive pressure increases upper airway collapsibility in healthy subjects. Respir Physiol Neurobiol 2008; 161:306–312.

52. Redolfi S, Yumino D, Ruttanaumpawan P, et al. Relationship between overnight rostral fluid shift and obstructive sleep apnea in non-obese men. Am J Respir Crit Care Med 2009; 179:241–246.

53. Wellman A, Jordan AS, Malhotra A, et al. Ventilatory control and airway anatomy in obstructive sleep apnea. Am J Respir Crit Care Med 2004; 170:1225–1232.

54. MacDonald M, Fang J, Pittman SD, et al. The current prevalence of sleep disordered breathing in congestive heart failure patients treated with beta-blockers. J Clin Sleep Med 2008; 4:38–42.

55. Effect of metoprolol CR/XL in chronic heart failure: Metoprolol CR/XL Randomised Intervention Trial in Congestive Heart Failure (MERIT-HF). Lancet 1999; 353:2001–2007.

56. Pitt B, Zannad F, Remme WJ, et al. The effect of spironolactone on morbidity and mortality in patients with severe heart failure. Randomized Aldactone Evaluation Study investigators. N Engl J Med 1999; 341:709–717.

57. Khatri IM, Freis ED. Hemodynamic changes during sleep. J Appl Physiol 1967; 22:867–873.

58. White DP, Weil JV, Zwillich CW. Metabolic rate and breathing during sleep. J Appl Physiol 1985; 59:384–391.

59. Somers VK, Dyken ME, Mark AL, et al. Sympathetic-nerve activity during sleep in normal subjects. N Engl J Med 1993; 328:303–307.

60. Shepard JW Jr. Gas exchange and hemodynamics during sleep. Med Clin North Am 1985; 69:1243–1264.

61. Hornyak M, Cejnar M, Elam M, et al. Sympathetic muscle nerve activity during sleep in man. Brain 1991; 114(pt 3):1281–1295.

62. Furlan R, Guzzetti S, Crivellaro W, et al. Continuous 24-hour assessment of the neural regulation of systemic arterial pressure and RR variabilities in ambulant subjects. Circulation 1990; 81:537–547.

63. Young ME. The circadian clock within the heart: potential influence on myocardial gene expression, metabolism, and function. Am J Physiol Heart Circ Physiol 2006; 290:H1–H16.

64. Davies RJ, Belt PJ, Roberts SJ, et al. Arterial blood pressure responses to graded transient arousal from sleep in normal humans. J Appl Physiol 1993; 74:1123–1130.

65. Phillipson EA, Bowes G. Control of breathing during sleep. In: Cherniack NS, Widdicombe JG, eds. Handbook of Physiology. Vol 2: Control of Breathing. Bethesda, MD: American Physiology Society, William & Wilkins, 1986:649–849.

66. Orem J, Osorio I, Brooks E, et al. Activity of respiratory neurons during NREM sleep. J Neurophysiol 1985; 54:1144–1156.

67. Xie A, Wong B, Phillipson EA, et al. Interaction of hyperventilation and arousal in the pathogenesis of idiopathic central sleep apnea. Am J Respir Crit Care Med 1994; 150:489–495.

68. Guyenet PG, Koshiya N, Huangfu D, et al. Central respiratory control of A5 and A6 pontine noradrenergic neurons. Am J Physiol 1993; 264:R1035–R1044.

69. Orem J. Neuronal mechanisms of respiration in REM sleep. Sleep 1980; 3:251–267.

70. Remmers JE, deGroot WJ, Sauerland EK, et al. Pathogenesis of upper airway occlusion during sleep. J Appl Physiol 1978; 44:931–938.

71. Brown IG, Bradley TD, Phillipson EA, et al. Pharyngeal compliance in snoring subjects with and without obstructive sleep apnea. Am Rev Respir Dis 1985; 132:211–215.

72. Bradley TD, Brown IG, Grossman RF, et al. Pharyngeal size in snorers, nonsnorers, and patients with obstructive sleep apnea. N Engl J Med 1986; 315:1327–1331.

73. Magder SA, Lichtenstein S, Adelman AG. Effect of negative pleural pressure on left ventricular hemodynamics. Am J Cardiol 1983; 52:588–593.

74. Buda AJ, Pinsky MR, Ingels NB Jr., et al. Effect of intrathoracic pressure on left ventricular performance. N Engl J Med 1979; 301:453–459.

75. Hanly P, Sasson Z, Zuberi N, et al. ST-segment depression during sleep in obstructive sleep apnea. Am J Cardiol 1993; 71:1341–1345.

76. Robotham JL, Rabson J, Permutt S, et al. Left ventricular hemodynamics during respiration. J Appl Physiol 1979; 47:1295–1303.

77. Scharf SM, Graver LM, Balaban K. Cardiovascular effects of periodic occlusions of the upper airways in dogs. Am Rev Respir Dis 1992; 146:321–329.

78. Peters J, Fraser C, Stuart RS, et al. Negative intrathoracic pressure decreases independently left ventricular filling and emptying. Am J Physiol 1989; 257:H120–H131.

79. Tolle FA, Judy WV, Yu PL, et al. Reduced stroke volume related to pleural pressure in obstructive sleep apnea. J Appl Physiol 1983; 55:1718–1724.

80. Buda AJ, Schroeder JS, Guilleminault C. Abnormalities of pulmonary artery wedge pressures in sleep-induced apnea. Int J Cardiol 1981; 1:67–74.

81. Tilkian AG, Guilleminault C, Schroeder JS, et al. Hemodynamics in sleep-induced apnea. Studies during wakefulness and sleep. Ann Intern Med 1976; 85:714–719.

82. Chan HS, Chiu HF, Tse LK, et al. Obstructive sleep apnea presenting with nocturnal angina, heart failure, and near-miss sudden death. Chest 1991; 99:1023–1025.

83. Chaudhary BA, Nadimi M, Chaudhary TK, et al. Pulmonary edema due to obstructive sleep apnea. South Med J 1984; 77:499–501.

84. Franklin KA, Nilsson JB, Sahlin C, et al. Sleep apnoea and nocturnal angina. Lancet 1995; 345:1085–1087.

85. Chaudhary BA, Ferguson DS, Speir WA Jr. Pulmonary edema as a presenting feature of sleep apnea syndrome. Chest 1982; 82:122–124.

86. Schroeder JS, Motta J, Guilleminault C. Hemodynamic studies in sleep apnea. In: Guilleminault C, Dement WC, eds. Sleep Apnea Syndromes. Kroc Foundation Series. Vol II. New York: Liss, 1978:177.

87. Stoohs R, Guilleminault C. Cardiovascular changes associated with obstructive sleep apnea syndrome. J Appl Physiol 1992; 72:583–589.

88. Dematteis M, Julien C, Guillermet C, et al. Intermittent hypoxia induces early functional cardiovascular remodeling in mice. Am J Respir Crit Care Med 2008; 177:227–235.

89. Chen L, Einbinder E, Zhang Q, et al. Oxidative stress and left ventricular function with chronic intermittent hypoxia in rats. Am J Respir Crit Care Med 2005; 172:915–920.

90. Chen L, Zhang J, Gan TX, et al. Left ventricular dysfunction and associated cellular injury in rats exposed to chronic intermittent hypoxia. J Appl Physiol 2008; 104:218–223.
91. Kusuoka H, Weisfeldt ML, Zweier JL, et al. Mechanism of early contractile failure during hypoxia in intact ferret heart: evidence for modulation of maximal Ca^{2+}-activated force by inorganic phosphate. Circ Res 1986; 59:270–282.
92. Cargill RI, Kiely DG, Lipworth BJ. Adverse effects of hypoxaemia on diastolic filling in humans. Clin Sci (Lond) 1995; 89:165–169.
93. Gilmartin GS, Tamisier R, Curley M, et al. Ventilatory, hemodynamic, sympathetic nervous system, and vascular reactivity changes after recurrent nocturnal sustained hypoxia in humans. Am J Physiol Heart Circ Physiol 2008; 295:H778–H785.
94. Somers VK, Mark AL, Zavala DC, et al. Contrasting effects of hypoxia and hypercapnia on ventilation and sympathetic activity in humans. J Appl Physiol 1989; 67:2101–2106.
95. Vongpatanasin W, Thomas GD, Schwartz R, et al. C-reactive protein causes down-regulation of vascular angiotensin subtype 2 receptors and systolic hypertension in mice. Circulation 2007; 115:1020–1028.
96. Kato M, Roberts-Thomson P, Phillips BG, et al. Impairment of endothelium-dependent vasodilation of resistance vessels in patients with obstructive sleep apnea. Circulation 2000; 102:2607–2610.
97. Ip MS, Lam B, Chan LY, et al. Circulating nitric oxide is suppressed in obstructive sleep apnea and is reversed by nasal continuous positive airway pressure. Am J Respir Crit Care Med 2000; 162:2166–2171.
98. Bedwell S, Dean RT, Jessup W. The action of defined oxygen-centred free radicals on human low-density lipoprotein. Biochem J 1989; 262:707–712.
99. Faller DV. Endothelial cell responses to hypoxic stress. Clin Exp Pharmacol Physiol 1999; 26:74–84.
100. El-Solh AA, Mador MJ, Sikka P, et al. Adhesion molecules in patients with coronary artery disease and moderate-to-severe obstructive sleep apnea. Chest 2002; 121:1541–1547.
101. Carlson JT, Rangemark C, Hedner JA. Attenuated endothelium-dependent vascular relaxation in patients with sleep apnoea. J Hypertens 1996; 14:577–584.
102. Fletcher EC, Lesske J, Culman J, et al. Sympathetic denervation blocks blood pressure elevation in episodic hypoxia. Hypertension 1992; 20:612–619.
103. Gleeson K, Zwillich CW, White DP. The influence of increasing ventilatory effort on arousal from sleep. Am Rev Respir Dis 1990; 142:295–300.
104. Hlavac MC, Catcheside PG, McDonald R, et al. Hypoxia impairs the arousal response to external resistive loading and airway occlusion during sleep. Sleep 2006; 29:624–631.
105. Kimoff RJ, Makino H, Horner RL, et al. Canine model of obstructive sleep apnea: model description and preliminary application. J Appl Physiol 1994; 76:1810–1817.
106. Bradley TD, Phillipson EA. Pathogenesis and pathophysiology of the obstructive sleep apnea syndrome. Med Clin North Am 1985; 69:1169–1185.
107. Somers VK, Mark AL, Zavala DC, et al. Influence of ventilation and hypocapnia on sympathetic nerve responses to hypoxia in normal humans. J Appl Physiol 1989; 67:2095–2100.
108. Morgan BJ, Denahan T, Ebert TJ. Neurocirculatory consequences of negative intrathoracic pressure vs. asphyxia during voluntary apnea. J Appl Physiol 1993; 74:2969–2975.
109. Hedner J, Ejnell H, Sellgren J, et al. Is high and fluctuating muscle nerve sympathetic activity in the sleep apnoea syndrome of pathogenetic importance for the development of hypertension? J Hypertens Suppl 1988; 6:S529–S531.
110. Seals DR, Suwarno NO, Dempsey JA. Influence of lung volume on sympathetic nerve discharge in normal humans. Circ Res 1990; 67:130–141.
111. Somers VK, Dyken ME, Skinner JL. Autonomic and hemodynamic responses and interactions during the Mueller maneuver in humans. J Auton Nerv Syst 1993; 44:253–259.

112. Ringler J, Basner RC, Shannon R, et al. Hypoxemia alone does not explain blood pressure elevations after obstructive apneas. J Appl Physiol 1990; 69:2143–2148.
113. Lorenzi-Filho G, Dajani HR, Leung RS, et al. Entrainment of blood pressure and heart rate oscillations by periodic breathing. Am J Respir Crit Care Med 1999; 159:1147–1154.
114. O'Donnell CP, King ED, Schwartz AR, et al. Relationship between blood pressure and airway obstruction during sleep in the dog. J Appl Physiol 1994; 77:1819–1828.
115. Carlson JT, Hedner J, Elam M, et al. Augmented resting sympathetic activity in awake patients with obstructive sleep apnea. Chest 1993; 103:1763–1768.
116. Narkiewicz K, van de Borne PJ, Cooley RL, et al. Sympathetic activity in obese subjects with and without obstructive sleep apnea. Circulation 1998; 98:772–776.
117. Narkiewicz K, Kato M, Phillips BG, et al. Nocturnal continuous positive airway pressure decreases daytime sympathetic traffic in obstructive sleep apnea. Circulation 1999; 100: 2332–2335.
118. Xie A, Skatrud JB, Puleo DS, et al. Exposure to hypoxia produces long-lasting sympathetic activation in humans. J Appl Physiol 2001; 91:1555–1562.
119. Arabi Y, Morgan BJ, Goodman B, et al. Daytime blood pressure elevation after nocturnal hypoxia. J Appl Physiol 1999; 87:689–698.
120. Hui AS, Striet JB, Gudelsky G, et al. Regulation of catecholamines by sustained and intermittent hypoxia in neuroendocrine cells and sympathetic neurons. Hypertension 2003; 42:1130–1136.
121. Narkiewicz K, van de Borne PJ, Montano N, et al. Contribution of tonic chemoreflex activation to sympathetic activity and blood pressure in patients with obstructive sleep apnea. Circulation 1998; 97:943–945.
122. Serizawa N, Yumino D, Kajimoto K, et al. Impact of sleep-disordered breathing on life-threatening ventricular arrhythmia in heart failure patients with implantable cardioverter-defibrillator. Am J Cardiol 2008; 102:1064–1068.
123. Hung J, Whitford EG, Parsons RW, et al. Association of sleep apnoea with myocardial infarction in men. Lancet 1990; 336:261–264.
124. Galatius-Jensen S, Hansen J, Rasmussen V, et al. Nocturnal hypoxaemia after myocardial infarction: association with nocturnal myocardial ischaemia and arrhythmias. Br Heart J 1994; 72:23–30.
125. Garpestad E, Parker JA, Katayama H, et al. Decrease in ventricular stroke volume at apnea termination is independent of oxygen desaturation. J Appl Physiol 1994; 77:1602–1608.
126. Loui WS, Blackshear JL, Fredrickson PA, et al. Obstructive sleep apnea manifesting as suspected angina: report of three cases. Mayo Clin Proc 1994; 69:244–248.
127. Kuniyoshi FH, Garcia-Touchard A, Gami AS, et al. Day-night variation of acute myocardial infarction in obstructive sleep apnea. J Am Coll Cardiol 2008; 52:343–346.
128. Marin JM, Carrizo SJ, Vicente E, et al. Long-term cardiovascular outcomes in men with obstructive sleep apnoea-hypopnoea with or without treatment with continuous positive airway pressure: an observational study. Lancet 2005; 365:1046–1053.
129. Young T, Peppard P, Palta M, et al. Population-based study of sleep-disordered breathing as a risk factor for hypertension. Arch Intern Med 1997; 157:1746–1752.
130. Stamler J, Stamler R, Neaton JD. Blood pressure, systolic and diastolic, and cardiovascular risks. US population data. Arch Intern Med 1993; 153:598–615.
131. Peppard PE, Young T, Palta M, et al. Prospective study of the association between sleep-disordered breathing and hypertension. N Engl J Med 2000; 342:1378–1384.
132. Brooks D, Horner RL, Kozar LF, et al. Obstructive sleep apnea as a cause of systemic hypertension. Evidence from a canine model. J Clin Invest 1997; 99:106–109.
133. Fletcher EC, Lesske J, Qian W, et al. Repetitive, episodic hypoxia causes diurnal elevation of blood pressure in rats. Hypertension 1992; 19:555–561.

134. Fletcher EC, Lesske J, Behm R, et al. Carotid chemoreceptors, systemic blood pressure, and chronic episodic hypoxia mimicking sleep apnea. J Appl Physiol 1992; 72:1978–1984.

135. Carlson JT, Hedner JA, Ejnell H, et al. High prevalence of hypertension in sleep apnea patients independent of obesity. Am J Respir Crit Care Med 1994; 150:72–77.

136. Hoffstein V. Blood pressure, snoring, obesity, and nocturnal hypoxaemia. Lancet 1994; 344:643–645.

137. Miller WP. Cardiac arrhythmias and conduction disturbances in the sleep apnea syndrome. Prevalence and significance. Am J Med 1982; 73:317–321.

138. Mehra R, Benjamin EJ, Shahar E, et al. Association of nocturnal arrhythmias with sleep-disordered breathing: The Sleep Heart Health Study. Am J Respir Crit Care Med 2006; 173:910–916.

139. Nakashima H, Katayama T, Takagi C, et al. Obstructive sleep apnoea inhibits the recovery of left ventricular function in patients with acute myocardial infarction. Eur Heart J 2006; 27:2317–2322.

140. Kim SH, Cho GY, Shin C, et al. Impact of obstructive sleep apnea on left ventricular diastolic function. Am J Cardiol 2008; 101:1663–1668.

141. Arias MA, Garcia-Rio F, Alonso-Fernandez A, et al. Obstructive sleep apnea syndrome affects left ventricular diastolic function: effects of nasal continuous positive airway pressure in men. Circulation 2005; 112:375–383.

142. Arai M, Alpert NR, MacLennan DH, et al. Alterations in sarcoplasmic reticulum gene expression in human heart failure. A possible mechanism for alterations in systolic and diastolic properties of the failing myocardium. Circ Res 1993; 72:463–469.

143. Usui K, Parker JD, Newton GE, et al. Left ventricular structural adaptations to obstructive sleep apnea in dilated cardiomyopathy. Am J Respir Crit Care Med 2006; 173:1170–1175.

144. Shivalkar B, Van de Heyning C, Kerremans M, et al. Obstructive sleep apnea syndrome: more insights on structural and functional cardiac alterations, and the effects of treatment with continuous positive airway pressure. J Am Coll Cardiol 2006; 47:1433–1439.

145. Bradley TD, Tkacova R, Hall MJ, et al. Augmented sympathetic neural response to simulated obstructive apnoea in human heart failure. Clin Sci (Lond) 2003; 104:231–238.

146. Reiken S, Gaburjakova M, Gaburjakova J, et al. Beta-adrenergic receptor blockers restore cardiac calcium release channel (ryanodine receptor) structure and function in heart failure. Circulation 2001; 104:2843–2848.

147. Lehnart SE, Wehrens XH, Marks AR. Calstabin deficiency, ryanodine receptors, and sudden cardiac death. Biochem Biophys Res Commun 2004; 322:1267–1279.

148. Kaye DM, Lefkovits J, Jennings GL, et al. Adverse consequences of high sympathetic nervous activity in the failing human heart. J Am Coll Cardiol 1995; 26:1257–1263.

149. Daly PA, Sole MJ. Myocardial catecholamines and the pathophysiology of heart failure. Circulation 1990; 82:I35–I43.

150. Ross J Jr., Covell JW, Mahler F. Contractile responses of the left ventricle to acute and chronic stress. Eur J Cardiol 1974; 1:325–332.

151. Ross J Jr. Afterload mismatch and preload reserve: a conceptual framework for the analysis of ventricular function. Prog Cardiovasc Dis 1976; 18:255–264.

152. Scharf SM, Bianco JA, Tow DE, et al. The effects of large negative intrathoracic pressure on left ventricular function in patients with coronary artery disease. Circulation 1981; 63:871–875.

153. Hall MJ, Ando S, Floras JS, et al. Magnitude and time course of hemodynamic responses to Mueller maneuvers in patients with congestive heart failure. J Appl Physiol 1998; 85: 1476–1484.

154. Yumino D, Wang H, Floras JS, et al. Relationship between sleep apnea and mortality in patients with ischemic heart failure. Heart 2009; 95(10):819–824.

155. Francis GS. Development of arrhythmias in the patient with congestive heart failure: pathophysiology, prevalence and prognosis. Am J Cardiol 1986; 57:3B–7B.

156. Middlekauff HR, Stevenson WG, Stevenson LW, et al. Syncope in advanced heart failure: high risk of sudden death regardless of origin of syncope. J Am Coll Cardiol 1993; 21:110–116.
157. Shepard JW Jr. Hypertension, cardiac arrhythmias, myocardial infarction, and stroke in relation to obstructive sleep apnea. Clin Chest Med 1992; 13:437–458.
158. Hedner J, Ejnell H, Caidahl K. Left ventricular hypertrophy independent of hypertension in patients with obstructive sleep apnoea. J Hypertens 1990; 8:941–946.
159. Vasan RS, Larson MG, Levy D, et al. Distribution and categorization of echocardiographic measurements in relation to reference limits: the Framingham Heart Study: formulation of a height- and sex-specific classification and its prospective validation. Circulation 1997; 96:1863–1873.
160. Ruttanaumpawan P, Gilman MP, Usui K, et al. Sustained effect of continuous positive airway pressure on baroreflex sensitivity in congestive heart failure patients with obstructive sleep apnea. J Hypertens 2008; 26:1163–1168.
161. Yumino D, Bradley TD. Central sleep apnea and Cheyne-Stokes respiration. Proc Am Thorac Soc 2008; 5:226–236.
162. Hall MJ, Xie A, Rutherford R, et al. Cycle length of periodic breathing in patients with and without heart failure. Am J Respir Crit Care Med 1996; 154:376–381.
163. Solin P, Bergin P, Richardson M, et al. Influence of pulmonary capillary wedge pressure on central apnea in heart failure. Circulation 1999; 99:1574–1579.
164. Phillipson EA. Control of breathing during sleep. Am Rev Respir Dis 1978; 118:909–939.
165. Javaheri S. A mechanism of central sleep apnea in patients with heart failure. N Engl J Med 1999; 341:949–954.
166. Solin P, Roebuck T, Johns DP, et al. Peripheral and central ventilatory responses in central sleep apnea with and without congestive heart failure. Am J Respir Crit Care Med 2000; 162:2194–2200.
167. Hanly P, Zuberi N, Gray R. Pathogenesis of Cheyne-Stokes respiration in patients with congestive heart failure. Relationship to arterial PCO_2. Chest 1993; 104:1079–1084.
168. Naughton M, Benard D, Tam A, et al. Role of hyperventilation in the pathogenesis of central sleep apneas in patients with congestive heart failure. Am Rev Respir Dis 1993; 148:330–338.
169. Yu J, Zhang JF, Fletcher EC. Stimulation of breathing by activation of pulmonary peripheral afferents in rabbits. J Appl Physiol 1998; 85:1485–1492.
170. Lorenzi-Filho G, Azevedo ER, Parker JD, et al. Relationship of carbon dioxide tension in arterial blood to pulmonary wedge pressure in heart failure. Eur Respir J 2002; 19:37–40.
171. Paintal AS. Vagal sensory receptors and their reflex effects. Physiol Rev 1973; 53:159–227.
172. Bradley TD, Phillipson EA. Central sleep apnea. Clin Chest Med 1992; 13:493–505.
173. Xie A, Skatrud JB, Puleo DS, et al. Apnea-hypopnea threshold for CO_2 in patients with congestive heart failure. Am J Respir Crit Care Med 2002; 165:1245–1250.
174. Xie A, Skatrud JB, Khayat R, et al. Cerebrovascular response to carbon dioxide in patients with congestive heart failure. Am J Respir Crit Care Med 2005; 172:371–378.
175. Bradley TD. Crossing the threshold: implications for central sleep apnea. Am J Respir Crit Care Med 2002; 165:1203–1204.
176. Nakayama H, Smith CA, Rodman JR, et al. Effect of ventilatory drive on carbon dioxide sensitivity below eupnea during sleep. Am J Respir Crit Care Med 2002; 165:1251–1260.
177. Javaheri S. Acetazolamide improves central sleep apnea in heart failure: a double-blind, prospective study. Am J Respir Crit Care Med 2006; 173:234–237.
178. Cherniack NS, Longobardo GS. Cheyne-Stokes breathing. An instability in physiologic control. N Engl J Med 1973; 288:952–957.
179. Longobardo GS, Cherniack NS, Fishman AP. Cheyne-Stokes breathing produced by a model of the human respiratory system. J Appl Physiol 1966; 21:1839–1846.

180. Alex CG, Onal E, Lopata M. Upper airway occlusion during sleep in patients with Cheyne-Stokes respiration. Am Rev Respir Dis 1986; 133:42–45.
181. Tkacova R, Niroumand M, Lorenzi-Filho G, et al. Overnight shift from obstructive to central apneas in patients with heart failure: role of PCO2 and circulatory delay. Circulation 2001; 103:238–243.
182. Crowell JW, Guyton AC, Moore JW. Basic oscillating mechanism of Cheyne-Stokes breathing. Am J Physiol 1956; 187:395–398.
183. Datta AK, Shea SA, Horner RL, et al. The influence of induced hypocapnia and sleep on the endogenous respiratory rhythm in humans. J Physiol 1991; 440:17–33.
184. Nopmaneejumruslers C, Kaneko Y, Hajek V, et al. Cheyne-Stokes respiration in stroke: relationship to hypocapnia and occult cardiac dysfunction. Am J Respir Crit Care Med 2005; 171:1048–1052.
185. Ruttanaumpawan P, Logan AG, Floras JS, et al. Effect of continuous positive airway pressure on sleep structure in heart failure patients with central sleep apnea. Sleep 2009; 32:91–98.
186. Tarasiuk A, Scharf SM. Cardiovascular effects of periodic obstructive and central apneas in dogs. Am J Respir Crit Care Med 1994; 150:83–89.
187. Yasuma F, Kozar LF, Kimoff RJ, et al. Interaction of chemical and mechanical respiratory stimuli in the arousal response to hypoxia in sleeping dogs. Am Rev Respir Dis 1991; 143:1274–1277.
188. Harrison TR, King CE, Calhoun JA, et al. Congestive heart failure: Cheyne-Stokes respiration as the cause of dyspnea at the onset of sleep. Arch Int Med 1934; 53:891–910.
189. Berssenbrugge A, Dempsey J, Iber C, et al. Mechanisms of hypoxia-induced periodic breathing during sleep in humans. J Physiol 1983; 343:507–526.
190. Khoo MC, Kronauer RE, Strohl KP, et al. Factors inducing periodic breathing in humans: a general model. J Appl Physiol 1982; 53:644–659.
191. Franklin KA, Sandstrom E, Johansson G, et al. Hemodynamics, cerebral circulation, and oxygen saturation in Cheyne-Stokes respiration. J Appl Physiol 1997; 83:1184–1191.
192. Sasayama S, Izumi T, Seino Y, et al. Effects of nocturnal oxygen therapy on outcome measures in patients with chronic heart failure and cheyne-stokes respiration. Circ J 2006; 70:1–7.
193. Bradley TD, Floras JS. Sleep apnea and heart failure: part II: central sleep apnea. Circulation 2003; 107:1822–1826.
194. van de Borne P, Oren R, Abouassaly C, et al. Effect of Cheyne-Stokes respiration on muscle sympathetic nerve activity in severe congestive heart failure secondary to ischemic or idiopathic dilated cardiomyopathy. Am J Cardiol 1998; 81:432–436.
195. Naughton MT, Benard DC, Liu PP, et al. Effects of nasal CPAP on sympathetic activity in patients with heart failure and central sleep apnea. Am J Respir Crit Care Med 1995; 152:473–479.
196. Leung RS, Floras JS, Lorenzi-Filho G, et al. Influence of Cheyne-Stokes respiration on cardiovascular oscillations in heart failure. Am J Respir Crit Care Med 2003; 167:1534–1539.
197. Ponikowski P, Anker SD, Chua TP, et al. Oscillatory breathing patterns during wakefulness in patients with chronic heart failure: clinical implications and role of augmented peripheral chemosensitivity. Circulation 1999; 100:2418–2424.
198. Trinder J, Merson R, Rosenberg JI, et al. Pathophysiological interactions of ventilation, arousals, and blood pressure oscillations during cheyne-stokes respiration in patients with heart failure. Am J Respir Crit Care Med 2000; 162:808–813.
199. Hayano J, Yasuma F, Okada A, et al. Respiratory sinus arrhythmia. A phenomenon improving pulmonary gas exchange and circulatory efficiency. Circulation 1996; 94:842–847.
200. Leung RS, Diep TM, Bowman ME, et al. Provocation of ventricular ectopy by cheyne-stokes respiration in patients with heart failure. Sleep 2004; 27:1337–1343.

201. Leung RS, Huber MA, Rogge T, et al. Association between atrial fibrillation and central sleep apnea. Sleep 2005; 28:1543–1546.
202. Leung RS, Bowman ME, Diep TM, et al. Influence of Cheyne-Stokes respiration on ventricular response to atrial fibrillation in heart failure. J Appl Physiol 2005; 99:1689–1696.
203. Mansfield D, Kaye DM, Brunner La Rocca H, et al. Raised sympathetic nerve activity in heart failure and central sleep apnea is due to heart failure severity. Circulation 2003; 107:1396–1400.
204. Kara T, Novak M, Nykodym J, et al. Short-term effects of cardiac resynchronization therapy on sleep-disordered breathing in patients with systolic heart failure. Chest 2008; 134:87–93.
205. Arzt M, Floras JS, Logan AG, et al. Suppression of central sleep apnea by continuous positive airway pressure and transplant-free survival in heart failure: a post hoc analysis of the Canadian Continuous Positive Airway Pressure for Patients with Central Sleep Apnea and Heart Failure Trial (CANPAP). Circulation 2007; 115:3173–3180.
206. Pepperell JC, Maskell NA, Jones DR, et al. A randomized controlled trial of adaptive ventilation for Cheyne-Stokes breathing in heart failure. Am J Respir Crit Care Med 2003; 168:1109–1114.
207. Teschler H, Dohring J, Wang YM, et al. Adaptive pressure support servo-ventilation: a novel treatment for Cheyne-Stokes respiration in heart failure. Am J Respir Crit Care Med 2001; 164:614–619.

18
Prevalence and Prognostic Significance of Obstructive and Central Sleep Apnea in Heart Failure

PAOLA A. LANFRANCHI
University of Montreal, Montreal, Quebec, Canada

I. Introduction

Both obstructive sleep apnea (OSA) and central sleep apnea (CSA) are frequently encountered in congestive heart failure (HF) and have recently been gaining recognition as potential factors implicated in the development and progression of HF (1). As discussed extensively elsewhere in this book, OSA is a risk factor for cardiovascular morbidity and mortality among the general population (2–5). OSA would also appear to contribute to the development of HF (6,7). In the Sleep Heart Health Study, the presence of OSA was associated with more than twofold greater odds for HF independently of known cardiovascular risk factors (7). Hypoxia and hemodynamic changes, along with sleep loss and sleep fragmentation, are common features of this condition and are important triggers for a wide variety of autonomic, hemodynamic, inflammatory, and neuroendocrine responses (6,8), potentially contributing to both the development of HF and the further deterioration of a failing heart. However, CSA, with its typical periodic pattern of Cheyne–Stokes respiration (CSR), likely occurs secondarily to the condition of HF itself (9).

Almost one century ago CSA-CSR was already recognized in the medical text books as a typical feature of HF (10), especially occurring with sleep onset and associated with sleep disorders in patients in end-stage HF (11). What has become evident in the past decades is that this breathing disorder is highly prevalent, not only in patients in end-stage HF, but also in those with relatively preserved functional class (Table 1). CSA appears to be related to the severity of the hemodynamic compromise in HF (12–14). However, its presence may lead to several additional unfavorable consequences related to cyclic hypoxia, arousal from sleep with sleep fragmentation, and sympathetic activation, all factors potentially harmful to a failing heart (15).

In this chapter, we will focus on the clinical relevance of OSA and CSA, primarily examining the prevalence of these sleep-disordered breathing (SDB) in HF and the current evidence suggesting or refuting their impact on mortality.

II. Prevalence of CSA and OSA in HF and Left Ventricular Systolic Dysfunction

Table 1 summarizes the studies addressing SDB in congestive HF and left ventricular systolic dysfunction published in the past and current decades (13,14,16–24). In clinically stable patients with HF due to left ventricular systolic dysfunction the following

Table 1 Prevalence of OSA and CSA in Patients with Congestive Heart Failure

Author, year	Subjects n (% F)	Age	LVEF (%)	NYHA	β-Blockers (%)	Diagnostic criteria	no SDB n (%)	OSA n (%)	CSA n (%)
Lofaso, 1994 (16)	20 (15)	49	<25	–	–	AHI ≥ 10/hr	11 (55)	1 (5)	8 (40)
Javaheri, 1998 (13)	81 (0)	62	25	I–III	–	AHI ≥ 15/hr	40 (50)	9 (11)	32 (40)
Sin, 1999 (17)	450 (15)	57	27	II–IV	–	AHI ≥ 10/hr	134 (30)	168 (37)	148 (33)
Retrospective study									
Lanfranchi, 1999 (14)	66 (2)	57	23	II–III	–	AHI ≥ 10/hr	16 (24)	4 (6)	46 (70)
Tremel, 1999 (18)	34 (0)	62	30	II–III	–	AHI ≥ 15/hr	6 (18)	7 (20)	21 (62)
Ferrier, 2005 (19)	53 (23)	60	34	I–IV	31	AHI ≥ 10/hr	17 (32)	28 (53)	8 (15)
Oldenburg, 2007 (20)	700 (20)	64	28	II–IV	85	AHI ≥ 6/hr	169 (12)	253 (36)	278 (40)
Schultz, 2007 (21)	203 (25)	65	28	II–III	90	AHI ≥ 10/hr	58 (29)	88 (43)	57 (28)
Vazir, 2007 (22)	55 (0)	61	31	II	78	AHI ≥ 15/hr	26 (47)	8 (15)	21 (38)
Wang, 2007 (23)	218 (20)	55	26[a]	II–IV	81	AHI ≥ 15/hr	113 (52)	56 (26)	45 (21)
Macdonald, 2008 (24)	108 (15)	57	20	II–IV	82	AHI ≥ 15/hr	42 (39)	32 (30)	34 (31)

[a]Mean LVEF of OSA and subjects without sleep disordered breathing.

Abbreviations: LVEF, left ventricular ejection fraction; NYHA, New York Heart Association; SDB, sleep-disordered breathing; OSA, obstructive sleep apnea; CSA, central sleep apnea.

characteristics emerge. Firstly, the prevalence of SDB is extremely high, ranging from 45% to 85%, even in patients receiving maximal medical therapy. Secondly, the prevalence of CSA varies greatly from study to study (15–75%), with a higher prevalence among samples including exclusively or predominantly men (13,14,22) and lower prevalence among samples on β-blocker therapy and including a significant proportion of women (19,21,23). Thirdly, while initial studies suggested a similar prevalence of OSA in HF patients as in the general population (13,25), more recent studies in β-blocker-treated patients (20–24) and in selected HF patients with suspect sleep apnea (17) report a higher prevalence of OSA.

The first prospective evaluation of the prevalence and clinical correlates of CSA in stable HF patients was that of Javaheri et al. (13). In this study, involving 81 consecutive male outpatients who underwent full in-hospital polysomnography, 51% had significant SDB (defined as AHI $\geq$ 15/hr), predominantly CSA (40%), with fewer having OSA (11%). Patients with SDB (CSA and OSA), compared with those without SDB, had lower ejection fraction of the left ventricle (LVEF) (22% vs. 27%), and a higher prevalence of both atrial fibrillation (22% vs. 5%) and premature ventricular complexes. In a larger sample of 100 patients (including the first 81 patients noted above), Javaheri found that patients with CSA ($n = 37$) had a lower LVEF and more advanced New York Heart Association (NYHA) class compared to the other groups (26). No significant differences in LVEF, NYHA, and arrhythmias were found in OSA patients compared with patients without SDB. A higher body mass index was the only hallmark of patients with OSA.

A very high prevalence of CSA (70%) and a low prevalence of OSA (6%) were observed by Lanfranchi et al. (14) in a cohort of 66 lean predominantly male patients in sinus rhythm. In this study, aimed to assess the relationship between CSA and mortality, more severe AHI (>30/hr) was associated with echocardiographic indices of poorer systolic and diastolic function, poorer functional class, and more profound autonomic derangements.

In a large retrospective analysis of 450 consecutive HF patients (15% women) who were referred to the sleep laboratory for suspected sleep apnea, Sin et al. reported a much higher proportion of OSA (38%) (17). This study allowed identification of the risk factors for both CSA and OSA among HF patients with SDB. Left ventricular ejection fraction was linked to CSA as defined by AHI $\geq$10. Conversely, along with atrial fibrillation and daytime hypocapnia, male sex and age also emerged as additional independent risk factors for CSA. Male sex was associated with fourfold greater risk for CSA relative to female sex, and age $\geq$60 years was associated with a 2.4-fold risk for CSA relative to younger individuals. Higher BMI emerged as the sole risk factor for OSA in men with HF, whereas age was the sole risk factor for OSA in women with HF.

Six studies published between 2005 and 2008 have addressed the prevalence and characterization of SDB in HF in patients receiving maximal medical therapy according to current HF recommendations that include, in particular, the extensive use of β-blockers (19–24). Some of these studies also included patients possessing a biventricular pacemaker for cardiac resynchronization therapy (20,21), which has the potential to reduce CSA (27); however, the number of patients was either small (21) or not specified (20). All but one study (22) included females, although in a percentage slightly lower compared to the percentage of females participating to major clinical trials of HF with left ventricular systolic dysfunction (28). The overall SDB prevalence in these studies is remarkably high, ranging from 53% to 76% with the highest prevalence occurring in the largest study implicating 700 patients in NYHA class II to IV, and using a low diagnostic threshold of AHI (20). When looking at the relative proportion of CSA and OSA, CSA emerged as the predominant SDB in one study (22), OSA was the most prevalent SDB in two studies (19,21), and the two forms of breathing disorders were almost equally represented in the remaining three studies (20,23,24).

Several reasons could potentially account for the differences in prevalence of SDB among the studies, including the mentioned demographic characteristics, severity of HF, methodological factors (AHI cutoffs, full polysomnography vs. cardiorespiratory recordings, in-hospital vs. home-based studies) (29), and, most of all, the specific dynamic nature of OSA and CSA in the context of HF, i.e., the breathing pattern instability observed in some patients with HF and SDB whether or not on β-blockers. Tkacova et al. (30) first demonstrated that in some individuals with SDB, there is an overnight shift of the type of apnea from OSA to CSA during the same night, with OSA events predominating at the beginning of the night and CSA events at the end of the night. This overnight shift from OSA to CSA was associated with a lowering of Pco_2 and a progressive lengthening of the circulatory delay, stemming from a progressive deterioration of cardiac output and increasing filling pressures induced by OSA leading to CSA. In a subsequent retrospective analysis of 28 subjects with OSA and CSA who repeated a second sleep study on average seven months later, the same authors observed a shift of their dominant breathing pattern from obstructive to central or vice versa in a significant proportion (43%) of subjects (31). In these patients transcutaneous Pco_2 was lower (suggesting hyperventilation) and the periodic breathing cycle length was significantly longer (suggesting reduction of cardiac output) during the CSA phase compared to the OSA phase. This has led to the hypothesis that in some patients with HF due to left ventricular systolic dysfunction, OSA and CSA may represent a continuum of breathing alterations in which the deterioration of cardiac function leads to CSA and its improvement to a reversion to OSA (31). Finally, Vazir et al. (32) observed night-to-night breathing instability to occur in patients with less severe impairment of LVEF (34%) and mostly on β-blocker therapy (90%) over four-night sleep studies. Eight patients out of 19 (42%) shifted their type of SDB from one night to the other (3 subjects from CSA to OSA and 5 subjects from OSA to CSA). No significant daytime clinical or functional differences were present between patients with stable and unstable breathing patterns. It is possible that night-to-night breathing instability could also be a reflection of subtle hemodynamic changes and volume overload secondary to day-to-day variations in patient adherence to salt and liquid restriction, which is encountered commonly in chronic HF patients.

It is noteworthy that despite their overall beneficial effects on HF (33) and potential to reduce the incidence and severity of CSA in this condition, β-blockers have not been shown to significantly reduce the prevalence of CSA in HF. As in previous studies involving patients without β-blockers, patients with HF and CSA on β-blocker therapy are characterized by more severe left ventricular systolic dysfunction (19,20), impaired work capacity (24), more advanced NYHA class (20,24), and higher urinary norepinephrine excretion (24) compared to patients without SDB or OSA. It can be hypothesized that the lack of hemodynamic improvement with β-blockers in some HF patients might be responsible for the persistence of nocturnal CSA. Conversely, more severe CSA might theoretically overcome the benefit of β-blocker therapy. Unfortunately, the duration patients were treated with β-blockers was not specified in any of the above-mentioned studies. The hemodynamic benefit of β-blocker is time dependent and only becomes evident several months after the initiation of therapy (34). Preliminary data suggest that the benefit in reducing CSA is dose dependent in patients with HF (35). One cannot exclude that duration of treatment with β-blocker was too short in some patients, and suboptimal medication doses may also have been used. To date, no controlled studies examining the effect of the maximization of HF therapy on the evolution of CSA have been performed.

III. Prevalence of Sleep Disordered Breathing in Patients with Heart Failure and Preserved Systolic Function

Nearly 50% of subjects hospitalized for HF have preserved ejection fraction (36). In this population, impairment in left ventricular relaxation properties is believed to be the principal mechanism leading to HF symptoms (37). Data from several available registries indicate that subjects with diastolic HF are more likely to be older individuals, especially women, and suffer from hypertension, diabetes, and atrial fibrillation (38), all conditions known to be linked to OSA (3,18,39,40). Studies have shown that a dose-response relationship exists between OSA and impaired diastolic function, which appears to be related to both the degree of oxygen impairment and autonomic activation (41). An impairment of diastolic function has been observed in children with sleep apnea, independent of obesity and cardiac hypertrophy, and may be reversed following correction of the breathing disorder (42). Therefore, OSA would appear to play a primary or major contributing role in the ventricular filling abnormalities that lead to diastolic HF.

To date, only one study has examined the prevalence of SDB among patients with diastolic HF. In a small cohort of 20 individuals with HF and normal LVEF, Chan et al. detected OSA in seven subjects (35%) and CSA in four (20%) (43). Compared with patients without SDB, those with SDB (OSA and CSA pooled together) had similar blood pressure, body mass index, and Pco_2, but more profound diastolic impairment by echocardiography, suggesting a direct effect of OSA on ventricle mechanical properties independent of risk factors.

IV. Central Sleep Apnea and Mortality in Heart Failure

The independent link between CSA and mortality in patients with stable chronic HF remains a matter of debate, especially in the context of newer strategies for the treatment of advanced HF. Table 2 shows the studies addressing the prognostic value of CSA with both positive and negative results. The first report of an association between CSA and mortality, more than 20 years ago, was by Findley et al. who observed that 6/6 patients with HF and CSA died within six months versus 3/9 of the subjects without CSA (44). Hanly et al. (45) subsequently reported a three-year mortality of 56% in eight patients with HF and nocturnal CSA compared with 11% in eight patients without CSA, despite similar functional status and LVEF between the two groups. In a study examining the impact of SDB on long-term outcomes (17.5 years) in 353 elderly hospitalized men with and without HF, Ancoli-Israel et al. (46) observed greater mortality in patients who had

Table 2 Studies Examining the Relationship Between CSA and Prognosis

Author, year	Subjects n (% F)	Ischemic etiology (%)	LVEF (%)	β-Blockers (%)	CRS-CSA criteria	Primary endpoints	CRS-CSA is predictor
Findley, 1985 (44)	15 (0)	NA	31	–	AHI > 5/hr	Death	Yes
Hanly, 1996 (45)	16 (0)	100	23	–	Any	Death + Tx	Yes
Andreas, 1996 (50)	36 (14)	11	20	–	CSR/TST >20%	Death + Tx	No
Traversi, 1997 (51)	60 (3)	70	23	–	Any	Death + urgent Tx	No
Lanfranchi, 1999 (14)	62 (12)	53	23	–	AHI ≥ 30/hr	Cardiac death	Yes
Sin 2000 (47)	66 (12)	65	20	21	AHI ≥ 15/hr	Death + Tx	Yes
Roebuck, 2004 (52)	78 (22)	53	20	14	AHI > 5/hr	Death, Death + Tx	No
Corrà, 2006 (48)	133 (6)	64	23	53	AHI ≥ 30/hr	Cardiac death + urgent Tx	Yes
Javaheri, 2007 (49)	88 (0)	75	24	10	AHI ≥ 5/hr	Death	Yes

both HF and CSA relative to those with only HF at baseline (HR 1.66). Survival was more than 6.75 years in patients with CSA or OSA without HF, more than 4 years in HF patients, and only more than 2.5 years in patients with both HF and CSA.

Present evidence for an independent impact of CSA on mortality comes from four prospective studies. Lanfranchi et al. assessed the impact of CSA on cardiac mortality in 62 consecutive patients with and without CSA, most of whom had underlying ischemic heart disease (14). Over a mean follow-up of 28 months, 15 patients died of cardiac causes (24%). Univariate predictors of mortality included worse NYHA class, lower LVEF, indices of diastolic dysfunction, left atrial area, and several autonomic parameters. Multivariate regression analyses revealed severe AHI ($\geq$30/hr) to be the most powerful independent predictor of cardiac mortality. The cumulative one– and two–year cardiac mortalities were respectively 21.4% and 50% in patients with AHI $\geq$30/hr versus 5.4% and 26.2% in those with AHI < 30/hr (p < 0.01). Left atrial area was an additional and independent prognostic predictor of cardiac death. Interestingly, the risk of cardiac death increased progressively with increasing AHI and left atrial area: patients at very high risk for fatal outcomes were identified by an AHI $\geq$30/hr and significant left atrial dilatation (left atrial area $\geq$ 25 cm^2) (Fig. 1). However, patients with isolated left atrial dilatation without significant breathing disorders and, similarly, those with AHI $\geq$30/hr and lacking significant left atrial dilatation were at relatively low risk of death (Fig. 1). These data are suggestive of an interdependent relationship that may exist between left atrial size and AHI with respect to prognosis, with low left atrial size reflecting either relatively low left-sided filling pressures (although increased) or a short time since onset of HF and CSA.

The prognostic value of CSA was subsequently confirmed by Sin et al. (47), who investigated the effects of three months continuous positive airway pressure (CPAP)

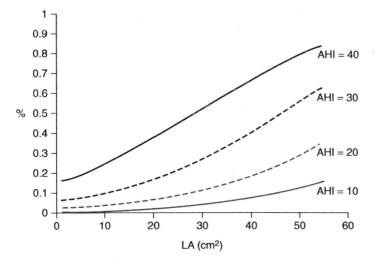

Figure 1 Occurrence of cardiac mortality according to AHI and left atrium size in patients with HF and CSA. The risk of cardiac death increased progressively with the value of AHI and left atrium size. *Source*: From Ref. 14.

treatment with CPAP on LVEF and long-term transplant-free survival in 66 HF subjects without ($n = 37$) and with ($n = 29$) CSA. An event rate of 32% was observed among subjects without CSA and 48% among those with CSA. The study showed that the presence of CSA confers a 2.5-fold increased risk for the combined endpoint of all-cause mortality and heart transplantion independently of CPAP use. Among patients with CSA, however, those who were randomized to CPAP and complied with this treatment had better survival than those who remained untreated.

Corrà et al. (48) investigated, in a larger study of 133 HF patients (53% on β-blocker and 34% on spironolactone), whether the occurrence of severe nocturnal CSA (AHI $\geq$ 30/hr) and exertional oscillatory ventilation alone or in association could affect outcome. Severe CSA was observed in 46% of the study sample and exertional oscillatory ventilation in 21%. Sixteen percent of the subjects had both breathing disorders. Over three years of follow-up, 30 patients died from cardiac causes and 1 patient required urgent heart transplantation. One and two-year actuarial cardiac mortality rates were respectively 9% and 15%. In multivariate analyses, severe AHI was found to be a strong predictor of cardiac death and urgent transplant (adjusted HR 3.7, 95% CI 1.5 to 9.5, $p <$ 0.01). A striking sixfold increased risk for cardiac death (adjusted HR 6.65, <0.01) was found when AHI $\geq$30/hr was associated with exercise-induced periodic breathing. The use of β-blockers conferred a better survival (HR 0.45, CI 95% 0.23 to 0.99, $p < 0.05$). It is important to underline that severe CSA remained an independent prognostic variable in this study, despite the fact that overall mortality was lower than that observed in previous studies, most certainly reflecting greater use of β-blockers and aldosterone antagonists.

Finally, Javaheri et al. (49) in a study, involving 88 subjects, found that even mild-moderate CSA confers a poorer long-term prognosis. Indeed, patients without CSA (AHI < 5/hr) had higher survival probability than patients with CSA (AHI > 5/hr) (HR 2.14, $p = 0.02$), over a median follow-up period of 51 months after adjusting for potential confounders. The median survival time of patients with and without CSA was 45 and 90 months, respectively. Additional factors independently linked to survival were right ventricular ejection fraction and diastolic blood pressure.

The concept of an independent prognostic value of CSA has been challenged by the results of three other studies. Andreas et al. (50) did not find CSA to predict mortality rates and urgent heart transplantation among 36 HF patients. In this study, CSA was quantified as the percentage of total sleep time in which Cheyne–Stokes respiration was present. No analyses were made using any of the AHI severity cutoffs used in other studies to assess relationships between SDB and heart disease. Negative results were also reported by Traversi et al. (51) who investigated the impact of CSA on cardiac mortality and urgent transplantation in 60 HF patients. In this cohort, during two years of follow-up, 7 patients underwent urgent cardiac transplant and 11 patients died. The only variable significantly predictive of unfavorable outcome was pulmonary wedge pressure. AHI, entered into the multivariate analyses as a continuous variable, was not found to be an independent prognostic factor. In this study, no AHI cutoff was used for the diagnostic and prognostic analyses. Furthermore it is not clear how patients with OSA were considered in the analysis.

Finally, Roebuck et al. (52) examined the effect of overall SDB (defined by AHI > 5/hr), as well as CSA and OSA separately, on outcome in a cohort of 78 patients with severe HF ($n = 33$ with CSA, $n = 22$ with OSA, 23 without SDB) referred for cardiac transplant assessment. During a median follow-up of 52 months, 31 patients underwent heart transplantation and 31 died (6 post transplantation). The percentages of patients experiencing the combined endpoints of all cause death and death + transplantation were similar across groups of patients with CSA, OSA, and patients without SDB. Although the cumulative survival was similar between groups, CSA, but not OSA, appeared to affect short-term survival and transplant-free survival. Indeed, mortality at 500 days was 30% in the CSA group and 13% in patients without SDB ($p < 0.05$). Multivariate analysis identified only heart transplantation as independently related to survival, whereas several acknowledged prognostic factors such as NYHA, LVEF, pulmonary capillary wedge pressure were not. Nonurgent heart transplantation, which occurred in 40% of the CSA group and presumably corrected the breathing disorder, may explain why CSA was not an independent predictor of survival among patients surviving past 500 days of follow-up in this highly selected population. A second major confounder of the study, which could have significantly affected the outcome, was the use of CPAP or supplemental O_2. These treatments were used for at least three months in more than one-third of the subjects and for over six months in a smaller subset. Unfortunately, these therapies were not included in the multivariate survival analyses.

In conclusion, the current evidence supporting the prognostic impact of CSA is stronger than the evidence against it. However several questions remain.

First, it is still uncertain as to whether CSA is a more refined marker of more severe HF or whether it per se carries an additional risk for poor prognosis. Marked neurohumoral activation secondary to repetitive hypoxia and arousal from sleep (15) with important repetitive surges in heart rate, blood pressure, and afterload could be implicated in inducing myocardial ischemia and remodeling, leading to further deterioration of ventricular function and a greater propensity to arrhythmias. Available data in the scientific literature do not allow us to make inferences regarding the mode of death and the potential mechanisms implicated in the relationship between CSA and death. Although patients with CSA and HF have more ventricular arrhythmias either in association with (13,53,54) or, in the daytime, independently of respiratory events (55), most studies conducted in HF patients with implantable cardioverter-defibrillators for both primary and secondary prevention have failed to demonstrate an association between CSA and lethal ventricular arrhythmia (56,57). However, in a recently published report from Japan, involving 71 patients with HF and an implanted defibrillator, followed for up to 180 days after polysomnography, the presence of sleep disordered breathing was common (66% of patients) and found to be an independent predictor of life-threatening arrhythmias. Importantly, these were more likely to occur during sleep (58).

Second, women are less frequently affected by CSA compared to men (17,20). For reasons that remain unclear, women with HF and left ventricular systolic dysfunction also have a better survival across the different HF etiologies (28). It is currently unknown whether the prognostic impact of CSA is similar in men and women.

Finally, it remains to be clarified as to whether the prognostic link between CSA and mortality remains in patients receiving maximal medical therapy with β-blockers and aldosterone antagonists, both of which are associated with improved survival in HF populations. As documented in the CANPAP trial, there was a significant time-dependent decline in mortality in all patients with CSA (59) as a result of advances in the treatment of HF during the course of the trial. In the study of Corrà et al. (48), the only study in which at least one-half of the patients were on β-blockers and one-third on spironolactone, β-blocker therapy was associated with improved survival in patients with and without CSA. Therefore, a question remains as to whether the maximization of HF therapies may attenuate those mechanisms by which CSA may accelerate the death rate among patients with HF (60).

V. OSA and Mortality in HF

Large observational cohort studies have shown that OSA is associated with higher risk for fatal and nonfatal cardiovascular events (4) and death from any cause (5) among the general population. OSA, by acting through various complex pathophysiological mechanisms that have been discussed extensively in previous chapters, may be particularly detrimental in patients with HF by worsening cardiac function, predisposing to arrhythmias, and potentiating neuroendocrine derangements that contribute to the progression of HF and potentially impair prognosis.

To date only two small observational studies have addressed the prognostic impact of OSA in HF with contrasting results. In the study of Roebuck et al. (52), which has been described above, the presence of mild-to-severe OSA as diagnosed by AHI >5/hr did not show any effect on long-term survival or transplant-free survival among 22 patients with OSA relative to 23 subjects without SDB during a median follow-up of 52 months. Overall 31 patients underwent heart transplantation and 31 died (6 posttransplantation). A similar 36% and 39% of deaths and 73 % and 72% of death + transplantation occurred in OSA and patients without SDB, respectively. As discussed above, in this study 27% of subjects with OSA were given a trial of CPAP and 14% continued CPAP for more than 6 months. The potential bias by the supplemental treatment was not taken into account in this study.

Conversely, a significant independent association between moderate-to-severe OSA (AHI ≥ 15/hr) and cumulative mortality has been reported more recently by Wang et al. (23), in a prospective observational study implicating subjects with untreated OSA ($n = 37$), treated OSA ($n = 14$), and mild to none sleep apnea (M-NSA) ($n = 113$). Patients classified as having untreated OSA were those who either did not initiate CPAP or quickly abandoned its use. Over a mean follow-up of 2.9 years (max 7.3 years), nine deaths were encountered among untreated OSA patients (24%, corresponding to a mortality rate of 8.7 per 100 person-years) and 14 (12%) in subjects without significant SDB (mortality rate of 4.2 per 100 person-year). All deaths were due to cardiac causes. No deaths were encountered among treated OSA patients. Multivariate survival analysis showed worse survival in HF patients with untreated OSA versus those with mild or no SDB (adjusted Hazard ratio 2.81, $p = 0.029$, Fig. 2). In this study, there was a statistical trend ($p = 0.07$) toward a lower mortality among patients with treated OSA compared to untreated OSA patients. It is noteworthy to mention that these patients did not report daytime sleepiness, which is a major complaint of OSA patients without HF and a common indication for their referral for a sleep study. Thus, in this group of HF patients who ordinarily might not be referred for a sleep study, untreated OSA has an adverse impact on outcome (23).

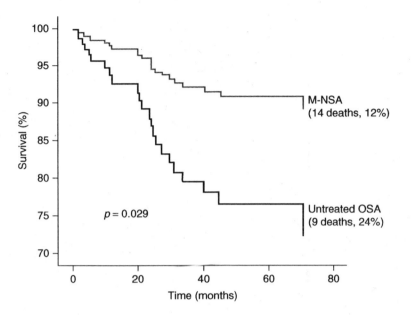

Figure 2 Multivariate Cox proportional Hazards plots for patients with untreated OSA versus patients with mild to none sleep apnea (M-NSA). Adjusted survival was worse in patients with untreated OSA than in patients with M-NSA. *Source*: From Ref. 23.

VI. Conclusions

1. The prevalence of CSA is very high in patients with stable HF and left ventricular systolic dysfunction and continues to remain high despite optimal medical therapy according to current recommendations.
2. Studies conducted prior to the extensive use of β-blockers support the independent prognostic impact of CSA in patients with HF and left ventricular systolic dysfunction.
3. OSA is also highly prevalent in patients with stable HF and left ventricular systolic dysfunction.
4. Asymptomatic OSA in HF patients seems to be associated with increased mortality.
5. Future studies are needed to clarify: firstly, as whether CSA still carries a prognostic information in the current HF population receiving maximal medical therapy and in women and secondly, the potential mechanisms eventually linking CSA and death.
6. More data are also needed to assess prevalence and clinical impact of SDB in HF with preserved left ventricular ejection fraction, a condition with a growing prevalence due to the aging of our society and is associated with a high rate of hospitalization and mortality.

References

1. American College of Cardiology/American Heart Association Task force. ACC/AHA Guidelines for the evaluation and management of chronic heart failure in the adult: executive summary. A report of the American College of Cardiology/American Heart Association Task Force on Practice Guidelines (committee to revise the 1995 guidelines for the evaluation and management of heart failure). Circulation 2001; 104:2996–3007.
2. Nieto FJ, Young TB, Bonnie KL, et al., for the Sleep Heart Health Study. Association of sleep-disordered breathing, sleep apnea, and hypertension in a large community-based study. JAMA 2000; 283:1829–1836.
3. Peppard PE, Young T, Palta M, et al. Prospective study of the association between sleep-disordered breathing and hypertension. N Engl J Med 2000; 342:1378–1384.
4. Marin JM, Carrizo SJ, Vicente E, et al. Long-term cardiovascular outcomes in men with obstructive sleep apnoea-hypopnoea with or without treatment with continuous positive airway pressure: an observational study. Lancet 2005; 365:1046–1053.
5. Yaggi HK, Concato J, Kernan WN, et al. Obstructive sleep apnea as a risk factor for stroke and death. N Engl J Med 2005; 353;2034–2041.
6. Bradley TD, Floras JS. Sleep apnea and heart failure: part I. Obstructive sleep apnea. Circulation 2003; 107:1671–1678.
7. Shahar E, Whithney CW, Redline S, et al., for the Sleep Heart Heath Study Research Group. Sleep-disordered breathing and cardiovascular disease. Am J Respir Crit Care Med 2001; 163:19–25.
8. Shamsuzzaman AS, Gersh BJ, Somers VK. Obstructive sleep apnea: implications for cardiac and vascular disease. JAMA 2003; 290(14):1906–1914.
9. Bradley TD, Floras JS. Sleep apnea and heart failure: part II. Central sleep apnea. Circulation 2003; 107:1822–1826.
10. Osler W. The Principle and Practice of Medicine. New York: Appleton, 1918.
11. Mackenzie J. Diseases of the Heart. 4th ed. New York: Oxford University Press, 1923.
12. Solin P, Bergin P, Richardson M, et al. Influence of pulmonary capillary wedge pressure on central apnea in heart failure. Circulation 1999; 99:1574–1579.
13. Javaheri S, Parker TJ, Liming JD, et al. Sleep apnea in 81 ambulatory male patients with stable heart failure. Types and their prevalences, consequences, and presentations. Circulation 1998; 97:2154–2159.
14. Lanfranchi PA, Braghiroli A, Bosimini E, et al. Prognostic value of nocturnal Cheyne-Stokes respiration in chronic heart failure. Circulation 1999; 99:1435–1440.
15. Leung RST, Bradley DT. Sleep and cardiovascular disease. Am J Respir Crit Care Med 2001; 164:2147–2165.
16. Lofaso F, Verscheuren P, Dubois Rande JL, et al. Prevalence of sleep-disordered breathing in patients on a heart transplant waiting list. Chest 1994; 106:1689–1694.
17. Sin DD, Fitzgerald F, Parker JD, et al. Risk factors for central and obstructive sleep apnea in 450 men and women with congestive heart failure. Am J Respir Crit Care Med 1999; 160: 1101–1106.
18. Tremel F, Pepint JL, Veale D, et al. High prevalence and persistence of sleep apnea in patients referred for acute left ventricular failure and medically treated over 2 months. Eur Heart J 1999; 20:1201–1209.
19. Ferrier K, Campbell A, Yee B, et al. Sleep-disordered breathing occurs frequently in stable outpatients with congestive heart failure. Chest 2005; 128(4):2116–2122.
20. Oldenburg O, Lamp B, Faber L, et al. Sleep-disordered breathing in patients with symptomatic heart failure: a contemporary study of prevalence in and characteristics of 700 patients. Eur J Heart Fail 2007; 9(3):251–257.
21. Schulz R, Blau A, Börgel J, et al., and the working group Kreislauf und Schlaf of the German Sleep Society (DGSM). Sleep apnoea in heart failure. Eur Respir J 2007; 29(6):1201–1205.

22. Vazir A, Hastings PC, Dayer M, et al. A high prevalence of sleep disordered breathing in men with mild symptomatic chronic heart failure due to left ventricular systolic dysfunction. Eur J Heart Fail 2007; 9(3):243–250.
23. Wang H, Parker JD, Newton GE, et al. Influence of obstructive sleep apnea on mortality in patients with heart failure. J Am Coll Cardiol 2007; 49(15):1625–1631.
24. MacDonald M, Fang J, Pittman SD, et al. The current prevalence of sleep disordered breathing in congestive heart failure patients treated with beta-blockers. J Clin Sleep Med 2008; 4(1):38–42.
25. Young T, Palta M, Dempsey J, Skarrud J, et al. The occurrence of sleep-disordered breathing among middle-aged adults. N Engl J Med 1993; 328:1230–1235.
26. Javaheri S. Sleep disorders in systolic heart failure: a prospective study of 100 male patients. The final report. Int J Cardiol 2006; 106(1):21–28.
27. Gabor JY, Newman DA, Barnard-Roberts V, et al. Improvement in Cheyne-Stokes respiration following cardiac resynchronization therapy. Eur Respir J 2005; 26:95–100.
28. Frazier CG, Alexander KP, Newby LK, et al. Association of gender and etiology with outcomes in heart failure with systolic dysfunction. A pooled analysis of 5 randomized control trials. J Am Coll Cardiol 2007; 49(13):1450–1458.
29. Smith LA, Chong DW, Vennelle M, et al. Diagnosis of sleep-disordered breathing in patients with chronic heart failure: evaluation of a portable limited sleep study system. J Sleep Res 2007; 16(4):428–435.
30. Tkacova R, Niroumand M, Lorenzi-Filho G, Bradley DT. Overnight shift from obstructive to central sleep apneas in patients with heart failure. Role of PCO2 and circulatory delay. Circulation 2001; 103:238–243.
31. Tkacova R, Wang H, Bradley TD. Night-to-night alterations in sleep apnea type in patients with heart failure. J Sleep Res 2006; 15(3):321–328.
32. Vazir A, Hastings PC, Papaioannou I, et al. Variation in severity and type of sleep-disordered breathing throughout 4 nights in patients with heart failure. Respir Med 2008; 102(6):831–839.
33. Lechat P, Packer M, Chalon S, et al. Clinical effects of beta-adrenergic blockade in chronic heart failure: a meta-analysis of double-blind, placebo-controlled, randomized trials. Circulation 1998; 98(12):1184–1191.
34. Hall SA, Cigarroa CG, Marcoux L, et al. Time course of improvement in left ventricular function, mass and geometry in patients with congestive heart failure treated with beta-adrenergic blockade. J Am Coll Cardiol 1995; 25:1154–1161.
35. Tamura A, Kawano Y, Naono S, et al. Relationship between β-blocker treatment and the severity of central sleep apnea in chronic heart failure. Chest 2007; 131:130–135.
36. Owan TE, Redfield MM. Epidemiology of diastolic heart failure. Prog Cardiovasc Dis 2005; 47(5):320–332.
37. Brutsaert DL, Sys SU, Gillebert TC. Diastolic failure: pathophysiology and therapeutic implications. J Am Coll Cardiol 1993; 22:318–325.
38. Bhatia RS, Tu JV, Lee DS, et al. Outcome of heart failure with preserved ejection fraction in a population-based study. N Engl J Med 2006; 355(3):260–269.
39. Tasali E, Mokhlesi B, Van Cauter E. Obstructive sleep apnea and type 2 diabetes: interacting epidemics. Chest 2008; 133(2):496–506.
40. Kanagala R, Murali NS, Friedman PA, et al. Obstructive sleep apnea and the recurrence of atrial fibrillation. Circulation 2003; 107:2589–2594.
41. Cargill RI, Kiely DG, Lipworth BJ. Adverse effects of hypoxemia on diastolic filling in humans. Clin Sci 1995; 89:165–169.
42. Amin RS, Kimball R, Lalra M, et al. Left ventricular function in children with sleep-disordered breathing. Am J Cardiol 2005; 95:801–804.
43. Chan JJ, Sanderson J, Chan W, et al. Prevalence of sleep-disordered breathing in diastolic heart failure. Chest 1997; 111:1488–1493.

44. Findley LJ, Zwillich CW, Ancoli-Israel S, et al. Cheyne-Stokes breathing during sleep in patients with left ventricular heart failure. South Med J 1985; 78:11–15.
45. Hanly PJ, Zuberi-Khokhar NS. Increased mortality associated with Cheyne-Stokes respiration in patients with congestive heart failure. Am J Respir Crit Care Med 1996; 153:272–276.
46. Ancoli-Israel S, DuHamel ER, Stepnowsky C, et al. The relationship between congestive heart failure, sleep apnea, and mortality in older men. Chest 2003; 124(4):1400–1405.
47. Sin DD, Logan AG, Fitzgerald FS, et al. Effects of continuous positive airway pressure on cardiovascular outcomes in heart failure patients with and without Cheyne-Stokes respiration. Circulation 2000; 102:61–66.
48. Corrà U, Pistono M, Mezzani A, et al. Sleep and exertional periodic breathing in chronic heart failure. Prognostic importance and interdependence. Circulation 2006; 113:44–50.
49. Javaheri S, Shukla R, Zeigler H, et al. Central sleep apnea, right ventricular dysfunction, and low diastolic blood pressure are predictors of mortality in systolic heart failure. J Am Coll Cardiol 2007; 49(20):2028–2034.
50. Andreas S, Hagenah G, Moller C, et al. Cheyne-Stokes respiration and prognosis in congestive heart failure. Am J Cardiol 1996; 78:1260–1264.
51. Traversi E, Callegari G, Pozzoli M, et al. Sleep disorders and breathing alterations in patients with chronic heart failure. G Ital Cardiol 1997; 27(5):423–429.
52. Roebuck T, Solin P, Kaye DM, et al. Increased long-term mortality in heart failure due to sleep apnoea is not yet proven. Eur Respir J 2004; 23:735–740.
53. Leung RS, Diep TM, Bowman ME, et al. Provocation of ventricular ectopy by cheyne-stokes respiration in patients with heart failure. Sleep 2004; 27(7):1337–1343.
54. Fitcher J, Bauer D, Arampatzis S, et al. Sleep-related breathing disorders are associated with ventricular arrhythmias in patients with an implantable cardioverter–defibrillator. Chest 2002; 122:558–561.
55. Lanfranchi PA, Somers VK, Braghiroli A, et al. Central sleep apnea in left ventricular dysfunction: prevalence and implications for arrhythmic risk. Circulation 2003; 107(5):727–732.
56. Fries R, Bauer D, Heisel A, et al. Clinical significance of sleep-related breathing disorders in patients with implantable cardioverter defibrillators. Pacing Clin Electrophysiol 1999; (1 Pt 2): 223–227.
57. Staniforth AD, Sporton SC, Wedzicha JA, et al. Ventricular arrhythmia, Cheyne-Stokes respiration and death: observations from patients with defibrillators. Heart 2005; 91:1418–1422.
58. Serizawa N, Yumino D, Kajimoto K, et al. Impact of sleep-disordered breathing on life-threatening ventricular arrhythmias in heart failure patients with implantable cardioverter-defibrillator. Am J Cardiol 2008; 102:1064–1068.
59. Bradley TD, Logan AG, Kimoff RJ, et al., CANPAP Investigators. Continuous positive airway pressure for central sleep apnea and heart failure. N Engl J Med 2005; 353(19):2025–2033.
60. Somers VK. Sleep-A new cardiovascular frontier. New Eng J Med 2005; 353:2070–2073.

19
Treatment of Obstructive and Central Sleep Apnea in Patients with Heart Failure

MATTHEW T. NAUGHTON
Alfred Hospital and Monash University, Melbourne, Australia

MICHAEL ARZT
University of Regensburg, Regensburg, Germany

I. Introduction

The prevalence of either obstructive sleep apnea (OSA) or central sleep apnea (CSA), or a combination of both, is in excessive of 50% of heart failure (HF) patients. Untreated OSA is thought to be detrimental toward the failing heart, whereas CSA is considered a result of advanced HF. The effectiveness of OSA treatment in HF populations is indicated by short- and medium-term studies that show OSA reversal with continuous positive airway pressure (CPAP) is associated with improvements in objective and subjective measures of HF. In the case of CSA and HF, most treatments directed toward HF have a beneficial effect upon the severity of CSA, suggesting HF and CSA severity change in parallel with each other. Nevertheless, it has also been shown that therapies directed toward relieving CSA, especially CPAP, can improve objective measures of cardiovascular function. Consequently, it would appear that CSA may have adverse effects on cardiovascular function, independent of HF status. Thus, the identification of OSA and CSA, the pathophysiological links between sleep apnea and HF, and the projected aims of therapy may vary between the two apnea types. This review will attempt to clarify indications for treatment, goals of therapy, and treatment modalities tried for OSA and CSA in the HF population.

II. Heart Failure with Obstructive Sleep Apnea
A. Indications for Therapy

HF is a common and disabling condition with high morbidity and mortality. Approximately 5% to 20% of the general community is estimated to have either systolic or diastolic HF, respectively (1). The five-year mortality from HF is estimated to be 20% for diastolic and 50% for systolic HF (2), on par with many malignancies. OSA is also common in the general non-HF community population (10%), whereas in an HF population the prevalence ranges between 11% and 38% (3–6).

OSA is thought to precede or contribute to the development of HF through several mechanisms. Large, negative intrathoracic pressure swings due to repetitive inspiratory efforts against the occluded pharynx (7), combined with apnea-related hypoxemia and hypercapnia and apnea-terminating arousals associated with sympathetic surge [illustrated by tachycardia and upward swings in systemic blood pressure (BP)], occur up to 800 times/night (8,9). Negative intrathoracic pressure swings increase left ventricular (LV) afterload (as do the positive systemic BP swings) and venous return to the right atrium and ventricle, thus increasing right ventricular preload and causing leftward displacement of the intraventricular septum during diastole (10). Hypoxemia and hypercapnia activate the sympathetic nervous system, contributing to systemic hypertension and tachycardia. Tachycardia in the setting of hypoxemia results in impaired myocardial relaxation (i.e., diastolic dysfunction) and contractility (i.e., systolic dysfunction) in addition to myocardial ischemia, leading to an elevation of pulmonary capillary wedge pressure (PCWP), ischemia, and arrhythmias. Hypercapnia results in reduced contractility and elevation of LV filling pressures (11).

Medium-term human studies have indicated OSA is associated with systemic hypertension and premature atherosclerosis (12–15). There is also growing evidence of OSA being associated with increased risk of fatal and nonfatal cardiovascular events (16–19). Randomized trials have also shown that reversal of OSA by CPAP reduces systemic BP and ameliorates early signs of atherosclerosis, providing further evidence that OSA contributes to the development of cardiovascular diseases (12,20–22).

In the non-HF population, the indications for OSA therapy generally require at least two hallmark features of OSA, sleepiness and a significant severity of OSA based on overnight monitoring. Sleepiness can be simplistically measured by a questionnaire, the Epworth Sleepiness Score (ESS), where eight potential scenarios of sleepiness are graded from 0 to 3 (23,24), with a maximum score of 24. Pathological sleepiness has been arbitrarily defined as ESS > 10. Severity of OSA has been assessed based on the frequency of apneas and hypopneas [the apnea-hypopnea index (AHI)] and the degree of hypoxemia. Mild OSA defined by AHI $\geq$5 to 15 episodes per hour (eph) with minimum SpO_2 values of >90%, moderate AHI $\geq$15 to 30 eph and minimum SpO_2 80% to 90%, and severe OSA (AHI $\geq$ 30 eph) and minimum SpO_2 <80% have been used as a guide. AHI $\geq$5 eph and total sleep time SpO_2 <90% are risk factors for the development of cardiovascular disease (15,25,26). Note that AHI and minimum SpO_2 are dependent on the techniques and equipment used to monitor patients in addition to the patients' sleep-stage architecture, body position, and other factors that might aggravate OSA (alcohol, nasal resistance, sleep deprivation). Indications to administer treatment are usually limited to symptomatic patients with moderate to severe OSA. Coexistent cardiovascular disease (such as coexistent systemic hypertension, type 2 diabetes) may influence the decision to treat at a lower AHI, oxygen saturation, or ESS threshold.

However, in the HF population, indications for OSA therapy are less clear. Most clinical trials have been limited to patients aged <80 years with symptomatic HF [New York Heart Association (NYHA) II or worse] and AHI thresholds $\geq$5 to 20 eph based on in-laboratory attended polysomnography. The utility of the ESS in the HF population has been placed in doubt by Arzt et al. (27), who evaluated subjective sleepiness (ESS) in 155 HF patients and a large community sample (Fig. 1). They demonstrated that patients with advanced HF have less subjective daytime sleepiness compared with individuals from a community sample, despite significantly reduced sleep time, whether or not they have OSA (27).

Therefore, which patients with HF and suspected HF should proceed to testing and a trial of treatment? Patients with established HF in whom loud or habitual snoring is witnessed (>3 nights/wk) that continues despite conservative management (attempted weight loss, cautious alcohol consumption, nasal decongestants, sleeping in lateral

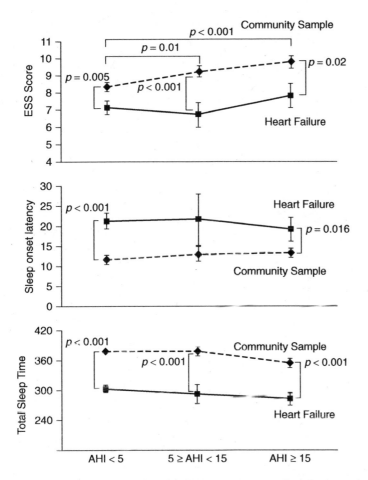

Figure 1 Sleepiness and sleep in HF patients (■, $n = 155$) and community group (♦, $n = 1139$) divided by AHI. Patients with HF had lower mean ESS [±SE] (7.1±0.4 vs. 8.3±0.2, 6.7±0.7 vs. 9.2±0.3, and 7.8+0.7 vs. 9.8±0.4) and longer sleep onset latencies (21.5±2.0 vs. 13.4±0.8 minutes, 21.9±6.5 vs. 13.2±1.9 minutes, and 19.4±2.9 vs.11.6±1.1 minutes) compared to a community sample with no history of HF in all AHI categories indicating less sleepiness despite sleeping less (total sleep time: 306±7 vs. 384±2 minutes, 295±19 vs. 384±5 minutes, and 285±13 vs. 359±7 minutes). In the community sample, mean ESS scores increased significantly with increasing AHI category. In contrast, there were no significant differences in ESS score in HF patients with increasing AHI category. *Abbreviations*: AHI, apnea-hypopnea index; ESS, Epworth sleepiness scores. *Source*: From Ref. 16.

position) should be considered for overnight monitoring. Patients with established HF, but without a bed partner, should be assessed if "high pretest probability of OSA" based on upper airway anatomy (e.g., high Mallampati score, retrognathia, nasal obstruction), body habitus (neck circumference >42 cm, BMI >30, systemic hypertension requiring >1 drug), and symptoms of fragmented sleep. Additional symptoms of poorly controllable HF (frequent hospitalizations for HF, orthopnea, paroxysmal nocturnal dyspnea, nocturia without daytime urinary frequency) should also alert the clinician to the possibility of underlying OSA.

B. Goals of OSA Therapy in HF

Reduction in mortality and improved quality of life are the two key end points one should strive for in long-term OSA and HF intervention–based clinical trials. Randomized controlled intervention trials in OSA-HF populations with sufficient patient numbers for a sufficient duration of time to determine mortality reduction have not been undertaken.

Quality of life has been measured in several smaller medium-term trials and can be measured by general and disease-specific symptom scores in addition to an overall patient assessment. For the assessment of treatment outcomes, the frequency and duration of HF hospitalizations, community participation (e.g., working status), plus any change in the status of accommodation (e.g., supported accommodation) are important to most patients as well as health economists.

Symptoms of general health, HF, and OSA have been used as end points for OSA-HF studies (28). General health has been assessed with the Short Form-36 (SF-36) questionniare, which assesses eight domains, namely, physical function, physical role, bodily pain, general health, vitality, social function, emotion, and mental health. The SF-36 (both baseline and response to therapy) can be used to compare normal healthy age–related populations, and other chronic illnesses plus assessment for the assessment of therapies.

Symptoms of HF have been self-classified using NYHA classes: class 1—asymptomatic but able to walk any distance without limitation; class 2—mild dyspnea but able to complete most activities of daily living; class 3—moderate dyspnea but able to carry out most activities of daily living; and class 4—severe dyspnea on minimal exertion.

Subjective sleepiness has been crudely assessed by the ESS questionnaire, but because most HF patients with OSA seem not to have subjective sleepiness, the absence of subjective sleepiness on the ESS or objective testing does not rule out OSA (27). Objective assessment of daytime sleepiness, for example, by the multiple sleep latency test or a test of alertness (e.g., the Osler test) may provide a more robust measure of sleepiness or alertness and may be used to assess the effects of treating OSA (29,30).

The primary objective end points of clinical trials of OSA treatment in HF have been structural and functional markers of HF. Most commonly, left ventricular ejection fraction (LVEF) measured either by transthoracic echocardiography or red cell technetium-labeled nucleotide scanning has been used at baseline and also the change over a one- to three-month treatment period. The change in LVEF (baseline to three months) has been shown to correlate with survival in large HF populations (31). Finally, LVEF has proven useful because it has a narrow day-to-day variability and may assist in the clinical assessment of an HF patient where the cause of dyspnea may not be entirely due to HF (i.e., may reflect deconditioning).

Structure, function, and chamber size of the heart have been used as objective end points. These include the degree of mitral regurgitation reflecting mitral annulus diameter and therefore LV end-diastolic diameter. The mitral regurgitant fraction can be assessed using nuclear techniques. Cardiac chamber size based on echocardiography or magnetic resonance imaging, in particular the LV end-diastolic dimension, has proven a sensitive marker of improved cardiac performance. Biological markers of cardiac chamber stretch [e.g., b-type natriuretic peptide (BNP)] have also been used in clinical trials.

Cardiopulmonary exercise testing has been utilized as an objective end point. Exercise testing can provide two of the most important markers for estimating prognosis and estimating optimal timing for heart transplantation in HF populations. These markers are the maximum oxygen consumption (peakVO_2, via cyclergometry or treadmill) and ventilatory efficiency during exercise (VE/VCO_2-slope) (32,33). Additional valuable parameters are maximal heart rate, BP changes, minute ventilation (VE), and CO_2 production (VCO_2). Although changes in these parameters are small following training or therapies (i.e., <10% even in highly trained athletes), they can be of use to assess subtle changes in pathophysiology, such as a fall in VE/VCO_2 ratio, which indicates a fall in the ventilatory response, a feature characteristic of improved HF.

More practical markers of exercise performance include the six-minute walk distance, shuttle test, and actigraphy. Of these, the six-minute walk distance appears to be the most sensitive to change. The average six-minute walk distance in HF ranges from 310 m in those with an LVEF of 20% (34) up to 427 m in those with mild disease (LVEF 53%) (35).The six-minute walk distance has an inverse relationship with the NYHA functional class and a weak inverse correlation with quality of life (36,37). The six-minute walk distance is strongly correlated with peakVO_2 (38,39). Despite these relationships, the utility of the six-minute walk distance as a predictor of survival in HF is not clear. A six-minute walk distance of less than 300 m is generally considered a strong indicator of increased mortality (36).

Secondary objective markers of cardiac response to CPAP in OSA-HF trials have included markers of sympathoneural activity: mean resting heart rate (21,28), resolution of arrhythmias (40), baroreflex sensitivity (41) time and power spectral analysis of heart rate variability (42), plasma and overnight urinary cathecholamines (mainly norepinephrine) (43), plasma skeletal muscle sympathetic nerve microneurography (44), and tritiated norepinephrine spillover (45).

Data from polysomnography is important: the quality and quantity of sleep [greater sleep efficiency, slow-wave sleep, and rapid eye movement (REM) sleep] in addition to a reduction in the frequency of arousals, apneas, and hypopneas and improved SpO_2 levels should be sought. Additional variables that are included are the mean sleep heart rate (and arrhythmias) and, in the setting of transcutaneous CO_2 monitoring, a $PaCO_2$ value closer to normal (40–45 mmHg). Observational data including the number of pillows and close scrutiny to body position (i.e., supine sleep) should also be sought.

No published randomized controlled study to date has included mortality as a primary end point. In observational studies of OSA performed to date, untreated severe OSA (AHI ≥ 30 eph) and mild OSA (AHI ≥5–30 eph) have been associated with greater mortality in both non-HF and HF populations (17–19). However, these studies have been limited by the lack of adequate control groups. Moreover, the untreated OSA patients were nonadherent patients by virtue of poor CPAP adherence and may have been poorly adherent to other cardiovascular therapies. The inclusion of heart transplantation to mortality is vexed: although patients with severe HF are listed for transplant, it is well recognized that transplantation is limited to patients with single-organ problems, of relatively young age (<65 years), with good social and mental health, and of appropriate religious beliefs.

C. Choice of Therapies for OSA
Positional Therapy
Body position changes can affect upper airway stability, although studies have been limited to patients without known HF. In patients with OSA, Cartwright (46) reported 58% of 24 males with OSA (mean AHI, 47.5 eph) to have positional OSA (defined by a

more than twofold difference in AHI, supine to side), of whom most were nonobese, with 33% of patients having no OSA in the lateral position. Oksenberg and colleagues (47) reported 56% of 574 consecutive sleep clinic patients with suspected OSA to have positional OSA. The positional patients were younger (53 vs. 55 years), were less obese (29 vs. 32 kg/m^2), and had less severe OSA overall (AHI 28 vs. 44 eph and minimal SpO$_2$ 81 vs. 73%) compared with nonpositional OSA patients. In a further study, Oksenberg et al. (48) reported longer apneas (27 vs. 23 seconds), greater desaturation (min SpO$_2$ 82 vs. 86%), and greater autonomic arousal (9 vs. 7 changes in heart rate with arousal) with supine compared with lateral apneas in 30 patients with severe OSA. Therapeutic CPAP was estimated to be 2.6 cmH$_2$O higher in the supine position compared with the lateral position (49). Penzel et al. (50) showed that the supine position increased the closing pressure compared with the lateral position. This rotational (changes from supine to the lateral body position) effect was tested by Berger et al. (51), who reported a fall in 24-hour systemic BP (from 133/78 to 127/75 mmHg) with positional therapy in 13 OSA patients, 6 of whom had hypertension.

Weight Loss

Although it is likely that the impact of changes in body weight would have a marked impact on OSA and cardiac function in clinical practice, there is a relative paucity of confirmatory published scientific data. Peppard et al. (52) studied 690 community dwellers with polysomnography and accurate weight assessment at baseline and again at four years. They reported that as a group, weight increased by approximately 1 kg/annum (or 1 BMI unit over four years). Moreover, a 10% weight increase was associated with a 32% increase in AHI and a sixfold greater chance of moderate to severe OSA. Conversely, a 10% weight loss was associated with a 26% reduction in AHI (52). However, Arzt et al. (27) found no relationship between weight and severity of OSA in an HF population, suggesting factors other than weight are playing an important role. Moreover, weight loss in an HF population is a sign of poor prognosis (53). Therefore, the relationship between weight and OSA in an HF population may differ from that of a non-HF population.

Dixon et al. (54) undertook a before and after analysis of 123 patients with obesity undergoing surgically assisted weight loss (gastric banding). The group mean BMI fell from 46 to 35 kg/m^2 (130 to 99 kg), paralleled by a fall in the symptoms of habitual snoring (82 to 14%), witnessed apneas (33 to 2%), and proportion of the group with excessive daytime sleepiness (39 to 4%). Unfortunately, polysomnography results at baseline were not reported nor was follow-up polysomnography undertaken in this study, so the effect of weight loss on AHI could not be assessed.

Obesity and the development of HF were assessed in the Framingham data series (55). Over a 14-year follow-up, 8.4% of the 5881 community dwellers, mean age 55 years, developed HF. The risk of HF rose for every BMI unit rise by 5% in women and 7% in men, independent of other known risk factors.

To understand the comparative influence of obesity-related complications [hypertension, diabetes, and sleep apnea (AHI $\geq$ 5 eph)] on cardiac function, Avelar et al. (56) studied 455 morbidly obese patients (BMI range 33 to 92 kg/m^2) and 59 nonobese (BMI $<$ 30 kg/m^2) controls with overnight cardiopulmonary monitoring, echocardiogram, office BP, and detailed blood tests [fasting glucose, insulin, hemoglobin A1$_C$ (HbA1$_C$), lipids]. LV hypertrophy was present in 78% of the obese subjects compared with 40% of nonobese control subjects and was best explained (using multivariate analysis) in descending order by mean nocturnal SpO_2, systolic BP, and BMI, whereas age, log AHI, glucose, and $HbA1_C$ were not predictive.

Scientific publications describing the effects of weight loss on cardiac function are limited. Alpert et al. (57) reported 14 obese HF patients in whom weight fell with bariatric surgery from 128 to 84 kg, associated with an improvement in transthoracic echocardiographic fractional shortening from 23% to 28% (normal > 28%) and with 12 of 14 patients having an improvement in the NYHA class.

Recently, two large trials of surgically assisted weight loss have been reported. The first, a large Swedish prospective controlled multicentered trial (58) of surgically assisted weight loss (gastric bypass, vertical gastroplasty, and gastric banding, $n = 4047$ subjects, mean follow-up 11 years) reported weight losses of 14% (banding), 16% (vertical gastroplasty), and 25% (gastric bypass) compared with no weight change in the untreated control group at 10 years follow-up. The all-cause mortality was significantly lower ($p = 0.04$) with weight loss; myocardial infarction and cancer were the main causes of death. There was a strong trend for a reduction in death related to HF. Although ~25% of the subjects had a positive questionnaire diagnosis of OSA, follow-up questionnaire data regarding OSA or polysomnography data (baseline or follow-up) were not reported.

The second was a larger retrospective controlled single-center trial (59) of 7925 obese patients undergoing gastric bypass who were followed up for seven years. All-cause mortality was 40% lower in the surgically assisted weight loss group compared with age and BMI-matched controls, who did not lose weight. Mortality due to coronary artery disease, HF, and cancer were both lower (56%, 70%, and 60%, respectively); however, the risk of death due to accidents and suicide was 58% greater. There have been no randomized controlled studies that have addressed the mechanisms and effectiveness of weight loss on HF combined with OSA.

Oral Appliances

Assessments of oral appliances (OAs) to advance the mandible to treat OSA are numerous, but there are none that assess cardiac function or the OSA-HF population. One study has assessed systemic BP. Gotsopoulos et al. (60) demonstrated a fall in awake systolic and diastolic BP (3.3 mmHg and 3.4 mmHg, respectively) and 24-hour mean diastolic BP (1.8 mmHg) in a randomized controlled crossover design study with OAs. This study involved 24-hour ambulatory BP monitoring in 61 non-HF patients (selected from 74 eligible patients), with AHI 26 eph, minimum SpO_2 85%, BMI 29 kg/m^2, of whom 39% were hypertensive.

Upper Airway Surgery

The effect of nasal, palatal, or bony surgery to overcome OSA and improve cardiac function has not been widely described. In children with OSA due to tonsillar enlargement, the impact of tonsillectomy on cardiac function has been assessed in a small controlled case series (61). Gorur and colleagues reported right and LV size and wall hypertrophy in children with OSA compared with non-OSA control children. In four children with OSA and abnormal echocardiography, reversal of OSA with tonsillectomy was associated with normalization of the cardiac dimensions.

Amin and coworkers (62) similarly reported impaired diastolic LV function in 10 children (mean age 12 years, AHI 25 eph, BMI 31 kg/m^2), which improved by 18%

(and all to normal values), one year following treatment for OSA (7 with tonsillectomy and 3 with CPAP).

The benefits of tracheostomy were initially described in adult patients with OSA and advanced right HF. Abolition of OSA in such patients was accompanied by improvements in oxygenation and clinical features of right HF (63), arrhythmias (64), and overnight urinary norepinephrine (65). However, no studies have assessed the effects of upper airway surgery on cardiac function in the OSA-HF population.

Positive Airway Pressure

CPAP is a unique form of therapy for HF that reduces LV preload and afterload, increases lung volume, and stabilizes the upper airway. The precise modes of action vary depending on the etiology and severity of HF.

First, CPAP provides an upper airway pneumatic splint that overcomes upper airway instability and thereby overcomes the negative effects of OSA (large, negative intrathoracic pressures, hypoxemia, hypercapnia, and surges in sympathetic activity). This effect is similar to that of a tracheostomy or (possibly) OA therapy. However, in contrast to tracheostomy and OA therapy, CPAP provides an additional positive intrathoracic pressure.

Second, CPAP provides positive intrathoracic pressure, which results in a reduction in preload. As patients with severe HF are often fluid-overloaded, with elevated filling pressures (PCWP, right atrial and jugular venous pressures), factors that might impede the venous return to the left ventricle may be beneficial. In contrast to a normal patient's Starling curve, in which stroke volume is linearly related to the "preload," in HF there is a "descending limb" at high preload values such that further elevations in preload result in a reduced stroke volume. Thus, a reduction in preload may result in a rise in stroke volume in HF patients with a very high preload probably due to reversal of adverse ventricular interactions.

Third, CPAP reduces LV afterload (66). The LV afterload is explained by the LaPlace relationship in which LV transmural pressure (PLVtm) equals systolic BP minus intrathoracic pressure (SBP – ITP) multiplied by the LV radius divided by LV wall thickness. Thus CPAP-induced afterload reduction is achieved by placing a positive pressure around the left ventricle, causing PLVtm to fall. Studies have also shown that the end-diastolic left ventricle volume falls with CPAP therapy (67). A case series of 25 OSA patients with preserved systolic ventricular function suggested that CPAP significantly reduced wall thickness of the interventricular septum (from 1.3 to 1.0 cm) (68). As such, for the above reasons, it is believed that cardiac work falls (69) and sympathetic activity required by the heart falls with CPAP (70). Yoshinaga and colleagues have reported an increase in cardiac metabolic efficiency after six weeks of CPAP treatment of HF patients with OSA (71), indicating that CPAP may prevent the energy depletion of the failing ventricle.

Fourth, CPAP success in OSA-HF may also relate to the pulmonary aspects. Patients with HF often have a reversible restrictive and obstructive ventilatory defect—restriction due to cardiomegaly, pleural effusions, respiratory muscle weakness, and a congested edematous abdomen splinting the diaphragm; and obstruction due to bronchial wall edema (72). Light et al. (73) observed a predominantly restrictive pattern on baseline lung function testing (spirometry, lung volumes, and diffusing capacity) in 28 patients (mean age 62 years) with severe HF. Following intensive medical therapy (initial diuresis ~ 8 kg) over eight weeks, total lung capacity and forced expiratory vital

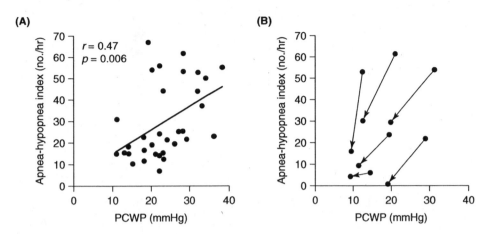

Figure 2 Effects of intensive medical HF therapy on pulmonary capillary wedge pressure and CSA. PCWP is elevated in heart failure patients with central sleep apnea compared with those with obstructive sleep apnea or without sleep apnea. (A) In patients with CSA PCWP correlated with the frequency and severity of CSA. (B) In patients with CSA and high PCWP, intensive medical therapy reduced both PCWP (29 ± 3 to 22 ± 2 mmHg; $p < 0.001$) and the frequency of (central) apneas and hypopneas (AHI, 39 ± 8 to 19 ± 5 events per hour of sleep; $p = 0.005$). Arrows indicate direction of change with time and therapy. *Abbreviations*: CSA, central sleep apnea; PCWP, pulmonary capillary wedge pressure; AHI, apnea-hypopnea index. *Source*: From Ref. 5.

capacity (FVC) increased by ~20% and 30%, respectively. Hosenpud et al. (74) reported increases in forced expiratory volume in one second (FEV_1) and FVC by 12% and 16%, respectively, in 17 patients (aged 42 years) before and 15 months post–heart transplant. The restrictive pattern could be statistically attributed to the reduction in cardiac volume. Naum et al. (75) confirmed a predominantly restrictive pattern in 56 patients with severe HF (LVEF 18%, aged 50 years) and also showed a significant direct correlation between PCWP and diffusing capacity, such that a low PCWP inferred a low diffusing capacity (Fig. 2). This later observation could be explained by the alveolar-capillary membrane interstitial fibrosis observed in animal models of acute HF (76,77). Thus treatments that increase lung volume might be helpful in HF by increasing the pulmonary oxygen reservoir and improving V/Q matching. It is known that 10 cmH$_2$O CPAP increases lung volumes acutely by 500 to 1000 mL (78) and thereby increases oxygen stores within the lungs (79). Although HF patients are rarely hypoxic awake at rest, during apneas the minimum SpO2 will often fall to values of <80% in OSA and percent total sleep time spent with SpO2 <90% values of 5% to 10% (43).

CPAP will increase alveolar pressure and thereby prevent alveolar collapse due to alveolar edema. This would have an effect to improve gas exchange and prevent pulmonary crepitations, predominantly during episodes of acute or subacute pulmonary edema.

Finally, CPAP also increases airway diameter by overcoming bronchial wall edema (80). For these immediate reasons, respiratory work falls with CPAP in stable, severe HF patients, both during wakefulness (66) and during sleep in those with OSA (9). A reduction in respiratory and cardiac work with CPAP is thereby likely to result in a reduction of cardiac sympathetic tone and oxygen consumption required by the myocardium (69,81).

There have been no studies on the efficacy of treating OSA in patients with overt diastolic HF. However, in one study involving patients with OSA, asymptomatic LV diastolic dysfunction was observed in 56% ($n = 27$) compared with only 20% of a non-OSA control group ($n = 15$). In a randomized crossover (12 weeks each arm) designed trial, markers of diastolic function (measured echocardiographically by the E/A ratio, deceleration, and isovolemic relaxation time) improved significantly with CPAP (82). Whether OSA can contribute to overt diastolic HF, and whether such HF will respond to treatment of OSA, remains to be determined.

In a before and after study lasting one month, 12 patients with HF due to systolic dysfunction received CPAP (7). After one month of CPAP, there was a striking improvement in LVEF (37 to 49%). Thereafter two randomized controlled trials were undertaken. The first by Kaneko et al. (21) involved 24 patients with HF (LVEF < 45%) and OSA (AHI $\geq$ 20 eph) followed for one month, and it showed that CPAP applied at a mean pressure of 8.9 cmH$_2$O for an average of 6.2 hr/night caused significant improvements in LVEF (25 to 34%), falls in systolic BP (126 to 116 mmHg), and a reduction in LV systolic but not diastolic dimension compared to the control group. Data from the same group also indicated that CPAP caused a reduction in muscle sympathetic activity (44), a reduction in the rate of ventricular ectopy during sleep (40), increased cardiac parasympathetic activity as manifested by an increase in heart rate variability (42), and baroreflex sensitivity (41). In another observational study, Wang et al. (18) reported a significantly higher mortality rate in 164 HF patients with untreated OSA compared with a non-OSA control group (8.7 vs. 4.2 deaths per 100 patient years, $p = 0.029$) followed for a maximum of 7.3 years. There was also a trend toward lower mortality in a subset of patients whose OSA was treated with CPAP ($p = 0.07$) (18).

In the second trial (28), 156 patients were screened to provide 55 patients with OSA-HF (AHI > 5 eph and LVEF < 55%) who were randomized, of whom 15 dropped out (6 controls and 9 CPAP). In the 40 patients who completed the study, the group randomized to CPAP (8.8 cmH$_2$O for 5.6 hr/night) achieved an improvement in LVEF (38 to 43%) as well as an improvement in the quality of life and a fall in sympathetic activity (urinary norepinephrine). However, there was no change in maximal exercise capacity (VO$_2$ max) measured by cycle ergometry. Of importance, however, were two deaths, both occurring in the CPAP-treated group: one sudden death and the other as a complication of an elective pacemaker lead reinsertion.

A single randomized controlled trial with parallel design of autotitrating positive airway pressure (APAP) (vs. sham APAP of <1 cmH$_2$O) was undertaken in 23 patients with OSA (AHI > 15 eph) and HF (LVEF < 45%) over a six-week period. APAP (mean CPAP 7 cmH$_2$O) and sham APAP usage were ~3.4 and 3.3 hr/night, respectively (83). A total of 349 patients were screened to achieve randomization in 26, of whom 23 completed the study. In those randomized to APAP, a significant improvement was noted in sleepiness but not in quality of life or LVEF. Follow-up sleep studies were also not performed, and therefore it was not proven that APAP abolished their OSA.

III. Heart Failure with Central Sleep Apnea

CSA also occurs commonly in approximately 30% of patients with HF (4–6). Characteristically, it is a waxing and waning pattern of respiration associated with periods of hyperventilation lasting approximately 30 seconds followed by apneas lasting about

30 seconds usually during stages 1 and 2 non-REM sleep: the so-called Cheyne–Stokes pattern of respiration. An arousal (or state change) often occurs two or three breaths after apnea termination, propagating the cyclic breathing. In contrast to OSA, CSA is caused by respiratory control instability. The primary stimulation for ventilation while asleep is $PaCO_2$ (84). One hallmark of HF patients with CSA is chronic hyperventilation that is likely an effect of (*i*) elevated sympathetic activity upon the carotid body and brainstem, which are responsible for ventilatory response to CO_2, (*ii*) pulmonary vagal irritant receptor stimulation by pulmonary congestion (Fig. 2A) (6,85,86), and (*iii*) increases in central and peripheral chemosensitivity for CO_2 (87,88). In addition, there is a tendency for an exaggerated fall in SpO_2 for a given apnea length, related to an underlying restrictive ventilatory defect (73,75,89) due to cardiomegaly and pulmonary edema. Another factor promoting ventilatory instability is a circulatory delay from the pulmonary signal ($PaCO_2$) reaching the carotid body (peripheral chemoreceptor) secondary to poor cardiac output (90). This results in a positive rather than negative feedback loop.

Like OSA, CSA causes intermittent nocturnal hypoxia and surges in sympathetic nervous system activity and BP (91). In contrast to OSA, however, CSA does not cause generation of large, negative intrathoracic pressure swings. Thus the impact of CSA on LV preload and afterload is less than in OSA.

In contrast to the OSA-HF population, the CSA-HF population is less likely to present with loud habitual snoring; therefore, bed partners will less often witness apneas. Similar to OSA-HF, studies have shown that CSA in severe HF is not associated with self-reported sleepiness (4,29,92). However, objectively assessed sleepiness by the maintenance of wakefulness test was found to be significantly increased in HF patients with sleep apnea compared with those without (29). Their symptom burden is usually dominated by those caused by advanced HF: namely, orthopnea, paroxysmal nocturnal dyspnea, frequent hospitalizations for HF, atrial fibrillation, fragmented sleep, lethargy, and reduced exercise capacity. Patients are typically male, with moderate to severe HF.

A. Indications for CSA Therapy

The indications for therapy in CSA-HF patients are symptoms of HF refractory to optimization of medical and device therapies or sleep apnea–related symptoms. Reevaluation of indication for therapy after a trial of positive airway pressure (PAP) therapy is advisable. A general recommendation for treatment of CSA with PAP therapy to reduce cardiac morbidity and to prolong life is not supported by the current literature.

B. Goals of CSA Therapy

Given that the symptoms of CSA-HF are that of severe HF, so too are the goals of therapy: to improve both symptoms and objective measures of HF. These include markers of ventricular performance and rhythm plus improvements in autonomic control. Markers of LV performance include the LVEF, LV fractional shortening, LV and left atrial dimensions, and LV end-diastolic and systolic pressures. Invasive right heart catheter monitoring can measure right-sided pressures, including pulmonary artery pressures, right atrial pressure, and PCWPs to determine whether or not elevated right-sided pressures are secondary to elevated left-sided pressures from the failing left ventricle. Biochemical markers of LV filling pressure include BNP; however, this becomes less reliable in the elderly (>70 years) and those with renal failure.

Cardiac rhythm is an important variable to observe. Maintenance of sinus rhythm is paramount in patients with HF, as cardiac output falls ~20% with loss of atrial contraction, as occurs with atrial fibrillation (93). Ventricular ectopy and runs of ventricular tachycardia are important variables, as they reflect impaired LV function and excessive sympathetic activity. Neurohumoral activity can be assessed with mean sleep heart rate, heart rate variability, plasma norepinephrine, and urinary norepinephrine.

Similar to HF patients with OSA, degree of sleepiness and/or alertness can be assessed either by subjective evaluation (e.g., ESS) or by objective assessments such as by the multiple sleep latency test, the maintenance of wakefulness test, or the Osler test (29,30,92).

C. Choice of Therapies for CSA
Optimization of Usual HF Medical Therapy
The initial approach to the CSA-HF patient should be to ensure that they are on, or have trialled, appropriate pharmacological therapy, which should include diuretics, angiotensin-converting enzyme inhibitors, angiotensin II receptor blockers, β-blockers, and digoxin. However, this recommendation is based on HF management per se rather than evidence that these agents ameliorate CSA. In an uncontrolled study, six patients with decompensated HF who were treated with a combination of anti-HF medications (diuretics, inotropes, and oxygen) underwent cardiopulmonary monitoring overnight and were reassessed ~42 days later: the AHI fell from 34 to 11 eph (94). In another uncontrolled study, eight patients with HF were treated with captopril for one month and the AHI fell from 35 to 20 eph (95). While systematic evidence from randomized controlled trials is lacking, small case series report that intensification of medical therapy for HF and thus hemodynamic improvement was accompanied by significant reductions or even full suppression of central respiratory events during sleep (Fig. 2B). The role of β-blockers in CSA has not been studied systematically. However, in a single-center HF clinic population ($n = 108$), 82% of whom were taking β-blockers, 31% still had CSA (96). The use of β-blockers did not predict the presence or absence of CSA. Similar findings were reported in a recent study (97).

Anemia occurs in about a third of patients with HF and is a risk factor for mortality, independent of HF severity (PCWP), BMI, and renal function (96). Reversal of anemia alleviates HF symptoms and improves objective markers of cardiac dysfunction in HF. Recently, Zilberman and colleagues (98) reported 38 HF patients with anemia (Hb < 12 gm/dL) had a 62% prevalence of pure CSA. Moreover, treatment of the HF-related anemia with a combination of erythropoietin and iron over three months resulted in a rise in hemoglobin (10.3 to 12.3 gm/dL) and a fall in AHI from 27 to 18 eph accompanied by alleviation of symptoms of HF and sleepiness.

Thus although usual medical therapy for HF should be the first line in those with CSA, a view based on expert HF opinion, there is an absence of randomized trial evidence to support this opinion in HF populations with CSA.

Cardiac Pacing: Atrial Overdrive Pacing and Cardiac Resynchronization Therapy (Table 1)
The possibility that atrial overdrive pacing (AOP) may alleviate sleep apnea was tested in a small study by Kato and colleagues (109). Two of six HF patients who demonstrated CSA had an AOP inserted for sinus node disease or third-degree atrioventricular block.

Table 1 Effect of Pacemakers (AOP and CRT) on OSA and CSA

Author	Rx	Study (N)	Rhythm	LVEF	Duration	Outcomes
Kato et al. (99)	AOP	B+A (6)	Brady	N	1 W	CSA in 2 of 6↓ (AHI 38 to 21)
Garrigue et al. (100)	AOP+15	B+A (15)	Brady	54%	1D	↓ AHI (OSA + CSA) + PSG
Simantirakis et al. (101)	AOP+15	X over (16)	Brady	N	1D, 1M	↓ AHI (OSA) & PSG with CPAP, not AOP
Pepin (102)	AOP+15	X over (17)	Brady	64%	1M	no Δ AHI (OSA) or PSG
Luthje et al. (103)	AOP+7,+15	RCT-X (20)	Brady	47%	1D	no Δ AHI (OSA) or PSG
Unterberg et al. (104)	AOP+15 vs. CPAP	RCT-X (10)	N	N	1D	↓AHI (OSA) & PSG with CPAP, no Δ with AOP
Krahn et al. (2006) (105)	AOP	RCT-X (15)	N	N	1N	(HR 65 to 77 bpm) No effect on AHI or hypoxic time
Sinha et al. (106)	CRT	B+A (24)	LBBB	HF	17W	CSA in 14/24. ↓ CAI 19 →5/hr
Gabor et al. (107)	CRT	B+A (10)	LBBB	HF	7M	CSA diminished in 6/10 patients, no ΔCO_2 or CT
Stanchina et al. (108)	CRT vs. AOP+15	RCT (13)	LBBB	HF	1W	OSA in 13/24. CRT: ↓AHI (OSA) 41 → 30/hr & LVEF 22→34%; AOP: No Δ in OSA

AOP: +7 or +15 indicates set at 7 or 15 beats above mean nocturnal heart rate.

Abbreviations: AOP, atrial overdrive pacemaker; CRT, cardiac resynchronization therapy; OSA, obstructive sleep apnea; CSA, central sleep apnea; LVEF, left ventricular ejection fraction; RCT, randomized controlled trial; N, subject number; B+A, before and after; Brady, bradycardia; LBBB, left bundle branch block; CT, circulation time (lung-to-finger CT measured by oximeter); PSG, polysomnography.

This resulted in an improvement in, but not the cure of, CSA (mean AHI 38 to 21 eph) with AOP. Garrigue and colleagues (100) reported in a study of 15 patients with CSA as well as OSA, who had pacemakers implanted for symptomatic bradyarrhythmias, greater than 50% improvement in the overall (central and obstructive) AHI after AOP to 15 beats per minute (bpm) above the intrinsic heart rate (57 to 72 bpm).

Although the patients reported by Garrigue et al. (100) did not have overt HF, all had bradyarrhythmias and, presumably, reduced cardiac output. In the recumbent position, it is possible that in addition to low cardiac output, they may have developed subtle pulmonary congestion, both of which can destabilize the respiratory control system and facilitate the development of CSA (6,85). Consequently, the most likely mechanism whereby AOP alleviated CSA was by augmenting cardiac output and reducing pulmonary congestion, thereby stabilizing the respiratory control system. However, it is not clear how this mechanism would alleviate obstructive events, as respiratory control system instability generally plays a less prominent role in the pathogenesis of OSA than of CSA (110,111).

Indeed, several subsequent studies (101–104,112) did not confirm Garrigue et al.'s (100) finding that AOP attenuated obstructive apneas and hypopneas. However, all these studies had in common that the majority of patients had preserved LV function and that pacemakers or cardioversion defibrillators with pacing function were also implanted for a variety of indications other than bradyarrhythmias. Thus, in these studies the potential to increase cardiac output by AOP was less than in the bradyarrhythmic patients in the trial of Garrigue et al. (100). In a study by Krahn et al. (113), 15 patients with OSA who were intolerant of CPAP were randomized to a single night of AOP or no AOP. None of these patients had HF, arrhythmias, or heart block. Increasing heart rate from 65 to 77 bpm did not alter the AHI or markers of oxygenation (108). Patients with HF and CSA with low cardiac output are patients most likely to benefit from AOP, since in them it may augment cardiac output and thereby stabilize ventilatory control. However, this has not yet been studied with randomized controlled trials.

Another form of cardiac pacing, cardiac resynchronization therapy (CRT) by biventricular pacing, has been shown to improve LV function, exercise capacity, and reduce the composite end point of death and hospitalization (114,115) or death from any cause (116) in suitable HF patients with intraventricular conduction delay. This technique improves cardiac pump function through mechanical resynchronization of abnormal ventricular contraction by pacing both the left and right ventricles in synchrony to prevent leftward shift of the interventricular septum. Ideal patients have a left bundle branch block, LVEF < 35%, with class 3 or 4 NYHA symptoms and sinus rhythm (114–116).

Three investigator groups who studied the effects of CRT in 26 patients with concomitant CSA with "before and after" designed trials showed a 50 to 70% reduction in AHI over one-week to seven-month time spans (106,107,109). This improvement in CSA was associated with an increase of LVEF (24 to 34%), peak oxygen consumption during exercise (10.1 to 13.3 mL/min·kg) (106), and a reduction in mitral regurgitation (109). These data suggested that the improvement in cardiac function contributed significantly to stabilization of respiratory control and alleviation of CSA.

Interestingly, in another case series of HF patients with CSA, CRT also caused a significant 25% reduction of CSA AHI (but not OSA AHI) in conjunction with an improvement of cardiac function (107). The addition of increased rate pacing (15 bpm above the baseline sleeping heart rate) to the CRT group had no additional effect on the AHI and circulation time (107).

However, long-term cardiac pacing in HF patients who have no established pacemaker indication may cause harm by promoting pacing-induced arrhythmias (117). In addition, the implantation of biventricular pacing wires into the coronary sinus is associated with a 2 to 4% implantation/activation failure rate and a 2 to 12% rate of serious adverse events such as infection, pocket erosion, lead displacement, coronary sinus erosion, and pneumothorax (114,116). Thus, CSA or OSA itself cannot constitute an indication for AOP or CRT in HF patients as long as there is no evidence that these interventions improve clinical outcome in HF patients with either CSA or OSA, without other indications for cardiac pacing. To date the indication for CRT is limited to the subgroup of HF patients in sinus rhythm, with significant ventricular conduction delay as well as severely impaired LVEF and exercise capacity.

Cardioversion
Reversion from atrial fibrillation to sinus rhythm is associated with up to 40% improvement in cardiac output (118). Whether reversal of atrial fibrillation to sinus rhythm in HF patients will alter the OSA or CSA severity is yet to be reported; however, if it is successful and if cardiac output improves subsequently, then one would expect an improvement in CSA.

Mitral Valve Surgery and Heart Transplantation
A few case reports have documented alleviation of CSA following surgical repair of severe mitral regurgitation (119,120). In a series of 13 patients with HF who underwent heart transplantation, restoration of LV function was accompanied by a significant reduction in the severity of CSA (121). More than six months after heart transplantation, six patients had no sleep apnea, four patients converted to OSA, and three patients had some residual CSA, although with a shorter apnea-hyperpnea cycle length (65 seconds vs. 31 seconds), suggesting marked improvement in cardiac output. While CSA is rare after heart transplantation, OSA is highly prevalent in such patients (33%) and was found in association with pronounced posttransplant weight gain and arterial hypertension (16 vs. 9 kg and 88 vs. 50% in the OSA and non-OSA groups, respectively) (122).

These data provide further evidence that impaired LV function contributes to the pathogenesis of CSA, and therefore, the first step to treat CSA in patients with HF should be optimizing the treatment of LV failure before targeting ventilation directly.

Positional Therapy
Attention to the body position in HF has important implications in terms of diagnostic symptoms (e.g., orthopnea) as well as therapeutics (e.g., seated position for HF). Vertical (i.e., upright vs. supine) and transverse rotational (i.e., right or left lateral position vs. supine) changes have been independently studied in HF and non-HF populations.

Vertical body position changes (i.e., head up vs. head down) have an impact on breathing patterns of HF populations due to fluid redistribution and altered ventilation perfusion matching. Over half a century ago, the effects of vertical changes in body position on Cheyne–Stokes respiration in patients with HF while awake were studied by Altschule and Iglauer (123). They showed a clear-cut reduction in Cheyne–Stokes respiration with elevation of the head to 45° compared with lying flat in bed. One possible explanation for this effect is that, compared to the supine position, the gravitational effect of moving to the upright position would reduce venous return to the right heart, thereby reducing LV filling pressures, pulmonary congestion, and the tendency to hyperventilate (124).

More recently, Sahlin and coworkers (125) reported that the severity of CSA decreased with a change from the supine to the lateral position (AHI 41 to 26 eph) in 20 HF patients. Szollosi et al. (126) reported a lower central apnea index (19 vs. 7 eph) and higher minimum SpO_2 (91.5 vs. 92.9%) in 20 consecutive HF patients in the nonsupine position compared with the supine position. Significant differences in AHI between right and left positions were not identified (126). The mechanisms for reduced severity of CSA and in the decubitus than in the supine position have not been identified.

Oxygen

Although oxygen has been used ubiquitously within cardiac wards for decades, its use has rarely been subject to scrutiny. Two studies have shown that the acute application of moderate- to high-flow oxygen to normoxic patients with stable HF is associated with a fall in cardiac output and a rise in systemic vascular resistance, PCWP (127), and LV end-diastolic pressure (128).

In patients with acute myocardial infarction, supplemental oxygen has not been shown to be of clinical benefit in normoxic patients. In patients undergoing coronary angiography, administration of oxygen prevents acetylcholine-induced, endothelial-dependent coronary vasodilation but instead causes vasoconstriction (129). This observation suggests that hyperoxia abolishes endothelial-derived vasodilation by endogenous nitric oxide. More importantly, Rawles and Kenmure (130) undertook a randomized controlled trial in 157 uncomplicated patients with myocardial infarction using oxygen at 6 L/min. The oxygen-treated group developed a higher serum aspartate aminotransferase level (AST, indicating greater myocardial damage) and had greater mortality (11% vs. 4%), indicating that supplemental oxygen had adverse effects.

With respect to CSA in patients with HF, in general, oxygen therapy attenuates CSA, but to a variable degree, as shown in Table 2. In acute studies (131), high-flow oxygen was required to diminish AHI (19% reduction) with rises in PCO_2 accompanying these changes. Nearly all trials of oxygen therapy (Table 2) have used the central AHI and oxygen levels as the outcome variables. Only two trials studied also the effects of oxygen on cardiovascular function or ventilation during exercise in HF patients with CSA. Andreas et al. (136) reported that administration of nocturnal oxygen for seven days to 22 HF patients improved peak oxygen consumption (peakVO$_2$) and ventilatory efficiency during exercise (VE/VCO$_2$ slope), but had no effect on quality of life. In subsequent publications, Andreas and colleagues showed that supplemental oxygen was associated with a rise in $PaCO_2$ and a decrease in heart rate, whereas sympathetic activity did not change (139,140). Arzt et al. (138) allocated 10 consecutive patients to nocturnal oxygen and the next 16 consecutive patients to CPAP at 8 cmH$_2$O to 10 cmH$_2$O. The oxygen- and CPAP-treated groups experienced similar reductions in AHI of 70% and 66%, respectively. There was no change in peakVO$_2$ after three months in both treatment arms. In contrast to supplemental oxygen, CPAP significantly improved the VE/VCO$_2$ slope and LVEF (138). No trial has tested the effects of oxygen on morbidity and mortality in HF patients with CSA. Taken together, there are insufficient data to recommend oxygen as a therapy for CSA in patients with HF.

Respiratory Stimulant Therapy

Acetazolamide is a respiratory stimulator by virtue of its carbonic anhydrase inhibition and resultant metabolic acidosis. In a before and after study over a one-month period in CSA patients without known HF, a reduction in central AHI with acetazolamide was

Table 2 Effects of Supplemental Oxygen in HF Patients with CSA

Author	N	Time	Dose (L/min)	Reduction of AHI (%)	Reduction of AHI (eph)
Lorenzi-Filho (131)	10	10 min	variable	19	43→35
Krachman (132)	14	1 night	2	59	44→18
Hanly (133)	9	1 night	2–3	37	30→19
Javaheri (134)	36	1 night	2–4	62	49→29
Franklin (135)	20	1 night	28–60%	85	34→5
Andreas (136)	22	1 wk	4	62[a]	26→10
Staniford (137)	11	4 wk	2	70[b]	13→4 (central)
Arzt (138)	10	12 wk	2	70[c]	29→9

[a]Associated with an increase in peakVO$_2$ from 835 to 960 L/min.
[b]Associated with a fall in urinary norepinephrine from 8.3 to 4.1 nmol/mmol creatinine.
[c]Associated with no change in peakVO$_2$ from 15.4 to 15.6 mL/kg/min and no significant change in LVEF from 30.9 ± 2.4 to 32.5 ± 2.5%.
Abbreviations: HF, heart failure; CSA, central sleep apnea; AHI, apnea-hypopnea index; eph, episodes per hour; LVEF, left ventricular ejection fraction.

noted (141). In 12 patients with HF and CSA, a randomized controlled trial of aceta-zolamide for six days reduced CSA severity (AHI fell by 38%) (142), but no cardio-vascular end points were assessed. Until larger trials involving cardiac end points is undertaken, acetazolamide should be used with caution.

Theophylline is a central respiratory stimulant and weak positive inotrope. In a randomized controlled trial of 15 patients with CSA and HF, five days of theophylline resulted in a fall in AHI; however, there was no change in cardiac function (143). Moreover, a significant rise in arrhythmic side effects was noted. Thus theophylline induced arrhythmogenicity, and a lack of improved cardiac function would preclude its use in clinical management of CSA in HF.

Positive Airway Pressure
Continuous Positive Airway Pressure
The impact of CPAP varies depending on the clinical scenario. In the acute cardiogenic pulmonary edema setting, CPAP, plus oxygen and medical therapy, has been shown to improve physiological variables (heart and respiratory rate, stroke volume) and arterial blood gases faster than oxygen and medical therapy alone and to reduce the intubation rate (144). Meta-analysis of randomized trials suggests that CPAP and bilevel PAP (BPAP) are equipotent (despite 25–50% of acute patients being hypercapnic at presentation) and that the response is usually present within the first 12 hours of CPAP use (145,146).

The effects of CPAP in HF patients with CSA have been tested in several short-term single-center, randomized trials of one to three months' duration. CPAP caused improvements in LVEF and quality of life and reductions in sympathetic activity, mitral regurgitation, and biomarkers of HF (e.g., atrial natriuretic peptide) (70,147–149). Importantly, minute ventilation during sleep fell, and PaCO$_2$ levels rose with CPAP (150), suggesting a marked reduction in the drive to breathe, presumably secondary to unloading of pulmonary vagal irritant receptors by reductions in PCWP and pulmonary congestion.

The only long-term, multicenter randomized controlled trial of CPAP in patients with HF and CSA was the Canadian Positive Airway Pressure for Heart Failure and Central Sleep Apnea trial (CANPAP) (151) (Table 3), where the combined mortality and heart transplantation rate was the primary outcome. Eleven centers recruited 258 optimally medicated patients with LVEF <40% and AHI >15 eph with >50% central in type on attended polysomnography. The trial was terminated by the executive committee after an interim analysis because of a fall in the primary event rate, and an early divergence of event rates favoring the control group, such that the revised estimate of patient numbers needed to see or rule out a beneficial effect was significantly greater than was estimated at the time of study design.

Upon final analysis of the trial, several observations could be made. First, the overall combined death and heart transplant rate fell from 20 to 4 events per 100 person years between 1998 and 2004. This was partly attributed to the greater use of β-blockers and spironolactone over the course of the trial. Second, patients tolerated CPAP well and used it for a mean of 4 to 5 hr/night at a mean pressure of 9 cmH$_2$O, similar to that observed by earlier single-center trials (139,140). Only 15% dropped out of the CPAP arm, which was the same as in the control arm. However, CPAP only led to a 53% reduction in AHI (Fig. 3). Third, LVEF and exercise capacity (six-minute walk distance) increased, while sympathetic activity (plasma norepinephrine) fell consistent with previous studies. Hospitalizations and quality of life were unaltered by CPAP. Fourth, and most important, the heart transplant–free survival was identical in the CPAP and controlled groups (~85% in each after a mean follow-up of 2.2 years) over the entire trial period, and the trend toward lower heart transplant–free survival observed during the first 18 months of the trial crossed over to favor the CPAP group after 18 months, suggesting that there were two different groups with respect to their response to CPAP (Fig. 4).

Indeed, a post hoc analysis (154) indicated that in 210 patients (of 258 total) in whom a polysomnography was performed three months after randomization, patients whose AHI was suppressed below 15 eph, the threshold above which subjects were eligible to be enrolled, had a significantly greater improvement in LVEF and transplant-free survival compared with those with AHI >15 on CPAP and the control group (Fig. 5).

Thus an appropriate approach that could be taken is that in HF patients with CSA, a trial of CPAP could be initiated, with a follow-up polysomnogram performed within three months: if the follow-up AHI is <15 eph, then the patients could be advised to continue with it. If, on the other hand, AHI was ≥15 eph, then the patients could be advised to discontinue it or switch to another form of PAP [e.g., adaptive servoventilation (ASV)].

Bilevel Positive Airway Pressure

Other forms of PAP have been developed to achieve a more effective intervention in patients whose CSA is not sufficiently suppressed by conventional CPAP or who do not tolerate CPAP. While it has been demonstrated that bilevel PAP support with backup rate (BPAPbr) (152,155) and ASV (152,153,155,156) can effectively suppress CSA that is refractory to CPAP, data on mid- or long-term cardiovascular outcomes of HF with sleep apnea are sparse (Table 3).

BPAP was originally designed as a pressure support ventilator to treat hypercapnic respiratory failure. To this end, expiratory positive pressure (EPAP) is applied at a low

Table 3 Randomized Trials of PAP Support in HF Patients with OSA or CSA Measuring Cardiovascular Outcomes

Study	Treatment	Follow-up (mo)	N	Baseline AHI (/hr)	Baseline LVEF (%)	AHI	BPsys	HR	SNA	LVEF	ExC	QoL	Death/HTX
OSA													
Kaneko (21)	CPAP	1	24	41	27	↓↓↓	↓↓	→	NA	↑↑	NA	NA	NA
Usui (44)	CPAP	1	17	40	30	↓↓↓	↓↓	→	→	↑	NA	NA	NA
Ryan (40)	CPAP	1	18	42	30	↓↓↓	↓↓	→	NA	↑↑	NA	NA	NA
Mansfield (28)	CPAP	3	40	26	36	↓↓↓	↓↑	NA	NA	↑	↕	↑	NA
Smith (83)	APAP	1.5	26	36	29	NA	NA	NA	NA	↕	↕	(↑)	NA
CSA													
Naughton (147)	CPAP	3	29	39	20	↓↓	NA	NA	→	↑↑	NA	↑	NA
Sin (148)	CPAP	3/26	29	39	20	↓↓	NA	NA	NA	↑↑	NA	NA	(↓)
Bradley (151)	CPAP	24	258	40	24	↓↑	NA	NA	→	↑←	↑	↑↓	↑
Fietze (152)	BPAPbr	1.5	37	35	26	↓↓↓	NA	↕	NA	↑	NA	NA	NA
Pepperell (30)	ASV	1	30	20	35	NA	NA	NA	NA	↕	NA	↕	NA
Phillipe (153)	ASV	6	25	44	30	↓↓↓	NA	NA	NA	(↑)	NA	↑	NA
Fietze (152)	ASV	1.5	37	32	25	↓↓↓	NA	↕	NA	↑	NA	NA	NA

Abbreviations: AHI, apnea-hypopnea index; BPsys, systolic arterial blood pressure; HR, heart rate; SNA, sympathetic nerve activity; LVEF, left ventricular ejection fraction; ExC, exercise capacity (six-minute walk distance or peakVO$_2$); QoL, quality of life; HTX, heart transplantation; NA, not applicable; PAP, positive airway pressure; CPAP, continuous positive airway pressure; BPAP, bilevel positive airway pressure; HF, heart failure; OSA, obstructive sleep apnea; CSA, central sleep apnea; BPAPbr, BPAP backup rate; ASV, adaptive servoventilation; APAP, Autotitrating positive airway pressure.

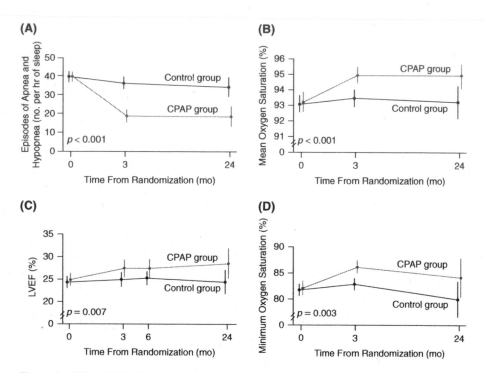

Figure 3 Effect of CPAP on the frequency of episodes of apnea and hypopnea, mean and minimal nocturnal oxygen saturation, and left ventricular ejection fraction. CPAP caused significant long-term reductions in the AHI (Panel A), and increases in mean and minimum nocturnal oxygen saturation (Panel A and D), and left ventricular ejection fraction (LVEF, Panel P). p-Values represent time-treatment interactions over the entire trial. Data represented are mean (circles) and 95% confidence interval (vertical bars). *Abbreviations*: CPAP, continuous positive airway pressure; AHI, apnea-hypopnea index. *Source*: From Ref. 13.

level to maintain lung volume and V/Q matching, upon which a higher level of inspiratory pressure (IPAP) is applied to augment ventilation. In the setting of OSA with hypercapnia, EPAP is usually set to the lowest level maintaining upper airway patency, thus suppressing obstructive apneas and hypopneas, while IPAP is set to increase ventilation and maintain oxygenation. BPAP can be applied with or without a backup rate.

BPAP has also been used to treat CSA in patients with HF. In one randomized crossover trial of two weeks' duration ($n = 16$), Kohnlein and colleagues (157) found that BPAP (without backup rate, mean 8.5/3 cmH$_2$O) and CPAP (mean 8.5 cmH$_2$O) led to a similar suppression of CSA: the pretreatment AHI of 27 was significantly reduced by CPAP and BPAP to 8 eph and 7 eph, respectively.

In another trial involving HF patients with CSA, BPAPbr suppressed CSA more effectively than CPAP during one night of treatment (AHI was 45 eph in the untreated state, 27 eph on CPAP, and 15 eph on BPAPbr) (155). CPAP and ASV led to a significant increase in capillary PCO$_2$ (by 4.3 mmHg and 3.6 mmHg, respectively) from the evening before to the morning after treatment, while with BPAPbr (set at the patients' spontaneous awake respiratory rate less 2 breaths/min), PCO$_2$ did not change overnight

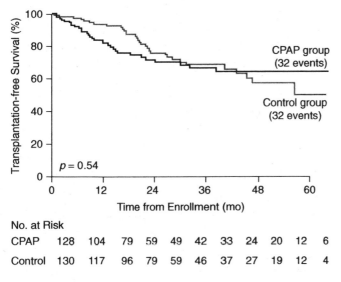

No. at Risk

CPAP	128	104	79	59	49	42	33	24	20	12	6
Control	130	117	96	79	59	46	37	27	19	12	4

Figure 4 CANPAP: Heart-transplantation–free survival. There was no difference in transplant free survival rates between the control and CPAP groups (Hazard ratio [HR] = 1.16, p = 0.54). However, there was an early divergence of event rates favouring the control group (HR = 1.5, p = 0.02) that crossed over after 18 months in favour of CPAP (HR = 0.66, p = 0.06). *Abbreviations*: CANPAP, canadian positive airway pressure for heart failure and central sleep apnea trial; CPAP, continuous positive airway pressure. *Source*: From Ref. 13.

(155), indicating that hyperventilation is maintained with this treatment. In the only randomized trial in which a cardiac physiological outcome was measured, Fietze et al. (152) compared the effects of BPAPbr to those of ASV in 37 HF patients with CSA during a six-week treatment period. While in the ASV group a modest nonsignificant improvement in LVEF was observed (24.6 to 26.5%), LVEF increased significantly in the BPAPbr group (25.5 to 31.1%, p < 0.01). In both groups suppression of CSA was similar. There was no obvious explanation for the different effects of the two interventions on LVEF.

Adaptive Pressure Support Servoventilation

ASV has been applied to HF patients with CSA with 4 to 5 cmH$_2$O EPAP and a minimum of 8 cmH$_2$O end-IPAP support during regular breathing. When a central apnea is detected, IPAP support increases up to 15 cmH$_2$O to maintain minute ventilation at 90% of the long-term average ventilation. Because the device provides minimal positive pressure during normal breathing and IPAP support on top of a relatively low EPAP only in the presence of respiratory events, the average pressure is lower than CPAP of 8 to 12.5 cmH$_2$O (155).

Teschler et al. (155) compared the effects of a single night each of supplemental oxygen (2 L/min), CPAP (mean 9.3 cmH$_2$O), BPAP (mean 13.5/5.2 cmH$_2$O), and ASV (mean IPAP 11–15 cmH$_2$O and EPAP 4–6 cmH$_2$O) on CSA and sleep quality on five consecutive nights in random order in 14 HF patients. The AHI decline from 45 (untreated) to 6 eph with ASV was significantly greater compared to all other tested therapies. Improvements in sleep structure characterized by increases in slow-wave and REM sleep

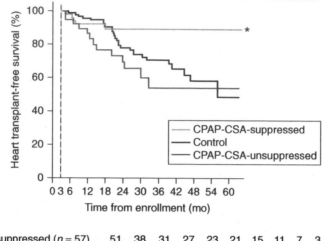

No. at Risk

CPAP-CSA-suppressed ($n = 57$)	51	38	31	27	23	21	15	11	7	3
Control ($n = 110$)	99	83	71	50	41	33	22	15	9	3
CPAP-CSA-unsuppressed ($n = 43$)	36	27	22	18	12	9	6	6	4	2

Figure 5 CANPAP: Heart-transplantation–free survival according to the suppression of CSA by CPAP. Kaplan-Meier survival plots demonstrating that compared to the control group, the CPAP-CSA-suppressed group (AHI<15 events per hour after 3 months) had significantly improved heart transplant-free survival (*unadjusted $p = 0.043$; adjusted for age and AHI at baseline $p = 0.034$), while the CPAP-CSA-unsuppressed group (AHI<15 events per hour after 3 months) did not (unadjusted and adjusted $p > 0.05$). *Abbreviations*: CANPAP, canadian positive airway pressure for heart failure and central sleep apnea trial; CSA, central sleep apnea; CPAP, continuous positive airway pressure. *Source*: From Ref. 100.

time occurred only with ASV. Although each treatment was applied for one night only, the effects on CSA were comparable to studies with longer treatment periods of CPAP (151), BPAPbr, and ASV (152). However, no clinical or cardiovascular outcomes were assessed.

In another trial by Arzt and colleagues (156), ASV was evaluated in a sample of 14 HF patients who had substantial residual CSA (mean AHI 22 eph) after a mean treatment period of 27 weeks on CPAP (8.3 cmH$_2$O)/BPAP (13.5/7.6 cmH$_2$O) therapy. ASV (8.0/6.5 cmH$_2$O) suppressed CSA to an AHI of 4 eph, indicating that ASV suppresses CSA that is refractory to conventional PAP therapy (CPAP or BPAP) using lower pressures (156). However, no cardiovascular outcomes were assessed.

Philippe et al. (153) found in a six-month parallel randomized trial of ASV and CPAP in 25 HF patients with CSA that treatment adherence (5.5 vs. 3.8 hr/night) and improvements in quality of life (Minesota Living with HF Questionnaire) at six months were significantly greater in the ASV group. Although LVEF was not systematically evaluated, it improved significantly more in a subset of seven patients treated with ASV versus a subset of six patients treated with CPAP. These results are difficult to interpret, since no attempt was made to titrate CPAP to an optimum level. Pepperell and colleagues (30) performed a randomized trial of therapeutic versus subtherapeutic ASV over one month in 30 stable HF patients with CSA with mild daytime hypersomnolence. The therapeutic and subtherapeutic ASV delivered 8.0 to 15.0 cmH$_2$O and 2.5 to 4.5 cmH$_2$O IPAP support, respectively. Nocturnal urinary metadrenaline and daytime brain natriuretic peptide concentrations were reduced, and daytime alertness increased significantly more by therapeutic than subtherapeutic ASV. LVEF was not systematically evaluated but, where measured, did not improve on ASV. While the effects of ASV on LVEF have been inconsistent (153), and its long-term cardiovascular effects in HF patients with CSA remain uncertain, ASV is currently being subjected to large-scale, long-term randomized trials (e.g., SERVE-HF; http://servehf.com) to evaluate such effects.

IV. Summary

OSA and CSA are common in HF patients and likely contribute to HF severity, symptoms, and prognosis. As their pathogeneses differ, so too do the treatment options. In the setting of OSA-HF, the main objective is to maintain upper airway patency and prevent "downstream effects" on the heart. CPAP best accomplishes this and causes improvements in cardiovascular function. However, most HF patients with OSA do not complain of excessive daytime sleepiness and therefore lack the usual indication to be treated. It therefore remains unclear whether alleviation of OSA in such patients improves symptoms or quality of life. Moreover, CPAP's effects on morbidity and mortality have not been tested in a randomized trial, and it is therefore not clear whether short-term improvements in cardiovascular function induced by CPAP translate into reduced morbidity or mortality. In contrast, in the setting of CSA-HF, identification of the cause of HF (pump, valve, rhythm) is crucial. Following usual targeted management of HF, patients with residual CSA in whom refractory and unstable HF is suspected or sleep apnea–related symptoms persist should be considered for a trial of CPAP, titrated carefully (e.g., from 5 to 10 cmH$_2$O) over several days, with a repeat sleep study on CPAP within three months. On the basis of that study, if AHI is <15 eph, patients should consider long-term CPAP, as it appears to carry with it a survival benefit. In those patients with AHI >15 eph at three months on CPAP, CPAP should be stopped and alternative devices (e.g., ASV or BPAP) could be considered. As with OSA, large-scale randomized trials will be required to determine whether alleviation of CSA will reduce morbidity and mortality in patients with HF.

References

1. Redfield MM, Jacobsen SJ, Burnett JC Jr., et al. Burden of systolic and diastolic ventricular dysfunction in the community: appreciating the scope of the heart failure epidemic. JAMA 2003; 289(2):194–202.
2. Levy D, Kenchaiah S, Larson MG, et al. Long-term trends in the incidence of and survival with heart failure. N Engl J Med 2002; 347(18):1397–1402.
3. Arzt M, Bradley TD. Treatment of sleep apnea in heart failure. Am J Respir Crit Care Med 2006; 173(12):1300–1308.
4. Javaheri S, Parker TJ, Liming JD, et al. Sleep apnea in 81 ambulatory male patients with stable heart failure. Types and their prevalences, consequences, and presentations. Circulation 1998; 97(21):2154–2159.
5. Sin DD, Fitzgerald F, Parker JD, et al. Risk factors for central and obstructive sleep apnea in 450 men and women with congestive heart failure. Am J Respir Crit Care Med 1999; 160(4): 1101–1106.

6. Solin P, Bergin P, Richardson M, et al. Influence of pulmonary capillary wedge pressure on central apnea in heart failure. Circulation 1999; 99(12):1574–1579.
7. Malone S, Liu PP, Holloway R, et al. Obstructive sleep apnoea in patients with dilated cardiomyopathy: effects of continuous positive airway pressure. Lancet 1991; 338(8781): 1480–1484.
8. Somers VK, Dyken ME, Clary MP, et al. Sympathetic neural mechanisms in obstructive sleep apnea. J Clin Invest 1995; 96(4):1897–1904.
9. Tkacova R, Rankin F, Fitzgerald FS, et al. Effects of continuous positive airway pressure on obstructive sleep apnea and left ventricular afterload in patients with heart failure. Circulation 1998; 98(21):2269–2275.
10. Tolle FA, Judy WV, Yu PL, et al. Reduced stroke volume related to pleural pressure in obstructive sleep apnea. J Appl Physiol 1983; 55(6):1718–1724.
11. Wexels JC, Mjos OD. Effects of carbon dioxide and pH on myocardial function in dogs with acute left ventricular failure. Crit Care Med 1987; 15(12):1116–1120.
12. Becker HF, Jerrentrup A, Ploch T, et al. Effect of nasal continuous positive airway pressure treatment on blood pressure in patients with obstructive sleep apnea. Circulation 2003; 107(1):68–73.
13. Drager LF, Bortolotto LA, Lorenzi MC, et al. Early signs of atherosclerosis in obstructive sleep apnea. Am J Respir Crit Care Med 2005; 172(5):613–618.
14. Minoguchi K, Yokoe T, Tazaki T, et al. Increased carotid intima-media thickness and serum inflammatory markers in obstructive sleep apnea. Am J Respir Crit Care Med 2005; 172(5): 625–630.
15. Peppard PE, Young T, Palta M, et al. Prospective study of the association between sleep-disordered breathing and hypertension. N Engl J Med 2000; 342(19):1378–1384.
16. Arzt M, Young T, Finn L, et al. Association of sleep-disordered breathing and the occurrence of stroke. Am J Respir Crit Care Med 2005; 172(11):1447–1451.
17. Marin JM, Carrizo SJ, Vicente E, et al. Long-term cardiovascular outcomes in men with obstructive sleep apnoea-hypopnoea with or without treatment with continuous positive airway pressure: an observational study. Lancet 2005; 365(9464):1046–1053.
18. Wang H, Parker JD, Newton GE, et al. Influence of obstructive sleep apnea on mortality in patients with heart failure. J Am Coll Cardiol 2007; 49(15):1625–1631.
19. Yaggi HK, Concato J, Kernan WN, et al. Obstructive sleep apnea as a risk factor for stroke and death. N Engl J Med 2005; 353(19):2034–2041.
20. Drager LF, Bortolotto LA, Figueiredo AC, et al. Effects of continuous positive airway pressure on early signs of atherosclerosis in obstructive sleep apnea. Am J Respir Crit Care Med 2007; 176(7):706–712.
21. Kaneko Y, Floras JS, Usui K, et al. Cardiovascular effects of continuous positive airway pressure in patients with heart failure and obstructive sleep apnea. N Engl J Med 2003; 348(13): 1233–1241.
22. Pepperell JC, Ramdassingh-Dow S, Crosthwaite N, et al. Ambulatory blood pressure after therapeutic and subtherapeutic nasal continuous positive airway pressure for obstructive sleep apnoea: a randomised parallel trial. Lancet 2002; 359(9302):204–210.
23. Johns MW. Reliability and factor analysis of the Epworth Sleepiness Scale. Sleep 1992; 15(4): 376–381.
24. Johns MW. Sleepiness in different situations measured by the Epworth Sleepiness Scale. Sleep 1994; 17(8):703–710.
25. Javaheri S, Shukla R, Zeigler H, et al. Central sleep apnea, right ventricular dysfunction, and low diastolic blood pressure are predictors of mortality in systolic heart failure. J Am Coll Cardiol 2007; 49(20):2028–2034.
26. Nieto FJ, Young TB, Lind BK, et al. Association of sleep-disordered breathing, sleep apnea, and hypertension in a large community-based study. Sleep Heart Health Study. JAMA 2000; 283(14):1829–1836.

27. Arzt M, Young T, Finn L, et al. Sleepiness and sleep in patients with both systolic heart failure and obstructive sleep apnea. Arch Intern Med 2006; 166(16):1716–1722.
28. Mansfield DR, Gollogly NC, Kaye DM, et al. Controlled trial of continuous positive airway pressure in obstructive sleep apnea and heart failure. Am J Respir Crit Care Med 2004; 169(3): 361–366.
29. Hastings PC, Vazir A, O'Driscoll DM, et al. Symptom burden of sleep-disordered breathing in mild-to-moderate congestive heart failure patients. Eur Respir J 2006; 27(4):748–755.
30. Pepperell JC, Maskell NA, Jones DR, et al. A randomized controlled trial of adaptive ventilation for Cheyne-Stokes breathing in heart failure. Am J Respir Crit Care Med 2003; 168(9):1109–1114.
31. Cintron G, Johnson G, Francis G, et al. Prognostic significance of serial changes in left ventricular ejection fraction in patients with congestive heart failure. The V-HeFT VA Cooperative Studies Group. Circulation 1993; 87(6 suppl):VI17–VI23.
32. Mancini DM, Eisen H, Kussmaul W, et al. Value of peak exercise oxygen consumption for optimal timing of cardiac transplantation in ambulatory patients with heart failure. Circulation 1991; 83(3):778–786.
33. Ponikowski P, Francis DP, Piepoli MF, et al. Enhanced ventilatory response to exercise in patients with chronic heart failure and preserved exercise tolerance: marker of abnormal cardiorespiratory reflex control and predictor of poor prognosis. Circulation 2001; 103(7): 967–972.
34. Cahalin LP, Mathier MA, Semigran MJ, et al. The six-minute walk test predicts peak oxygen uptake and survival in patients with advanced heart failure. Chest 1996; 110(2): 325–332.
35. Rostagno C, Olivo G, Comeglio M, et al. Prognostic value of 6-minute walk corridor test in patients with mild to moderate heart failure: comparison with other methods of functional evaluation. Eur J Heart Fail 2003; 5(3):247–252.
36. Bittner V, Weiner DH, Yusuf S, et al. Prediction of mortality and morbidity with a 6-minute walk test in patients with left ventricular dysfunction. SOLVD Investigators. JAMA 1993, 270(14):1702–1707.
37. Demers C, McKelvie RS, Negassa A, et al. Reliability, validity, and responsiveness of the six-minute walk test in patients with heart failure. Am Heart J 2001; 142(4):698–703.
38. Riley M, McParland J, Stanford CF, et al. Oxygen consumption during corridor walk testing in chronic cardiac failure. Eur Heart J 1992; 13(6):789–793.
39. Zugck C, Kruger C, Durr S, et al. Is the 6-minute walk test a reliable substitute for peak oxygen uptake in patients with dilated cardiomyopathy? Eur Heart J 2000; 21(7):540–549.
40. Ryan CM, Usui K, Floras JS, et al. Effect of continuous positive airway pressure on ventricular ectopy in heart failure patients with obstructive sleep apnoea. Thorax 2005; 60(9): 781–785.
41. Ruttanaumpawan P, Gilman MP, Usui K, et al. Sustained effect of continuous positive airway pressure on baroreflex sensitivity in congestive heart failure patients with obstructive sleep apnea. J Hypertens 2008; 26(6):1163–1168.
42. Gilman MP, Floras JS, Usui K, et al. Continuous positive airway pressure increases heart rate variability in heart failure patients with obstructive sleep apnoea. Clin Sci (Lond) 2008; 114(3):243–249.
43. Solin P, Kaye DM, Little PJ, et al. Impact of sleep apnea on sympathetic nervous system activity in heart failure. Chest 2003; 123(4):1119–1126.
44. Usui K, Bradley TD, Spaak J, et al. Inhibition of awake sympathetic nerve activity of heart failure patients with obstructive sleep apnea by nocturnal continuous positive airway pressure. J Am Coll Cardiol 2005; 45:2008–2011.
45. Mansfield D, Kaye DM, Brunner La Rocca H, et al. Raised sympathetic nerve activity in heart failure and central sleep apnea is due to heart failure severity. Circulation 2003; 107(10):1396–1400.

46. Cartwright RD. Effect of sleep position on sleep apnea severity. Sleep 1984; 7(2):110–114.
47. Oksenberg A, Silverberg DS, Arons E, et al. Positional vs nonpositional obstructive sleep apnea patients: anthropomorphic, nocturnal polysomnographic, and multiple sleep latency test data. Chest 1997; 112(3):629–639.
48. Oksenberg A, Khamaysi I, Silverberg DS, et al. Association of body position with severity of apneic events in patients with severe nonpositional obstructive sleep apnea. Chest 2000; 118(4):1018–1024.
49. Oksenberg A, Silverberg DS, Arons E, et al. The sleep supine position has a major effect on optimal nasal continuous positive airway pressure: relationship with rapid eye movements and non-rapid eye movements sleep, body mass index, respiratory disturbance index, and age. Chest 1999; 116(4):1000–1006.
50. Penzel T, Moller M, Becker HF, et al. Effect of sleep position and sleep stage on the collapsibility of the upper airways in patients with sleep apnea. Sleep 2001; 24(1):90–95.
51. Berger M, Oksenberg A, Silverberg DS, et al. Avoiding the supine position during sleep lowers 24 h blood pressure in obstructive sleep apnea (OSA) patients. J Hum Hypertens 1997; 11(10):657–664.
52. Peppard PE, Young T, Palta M, et al. Longitudinal study of moderate weight change and sleep-disordered breathing. JAMA 2000; 284(23):3015–3021.
53. Davos CH, Doehner W, Rauchhaus M, et al. Body mass and survival in patients with chronic heart failure without cachexia: the importance of obesity. J Card Fail 2003; 9(1):29–35.
54. Dixon JB, Schachter LM, O'Brien PE. Sleep disturbance and obesity: changes following surgically induced weight loss. Arch Intern Med 2001; 161(1):102–106.
55. Kenchaiah S, Evans JC, Levy D, et al. Obesity and the risk of heart failure. N Engl J Med 2002; 347(5):305–313.
56. Avelar E, Cloward TV, Walker JM, et al. Left ventricular hypertrophy in severe obesity: interactions among blood pressure, nocturnal hypoxemia, and body mass. Hypertension 2007; 49(1):34–39.
57. Alpert MA, Terry BE, Mulekar M, et al. Cardiac morphology and left ventricular function in normotensive morbidly obese patients with and without congestive heart failure, and effect of weight loss. Am J Cardiol 1997; 80(6):736–740.
58. Sjostrom L, Narbro K, Sjostrom CD, et al. Effects of bariatric surgery on mortality in Swedish obese subjects. N Engl J Med 2007; 357(8):741–752.
59. Adams TD, Gress RE, Smith SC, et al. Long-term mortality after gastric bypass surgery. N Engl J Med 2007; 357(8):753–761.
60. Gotsopoulos H, Kelly JJ, Cistulli PA. Oral appliance therapy reduces blood pressure in obstructive sleep apnea: a randomized, controlled trial. Sleep 2004; 27(5):934–941.
61. Gorur K, Doven O, Unal M, et al. Preoperative and postoperative cardiac and clinical findings of patients with adenotonsillar hypertrophy. Int J Pediatr Otorhinolaryngol 2001; 59(1):41–46.
62. Amin RS, Kimball TR, Kalra M, et al. Left ventricular function in children with sleep-disordered breathing. Am J Cardiol 2005; 95(6):801–804.
63. Guilleminault C, Simmons FB, Motta J, et al. Obstructive sleep apnea syndrome and tracheostomy. Long-term follow-up experience. Arch Intern Med 1981; 141(8):985–988.
64. Tilkian AG, Guilleminault C, Schroeder JS, et al. Sleep-induced apnea syndrome. Prevalence of cardiac arrhythmias and their reversal after tracheostomy. Am J Med 1977; 63(3):348–358.
65. Fletcher EC, Miller J, Schaaf JW, et al. Urinary catecholamines before and after tracheostomy in patients with obstructive sleep apnea and hypertension. Sleep 1987; 10(1):35–44.
66. Naughton MT, Rahman MA, Hara K, et al. Effect of continuous positive airway pressure on intrathoracic and left ventricular transmural pressures in patients with congestive heart failure. Circulation 1995; 91(6):1725–1731.

67. Mehta S, Liu PP, Fitzgerald FS, et al. Effects of continuous positive airway pressure on cardiac volumes in patients with ischemic and dilated cardiomyopathy. Am J Respir Crit Care Med 2000; 161(1):128–134.
68. Shivalkar B, Van de Heyning C, Kerremans M, et al. Obstructive sleep apnea syndrome: more insights on structural and functional cardiac alterations, and the effects of treatment with continuous positive airway pressure. J Am Coll Cardiol 2006; 47(7):1433–1439.
69. Kaye DM, Mansfield D, Aggarwal A, et al. Acute effects of continuous positive airway pressure on cardiac sympathetic tone in congestive heart failure. Circulation 2001; 103(19): 2336–2338.
70. Naughton MT, Benard DC, Liu PP, et al. Effects of nasal CPAP on sympathetic activity in patients with heart failure and central sleep apnea. Am J Respir Crit Care Med 1995; 152(2): 473–479.
71. Yoshinaga K, Burwash IG, Leech JA, et al. The effects of continuous positive airway pressure on myocardial energetics in patients with heart failure and obstructive sleep apnea. J Am Coll Cardiol 2007; 49(4):450–458.
72. Gehlbach BK, Geppert E. The pulmonary manifestations of left heart failure. Chest 2004; 125(2):669–682.
73. Light RW, George RB. Serial pulmonary function in patients with acute heart failure. Arch Intern Med 1983; 143(3):429–433.
74. Hosenpud JD, Stibolt TA, Atwal K, et al. Abnormal pulmonary function specifically related to congestive heart failure: comparison of patients before and after cardiac transplantation. Am J Med 1990; 88(5):493–496.
75. Naum CC, Sciurba FC, Rogers RM. Pulmonary function abnormalities in chronic severe car diomyopathy preceding cardiac transplantation. Am Rev Respir Dis 1992; 145(6):1334–1338.
76. De Pasquale CG, Arnolda LF, Doyle IR, et al. Prolonged alveolocapillary barrier damage after acute cardiogenic pulmonary edema. Crit Care Med 2003; 31(4):1060–1067.
77. De Pasquale CG, Bersten AD, Doyle IR, et al. Infarct-induced chronic heart failure increases bidirectional protein movement across the alveolocapillary barrier. Am J Physiol Heart Circ Physiol 2003; 284(6):H2136–H2145.
78. Naughton MT, Bookman I, Floras JS, et al. Effect of CPAP on respiratory mechanics in heart failure. Am J Respir Crit Care Med 1995; 151(4):A706.
79. Krachman SL, Crocetti J, Berger TJ, et al. Effects of nasal continuous positive airway pressure on oxygen body stores in patients with Cheyne-Stokes respiration and congestive heart failure. Chest 2003; 123(1):59–66.
80. Barach AL, Swenson P. Effect of breathing gases under positive pressure on lumens of small and medium sized bronchi. Arch Int Med 1939; 63:946–948.
81. Kaye DM, Mansfield D, Naughton MT. Continuous positive airway pressure decreases myocardial oxygen consumption in heart failure. Clin Sci (Lond) 2004; 106(6):599–603.
82. Arias MA, Garcia-Rio F, Alonso-Fernandez A, et al. Obstructive sleep apnea syndrome affects left ventricular diastolic function: effects of nasal continuous positive airway pressure in men. Circulation 2005; 112(3):375–383.
83. Smith LA, Vennelle M, Gardner RS, et al. Auto-titrating continuous positive airway pressure therapy in patients with chronic heart failure and obstructive sleep apnoea: a randomized placebo-controlled trial. Eur Heart J 2007; 28(10):1221–1227.
84. Phillipson EA. Control of breathing during sleep. Am Rev Respir Dis 1978; 118(5):909–939.
85. Lorenzi-Filho G, Azevedo ER, Parker JD, et al. Relationship of carbon dioxide tension in arterial blood to pulmonary wedge pressure in heart failure. Eur Respir J 2002; 19(1):37–40.
86. Yu J, Zhang JF, Fletcher EC. Stimulation of breathing by activation of pulmonary peripheral afferents in rabbits. J Appl Physiol 1998; 85(4):1485–1492.
87. Javaheri S. A mechanism of central sleep apnea in patients with heart failure. N Engl J Med 1999; 341(13):949–954.

88. Solin P, Roebuck T, Johns DP, et al. Peripheral and central ventilatory responses in central sleep apnea with and without congestive heart failure. Am J Respir Crit Care Med 2000; 162(6):2194–2200.
89. Szollosi I, Thompson BR, Krum H, et al. Impaired pulmonary diffusing capacity and hypoxia in heart failure correlates with central sleep apnea severity. Chest 2008; 134:67–72.
90. Crowell JW, Guyton AC, Moore JW. Basic oscillating mechanism of Cheyne-Stokes breathing. Am J Physiol 1956; 187(2):395–398.
91. Leung RS, Floras JS, Lorenzi-Filho G, et al. Influence of Cheyne-Stokes respiration on cardiovascular oscillations in heart failure. Am J Respir Crit Care Med 2003; 167(11): 1534–1539.
92. Arzt M, Harth M, Luchner A, et al. Enhanced ventilatory response to exercise in patients with chronic heart failure and central sleep apnea. Circulation 2003; 107(15):1998–2003.
93. Pozzoli M, Cioffi G, Traversi E, et al. Predictors of primary atrial fibrillation and concomitant clinical and hemodynamic changes in patients with chronic heart failure: a prospective study in 344 patients with baseline sinus rhythm. J Am Coll Cardiol 1998; 32(1): 197–204.
94. Dark DS, Pingleton SK, Kerby GR, et al. Breathing pattern abnormalities and arterial oxygen desaturation during sleep in the congestive heart failure syndrome. Improvement following medical therapy. Chest 1987; 91(6):833–836.
95. Walsh JT, Andrews R, Starling R, et al. Effects of captopril and oxygen on sleep apnoea in patients with mild to moderate congestive cardiac failure. Br Heart J 1995; 73(3):237–241.
96. MacDonald M, Fang J, Pittman SD, et al. The current prevalence of sleep disordered breathing in congestive heart failure patients treated with beta-blockers. J Clin Sleep Med 2008; 4(1):38–42.
97. Yumino D, Wang H, Floras JS, et al. Prevalence and physiological predictors of sleep apnea in heart failure. J Cardiac Fail 2009; 15:279–285.
98. Zilberman M, Silverberg DS, Bits I, et al. Improvement of anemia with erythropoietin and intravenous iron reduces sleep-related breathing disorders and improves daytime sleepiness in anemic patients with congestive heart failure. Am Heart J 2007; 154(5):870–876.
99. Kato M, Phillips BG, Sigurdsson G, et al. Effects of sleep deprivation on neural circulatory control. Hypertension 2000; 35(5):1173–1175.
100. Garrigue S, Bordier P, Jais P, et al. Benefit of atrial pacing in sleep apnea syndrome. N Engl J Med 2002; 346(6):404–412.
101. Simantirakis EN, Schiza SE, Chrysostomakis SI, et al. Atrial overdrive pacing for the obstructive sleep apnea-hypopnea syndrome. N Engl J Med 2005; 353(24):2568–2577.
102. Pepin JL, Defaye P, Garrigue S, et al. Overdrive atrial pacing does not improve obstructive sleep apnoea syndrome. Eur Respir J 2005; 25(2):343–347.
103. Luthje L, Unterberg-Buchwald C, Dajani D, et al. Atrial overdrive pacing in sleep apnea patients with implanted pacemaker. Am J Respir Crit Care Med 2005; 172:118–122.
104. Unterberg C, Luthje L, Szych J, et al. Atrial overdrive pacing compared to CPAP in patients with obstructive sleep apnoea syndrome. Eur Heart J 2005; 26(23):2568–2575.
105. Krahn AD, Yee R, Erickson MK, et al. Physiologic pacing in patients with obstructive sleep apnea: a prospective, randomized crossover trial. J Am Coll Cardiol 2006; 47:379–383.
106. Sinha AM, Skobel EC, Breithardt OA, et al. Cardiac resynchronization therapy improves central sleep apnea and Cheyne-Stokes respiration in patients with chronic heart failure. J Am Coll Cardiol 2004; 44(1):68–71.
107. Gabor JY, Newman DA, Barnard-Roberts V, et al. Improvement in Cheyne-Stokes respiration following cardiac resynchronisation therapy. Eur Respir J 2005; 26(1):95–100.
108. Stanchina ML, Ellison K, Malhotra A, et al. The impact of cardiac resynchronization therapy on obstructive sleep apnea in heart failure patients: a pilot study. Chest 2007; 132(2):433–439.

109. Kato I, Shiomi T, Sasanabe R, et al. Effects of physiological cardiac pacing on sleep-disordered breathing in patients with chronic bradydysrhythmias. Psychiatry Clin Neurosci 2001; 55(3):257–258.

110. Bradley TD, Brown IG, Grossman RF, et al. Pharyngeal size in snorers, nonsnorers, and patients with obstructive sleep apnea. N Engl J Med 1986; 315(21):1327–1331.

111. Naughton M, Benard D, Tam A, et al. Role of hyperventilation in the pathogenesis of central sleep apneas in patients with congestive heart failure. Am Rev Respir Dis 1993; 148(2):330–338.

112. Sharafkhaneh A, Sharafkhaneh H, Bredikus A, et al. Effect of atrial overdrive pacing on obstructive sleep apnea in patients with systolic heart failure. Sleep Med 2007; 8(1):31–36.

113. Krahn AD, Yee R, Erickson MK, et al. Physiologic pacing in patients with obstructive sleep apnea: a prospective, randomized crossover trial. J Am Coll Cardiol 2006; 47(2):379–383.

114. Abraham WT, Fisher WG, Smith AL, et al. Cardiac resynchronization in chronic heart failure. N Engl J Med 2002; 346(24):1845–1853.

115. Bristow MR, Saxon LA, Boehmer J, et al. Cardiac-resynchronization therapy with or without an implantable defibrillator in advanced chronic heart failure. N Engl J Med 2004; 350(21):2140–2150.

116. Cleland JG, Daubert JC, Erdmann E, et al. The effect of cardiac resynchronization on morbidity and mortality in heart failure. N Engl J Med 2005; 352(15):1539–1549.

117. Himmrich E, Przibille O, Zellerhoff C, et al. Proarrhythmic effect of pacemaker stimulation in patients with implanted cardioverter-defibrillators. Circulation 2003; 108(2):192–197.

118. Reale A. Acute effects of countershock conversion of atrial fibrillation upon right and left heart hemodynamics. Circulation 1965; 32:214–222.

119. Rubin AE, Gottlieb SH, Gold AR, et al. Elimination of central sleep apnoea by mitral valvuloplasty: the role of feedback delay in periodic breathing. Thorax 2004; 59(2):174–176.

120. Yasuma F, Hayashi H, Noda S, et al. A case of mitral regurgitation whose nocturnal periodic breathing was improved after mitral valve replacement. Jpn Heart J 1995; 36(2): 267–272.

121. Mansfield DR, Solin P, Roebuck T, et al. The effect of successful heart transplant treatment of heart failure on central sleep apnea. Chest 2003; 124(5):1675–1681.

122. Javaheri S, Abraham WT, Brown C, et al. Prevalence of obstructive sleep apnoea and periodic limb movement in 45 subjects with heart transplantation. Eur Heart J 2004; 25(3): 260–266.

123. Altschule MD, Iglauer A. The effect of position on periodic breathing in chronic cardiac decompensation. N Engl J Med 1958; 259(22):1064–1066.

124. Churchill E, Cope O. The rapid shallow breathing resulting from pulmonary congestion and edema. J Exper Med 1929; 49:531–537.

125. Sahlin C, Svanborg E, Stenlund H, et al. Cheyne-Stokes respiration and supine dependency. Eur Respir J 2005; 25(5):829–833.

126. Szollosi I, Roebuck T, Thompson B, et al. Lateral sleeping position reduces severity of central sleep apnea/Cheyne-Stokes respiration. Sleep 2006; 29(8):1045–1051.

127. Haque WA, Boehmer J, Clemson BS, et al. Hemodynamic effects of supplemental oxygen administration in congestive heart failure. J Am Coll Cardiol 1996; 27(2):353–357.

128. Mak S, Azevedo ER, Liu PP, et al. Effect of hyperoxia on left ventricular function and filling pressures in patients with and without congestive heart failure. Chest 2001; 120(2): 467–473.

129. McNulty PH, King N, Scott S, et al. Effects of supplemental oxygen administration on coronary blood flow in patients undergoing cardiac catheterization. Am J Physiol Heart Circ Physiol 2005; 288(3):H1057–H1062.

130. Rawles JM, Kenmure AC. Controlled trial of oxygen in uncomplicated myocardial infarction. Br Med J 1976; 1(6018):1121–1123.

131. Lorenzi-Filho G, Rankin F, Bies I, et al. Effects of inhaled carbon dioxide and oxygen on Cheyne-Stokes respiration in patients with heart failure. Am J Respir Crit Care Med 1999; 159(5 pt 1):1490–1498.

132. Krachman SL, D'Alonzo GE, Berger TJ, et al. Comparison of oxygen therapy with nasal continuous positive airway pressure on Cheyne-Stokes respiration during sleep in congestive heart failure. Chest 1999; 116(6):1550–1557.

133. Hanly PJ, Millar TW, Steljes DG, et al. The effect of oxygen on respiration and sleep in patients with congestive heart failure. Ann Intern Med 1989; 111(10):777–782.

134. Javaheri S, Ahmed M, Parker TJ, et al. Effects of nasal O2 on sleep-related disordered breathing in ambulatory patients with stable heart failure. Sleep 1999; 22(8):1101–1106.

135. Franklin KA, Eriksson P, Sahlin C, et al. Reversal of central sleep apnea with oxygen. Chest 1997; 111(1):163–169.

136. Andreas S, Clemens C, Sandholzer H, et al. Improvement of exercise capacity with treatment of Cheyne-Stokes respiration in patients with congestive heart failure. J Am Coll Cardiol 1996; 27(6):1486–1490.

137. Staniforth AD, Kinnear WJ, Starling R, et al. Effect of oxygen on sleep quality, cognitive function and sympathetic activity in patients with chronic heart failure and Cheyne-Stokes respiration. Eur Heart J 1998; 19(6):922–928.

138. Arzt M, Schulz M, Wensel R, et al. Nocturnal continuous positive airway pressure improves ventilatory efficiency during exercise in patients with chronic heart failure. Chest 2005; 127(3):794–802.

139. Andreas S, Bingeli C, Mohacsi P, et al. Nasal oxygen and muscle sympathetic nerve activity in heart failure. Chest 2003; 123(2):366–371.

140. Andreas S, Plock EH, Heindl S, et al. Nasal oxygen effects on arterial carbon dioxide pressure and heart rate in chronic heart failure. Am J Cardiol 1999; 83(5):795–798, A10.

141. DeBacker WA, Verbraecken J, Willemen M, et al. Central apnea index decreases after prolonged treatment with acetazolamide. Am J Respir Crit Care Med 1995; 151(1):87–91.

142. Javaheri S. Acetazolamide improves central sleep apnea in heart failure: a double-blind, prospective study. Am J Respir Crit Care Med 2006; 173(2):234–237.

143. Javaheri S, Parker TJ, Wexler L, et al. Effect of theophylline on sleep-disordered breathing in heart failure. N Engl J Med 1996; 335(8):562–567.

144. Bersten AD, Holt AW, Vedig AE, et al. Treatment of severe cardiogenic pulmonary edema with continuous positive airway pressure delivered by face mask. N Engl J Med 1991; 325(26): 1825–1830.

145. Masip J, Roque M, Sanchez B, et al. Noninvasive ventilation in acute cardiogenic pulmonary edema: systematic review and meta-analysis. JAMA 2005; 294(24):3124–3130.

146. Peter JV, Moran JL, Phillips-Hughes J, et al. Effect of non-invasive positive pressure ventilation (NIPPV) on mortality in patients with acute cardiogenic pulmonary oedema: a meta-analysis. Lancet 2006; 367(9517):1155–1163.

147. Naughton MT, Liu PP, Bernard DC, et al. Treatment of congestive heart failure and Cheyne-Stokes respiration during sleep by continuous positive airway pressure. Am J Respir Crit Care Med 1995; 151(1):92–97.

148. Sin DD, Logan AG, Fitzgerald FS, et al. Effects of continuous positive airway pressure on cardiovascular outcomes in heart failure patients with and without Cheyne-Stokes respiration. Circulation 2000; 102(1):61–66.

149. Tkacova R, Liu PP, Naughton MT, et al. Effect of continuous positive airway pressure on mitral regurgitant fraction and atrial natriuretic peptide in patients with heart failure. J Am Coll Cardiol 1997; 30(3):739–745.

150. Naughton MT, Benard DC, Rutherford R, et al. Effect of continuous positive airway pressure on central sleep apnea and nocturnal PCO2 in heart failure. Am J Respir Crit Care Med 1994; 150(6 pt 1):1598–1604.

151. Bradley TD, Logan AG, Kimoff RJ, et al. Continuous positive airway pressure for central sleep apnea and heart failure. N Engl J Med 2005; 353(19):2025–2033.
152. Fietze I, Blau A, Glos M, et al. Bi-level positive pressure ventilation and adaptive servo ventilation in patients with heart failure and Cheyne-Stokes respiration. Sleep Med 2007; 9(6):652–659.
153. Philippe C, Stoica-Herman M, Drouot X, et al. Compliance with and effectiveness of adaptive servoventilation versus continuous positive airway pressure in the treatment of Cheyne-Stokes respiration in heart failure over a six month period. Heart 2006; 92(3):337–342.
154. Arzt M, Floras JS, Logan AG, et al. Suppression of central sleep apnea by continuous positive airway pressure and transplant-free survival in heart failure: a post hoc analysis of the Canadian Continuous Positive Airway Pressure for Patients with Central Sleep Apnea and Heart Failure Trial (CANPAP). Circulation 2007; 115(25):3173–3180.
155. Teschler H, Dohring J, Wang YM, et al. Adaptive pressure support servo-ventilation: a novel treatment for Cheyne-Stokes respiration in heart failure. Am J Respir Crit Care Med 2001; 164(4):614–619.
156. Arzt M, Wensel R, Montalvan S, et al. Effects of dynamic bilevel positive airway pressure support on central sleep apnea in men with heart failure. Chest 2008; 134(1):61–66.
157. Kohnlein T, Welte T, Tan LB, et al. Assisted ventilation for heart failure patients with Cheyne-Stokes respiration. Eur Respir J 2002; 20(4):934–941.

Index